Gastroenterology

Made Ridiculously Simple

Stephen Goldberg, M.D.
Professor Emeritus
University of Miami
Miller School of Medicine
Miami, Florida

Howard I. Baikovitz, M.D.
Gastroenterology & Hepatology Associates
of South Florida
Pembroke Pines, Florida

MEDMASTER

ISBN #978-1-962445-12-2
eISBN #978-1-962445-13-9

Made in the United States of America

Published by:
MedMaster, Inc.
3389 Sheridan St., #243
Hollywood, FL 33021

Inside Illustrations by Jordan Collver and Isabel Loureiro

Works by Stephen Goldberg

Books:
Clinical Anatomy Made Ridiculously Simple
Clinical Physiology Made Ridiculously Simple
Clinical Biochemistry Made Ridiculously Simple
Clinical Genetics Made Ridiculously Simple
Clinical Neuroanatomy Made Ridiculously Simple
Clinical Hematology Made Ridiculously Simple
Endocrinology Made Ridiculously Simple
The Four-Minute Neurologic Exam
Goldberg's Brain Model
Ophthalmology Made Ridiculously Simple
Jonah: The Anatomy of the Soul
The Jonah Principle: The Basis for Human and Machine Consciousness
Consciousness, Information, and Meaning: The Origin of the Mind
Consciousness: How the Mind Arises from the Brain
Anatomy of the Soul: Mind, God, and the Afterlife
Consciousness Made Ridiculously Simple
Is the Mind Immortal?: The Origin of Consciousness
Clinical Biostatistics and Epidemiology Made Ridiculously Simple
LiveCode Lite: Computer Programming Made Ridiculously Simple
War Against the Germs: Epidemics, Microorganisms, and Biowarfare
Neurology Made Ridiculously Simple
Med'Toons

Computer Programs:
Differential Diagnosis
Atlas of Human Diseases
Neurologic Localization
Atlas of Microbiology
Atlas of Ophthalmology
Atlas of Dermatology
Atlas of Orthopedics
Medsearcher

Preface

This book is for medical, nursing, and PA students, primary care physicians, and other health professionals, to provide a brief, practical overview of gastroenterology, its diseases, diagnostic methods, and treatments. Although the field is vast, the clinical focus is on diseases that are more probable, more serious if missed, and more likely to lead to an effective remedy.

Thanks to Phyllis Goldenberg for her excellent proofreading and advice.

Contents

Part II. Diseases of the Digestive System

Part I. Introduction

The digestive tract extends from the mouth to the anus. Gastroenterology, though, deals mainly from the esophagus down, leaving the mouth and pharynx to dentistry and otolaryngology. Gastroenterology, however, includes problems affecting offshoots of the GI tract, namely the liver, gall bladder, bile ducts, and pancreas, since they produce and deliver the bile and a number of digestive enzymes that act in the intestines (**Fig. 1-1**).

1

The GI Tract

Peristalsis, the series of wave-like muscle contractions that move food through the digestive tract, begins in the upper esophagus. The muscle in the upper third of the esophagus is mainly voluntary (skeletal), which is under conscious control and initiates swallowing. The muscle of the lower two-thirds of the esophagus is mainly involuntary (smooth) and generates peristalsis without conscious control.

The main function of the stomach is storage and mechanical digestion of food through churning, along with chemical digestion of protein through the secretion of gastrin, acid, and pepsinogen. The acid also helps kill potentially harmful organisms. The stomach, in addition, produces intrinsic factor, necessary for the absorption of vitamin B12. It can also absorb certain substances, like alcohol and some medications.

The main function of the small intestine is the digestion and absorption of nutrients from food along with water. The large intestine (colon) is important in the absorption of water and formation of feces. It also hosts many bacteria, which assist in digestion and synthesize certain vitamins (e.g., vitamin K and some B vitamins). The lymphoid tissue in the colon is important in enhancing immune function.

Digestive system

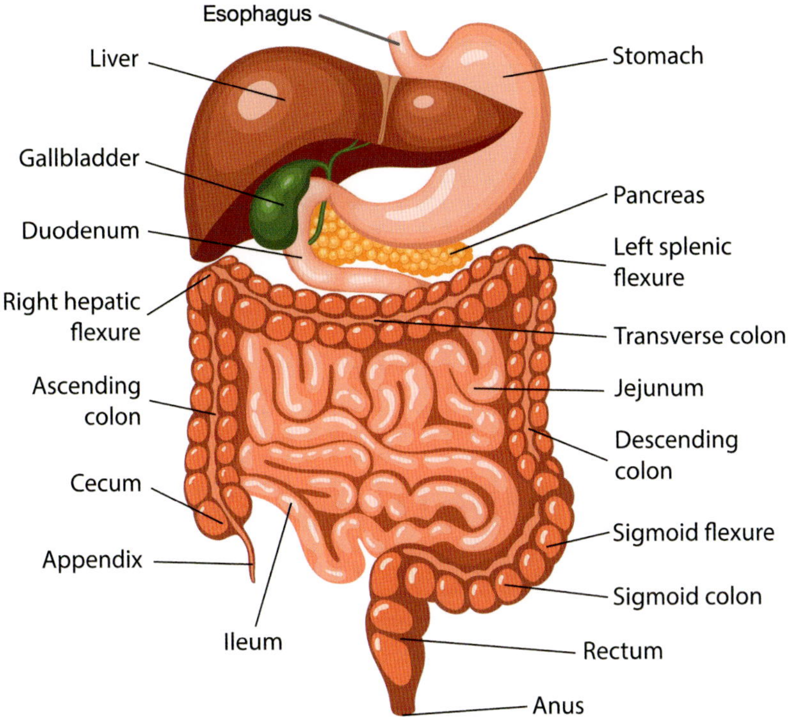

Figure 1-1 *The digestive system.*

2

Common Presenting Symptoms in Gastroenterology

Some of the more common presenting GI symptoms include:

- Abdominal Pain or Discomfort
- Heartburn and Acid Reflux
- Nausea and Vomiting
- Diarrhea
- Constipation
- Bloating and Gas
- Gastrointestinal Bleeding (oral or anal)
- Jaundice
- Altered Stool Appearance (fatty stools; change in stool color)
- Unintentional Weight Loss
- Difficulty Swallowing (dysphagia)
- Anorexia (loss of appetite)
- Anemia
- Ascites (fluid collection in the abdomen)

These symptoms may have many origins, some even outside the digestive system. **Figures 2-1** through **2-15** summarize the possible causes of GI symptoms.

FIGURE 2-1 CAUSES OF ABDOMINAL PAIN

Abdominal pain or discomfort occurs in many conditions, since the abdomen contains many organs, and pain can also be referred from the thorax and pelvis. The location of the pain in the abdomen provides an important diagnostic clue.

Upper Abdominal (Epigastric) Pain:
Gastroesophageal reflux disease (GERD)
Gastritis or peptic ulcer disease
Pancreatitis
Gallstones or cholecystitis (**right** side)
Perforated viscus (e.g., from peptic ulcer)
Subphrenic abscess (pus beneath the diaphragm)
Hepatitis or other liver disorders (**right** side)
Splenic pathology (e.g., infarct or rupture)(**left side**)
Pyelonephritis or renal colic (**right** or **left** side)
Myocardial ischemia or infarction (atypical presentation, especially in women)
Right or left lower lobe pneumonia or pleurisy (**right** or **left** abdominal pain respectively)

Periumbilical Pain:
Early appendicitis
Intestinal obstruction
Intestinal ischemia
Inflammatory bowel disease (Crohn's disease, ulcerative colitis)
Gastroenteritis

Lower Abdominal Pain
Urinary tract infection or inflammation
Appendicitis (**right** side usually)
Diverticulitis (**left** side usually in descending colon; cecal diverticulitis on **right**)
Crohn's disease (**right** side commonly, near the ileocecal valve between small and large intestine)
Colonic volvulus (Sigmoid - **left** side; Cecal – **right side**)
Ovarian torsion, ectopic pregnancy, or other gynecological conditions (**right** or **left** side)
Inguinal hernia (**right** or **left** side)
Testicular torsion (**right** or **left** side)

Diffuse Abdominal Pain:
Irritable bowel syndrome (IBS) (variable location)
Intestinal obstruction
Peritonitis
Gastroenteritis
Intestinal ischemia
Toxic megacolon
Metabolic disturbances (e.g., diabetic ketoacidosis, uremia, porphyria)
Sickle cell crisis (variable location)

FIGURE 2-2 CAUSES OF HEARTBURN
The origin of heartburn may lie in the esophagus, stomach, biliary tract, heart, lungs, or muscles, or it may be unknown (idiopathic). **Esophageal Causes of Heartburn:** Esophagitis (inflammation of the esophagus) due to infections, pills, or irritants Eosinophilic esophagitis (a chronic immune system disease) Esophageal motility disorders like achalasia or diffuse esophageal spasm Esophageal stricture or rings Esophageal cancer **Gastric Causes of Heartburn:** Gastroesophageal Reflux Disease (GERD) Gastritis (Inflammation of the stomach lining) Gastroparesis (delayed gastric emptying, often seen in diabetes) Peptic ulcer disease (gastric or duodenal ulcer) Gastric cancer **Cardiac Causes of Heartburn:** Angina or myocardial infarction Pericarditis (inflammation of the lining around the heart) **Biliary Tract Causes of Heartburn:** Biliary colic (with or without gallstones) Cholecystitis (inflammation of the gallbladder) **Pancreatic Causes of Heartburn:** Pancreatitis Pancreatic cancer **Pulmonary Causes of Heartburn:** Pulmonary embolism Pleurisy (inflammation of the pleura, the lining surrounding the lungs) Asthma (can be associated with GERD and can mimic some of its symptoms) **Musculoskeletal Causes of Heartburn:** Costochondritis (inflammation of rib cartilage) Muscle strain or chest wall pain **Functional Causes of Heartburn:** Functional heartburn (burning sensation in the chest without evidence of GERD on endoscopy or pH monitoring) Functional dyspepsia (chronic, recurring indigestion with no clear cause)

FIGURE 2-3 CAUSES OF NAUSEA AND VOMITING
Nausea and vomiting are nonspecific symptoms. The numerous causes include not only gastrointestinal, but neurologic, metabolic, endocrine, chemical-induced, infectious, cardiovascular and psychogenic.

Gastrointestinal Causes of Nausea and Vomiting:
Gastroenteritis (viral or bacterial)
Peptic ulcer disease
Gastroesophageal reflux disease (GERD)
Gastroparesis (delayed emptying of the stomach)
Intestinal obstruction (from adhesions, hernia, tumor, intussusception)
Cholecystitis (inflammation of the gallbladder), pancreatitis, or hepatitis
Appendicitis
Inflammatory bowel disease (Crohn's disease, ulcerative colitis)

Central Nervous System Causes of Nausea and Vomiting:
Migraine headaches
Intracranial pressure increase (from a tumor, hemorrhage, or hydrocephalus)
Meningitis or encephalitis
Vertigo and vestibular disorders (e.g., Meniere's disease, vestibular neuritis)

Metabolic and Endocrine Causes of Nausea and Vomiting:
Pregnancy (morning sickness)
Diabetic ketoacidosis
Uremia (from chronic kidney disease)
Hypercalcemia
Adrenal insufficiency (Addison's disease)
Thyroid disorders (hyperthyroidism or hypothyroidism)

Toxic and Drug-Induced Causes of Nausea and Vomiting:
Medications, e.g., chemotherapy, opioids, non-steroidal anti-inflammatory drugs (NSAIDs), antibiotics, etc.)
Alcohol or drug intoxication or withdrawal
Toxins (food poisoning from toxins such as staphylococcal enterotoxin or chemical poisoning)

Infectious Disease Causes of Nausea and Vomiting:
Viral infections (e.g., norovirus or rotavirus)
Bacterial infections (e.g., food poisoning from Salmonella, E. coli, etc.)
Parasitic infections (e.g., giardiasis)

Psychogenic Causes of Nausea and Vomiting:
Stress and anxiety
Eating disorders (anorexia nervosa, bulimia)
Psychosomatic disorders

Cardiovascular Causes of Nausea and Vomiting:
Myocardial infarction (especially inferior wall)
Heart failure

Other Causes of Nausea and Vomiting:
Postoperative nausea and vomiting
Radiation therapy
Concussion or head injury
Pyloric stenosis in infants

FIGURE 2-4 CAUSES OF DIARRHEA

Diarrhea is loose, watery stools occurring more frequently than usual. It may have infectious, medication-related, endocrine, food-related, GI disease-related, or other causes.

Infectious Causes of Diarrhea:
Viral infections (norovirus, rotavirus, adenovirus, and others)
Bacterial infections (*Escherichia coli, Salmonella, Shigella, Campylobacter, Clostridioides difficile*, and others)
Parasitic infections (*Giardia lamblia, Entamoeba histolytica, Cryptosporidium*, and others)

Medication Causes of Diarrhea:
Antibiotic-associated diarrhea
Laxative overuse
Antacids containing magnesium
Chemotherapy agents
NSAIDs (nonsteroidal anti-inflammatory drugs)

Gastrointestinal Causes of Diarrhea:
Inflammatory bowel diseases: Crohn's disease and ulcerative colitis.
Irritable bowel syndrome (IBS), especially IBS with predominant diarrhea (IBS-D).
Malabsorptive and maldigestive disorders: Celiac disease, pancreatic insufficiency, lactose intolerance
Colorectal cancer
Microscopic colitis (lymphocytic or collagenous colitis)
Bile acid malabsorption

Endocrine Causes of Diarrhea:
Hyperthyroidism
Addison's disease (adrenal insufficiency)
Carcinoid syndrome
Zollinger-Ellison syndrome
Diabetes mellitus (especially with autonomic neuropathy)

Functional Causes (symptoms with no clear origin) of Diarrhea:
Functional diarrhea

Toxin Causes of Diarrhea:
Heavy metals (e.g., arsenic or mercury)

Food Related Causes of Diarrhea:
Food poisoning (toxins produced by bacteria such as *Staphylococcus aureus* or *Bacillus cereus*)
Food allergies or intolerances (e.g., lactose intolerance, gluten sensitivity)
Artificial sweeteners (such as sorbitol or mannitol)

Systemic Disease Causes of Diarrhea:
HIV/AIDS
Systemic infections (such as sepsis)
Chronic liver disease
Chronic kidney disease

Post-Surgical Causes of Diarrhea:
Post-cholecystectomy syndrome
Gastric bypass surgery

Other Causes of Diarrhea:
Intestinal ischemia
Radiation enteritis
Intestinal tuberculosis (in endemic areas)
Intestinal lymphoma

FIGURE 2-5 CAUSES OF CONSTIPATION

Constipation is infrequent bowel movements or difficulty in passing stool, which may be hard, dry, and lumpy. It may have many causes, including diet, GI, endocrine, neurological, or psychological; or it may stem from medication, structural problems, systemic disorders, pregnancy, lifestyle, or other factors.

Dietary Causes of Constipation:
Inadequate dietary fiber intake
Insufficient fluid intake

Gastrointestinal Causes of Constipation:
Irritable bowel syndrome (IBS) with predominant constipation (IBS-C)
Intestinal obstruction or strictures
Anal fissure or hemorrhoids (leading to stool withholding due to pain)
Colonic inertia (slow colonic transit)
Rectal prolapse

Endocrine and Metabolic Causes of Constipation:
Hypothyroidism
Diabetes mellitus (especially if poorly controlled or with autonomic neuropathy)
Hypercalcemia
Hypokalemia
Uremia (due to chronic kidney disease)

Neurological Causes of Constipation:
Parkinson's disease
Multiple sclerosis
Spinal cord lesions or injury
Autonomic neuropathy

Psychological Causes of Constipation:
Depression
Anxiety
Eating disorders (e.g., anorexia nervosa)

Medication-Related Causes of Constipation:
Opioid analgesics
Anticholinergics
Calcium channel blockers
Iron supplements
Antidepressants (particularly tricyclics, due to anticholinergic effects)
Anticonvulsants
Antipsychotics

Structural Problems and Functional Causes of Constipation:
Pelvic floor dysfunction
Rectocele (bulging of the rectum into the vagina)
Hirschsprung disease (in children, congenital absence of enteric nervous system cells)
Functional constipation (normal tests but persistent symptoms)

Systemic Causes of Constipation:
Amyloidosis
Scleroderma and other connective tissue disorders

Lifestyle Causes of Constipation:
Physical inactivity
Disruption of regular routine (e.g., travel)
Ignoring the urge to have a bowel movement

Pregnancy Causes of Constipation:
Hormonal changes
Physical pressure from the growing uterus

Post-Surgical Causes of Constipation:
Postoperative ileus
Abdominal surgery complications
Anorectal surgery

FIGURE 2-6 CAUSES OF BLOATING AND GAS

Bloating and gas are common gastrointestinal symptoms that can have many causes, including diet, intrinsic disorders of GI function, infections, inflammation, endocrine abnormality, medications, psychological and other factors.

Dietary Causes of Bloating and Gas:
Lactose intolerance
Fructose intolerance
Celiac disease
Consumption of high-fiber foods
Carbonated beverages
Overeating
Swallowed air (aerophagia)

Functional Gastrointestinal Causes of Bloating and Gas:
Irritable bowel syndrome (IBS)
Functional dyspepsia

Gastrointestinal Motility Causes of Bloating and Gas:
Gastroparesis (delayed emptying of the stomach)
Chronic intestinal pseudo-obstruction (due to impaired intestinal nerve or muscle function rather than actual obstruction)

Malabsorption Causes of Bloating and Gas:
Celiac disease
Pancreatic insufficiency
Small intestinal bacterial overgrowth (SIBO)
Short bowel syndrome

Inflammatory Causes of Bloating and Gas:
Inflammatory bowel disease (Crohn's disease, ulcerative colitis)
Diverticulitis

Infection Causes of Bloating and Gas:
Gastroenteritis
Parasitic infections (e.g., Giardiasis)

Endocrine Causes of Bloating and Gas:
Diabetes mellitus (especially if associated with autonomic neuropathy)
Hypothyroidism
During phases of the menstrual cycle
Pregnancy

Medication Causes of Bloating and Gas:
Antibiotics (can alter gut flora)
Laxatives (excessive use)
Nonsteroidal anti-inflammatory drugs (NSAIDs, which can irritate the GI lining)
Opiates
Birth control pills (hormonal effect on GI motility)

Psychological Causes of Bloating and Gas:
Stress
Anxiety

Other Causes of Bloating and Gas:
Constipation
Intestinal obstruction or ileus
Ovarian cancer
Ascites due to liver disease, heart failure, or malignancy

FIGURE 2-7 CAUSES OF GI BLEEDING

Gastrointestinal (GI) bleeding can occur in any part of the digestive tract. GI bleeding is divided into two types based on the location: upper GI bleeding and lower GI bleeding. **Upper GI Bleeding** is usually characterized by **hematemesis** (vomiting blood) or **melena** (black, tarry stools). **Lower GI Bleeding** usually presents with **hematochezia** (bright red blood per rectum). The causes of GI bleeding include inflammation, ulcers, varices, tumors, coagulation disorders, medications, and trauma.

Upper GI Bleeding
Peptic ulcers (gastric or duodenal)
Gastritis (inflammation of the stomach lining)
Gastroesophageal reflux disease (GERD) with esophagitis
Esophageal varices (often due to cirrhosis and portal hypertension)
Mallory-Weiss tear (tear at the gastroesophageal junction caused by severe retching)
Arteriovenous malformations such as angiodysplasia
Gastric erosions (more superficial than gastric ulcers)
Gastric cancer
Dieulafoy's lesion (a rare, large-caliber arteriole, often in the stomach wall, that can bleed)
Aortoenteric fistula (a rare connection between the aorta and the gastrointestinal tract from aneurysm or aortic surgery)
Gastric antral vascular ectasia (GAVE): Neovascularization, particularly in the gastric antrum
Hemobilia (bleeding from the bile duct)
Hemosuccus pancreaticus (bleeding from the pancreatic duct)

Lower GI Bleeding
Diverticulosis
Colitis (inflammatory bowel disease, infectious colitis, ischemic colitis)
Anorectal diseases (hemorrhoids, anal fissures)
Polyps and colorectal cancer
Meckel's diverticulum (especially in children)
Radiation enteritis or colitis

Other Causes (of either upper or lower GI bleeding):
Coagulopathy (blood clotting disorders)
Medications that cause bleeding (such as NSAIDs, anticoagulants, and antiplatelet agents)
Post-polypectomy bleeding (after endoscopic polyp removal)
Ingestion of foreign bodies
Vascular abnormalities and systemic diseases affecting the GI tract

FIGURE 2-8 CAUSES OF JAUNDICE

Jaundice is due to high levels of bilirubin in the blood. It indicates an underlying disease affecting the liver, biliary system, or red blood cells. **Unconjugated (indirect) bilirubin** is normally produced from the breakdown of the heme pigment in red blood cells. It is not water-soluble and is instead transported bound to albumin in the blood; unconjugated bilirubin cannot be excreted by the kidney or liver. It becomes conjugated when it is taken up and processed by the liver. **Conjugated (direct) bilirubin** is water-soluble and can be excreted into the bile as well as the urine. Excess conjugated or unconjugated bilirubin can cause jaundice. The unconjugated form increases when the liver is unable to process it from the blood. Conjugated bilirubin builds up in liver diseases that affect bile excretion by the liver or blockage of the bile ducts. The differential diagnosis for jaundice can be categorized by prehepatic, hepatic, and posthepatic causes, indicating the place of origin of the jaundice.

Prehepatic (Hemolytic) Jaundice:
Hemolysis (increased breakdown of red blood cells), which could be due to:
- Hereditary spherocytosis or elliptocytosis
- Glucose-6-phosphate dehydrogenase (G6PD) deficiency
- Pyruvate kinase deficiency
- Sickle cell disease
- Autoimmune hemolytic anemia
- Drug-induced hemolysis
- Infections (e.g., malaria, babesiosis)
- Ineffective erythropoiesis (such as in thalassemia or pernicious anemia)
- Hemolytic disease of the newborn

Hepatic (Hepatocellular) Jaundice:
Viral hepatitis (hepatitis A, B, C, D, E)
Alcoholic liver disease (ranging from fatty liver disease to alcoholic hepatitis to cirrhosis to liver cancer)
Metabolic Associated Steatohepatitis (MASH)
Drug-induced liver injury
Autoimmune hepatitis
Wilson's disease (a disorder of copper metabolism)
Alpha-1 antitrypsin deficiency
Primary biliary cholangitis
Hemochromatosis (excess iron storage)
Cirrhosis of the liver from various causes
Acute liver failure from toxins like acetaminophen overdose
Liver cancer or metastatic cancer to the liver
Budd-Chiari syndrome (obstructed hepatic veins impairs blood flow from the liver, damaging the liver)
Ischemic hepatitis (from severe hypotension or heart failure)
Gilbert's syndrome (an inherited disorder of bilirubin processing)
Rotor syndrome (a benign hereditary disorder of hepatic storage and transport of bilirubin)
Dubin-Johnson syndrome (genetically impaired secretion of bilirubin into the bile)
Crigler-Najjar syndrome (genetically impaired processing of unconjugated bilirubin by the liver)

Posthepatic (Obstructive) Jaundice:
Gallstones causing obstruction of the bile duct (choledocholithiasis)
Strictures of the bile ducts
Cholangitis (inflammation of the bile ducts)
Pancreatic cancer at the head of the pancreas causing biliary obstruction
Cholangiocarcinoma (bile duct cancer)
Pancreatitis leading to biliary obstruction
Parasitic infections (e.g., ascariasis)
Primary sclerosing cholangitis

FIGURE 2-9 CAUSES OF CHANGE IN STOOL COLOR

Changes in stool color can be influenced by bleeding, diet, infections, malabsorption, decreased bile flow, foods and food coloring, medications, and various health conditions.

Black or Tarry Stools (Melena):
Upper gastrointestinal bleeding (e.g., from peptic ulcers, gastritis, esophageal varices)
Iron supplements
Bismuth-containing medications (like Pepto-Bismol)
Certain foods (such as large amounts of spinach or other leafy greens; black licorice)
Heavy metal poisoning (e.g., lead, bismuth)

Bright Red Stools (Hematochezia):
Lower gastrointestinal bleeding (e.g., from hemorrhoids, diverticulosis, anal fissures, colorectal cancer)
Ingestion of red-colored foods (beets, red food coloring)
Infectious gastroenteritis
Inflammatory bowel disease (e.g., Crohn's disease, ulcerative colitis)
Angiodysplasia (abnormal blood vessels in the gastrointestinal tract)

Green Stools:
Consumption of green foods (leafy vegetables, green food coloring)
Bacterial overgrowth
Diarrhea (rapid transit time)
Medications or supplements with green coloring

Yellow Stools:
Decreased bile production or blockage of bile flow (e.g., by gallstones or cholestasis)
Giardiasis (parasitic infection)
Fatty stools (steatorrhea), e.g., in celiac disease, cystic fibrosis, or chronic pancreatitis

Clay-Colored or Pale Stools:
Biliary obstruction (e.g., gallstones, pancreatic cancer, cholangiocarcinoma)
Hepatitis
Alcoholic liver disease
Cirrhosis

Orange Stools:
Foods with orange coloring (carrots, sweet potatoes)
Medications containing beta-carotene or aluminum hydroxide
Metabolic and digestive conditions that reduce bile salt (that can be caused by certain medications)

Dark Stools:
Upper GI bleeding
Foods that are dark purple or blue (e.g., blueberries)
Iron-rich foods
Certain medications, e.g., iron supplements, activated charcoal, Pepto-Bismol (bismuth subsalicylate)

Varied Colors:
Food dyes and colored foods
Medications (antibiotics can change stool color)
Supplements (some vitamins and minerals can alter stool hue)

FIGURE 2-10 CAUSES OF STEATORRHEA (FATTY STOOLS)

Steatorrhea, the excretion of abnormal quantities of fat with the feces (floating stools), is due to reduced absorption of fats from the intestine. It can be due to a range of conditions that affect the digestive tract or other related systems, including malabsorption syndromes, liver and biliary diseases, infection, GI surgery, infections, endocrine diseases, genetic disorders, dietary factors, and medication.

Malabsorption Causes of Steatorrhea:
Celiac disease: Gluten intolerance causing villous atrophy and malabsorption
Chronic pancreatitis: Insufficient pancreatic enzyme production with poor fat digestion
Cystic fibrosis: Thick secretions obstruct the pancreatic ducts, impairing enzyme delivery.
Pancreatic cancer: Tumors can obstruct the pancreatic duct or directly impair pancreatic function.

Biliary Causes of Steatorrhea:
Biliary atresia: Congenital absence or closure of the bile ducts
Primary sclerosing cholangitis: Chronic liver disease that leads to bile duct scarring
Cholecystectomy: Removal of the gallbladder can alter bile salt metabolism.
Cholestasis: Any condition that impairs the flow of bile, reducing fat digestion and absorption

Liver Causes of Steatorrhea:
Hepatitis: Inflammation of the liver affecting bile production
Cirrhosis: Scarring of the liver tissue can impact bile production and secretion.

Gastrointestinal Causes of Steatorrhea:
Crohn's disease: Inflammation and damage to the intestine, particularly the ileum, can impair fat absorption.
Short bowel syndrome: Less intestinal surface area for nutrient absorption due to surgical removal of a portion of the small intestine
Gastrectomy: Surgery to remove part or all of the stomach can affect digestive efficiency.
Gastric bypass surgery: Alters normal digestive processes and can lead to malabsorption

Infectious Causes of Steatorrhea:
Giardiasis: Parasitic infection that can lead to fat malabsorption
Whipple's disease: Rare bacterial infection affecting the intestinal lining
HIV/AIDS: Can lead to various GI tract infections and complications

Endocrine Causes of Steatorrhea:
Diabetes mellitus with autonomic neuropathy: Can affect GI motility and enzyme secretion
Hypothyroidism: Slowed metabolism can affect digestive processes.

Genetic Causes of Steatorrhea:
Abetalipoproteinemia: Rare condition affecting fat absorption and transport
Familial hypobetalipoproteinemia: Genetic disorder that affects lipoprotein production

Dietary Causes of Steatorrhea:
Overconsumption of certain oils or fats, particularly medium-chain triglycerides, that exceed the digestive system's capacity.

Medication Causes of Steatorrhea:
Orlistat: A drug used for weight loss that inhibits pancreatic lipase
Certain HIV medications
Chemotherapeutic agents

Other Causes of Steatorrhea
Zollinger-Ellison syndrome: Gastrin-secreting tumors (gastrinomas) lead to high acid production, which can inactivate pancreatic enzymes.
Intestinal lymphangiectasia: Lymphatic blockage preventing proper fat transport

FIGURE 2-11 CAUSES OF UNINTENDED WEIGHT LOSS

Weight loss, particularly when unintended, can be a sign of an underlying health issue. The differential diagnosis of unintended weight loss is extensive. It is classified based on etiologies such as gastrointestinal, endocrine, chronic infections, malignancy, psychiatric, neurologic, medication-related, and other miscellaneous causes.

Gastrointestinal Causes of Unintended Weight Loss:
Chronic liver disease (hepatitis, cirrhosis)
Inflammatory bowel disease (Crohn's disease, ulcerative colitis)
Malabsorption syndromes (celiac disease, tropical sprue, Whipple's disease)
Gastrointestinal malignancies (gastric cancer, colon cancer)
Pancreatic insufficiency
Peptic ulcer disease
Gastroparesis

Endocrine Causes of Unintended Weight Loss:
Diabetes mellitus (especially type 1 or poorly controlled type 2)
Hyperthyroidism
Adrenal insufficiency (Addison's disease)
Hyperparathyroidism

Infectious Causes of Unintended Weight Loss:
HIV/AIDS
Tuberculosis
Endocarditis
Chronic parasitic infections
Hepatitis

Malignancy Causes of Unintended Weight Loss:
Lymphoma
Leukemia
Solid organ cancers (pancreatic, lung, stomach, colorectal, etc.)
Metastatic cancer

Psychiatric Causes of Unintended Weight Loss:
Anorexia nervosa
Depression
Anxiety disorders
Substance abuse (alcohol, drugs)

Chronic Disease Causes of Unintended Weight Loss:
Chronic obstructive pulmonary disease (COPD)
Congestive heart failure
Rheumatoid arthritis and other chronic inflammatory conditions
Chronic kidney disease

Neurological Causes of Unintended Weight Loss:
Stroke
Parkinson's disease
Alzheimer's disease or other dementias

Medication Causes of Unintended Weight Loss:
Chemotherapy agents
Medications that cause nausea, gastrointestinal upset, or anorexia
Some psychiatric medications
Illicit drug use (cocaine, amphetamines, etc.)

Other Causes of Unintended Weight Loss:
Age-related changes in metabolism and taste
Socioeconomic factors (e.g., lack of food access)
Cachexia associated with chronic illness
Post-surgical states
End-stage organ failure

FIGURE 2-12 CAUSES OF DYSPHAGIA

Dysphagia (difficulty swallowing) can arise from a variety of conditions that affect the esophagus or the muscles and nerves responsible for swallowing. A differential diagnosis for dysphagia often considers the distinction between oropharyngeal dysphagia and esophageal dysphagia. **Oropharyngeal Dysphagia** is a problem with the initiation of swallowing and the transfer of food from the mouth to the esophagus. **Esophageal Dysphagia** is difficulty passing food through the esophagus to the stomach and can be caused by a problem with motility or obstruction. In general, esophageal motility disorders cause a problem with swallowing both liquids and solids; obstructive problems cause more difficulty with solids when the liquid can get around the obstruction. The origin of dysphagia includes mechanical blockage, neurologic, muscular, structural, inflammatory, or medication-related causes.

OROPHARYNGEAL DYSPHAGIA
Neurological Causes of Dysphagia:
Stroke
Parkinson's disease
Multiple sclerosis
Amyotrophic lateral sclerosis (ALS)
Myasthenia gravis
Cerebral palsy

Muscular Causes of Dysphagia:
Muscular dystrophy

Structural Causes of Dysphagia:
Zenker's diverticulum
Esophageal web (particularly occurs in the upper esophagus)
Tumors of the oropharynx or nasopharynx

Infectious Causes of Dysphagia:
Candidiasis
Herpes simplex virus
Human papillomavirus (HPV)-related growths

Inflammatory Causes of Dysphagia:
Eosinophilic esophagitis
Iatrogenic causes
Radiation therapy to the head and neck
Post-surgical changes

ESOPHAGEAL DYSPHAGIA
Structural Causes of Dysphagia:
Esophageal strictures or rings
Zenker's diverticulum
Esophageal web (particularly occurs in the upper esophagus)
Esophageal cancer
Peptic strictures (due to acid reflux)
External compression (e.g., from tumors or lymphadenopathy)

Motility Causes of Dysphagia:
Achalasia
Esophageal spasm (diffuse or nutcracker esophagus)
Scleroderma
Impaired muscle contractions
Radiation therapy
Degenerative neuromuscular diseases (e.g., amyotrophic lateral sclerosis, multiple sclerosis)
Secondary motility disorders due to systemic illnesses (e.g., diabetes, thyroid disease, Chagas disease)
Obstruction of esophagogastric junction outflow
Medications that affect smooth muscle function
Certain infections
Esophageal tumors

Esophagitis Causes of Dysphagia:
Gastroesophageal reflux disease (GERD)
Eosinophilic esophagitis
Infectious esophagitis (such as from Candida, herpes simplex virus, or cytomegalovirus, particularly in immunocompromised individuals)

Other Causes of Dysphagia:
Foreign body impaction
Pill-induced esophagitis
Caustic injury (from ingestion of corrosive substances)

Idiopathic

FIGURE 2-13 CAUSES OF ANOREXIA

Anorexia (decreased appetite) is a nonspecific symptom that could indicate a physical or psychological issue.

Psychological Causes of Anorexia:
Anorexia nervosa (a serious psychological disorder characterized by an intense fear of gaining weight and a distorted body image)

Depression
Anxiety disorders
Other psychiatric illnesses such as schizophrenia or bipolar disorder

Gastrointestinal Causes of Anorexia:
Chronic liver disease (hepatitis, cirrhosis)
Peptic ulcer disease
Gastritis
Gastroesophageal reflux disease (GERD)
Inflammatory bowel disease (Crohn's disease, ulcerative colitis)
Gastrointestinal malignancies
Postoperative (especially after abdominal surgery)

Endocrine and Metabolic Causes of Anorexia:
Diabetes mellitus (especially when poorly controlled)
Adrenal insufficiency
Thyroid disorders (hyperthyroidism or hypothyroidism)
Chronic kidney disease
Electrolyte imbalances

Infectious Causes of Anorexia:
HIV/AIDS
Tuberculosis
Hepatitis
Parasitic infections
Chronic infections

Neurological Causes of Anorexia:
Brain tumors
Cerebral infarction (stroke)
Dementia
Parkinson's disease
Multiple sclerosis

Cardiopulmonary Causes of Anorexia:
Chronic obstructive pulmonary disease (COPD)
Congestive heart failure

Medication and Substance-Related Causes of Anorexia:
Chemotherapy agents
Certain antibiotics
Opioid analgesics
Chronic alcoholism
Illicit drug use (cocaine, amphetamines, etc.)

Other Systemic Causes of Anorexia:
Cancer (especially advanced stages)
Chronic heart failure
Rheumatologic diseases (like rheumatoid arthritis or lupus)
Chronic fatigue syndrome

Idiopathic

FIGURE 2-14 CAUSES OF ANEMIA

Several types of anemia can be associated with GI causes, through blood loss, malabsorption, or inflammation. The most common GI-related cause of anemia is iron deficiency anemia from chronic blood loss.

Iron Deficiency Anemia:
Lack of iron in the diet
Peptic ulcers
Gastritis
Esophagitis
Esophageal varices
Hemorrhoids
Diverticulosis
Inflammatory bowel disease (Crohn's disease and ulcerative colitis)
Angiodysplasia (abnormal fragile blood vessels)
Colorectal polyps or cancer

Vitamin B12 Deficiency Anemia:
Lack of B12 in the diet (B12 is necessary for red blood cell production)
Pernicious anemia (lack of intrinsic factor, necessary for B12 absorption)
Crohn's disease
Gastrectomy or surgery that removes or bypasses the end of the small intestine
Atrophic gastritis (loss of intrinsic factor)
Celiac disease
Chronic pancreatitis (can interfere with the production of enzymes needed for vitamin B12 absorption)

Folate Deficiency Anemia:
Dietary insufficiency (folate deficiency impairs DNA synthesis of red blood cells in the bone marrow)
Malabsorption (celiac disease, tropical sprue, inflammatory bowel diseases, short bowel syndrome)

Anemia of Chronic Disease (Anemia of Inflammation):
Inflammatory bowel disease
Chronic liver disease (e.g., hepatitis and cirrhosis)

Infections
Viral (e.g., norovirus, rotavirus)
Bacterial (e.g., *Salmonella, Campylobacter, E. coli*)
Parasitic (e.g., hookworm, schistosomiasis, giardiasis)

Anemias of Non-GI Origin
Hemolytic anemias:
- Sickle cell
- Thalassemia
- Autoimmune hemolytic anemia
- Hereditary spherocytosis

Anemias due to deficient red blood cell (RBC) production:
- Aplastic anemia
- Myelodysplastic syndromes
- Leukemia and other cancers
- Anemia of chronic disease
- Renal anemia (lack of erythropoietin)
- Hypothyroidism (may lead to reduced RBC production)

FIGURE 2-15 CAUSES OF ASCITES

Ascites is the abnormal accumulation of fluid in the peritoneal cavity. Ascites may have abdominal or systemic origins.

Liver cirrhosis
Peritoneal carcinomatosis
Lymphoma
Primary liver cancers or hepatic metastases
Heart failure
Nephrotic syndrome
Infection
Pancreatic disease
Hypoalbuminemia
Budd-Chiari syndrome (thrombosis of the hepatic veins or inferior vena cava)
Myxedema in severe hypothyroidism (increased capillary permeability and reduced albumin synthesis) Chylous ascites (disruption of abdominal lymphatic vessel drainage)
Meigs' syndrome (ascites and pleural effusion associated with benign ovarian tumors)
Peritoneal dialysis
Vasculitis
Familial Mediterranean fever (peritoneal inflammation)
Sarcoidosis (with liver involvement or disruption of abdominal lymph drainage)
Congenital defects in children (e.g., congenital hepatic fibrosis)

3

Diagnostic Tools in Gastroenterology

There are many gastrointestinal diseases, but fortunately the gastroenterologist has many ways to diagnose them:

- History
- Physical Exam
- Blood and Urine Tests
- Stool Tests
- Endoscopy
- Imaging Studies
- Biopsy
- Other Tests

History

A careful patient history in gastroenterology, as in any medical field, not only provides clues as to diagnosis, but helps build a therapeutic relationship with the patient.

Chief Complaint (CC): Preferably described in the patient's own words

History of Present Illness (HPI): The *time of onset* of the symptoms, their *duration, intensity, character, frequency*, and what *aggravates or alleviates* the symptoms

Past Medical History (PMH): Information on the patient's past illnesses, surgeries, hospitalizations, injuries, allergies, and chronic conditions, e.g., previous GI diseases, liver diseases, pancreatitis

Medication History: A list of current and past medications, including over-the-counter drugs, prescriptions, herbal supplements, and any adverse reactions to them that might relate to the patient's symptoms

Family History (FH): Diseases within the family that might suggest a genetic predisposition to certain GI conditions, such as colorectal cancer, inflammatory bowel disease, celiac disease, or liver disease

Social History (SH): Includes lifestyle factors that can affect GI health, such as alcohol intake, smoking, diet, exercise, and occupation

Review of Systems (ROS): An inquiry about symptoms related to other body systems may reveal health issues that can impact the GI system.

Nutritional History: The patient's intake of fiber, fat, dairy products, caffeine, and other substances that may influence GI symptoms

Psychosocial History: Stress, anxiety, and depression can significantly impact GI symptoms and disorders.

Physical Exam

General Appearance: The patient's overall appearance, including signs of distress, nutritional status (obesity or cachexia), and any visible signs of GI disease (e.g., jaundice, spider angiomata (small spider-like blood vessels on the skin), or caput medusae (distended paraumbilical veins) in liver disease; pallor from anemia; dermatitis herpetiformis in celiac disease)

Vital Signs: Blood pressure, heart rate, respiratory rate, and temperature can provide clues to systemic involvement in gastrointestinal diseases.

Abdominal Examination includes:

- **Inspection:** Look for abdominal distension, scars, or skin changes (e.g., caput medusae in liver disease).
- **Auscultation:** Listen to bowel sounds to assess for hyperactivity (suggesting obstruction or gastroenteritis) or hypoactivity (indicating ileus or peritonitis), and bruits (vascular sounds that may indicate vascular disease).
- **Percussion:** Used to assess liver size, detect the presence of ascites (shifting dullness), and gas accumulation (tympanic sounds)
- **Palpation:** To identify areas of tenderness, masses, organomegaly, and the presence of ascites (e.g. fluid wave felt on opposite side of abdomen on tapping the abdomen). Palpation is performed last to avoid causing discomfort that might lead to guarding, which can interfere with the rest of examination or alter the exam results (e.g., stimulating bowel motility).

Rectal Examination: A digital rectal examination can assess the tone of the anal sphincter, presence of local masses, tenderness, and evaluate for occult blood, which can be a sign of gastrointestinal bleeding or colorectal cancer.

Cardiovascular and Respiratory Systems: Ischemic heart disease or pleuritis may result in referred pain to the abdomen; heart failure can result in liver enlargement and ascites.

Blood and Urine Tests

Complete Blood Count (CBC): Helps detect anemia (common in GI bleeding or malabsorption), infection, and inflammation.

Liver Function Tests (LFTs): Includes alanine aminotransferase (ALT), aspartate aminotransferase (AST), alkaline phosphatase (ALP), bilirubin, and gamma-glutamyl transferase (GGT). Abnormalities may suggest liver disease or bile duct obstruction.

Pancreatic Enzymes: Amylase and lipase levels can help diagnose acute pancreatitis and other pancreatic disorders.

Inflammatory Markers: C-reactive protein (CRP) and erythrocyte sedimentation rate (ESR) can indicate inflammation, which may be due to various GI conditions, such as inflammatory bowel disease (IBD).

Iron Studies: Including serum iron, ferritin, total iron-binding capacity (TIBC), and transferrin saturation. Useful in diagnosing iron deficiency anemia, which can result from chronic GI blood loss

Coagulation Profile: Including prothrombin time (PT) and partial thromboplastin time (PTT), as the liver produces clotting factors.

Serologic Tests for Celiac Disease: Tissue transglutaminase antibodies (tTG-IgA) and endomysial antibodies (EMA-IgA) help in the diagnosis of celiac disease, a gluten-sensitive enteropathy.

Tumor Markers: E.g., carcinoembryonic antigen (CEA) and CA 19-9. These can be elevated in certain GI cancers, like colorectal and pancreatic cancer, though not specific for those diseases.

Urinalysis: Can indirectly reflect GI diseases, especially through signs of dehydration or liver disease impacting kidney function. Bilirubin in the urine can indicate liver dysfunction or biliary obstruction.

5-Hydroxyindoleacetic Acid (5-HIAA): A breakdown product of serotonin. When elevated, as measured in a 24-hour urine test, this may indicate a carcinoid tumor, which can secrete serotonin and other substances causing the carcinoid syndrome, affecting both the GI tract and the liver

Stool Tests

Stool Occult Blood Testing: May indicate gastrointestinal bleeding, as from colorectal cancer

Stool Culture and Visualization: Can identify pathological bacteria, viruses, or parasites in the GI tract **Stool Antigen Test:** Can identify specific viral proteins in stool samples

Stool PCR Test: Can detect the genetic material of specific viruses in stool samples (e.g., norovirus, rotavirus)

Stool pH Test: Can indicate malabsorption (e.g., lactose intolerance) or other problems where stool pH changes

Stool Fat Test: Can help diagnose conditions where there is malabsorption of fat

Stool Calprotectin Test: Can help assess inflammatory bowel disease by measuring calprotectin, a protein that white blood cells release in response to inflammation

Stool DNA Test: Detects DNA abnormalities in the stool as a test for colorectal cancer

Endoscopy

Endoscopy provides a direct way of visualizing the wall of the digestive tract. In **upper endoscopy** (**Fig. 3-1**), a flexible endoscope tube with a light and camera at the end is inserted orally. It can look at the walls of the esophagus, stomach, and duodenum. With certain modifications (**push enteroscopy, single or double balloon enteroscopy, spiral enteroscopy, cap-assisted enteroscopy**), the endoscope can look further beyond the duodenum, even reaching the entire small intestine, especially if both an antegrade approach (through the mouth) and a retrograde approach (via the anus) are done.

In capsule endoscopy (**Fig. 3-2**) a small camera-containing capsule (about 23-25 mm [0.9-1I"] x 11 mm [0.4"]), which the patient swallows, sends pictures back to the examiner as it passes along the small intestine. It is sometimes used to examine the esophagus.

In **lower endoscopy** (**sigmoidoscopy** or **colonoscopy**), the examiner can view the rectum and large intestine. The **sigmoidoscope**, which is shorter than a **colonoscope**, can examine only the lower colon. The colonoscope can examine the entire colon, including the end of the small intestine in the region of the ileocecal valve (which connects the small and large intestine) (**Fig. 3-3**).

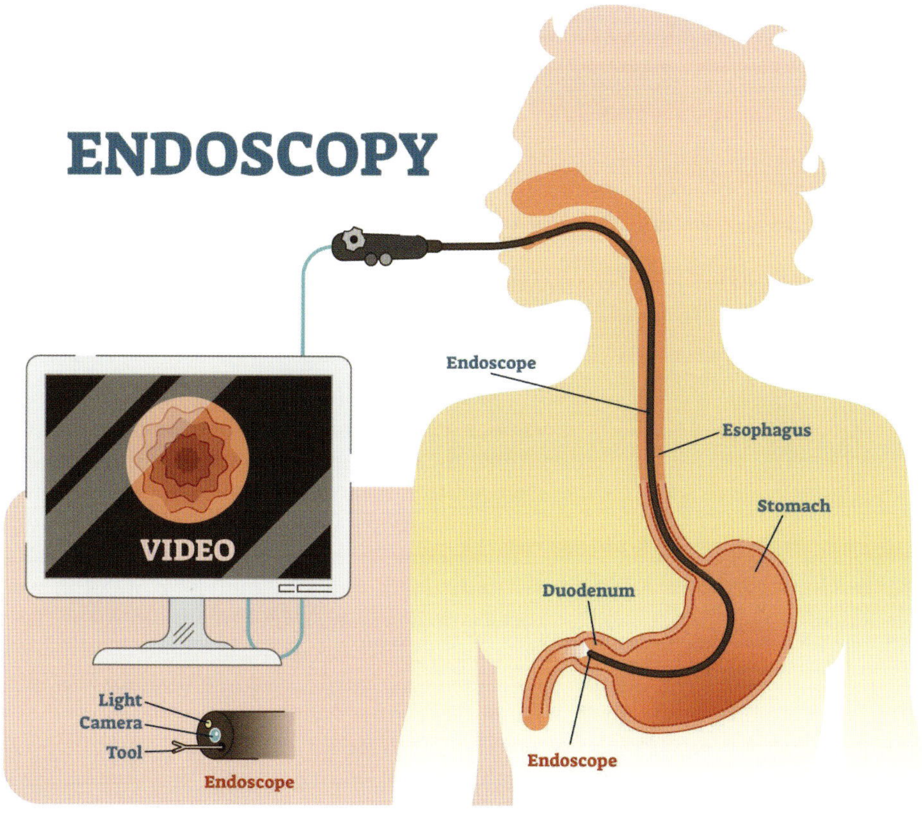

Figure 3-1 *Upper endoscopy.*

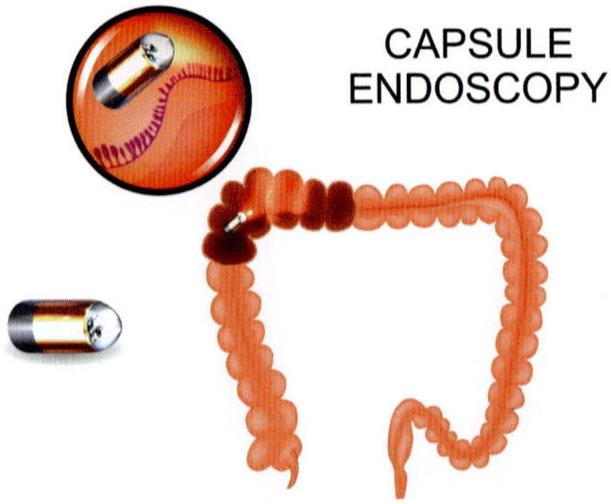

Figure 3-2 Capsule endoscopy.

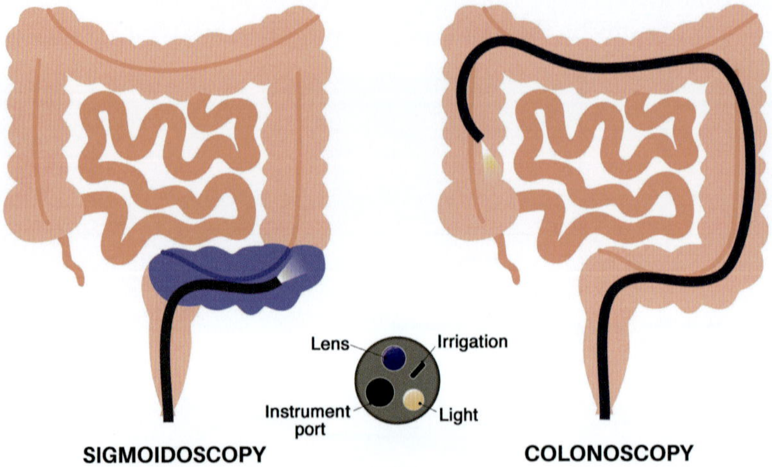

Figure 3-3 Sigmoidoscopy vs colonoscopy.

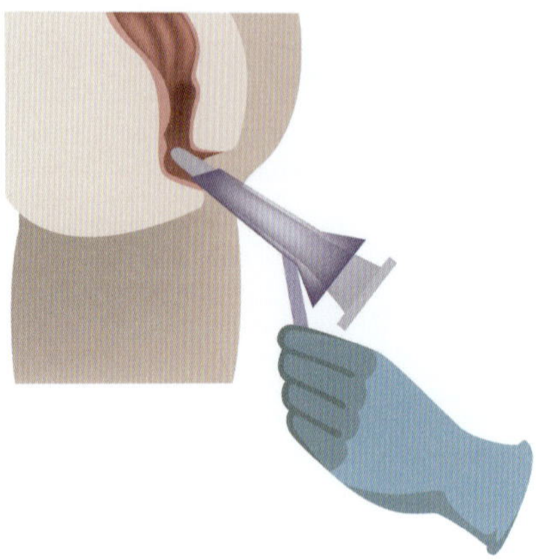

Figure 3-4 Anoscopy.

The shortest endoscope is an **anoscope (Fig. 3-4)**, which can examine the interior of the anus and lower rectum. A **proctoscope** is slightly longer and is used to examine the rectum.

Laparoscopy is a form of endoscopy where a **laparoscope** (a thin tube with a light and camera) is inserted through a small skin incision into the abdominal cavity, enabling the surgeon to view the internal organs of the abdomen and pelvis and perform surgical procedures that are less invasive than when done by open surgery.

The endoscope is more than just a fancy camera with a light source. It can have attached tools capable of biopsy and removal of polyps, stones, and other obstructions, and inject medications

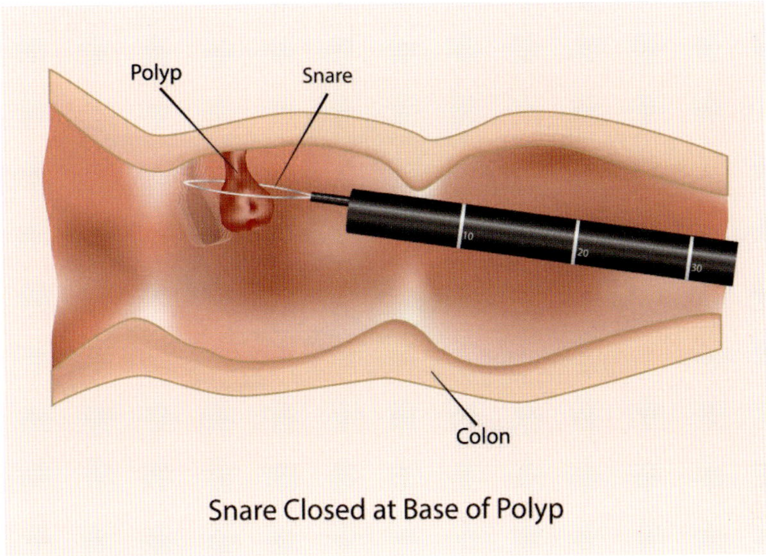

Figure 3-5 Polyp removal by colonoscopy.

(**Fig. 3-5**). It can dilate constrictions, place a stent to relieve an obstruction, and do certain kinds of surgery. It can have a microscope that directly visualizes the gut wall up close, sometimes with staining, like a histological slide. It can also make an abrupt turn and go into the bile duct and inject contrast that will outline the gallbladder and pancreas or remove stones in the bile or pancreatic ducts.

Imaging

Imaging provides an indirect way of looking inside the GI tract.

Plain X-rays are widely available and quick. They can often diagnose gastrointestinal obstructions, perforations, and some structural abnormalities.

Abdominal Ultrasound (AUS) can provide soft tissue detail of the liver, gallbladder, and kidneys and guide procedures like biopsies in real time. Ultrasound does not involve radiation and is relatively inexpensive.

Computerized Tomography (CT) scans are quick and can provide detailed information about soft tissue and bone. CT can identify tumors, inflammation, infections, and vascular problems. It involves radiation, though, and is more expensive than X-rays or ultrasound. It also may require the use of contrast agents, which in some people may cause allergic reactions.

Magnetic Resonance Imaging (MRI) is better than X-rays, ultrasound, and CT scan in outlining soft tissue. It can provide more details about tumors, inflammatory bowel disease, and liver disease, as well as functional information (e.g., the flow of bile, pancreatic juices, and blood). However, MRI is relatively expensive and time-consuming and is contraindicated in patients with metallic implants or significant claustrophobia.

Endoscopic Ultrasound (EUS) uses an ultrasound probe at the end of an endoscope, which the examiner advances either orally or rectally. This enables a closer analysis of the

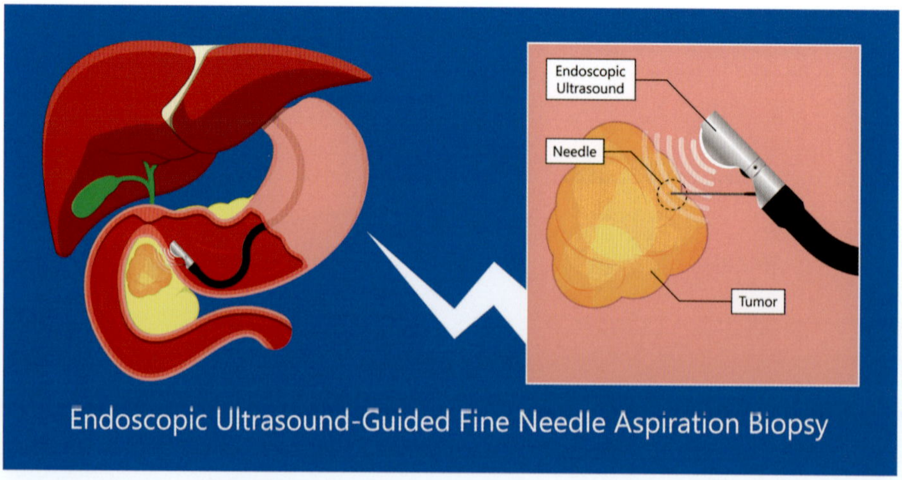

Figure 3-6

interior of the digestive tract. Unlike simple visualization of the gut lining, EUS can also assess the depth of a tumor invasion along with accompanying lymph nodes. It can also provide detailed images of the pancreas, bile duct and gallstones, bile duct obstruction and other abnormalities of the biliary system. EUS can also be used to guide fine-needle aspiration, or fine-needle biopsy in diagnosing cancer or other conditions. It is relatively non-invasive and can be used for both diagnosis and treatment (e.g., delivering medication and draining cysts) (**Fig. 3-6**).

Endoscopic Retrograde Cholangiopancreatography (ERCP) combines endoscopy and fluoroscopy in real time. It involves passing a small plastic tube or wire into the bile duct or pancreatic duct, with injection of a contrast dye that outlines the ducts and can be seen by fluoroscopy. ERCP is good at identifying bile duct stones, strictures, leaks, and pancreatic and bile duct cancer and is less invasive than open surgery. It can be used for biopsy or brushing suspicious areas to collect tumor cells for diagnosis. It can also be used to remove stones from the bile or pancreatic ducts, place stents or balloons to open narrowed or blocked ducts, or seal leaks in the bile or pancreatic ducts (**Fig. 3-7**).

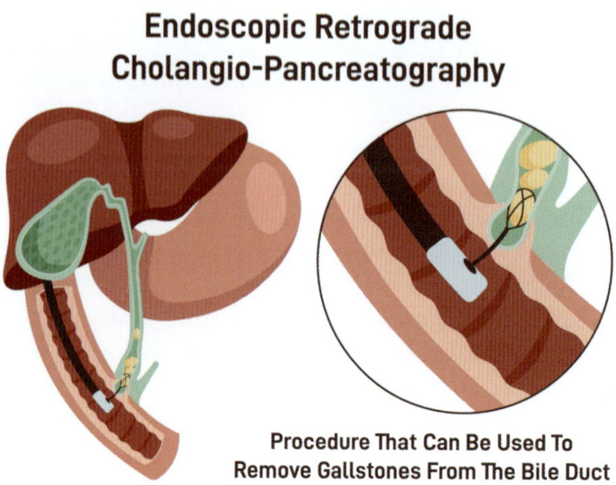

Figure 3-7

Magnetic Resonance Cholangiopancreatography (MRCP) Is a specific MRI technique that clearly shows fluid-filled structures (**Fig. 3-8**). This produces detailed pictures of the biliary and pancreatic ducts (with or without contrast material), revealing evidence of blockages, stones, tumors, and inflammation of the bile ducts and pancreas. It is less invasive than ERCP. However, it does not provide functional information (e.g., GI motility, secretion, absorption, and blood flow) and cannot take tissue samples or perform interventions. It might also miss very small ductal anomalies.

Techniques that provide **functional information** include fluoroscopy, barium swallow studies, ultrasound (e.g., blood flow), scintigraphy (uses radiopharmaceuticals to show tissue function), magnetic enterography (MRI with contrast material observed over time), manometry (measures pressure and movement changes over time), capsule endoscopy (observes the small intestine as the capsule passes through), pH monitoring over time, and breath tests.

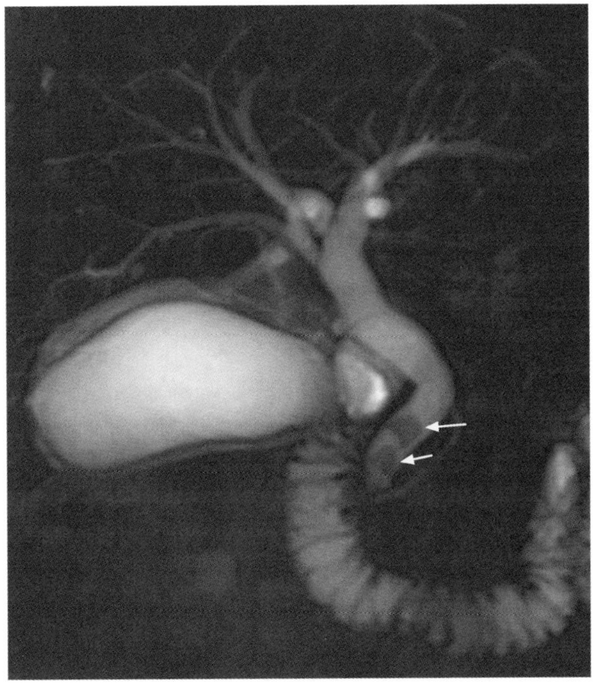

Figure 3-8 *Magnetic resonance cholangiopancreatography. Arrows are gallstones in distal common bile duct. Note bile duct dilation. (Image courtesy of Jordan Ditchek, M.D.)*

Barium X-ray Studies (such as a barium swallow or barium enema) use barium as a contrast material to outline the GI tract (**Figs. 3-9** and **3-10**). Such studies can detect motility problems as well as structural problems like blockages, anatomical variation, ulcers, and tumors. Barium studies are widely available, provide good visualization and are relatively cost-effective. However, they do involve radiation exposure and the pictures they provide are not as detailed as other imaging methods for evaluating soft tissue. They may also miss small lesions.

Chromoendoscopy (CE) is an endoscopic procedure that enhances visualization of the gut mucosa by applying special stains. It can find lesions missed by standard white-light endoscopy, such as precancerous polyps or cancer.

Optical Coherence Tomography (OCT) is an endoscopic procedure that uses near-infrared light waves to obtain high-resolution cross-sectional images of the GI tract, whether in the esophagus, colon, or pancreatic and biliary ducts, as can other imaging techniques. OCT, however, can also provide micron-level resolution. It can guide biopsies and may even eliminate the need for one. It is limited, though, by seeing through a depth of only about 1-2 mm.

Confocal Laser Endomicroscopy (CLE) is an endoscopic technique that uses a low-power laser to illuminate a small area of GI mucosa by exciting a systemically administered fluorescent dye that binds to specific targets so that the target emits light. This permits real-time microscopic cross-sectional examination of the GI wall at different mucosal depths, like a "virtual biopsy." It can identify abnormal cell patterns suggestive of cancer, Crohn's

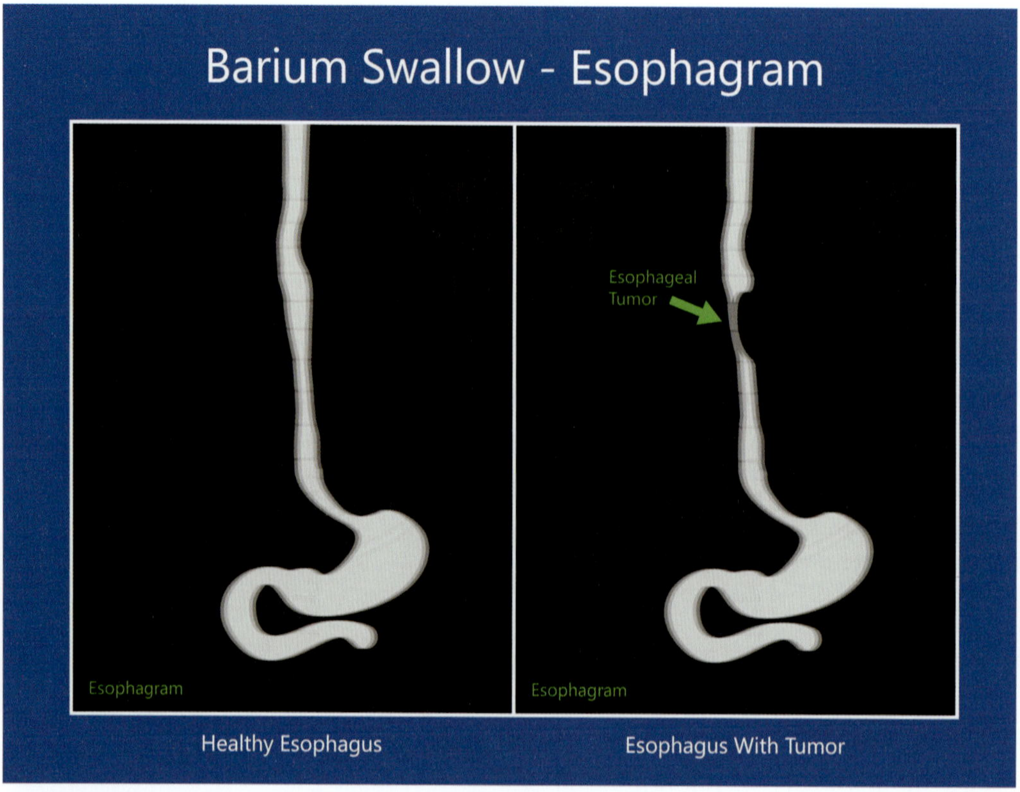

Figure 3-9

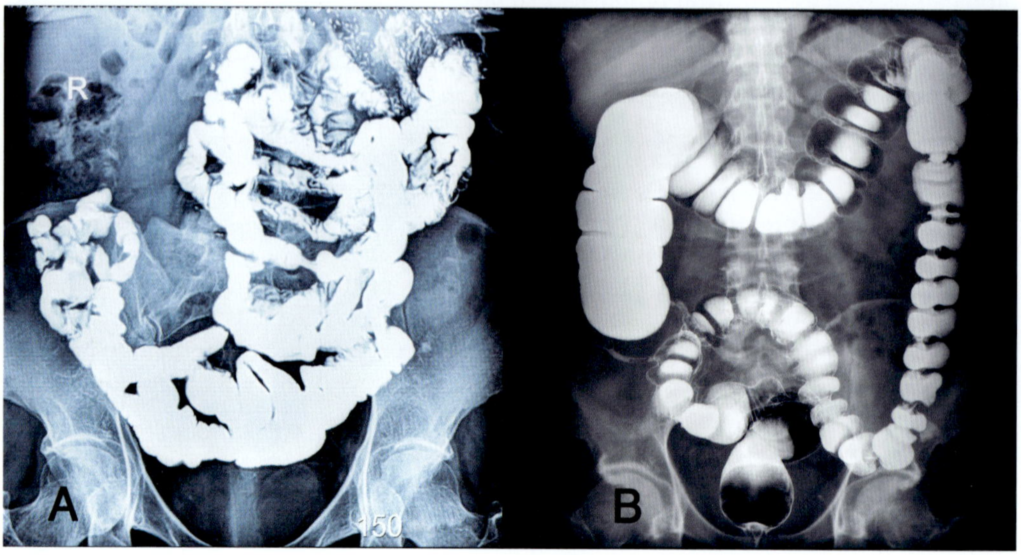

Figure 3-10 *A. Barium swallow small bowel follow-through. B. Barium enema, showing colon.*

disease, ulcerative colitis, Barrett's esophagus, and neoplastic vs non-neoplastic polyps. However, it can examine only small areas at once.

Scintigraphy (nuclear medicine scan) is an imaging technique that uses a radioactive tracer that can locate or treat problems by targeting specific tissues. E.g., it can be used for gastric emptying studies, detection of active bleeding, detection of tumors or cysts, bile leaks, and examining the adequacy of colonic transit. **Positron Emission Tomography (PET) Scan** is a scintigraphy technique that uses a radioactive tracer to detect tissue with a high metabolic rate, such as cancer cells, which show up in the form of hot spots on scanning. The **HIDA (Hepatobiliary Iminodiacetic Acid) Scan** is a form of scintigraphy in which a radioactive tracer injected into the bloodstream is absorbed by the liver and excreted into the bile. Progressive movement of the tracer through the liver, bile ducts, gallbladder, and small intestine is followed and provides a picture of how well bile is flowing. HIDA can help diagnose inflammation of the gallbladder, bile duct obstruction, and liver dysfunction. **Somatostatin receptor scintigraphy (OctreoScan)** uses a radioactive tracer bound to a synthetic form of somatostatin. The tracer has a high affinity for somatostatin receptors, which are found on the surface of certain kinds of tumors cells (e.g., neuroendocrine tumors). This allows visualization of those tumors and their metastases.

Liver Elastography is a non-invasive ultrasound-based technique to assess liver fibrosis.

Other Tests

Genetic Tests may be done for hereditary conditions like hereditary nonpolyposis colorectal cancer (Lynch syndrome) or familial adenomatous polyposis.

The **Hydrogen Breath Test** confirms carbohydrate malabsorption (such as lactose intolerance) or small intestinal bacterial overgrowth. The patient drinks a solution containing sugar, which normally is absorbed in the small intestine. If it's not absorbed, bacteria in the colon (which normally has far more bacteria than the small intestine) ferment the sugar, producing hydrogen. The hydrogen is absorbed into the bloodstream, where it can be measured in the patient's breath. Elevated breath hydrogen suggests either malabsorption of the sugar (e.g., lactose intolerance), bacterial overgrowth in the small intestine, or that the sugar is moving too fast through the small intestine to be absorbed and is being fermented in the colon.

The **Urea Breath Test** helps confirm *Helicobacter pylori* infection, a major cause of gastric and duodenal ulcers. The patient ingests radiolabeled urea. *H. pylori* produces an enzyme (urease) that breaks down urea into CO_2 and ammonia. If the exhaled labeled CO_2 is higher than normal, this suggests that the urea was broken down by *H. pylori*.

pH Monitoring using a **Bravo pH monitor** is used to measure acid in the esophagus and to diagnose gastroesophageal reflux disease (GERD). Bravo involves attachment of a small, wireless capsule to the lower esophageal wall. The capsule relays pH levels over several days to a small external receiver. The patient maintains a diary of meals and symptoms over that time, after which the capsule naturally detaches and is passed through the GI tract. The method is less invasive and more comfortable than the method using a traditional pH catheter.

Manometry: Esophageal Manometry is a test for measuring the pressure and movement of the esophagus, as in achalasia, where there is loss of peristaltic movement in the esophagus. **Anorectal Manometry** evaluates bowel muscle function in patients with constipation or fecal incontinence.

4

Treatments in Gastroenterology

The armamentarium of the gastroenterologist includes many treatment modalities:

Pharmacological Treatments

Antacids: Neutralize stomach acid for quick relief of acid reflux, e.g., *aluminum hydroxide/ magnesium hydroxide (Maalox, Mylanta), calcium carbonate (Tums), sodium bicarbonate (Alka-Seltzer), magnesium hydroxide (Milk of Magnesia).*

Proton Pump Inhibitors (PPIs): Prevent the stomach parietal cells from secreting acid by blocking their hydrogen-potassium ATPase pump (the proton pump), e.g., *omeprazole (Prilosec), esomeprazole (Nexium), lansoprazole (Prevacid), pantoprazole (Protonix), rabeprazole (Aciphex), dexlansoprazole (Dexilant). Vonoprazan [Voquezna]* is a more recent drug that interacts with the proton pump, but via a somewhat different mechanism than standard PPIs; *vonoprazan* does not require an acidic environment to be activated, has a faster onset of action than PPIs, and is longer-lasting, but there is less data regarding long-term safety.

H2 Blockers (histamine H2-receptor antagonists): Reduce stomach acid by blocking the action of histamine on H2 receptors of stomach parietal cells, thereby blocking the ability of histamine (a naturally occurring body chemical) to stimulate acid secretion, e.g., *ranitidine (Zantac), famotidine (Pepcid), cimetidine (Tagamet), mizatidine (Axid)*. H2 blockers act more quickly than proton pump inhibitors. However, they are not as potent or long-acting.

Antibiotics: To treat infections, such as *H. pylori*

Antispasmodics: To relieve symptoms of irritable bowel syndrome (IBS)

Antidiarrheals: To manage diarrhea

Laxatives: For constipation relief

Anti-inflammatory Drugs: E.g., aminosalicylates (e.g., *mesalamine*), corticosteroids, and immunosuppressants for inflammatory bowel diseases

Biologic Therapies: TNF inhibitors (e.g., *infliximab* [*Remicade*]) and integrin receptor antagonists (e.g., *veolizumab* [*Entyvio*]) target specific components of the immune system in the treatment of inflammatory bowel diseases.

Antiemetics: To control nausea and vomiting

Cholestyramine: Binds excess bile acids in the intestine, preventing bile acid diarrhea. It also reduces reabsorption of bile acids, preventing excess accumulation of bile acids in the bloodstream, which can cause marked pruritus (itching).

Pancreatic Enzyme Supplements: Aid digestion in conditions like chronic pancreatitis, where there is a deficiency in pancreatic digestive enzymes.

Hepatoprotective Drugs: Prevent damage to the liver and support its healing and regenerative processes, e.g., *silymarin* (*Milk Thistle*), *ursodeoxycholic acid* (*UDCA*), *n-acetylcysteine* (*NAC*), *s-adenosylmethionine* (*SAMe*), *L-Ornithine L-Aspartate* (*LOLA*), *phosphatidylcholine* (*Lecithin*), *vitamin E*, *Liv.52* (*Ayurvedic Medicine*).

Endoscopic Treatments

Polypectomy: Removal of polyps during a colonoscopy

Foreign body removal

Variceal Banding or Sclerotherapy: For eliminating varices

Argon Plasma Coagulation: To cauterize GI bleeds

Hemostasis: To control bleeding using clips, coagulation, or injection

Dilation of narrowed areas of the esophagus, stomach, or intestine, using balloons or dilators

Stent placement to relieve obstruction in the bile duct or GI tract

Endoscopic Mucosal Resection (EMR) for removal of superficial lesions, or **Endoscopic Submucosal Dissection (ESD)** for deeper lesions.

Percutaneous Endoscopic Gastrostomy (PEG): For long-term feeding in patients unable to take oral nutrition

Fecal Microbiota Transplant (FMT): For recurrent *Clostridioides difficile* infection

Radiofrequency Ablation (Stretta): The Stretta procedure involves the delivery of radiofrequency (RF) energy to the muscle tissue at the junction of the esophagus and stomach, specifically the lower esophageal sphincter (LES) and the gastric cardia to prevent gastric reflux.

Endoscopic plication (EsophyX): Reconstructs the lower esophageal sphincter with a fold that can be tightened to reduce GERD

Endoscopic retrograde cholangiopancreatography (ERCP) can both diagnose and treat problems in the bile and pancreatic ducts, e.g., stone removal and stent placement.

Endoscopic ultrasound (EUS) with fine needle aspiration to obtain tissue samples from the GI tract **Endoscopic suturing**

Part II. Diseases of the Digestive System

5

Diseases of the Esophagus

Gastroesophageal Reflux Disease (GERD)

Gastroesophageal reflux disease (GERD) is a chronic condition where stomach contents back up into the esophagus and irritate it. GERD is characterized by frequent heartburn. If untreated, it can lead to serious complications, such as esophagitis, esophageal strictures, and Barrett's esophagus (where the esophageal lining resembles that of the intestine). Barrett's increases the risk of developing esophageal cancer. GERD can be caused by weakening of the lower esophageal sphincter (LES); obesity, which increases the pressure on the stomach; pregnancy; conditions that slow down gastric emptying (gastroparesis); and certain medications and foods (e.g., spicy or fatty foods, chocolate, caffeine, alcohol or carbonated drinks). Hiatal hernia (**Fig. 6-2**) can contribute to GERD by altering the anatomy of the lower esophageal sphincter. Excess smoking relaxes the LES. There may also be genetic factors, as GERD often runs in families.

Diagnosis of GERD

History: The classic symptom of GERD is heartburn from acid reflux. Atypical symptoms may include cough, chest pain, laryngitis, asthma-like symptoms, and dental erosions. To get a better idea of what the patient is experiencing, ask about the frequency and severity of symptoms, exacerbating factors, response to over-the-counter medications, and impact on the quality of the patient's life.

Diagnostic Procedures: A trial of proton pump inhibitors (PPIs) may be given for symptomatic relief. If the patient improves, this supports the diagnosis of GERD.

- **Endoscopy** can identify esophageal mucosal damage or other complications like Barrett's esophagus.

- **pH Monitoring** over 24-hours using a Bravo capsule positioned above the lower esophageal sphincter can confirm abnormal acid reflux.
- **Esophageal Manometry** evaluates the function of the lower esophageal sphincter and esophageal motility.
- **Barium Swallow Radiography** is less commonly used but can show a hiatal hernia or other structural abnormality.

Treatment of GERD

Lifestyle Modifications:

- Weight loss if overweight
- Elevate the head of the bed.
- Avoid food triggers (e.g., fatty foods, caffeine, chocolate, spicy foods, and carbonated beverages).
- Avoid lying down within 2-3 hours after eating.
- Stop smoking, which can exacerbate GERD symptoms by increasing acid production, weaken the lower esophageal sphincter, and induce reflux through coughing and deep inspiration.

Pharmacological Treatment:

- **Antacids:** For immediate symptom relief.
- **H2 Receptor Antagonists:** For mild, infrequent heartburn
- **Proton Pump Inhibitors (PPIs):** Long-acting first-line therapy for more significant symptoms
- **Prokinetics** can be used in select cases to enhance gastric emptying and esophageal motility (e.g., *metoclopramide, domperidone, erythromycin*).
- **Alginate Therapy**, often combined with antacids, forms a floating gel in the stomach that reduces reflux and protects the esophageal lining (e.g., *Gaviscon, Peptac, Refluxil*).
- **Maintenance Therapy:** Long-term PPI therapy may be necessary for chronic symptoms and esophagitis healing.

Monitoring and Follow-Up:

- Monitoring for potential complications such as Barrett's esophagus
- Regular follow-up to assess symptom control and medication side effects

Surgical and Endoscopic Interventions (if necessary):

- **Nissen Fundoplication:** Surgical enhancement of lower esophageal sphincter pressure (**Fig. 5-1**), generally done laparoscopically.

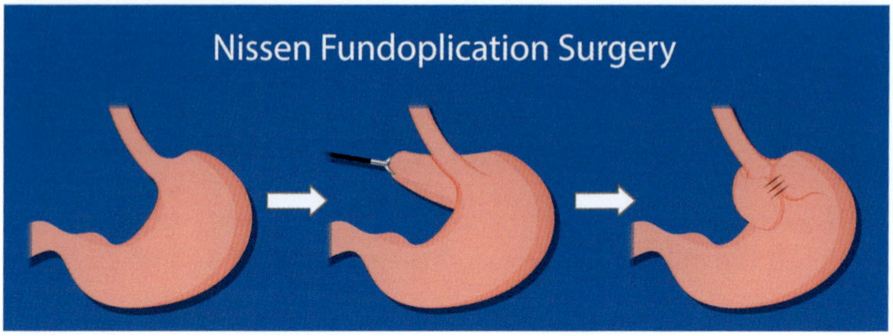

Figure 5-1

- **LINX device:** A ring of magnetic beads is placed around the lower esophageal sphincter (LES) to strengthen and close the LES (**Fig. 5-2**).
- **Radiofrequency Ablation (Stretta)** creates small burns in the LES muscle and upper stomach, reducing the tendency of the LES to relax inappropriately.
- **Transoral Incisionless Fundoplication (EsophyX)** creates an auxiliary valve mechanism at the gastroesophageal junction by creating a fold of stomach tissue around the lower end of the esophagus.

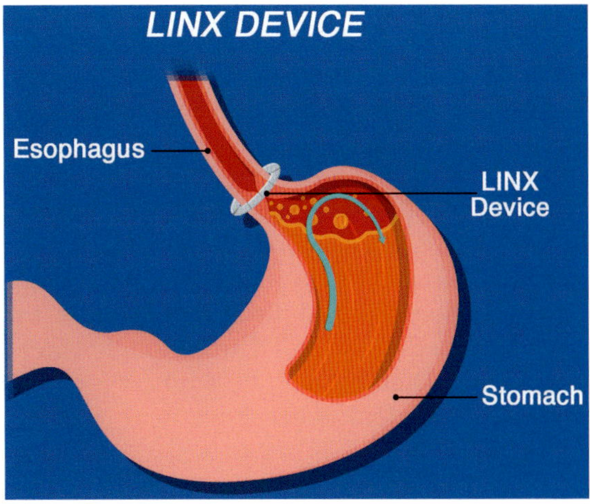

Figure 5-2

Esophagitis

Esophagitis (inflammation of the esophagus) most commonly results from acid reflux disease. However, it can also result from infections (e.g., herpes simplex, cytomegalovirus, candida), certain medications (e.g., bisphosphonates, tetracycline), allergies (eosinophilic esophagitis), chemical irritants (e.g., household cleaners), chronic vomiting, GI diseases (e.g., Crohn's disease), hiatal hernia, physical obstruction, or irradiation.

Diagnosis of Esophagitis

The patient may report **dysphagia** (difficulty swallowing), **odynophagia** (painful swallowing), chest pain, heartburn, or food impaction. Inquire about the patient's dietary habits, medication use (e.g., NSAIDs), past medical history, and potential exposure to infectious agents.

Endoscopy with Biopsy: Upper Gastrointestinal Endoscopy (EGD) can identify inflammation, ulcers, strictures, or other abnormalities. Biopsy samples may be taken during the endoscopy to look for eosinophils (suggestive of eosinophilic esophagitis), viral inclusions, fungal organisms, or cellular changes indicative of Barrett's esophagus, where the esophageal lining changes to tissue resembling the lining of the intestine, often resulting from chronic GERD. Barrett's esophagus is a risk factor for developing esophageal adenocarcinoma.

A **Barium Swallow X-ray** can show strictures or motility issues.

pH Monitoring or **pH-Impedance Testing** both test for gastric reflux. pH monitoring specifically tests for acidity, while pH-impedance testing also tests for non-acid reflux, which may also be irritating.

Blood Tests can check for anemia, inflammatory markers, or allergens.

Manometry evaluates the function of the esophageal muscles and sphincters.

In the **Bernstein** test, acid is instilled into the esophagus to see if it simulates the patient's symptoms.

Treatment of Esophagitis

GERD-Related Esophagitis employs the same treatment as for GERD.

Eosinophilic Esophagitis (EoE) is treated with elimination diets that remove the offending allergen. Swallowed steroids (*fluticasone* or *budesonide*) can reduce inflammation. Proton pump inhibitors can help in some cases.

Infectious Esophagitis: Antifungal medications are used for fungal infections like candidiasis. Antiviral medications are used for viral infections (e.g., *herpes simplex* or *cytomegalovirus*). Antibiotics are prescribed in some cases where there is a bacterial infection.

Medication-Induced Esophagitis: It is important to identify and discontinue the offending medication and drink enough water while favoring an upright position.

Dilation Therapy may be advised for strictures. **Surgery** may be needed for severe strictures or perforations.

Barrett's Esophagus

Barrett's esophagus is a common condition in which the lower esophagus lining changes, becoming more like the lining of the intestine, typically due to chronic acid exposure from GERD. It is a risk factor for esophageal adenocarcinoma.

Diagnosis of Barrett's Esophagus

Endoscopic Examination: Areas of suspected Barrett's tissue typically look redder than the normal pink.

Biopsy: Tissue samples from endoscopy confirms that the esophagus is non-neoplastic Barrett's or has dysplasia (pre-cancerous), whether low or high grade.

Other tests: pH monitoring may be done if GERD symptoms persist.

Treatment of Barrett's Esophagus

Acid Reduction can be accomplished with antacids, H2 receptor blockers or proton pump inhibitors.

Monitoring: Repeat endoscopy is done, which may include biopsy, typically every 3-5 years for those without dysplasia, every 6-12 months for low-grade dysplasia, and more frequently for high-grade dysplasia to determine progression of the disease, especially to esophageal adenocarcinoma.

Lifestyle Modifications are similar to GERD management, including weight loss if appropriate, dietary modifications, smoking cessation, and elevating the head of the bed.

Endoscopic Treatment (for dysplastic Barrett's esophagus):

- **Radiofrequency Ablation (RFA)** uses heat to remove abnormal tissue.
- **Cryotherapy** freezes the abnormal cells.
- **Endoscopic Mucosal Resection (EMR)** is less invasive than surgery. It removes superficial precancerous or cancerous cells or nodules via an endoscope.

Surgical Intervention: Esophagectomy, the surgical removal of part of the esophagus, is generally reserved for high-grade dysplasia or early-stage esophageal cancer.

Esophageal Varices

Esophageal varices are enlarged veins in the esophagus that occur mainly because of portal hypertension, often due to liver cirrhosis.

Diagnosis of Esophageal Varices

History and Physical may suggest cirrhosis, jaundice, ascites, spider angiomas, or splenomegaly.

Endoscopy enables direct visualization and grading of varices.

Imaging:

- **Ultrasound** with Doppler can assess portal vein flow.
- **CT scan** or **MRI** help evaluate portal hypertension. CT scan can see the vascular anatomy, view liver morphology that may suggest cirrhosis, measure spleen size, and detect ascites. MRI provides very good soft tissue contrast to visualize the liver's structure. **MRI angiography** can detect blockages in the portal venous system. **Hepatic elastography**, if available, can measure liver stiffness suggestive of fibrosis associated with portal hypertension.

Lab Tests: Liver function tests, complete blood count, and coagulation profile help assess liver disease and any other hematological abnormalities that may be associated with decreased hepatic function.

Treatment of Esophageal Varices

Primary Prophylaxis: Beta-blockers (e.g., *propranolol, carvedilol,* or *nadolol*) reduce the risk of bleeding by decreasing portal hypertension. **Endoscopic variceal ligation** (EVL) may be used for patients with contraindications to or side effects from beta-blockers.

Controlling Acute Variceal Hemorrhage:

- **Initial Stabilization** includes fluid resuscitation, blood transfusions, and correction of coagulopathy.
- **Vasoactive Drugs:** *Octreotide* and *vasopressin* reduce portal pressure. Vasopressin acts as a vasoconstrictor that reduces inflow of blood into the portal vein. Octreotide is a somatostatin analogue that has inhibitory effects on the digestive system, including reducing blood flow to the gastrointestinal tract, thereby reducing pressure in the portal veins.

Antibiotics may be prescribed to prevent infection.

Endoscopic Therapy: Endoscopic variceal ligation or **sclerotherapy** can control variceal bleeding. **Balloon tamponade** (e.g., **Sengstaken-Blakemore tube**) is a temporary measure for uncontrolled bleeding.

Transjugular Intrahepatic Portosystemic Shunt (TIPS) creates a shunt between the portal and systemic circulations, thereby reducing portal vein pressure.

Managing Underlying Liver Disease may include antiviral treatment for hepatitis, alcohol abstinence, or management of non-alcoholic fatty liver disease (weight loss, healthy diet, exercise, control of type 2 diabetes and cholesterol).

Esophageal Strictures

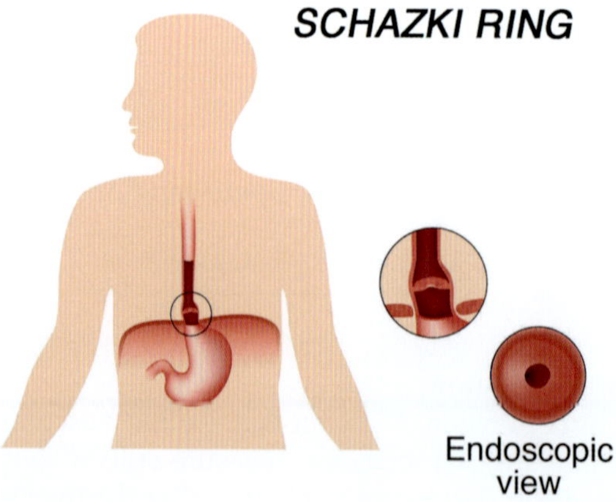

Figure 5-3

Esophageal stricture is a narrowing of the esophagus that can cause dysphagia (difficulty swallowing), food impaction and significant nutritional problems. It can result from chronic GERD, eosinophilic esophagitis, radiation therapy, ingestion of caustic chemicals, certain medications that get caught in the esophagus after swallowing, congenital abnormalities, tumors (benign or malignant, inside or outside the esophagus), esophageal webs (thin membranes that grow across the esophageal lumen), or Schatzki's rings (**Fig. 5-3**).

Diagnosis of Esophageal Strictures

Difficulty swallowing is the primary symptom. Pain on swallowing (odynophagia) and regurgitation of food may occur in some people.

Barium Swallow: The esophagus is viewed on X-ray as the patient swallows a radiopaque contrast liquid, containing barium sulfate. This can identify the area of the stricture.

Endoscopy allows direct visualization of the stricture and enables biopsy to determine if there is malignancy or eosinophilic esophagitis.

CT scan or **MRI** may help in specific cases, if there is suspicion of a tumor or extrinsic compression of the esophagus.

Manometry can help determine if there is a motility problem..

Treatment of Esophageal Strictures

Esophageal Dilation: Done with balloons or a bougie dilating instrument. Dilation may be needed on more than one occasion.

Medications:

- Proton pump inhibitors (PPIs) or other acid-reducing medications if GERD is the cause of the stricture
- Steroids for certain cases of inflammation. e.g., eosinophilic esophagitis. *Budesonide* is given topically by swallow. *Dupilumab* (*Dupixent*) is an anti-inflammatory agent given by subcutaneous injection and may be administered in patients not responding to topical corticosteroids.
- Antibiotics if infection is the cause

Stent Placement when dilation doesn't work, or if stricture is due to malignancy (**Fig. 5-4**)

Surgical Treatment: Esophagectomy or **stricturoplasty** (surgical widening), e.g., for cancer or strictures non-responsive to other measures

Nutritional Support: The patient may need a liquid diet. In refractory cases, the patient may need a surgically-placed percutaneous endoscopic gastrostomy (PEG) tube (a feeding tube is directly placed in the stomach) or a temporary nasogastric tube.

Esophageal Cancer

There are two main types of esophageal cancer: **squamous cell carcinoma** and **adenocarcinoma**, each with distinct risk factors and patterns of occurrence. **Squamous cell carcinoma** is more common in the upper and middle esophagus and is more common in East Asia and South Africa and in African American men. Risk factors include tobacco and alcohol use, drinking very hot liquids, poor nutrition, achalasia, and **tylosis** (a rare genetic skin disorder). **Adenocarcinoma** is more common in the lower esophagus and in Western countries, e.g., the U.S. and Western Europe, mainly in Caucasian men. Risk factors include GERD, obesity, Barrett's esophagus, smoking, and diets high in processed meat.

Diagnosis of Esophageal Cancer

Common symptoms include difficulty swallowing (dysphagia), unintentional weight loss, chest pain, chronic cough, and indigestion. Digestive symptoms often appear once the tumor grows large enough to restrict the esophagus. Some patients may develop a fistula between esophagus and trachea, leading to leakage of swallowed material into the lungs.

Endoscopy allows direct visualization and biopsy of the esophagus.

Barium Swallow X-ray outlines the esophagus.

Endoscopic Ultrasound can determine the depth of tumor invasion in the esophageal wall and assess the presence of nearby lymph nodes.

Computed Tomography (CT) Scan can determine local invasion and metastasis to the lungs, liver, and elsewhere.

Positron Emission Tomography (PET) Scan detects cancer spread by identifying areas of high metabolic activity.

Bronchoscopy may be done when there is suspicion of tumor involvement of the airways.

TNM Staging Esophageal Cancer:

- **T (Tumor size):** How deep has the tumor invaded the esophagus and surroundings?
- **N (Nodes):** Has the cancer spread to the lymph nodes?
- **M (Metastasis):** Has the cancer metastasized?

Treatment of Esophageal Cancer

Surgical Resection: Esophagectomy may include nearby lymph nodes.

Chemotherapy can shrink the tumor and may be given after surgery to clear up remaining tumor cells, or may be given alone if surgery is not feasible.

Radiation Therapy may be given with chemotherapy, immunotherapy, or surgery.

Laser Ablation burns away abnormal esophageal tissue mass.

Palliative Care may use a stent to relieve obstruction (**Fig. 5-4**); chemotherapy or radiation therapy may shrink tumors; pain management and nutritional and emotional support may be helpful.

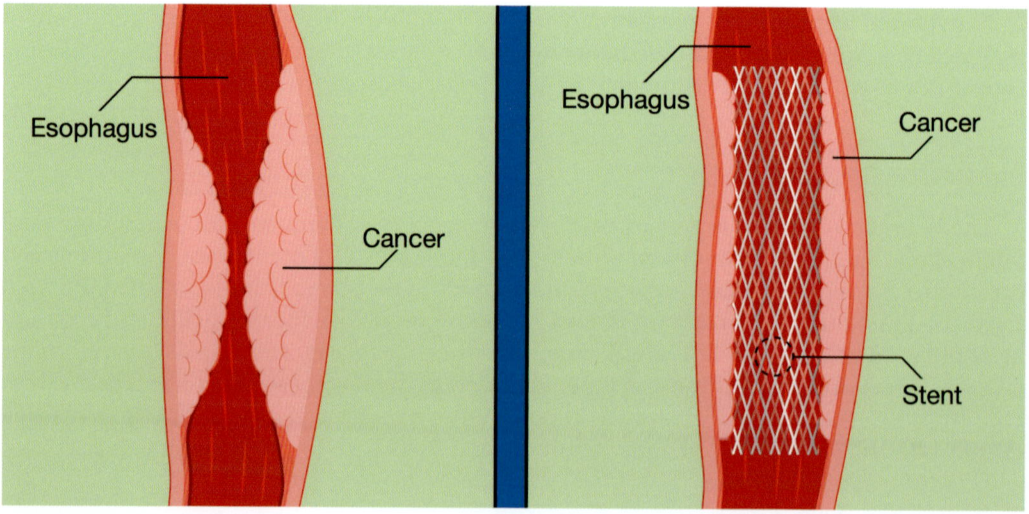

Figure 5-4 *Stent placement.*

Esophageal Ulcers

Esophageal ulcers can be caused by prolonged acid reflux (GERD), infections (e.g., *Candida, herpes simplex, cytomegalovirus*), medications, e.g., nonsteroidal anti-inflammatory drugs (NSAIDs), excess alcohol consumption, ingestion of caustic substances, and trauma from endoscopy.

Diagnosis of Esophageal Ulcers

Common symptoms include pain or difficulty swallowing, heartburn, chest pain, and sometimes bleeding (vomiting blood, or black, tarry stools).

Endoscopy allows direct esophageal visualization, biopsy for malignancy, and sampling for infections.

Barium Swallow X-ray can reveal irregularities or ulceration in the esophageal lining.

Lab Tests:

- Can check for anemia from bleeding
- Can check for *Helicobacter pylori* bacteria in a biopsy specimen, in stool antigen testing, and in PCR of the biopsy, stool or saliva. The **urea breath test** measure radiolabeled CO_2 in the breath after drinking a solution containing radiolabeled urea. *H. pylori* breaks down the urea, releasing the labeled CO_2, which is detected in the breath.

pH Monitoring: GERD pH monitoring over 24 hours can measure acid levels in the esophagus.

Treatment of Esophageal Ulcers

- Control bleeding. Esophageal bleeding may require endoscopic cauterization or clipping of bleeding vessels.

- Discontinue ulcerogenic medications like NSAIDs or, depending on the patient, corticosteroids.
- Reduce stomach acid, using proton pump inhibitors (PPIs), H2 receptor antagonists, or antacids.
- Treat the underlying cause, e.g., antifungal medication for *Candida* or antiviral drugs for *herpes* or *cytomegalovirus (CMV)*.

Endoscopic Dilation may be needed if strictures are significant.
Surgery may be done for perforation or bleeding unresponsive to other measures.

Lifestyle Modifications:

- Avoid foods that exacerbate reflux (e.g., spicy foods, alcohol, caffeine).
- Elevate the head during sleep to prevent nocturnal reflux.
- Lose weight if obese.

Achalasia

Achalasia is marked by the loss of esophageal peristalsis and inability of the lower esophageal sphincter to relax. This can result in difficulty swallowing solids and often liquids. The chronic stasis of food in the esophagus causes inflammation that is a risk factor, however small, for developing squamous cell carcinoma of the esophagus. Achalasia can be caused by damage to the esophageal nerves, particularly those that innervate the lower esophageal sphincter. It can also be due to an autoimmune reaction to esophageal cells (e.g., scleroderma), genetic factors, infection (e.g., the *Trypanosoma cruzi* parasite of *Chagas disease*, which is a risk factor for developing esophageal squamous cell cancer). Often the cause of achalasia remains unknown.

Diagnosis of Achalasia

The patient presents with dysphagia and regurgitation of undigested food, and sometimes chest pain and weight loss.

Barium Swallow X-ray: The esophagus appears dilated and tortuous, with a "bird's beak" sign at the lower esophageal sphincter (**Fig. 5-5**). This sign is due to dilation of the distal esophagus (bird's head) together with a narrowed lower esophageal sphincter (bird's beak).

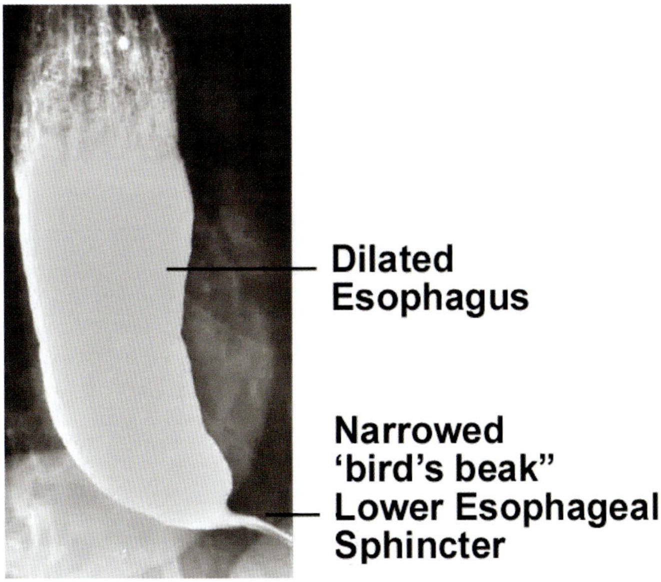

Figure 5-5 *Bird's beak sign in achalasia from tapering of the distal esophagus (by Farnoosh Farrokhi, Michael F. Vaezi. [CC BY 2.0], via Wikimedia Commons).*

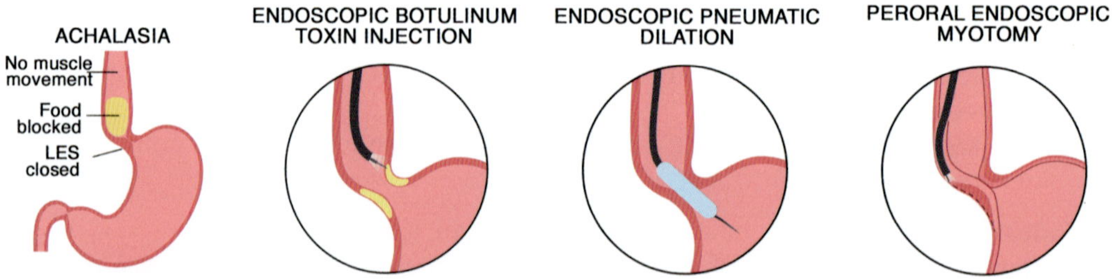

Figure 5-6 Treatments for achalasia.

Esophageal Manometry is a definitive test for achalasia. It shows elevated LES (lower esophageal sphincter) pressure with incomplete LES relaxation, along with loss of esophageal peristalsis.

Endoscopy determines if there is mechanical obstruction by retained food.

Esophageal pH Monitoring determines if there is GERD, which can mimic the symptoms of achalasia.

Treatment of Achalasia

Botulinum Toxin (Botox) Injection relaxes the LES by injecting botulinum toxin into it (**Fig. 5-6**).

Pneumatic Dilation uses a balloon to stretch the fibers of the LES to open it (**Fig. 5-6**).

Myotomy cuts the muscles of the LES to allow food to pass more easily into the stomach (**Fig. 5-6**).

Calcium Channel Blockers and **Nitrates** can decrease LES pressure by relaxing the smooth muscle of the LES.

Lifestyle Modifications include chewing food thoroughly and drinking lots of fluids with meals, as well as eating upright.

Esophagectomy (removal of part of the esophagus) is used in some advanced cases where the esophagus is hopelessly dilated and nonfunctional.

Esophageal Spasms

Esophageal spasms are abnormal contractions of the esophagus that can cause chest pain and difficulty swallowing. There are two main types: **diffuse esophageal spasms**, which are uncoordinated, and **nutcracker spasms**, which are coordinated but excessively intense. Both types of esophageal spasms can cause difficulty swallowing, chest pain (which can mimic a heart attack), regurgitation and the sensation of food stuck in the esophagus.

Diagnosis of Esophageal Spasm

Esophageal Manometry can detect abnormal esophageal contractions.

Barium Swallow X-ray can outline the abnormal areas of contraction.

Endoscopy can help rule out other causes of the symptoms, e.g., inflammation, stricture, or malignancy.

ECG and **Cardiac Evaluation** can help rule out a cardiac origin.

Treatment of Esophageal Spasms

Drugs:

- **Calcium channel blockers** and **nitrates** can relax the esophageal muscles and reduce contractions.
- **Antidepressants**, e.g., tricyclic antidepressants, can help reduce pain and anxiety.
- **Peppermint oil** can relax the smooth muscle of the esophagus and alleviate symptoms.

Diet and Lifestyle Changes: Avoid triggers such as very hot or cold foods; eat more slowly.

Endoscopic Therapy with Botox can temporarily paralyze the spastic areas of the esophagus.

Surgery: Severing the spastic muscles of the esophagus (myotomy) may be used in refractory cases.

Pain Management

Treatment of Reflux with proton pump inhibitors or H2 receptor blockers

Foreign Body Impaction

Sometimes a foreign body can get lodged in the esophagus, particularly in children (e.g., small toy parts, coins, button batteries, marbles) or the elderly (large pieces of inadequately chewed food, fish or chicken bones, partial dentures, large pills, or capsules), which may cause perforation, pain, infection, or airway compromise by pressure on the trachea.

Diagnosis of Esophageal Foreign Body Impaction

The patient may report the sensation of something stuck in their throat or chest, chest discomfort, or inability to swallow saliva. A child may be irritable or refuse to eat.

Physical Examination: There may be drooling, or airway sounds suggestive of aspiration.

Imaging:

- **X-ray** or **CT scan** of the neck and chest can identify radiopaque objects and mediastinal air-trapping or subcutaneous emphysema from esophageal perforation.
- **Endoscopy** can help locate a foreign body in the esophagus that is radiolucent to X-ray.

Treatment of Esophageal Foreign Body Impaction

Endoscopic Removal: Apart from using endoscopy to remove the impacted object, sometimes it can be used to push a bolus of food into the stomach.

Foley Catheter Technique: Sometimes a Foley catheter can be passed beyond the impacted object and pulled back to remove it.

Glucagon Administration: Glucagon relaxes the esophageal sphincter, which may help the object pass into the stomach.

Surgery may be needed if there is esophageal perforation or if attempted removal by endoscope does not work.

Simple Close Observation may sometimes be effective in itself, as the obstruction may spontaneously resolve with time.

Antibiotics may be prescribed if there is concern about perforation or if the obstruction has been present for a long time.

Infectious Esophagitis

Infectious esophagitis can be caused by fungi, viruses, bacteria, or parasites, most commonly *Candida, herpes simplex* virus (HSV), or *cytomegalovirus* (CMV). It occurs more commonly in people with compromised immune systems, e.g., in HIV/AIDS, cancer patients undergoing chemotherapy, or organ transplant recipients on immunosuppressive therapy.

Diagnosis of Infectious Esophagitis

The patient experiences painful, difficult swallowing; retrosternal chest pain; and, in some cases, fever and sore throat. Consider whether the patient is at risk for developing infections (e.g., immunosuppressive drugs, diabetes mellitus, long-term antibiotic use, chemotherapy).

Lab Tests:

- **Blood Tests** are done for HIV, diabetes, and overall immune assessment.
- **Cultures and Stains:** Throat swabs are used to detect the infectious organism.

Regular or Barium Swallow X-ray, or **CT Scan** can rule out other causes of esophageal symptoms.

Endoscopy is done for visual examination of the esophagus, sometimes with biopsy.

Cytology: Histological examination may identify the infectious agent.

PCR (Polymerase Chain Reaction) is used to identify DNA or RNA of the infectious agent.

Treatment of Infectious Esophagitis

Hydration

Alternative Nutritional Support is provided if swallowing is severely impaired.

Antimicrobial Therapy:

- ***Candida:*** Antifungal agents (e.g., *fluconazole*)
- ***HSV* (*Herpes Simplex Virus*):** Antiviral therapy (e.g., *acyclovir, valacyclovir, or famciclovir*)
- ***CMV* (*Cytomegalic Inclusion Virus*):** Antiviral agents (e.g., *ganciclovir, valganciclovir*)
- **Bacteria:** Broad-spectrum antibiotics
- **HIV/AIDS:** Antiretroviral therapy

Immunosuppressive Therapy Adjustment may involve reducing certain immunosuppressive medications.

Pain Management

Acid Suppression: Proton pump inhibitors (PPIs) or H2 blockers

Boerhaave Syndrome

Boerhaave syndrome is a spontaneous transmural perforation of the esophagus, commonly after forceful vomiting. It is a life-threatening condition and requires immediate medical attention. The patient experiences violent retching followed by severe chest pain and may exhibit **Mackler's triad** – intense vomiting, lower chest pain, and subcutaneous emphysema.

Diagnosis of Boerhaave Syndrome

Physical Exam may show tachycardia, fever, neck pain, dyspnea, and crepitus on palpation due to subcutaneous emphysema.

Imaging:

- **Chest X-ray** may show pneumomediastinum, subcutaneous emphysema, or pleural effusions.
- **CT Scan** can show the site of perforation as well as fluid accumulation outside the esophagus.
- **Contrast Esophagography:** The X-ray can show if administered contrast leaks out of the esophagus.

Blood Tests show an increased white blood cell count, suggesting inflammation or infection.

Treatment of Boerhaave Syndrome

The approach includes sealing the perforation, draining the contaminated area, and treating infection with broad-spectrum antibiotics.

Mallory-Weiss Syndrome

Mallory-Weiss syndrome results from a laceration of the mucosa near the gastroesophageal junction. It often follows marked or prolonged vomiting and may result in GI bleeding.

Diagnosis of Mallory-Weiss Syndrome

The patient has a history of severe vomiting or coughing with hematemesis (vomiting blood). It can also occur after a seizure or heavy alcohol intake.

Lab Tests: Complete Blood Count (CBC) assesses for anemia.

Endoscopy can confirm the source of bleeding,

Treatment of Mallory-Weiss Syndrome

Endoscopic Thermal Coagulation, Hemoclip, or **Banding**, which may include epinephrine injection to control hemorrhage

Blood Transfusion for significant bleeding

Medication, using proton pump inhibitors or H2 blockers

Preventive measures for conditions that may have led to severe vomiting, e.g. GERD, eating disorders, alcoholism, or certain medications that can cause vomiting.

Eosinophilic Esophagitis

Eosinophilic esophagitis (EoE), more common in young people, is a chronic immune-mediated esophageal disease with eosinophilic inflammation, often associated with allergies. The patient may have dysphagia, food impaction and chest pain, symptoms often found in other esophageal diseases.

Diagnosis of Eosinophilic Esophagitis

The patient reports dysphagia, particularly to solid foods, with food impaction, along with a personal or family history of allergic diseases (e.g., asthma, allergic rhinitis, atopic dermatitis).

Endoscopy shows rings, furrows, white plaques, or exudates, and narrowing of the esophagus.

Biopsy confirms the presence of eosinophils. There may also be eosinophilic microabscesses, epithelial changes, and fibrosis from the inflammation.

Allergy Testing

Blood Tests may show eosinophilia or elevated IgE levels.

Treatment of Eosinophilic Esophagitis

Allergy-Directed Diet depending on the allergy

Drugs:

- **Proton Pump Inhibitors (PPIs):** Although EoE is not caused by acid reflux, the patient may improve, suggesting either that there is coinciding GERD or that the patient has a particular form of EoE that is PPI-responsive.
- **Topical Steroids:** Swallowed topical corticosteroids in liquid or aerosol form (such as *fluticasone propionate* or *budesonide*) coat the esophageal lining and reduce esophageal inflammation without incurring the systemic side effects of standard oral steroids.
- **Biologic therapy** with *dupilumab* (*Dupixent*), a monoclonal antibody that targets and inhibits specific pathways in the inflammatory response

Endoscopic Dilation may help improve dysphagia in cases where there is significant stricture of the esophagus.

Zenker's Diverticulum

Zenker's diverticulum is a pouch that forms at the junction of the hypopharynx and esophagus (**Fig. 5-7**). Food can get caught there and result in dysphagia, regurgitation of undigested food, coughing, voice changes, sense of a lump in the throat, weight loss, and bad breath. It can also lead to an aspiration pneumonia.

Diagnosis of Zenker's Diverticulum

Barium Swallow X-ray Study and Careful Endoscopic Evaluation show the diverticulum, just above the esophagus.

Treatment of Zenker's Diverticulum

Surgical Closure by an open or endoscopic approach

Dietary modification toward softer foods, eaten slowly

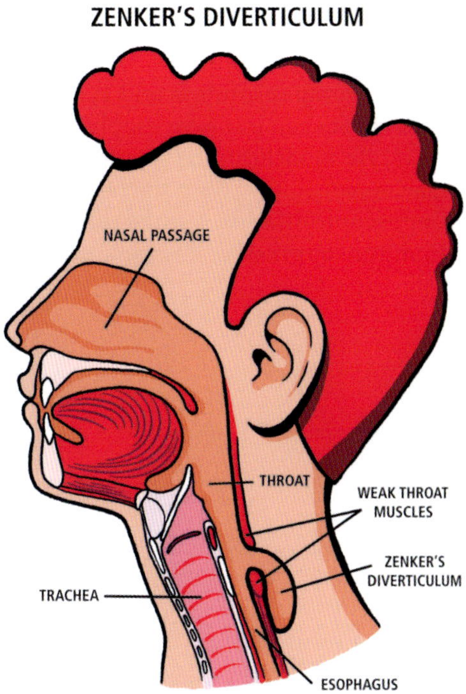

Figure 5-7

Scleroderma

Scleroderma is a chronic autoimmune connective tissue disease, characterized by the hardening and tightening of the skin and connective tissues. When it affects the esophagus, it replaces the smooth muscle fibers of the esophagus with fibrous tissue, reducing the ability of the esophagus to contract. The patient experiences dysphagia, acid reflux, and a sensation of food being stuck in the throat, from an inefficient gastroesophageal sphincter.

Scleroderma differs in mechanism from achalasia. Although both involve decreased esophageal motility, achalasia is a neurogenic disorder of esophageal peristalsis, while scleroderma is an autoimmune disorder with fibrosis and scarring of the esophagus. In achalasia, the LES fails to relax properly, creating an obstruction at the LES, where food can have difficulty passing into the stomach. In scleroderma, the opposite is true; the LES muscle is weakened and there is gastric reflux.

Diagnosis of Esophageal Scleroderma

Blood Tests can detect antibodies common in scleroderma (anti-Sci-70 topoisomerase I and anti-centromere antibodies).

Barium Swallow X-ray shows decreased esophageal motility, strictures, dilation, and gastroesophageal reflux.

Endoscopy can show signs of inflammation, fibrosis, signs of esophageal damage, or lower esophageal sphincter (LES) abnormality. It can also be used for biopsy to make the diagnosis and rule out other causes of esophageal symptoms.

24-hour pH Monitoring can evaluate GERD, a common complication of esophageal scleroderma.

Chest X-ray, CT Scan, or **MRI** are part of a broader workup of scleroderma. They can help identify systemic complications of scleroderma (e.g., lung fibrosis, aspiration pneumonia, soft tissue calcification).

Pulmonary Function Tests can help evaluate interstitial lung disease found in scleroderma.

Treatment of Esophageal Scleroderma

Since there is no cure for scleroderma, treatment is symptomatic:

Proton pump inhibitors and **H2 blockers** are prescribed to reduce acidity.

Prokinetics can improve esophageal motility and gastric emptying.

Lifestyle modifications include eating small, frequent meals, avoiding food that can aggravate reflux, elevating the head of the bed, and avoiding eating before bedtime.

Endoscopic dilation may be done for esophageal strictures.

Immunosuppressive Therapy may be used for systemic scleroderma.

6

Diseases of the Stomach

Gastrin, a hormone produced by G cells in the stomach antrum (**Fig. 6-1**), stimulates the stomach parietal cells, found particularly in the fundus and body of the stomach, to secrete gastric acid (HCl).

Gastric acid sterilizes the stomach contents. It also converts the enzyme **pepsinogen** (produced by chief cells mainly in the body and fundus of the stomach) into **pepsin**, a digestive enzyme that breaks down proteins into smaller peptides.

Mucus, produced by mucous cells, found in all areas of the stomach lining, protects the stomach epithelial lining from acid and smooths the passage of food.

Bicarbonate, also produced by mucous cells, guards against excessive stomach acid by helping neutralize it.

Intrinsic factor, produced by parietal cells along with gastric acid, is essential for absorbing vitamin B12 in the small intestine.

The combination of lower esophageal sphincter and pyloric sphincters (**Fig. 6-1**) keeps food in the stomach during digestion, preventing it from reflux back into the esophagus or entering prematurely into the duodenum. (There is also an upper esophageal sphincter at the junction between the pharynx and esophagus; it relaxes during swallowing and prevents backflow of esophageal contents, which might damage the larynx.)

Damage to the stomach or malsecretion of its digestive molecules can result in a number of digestive diseases.

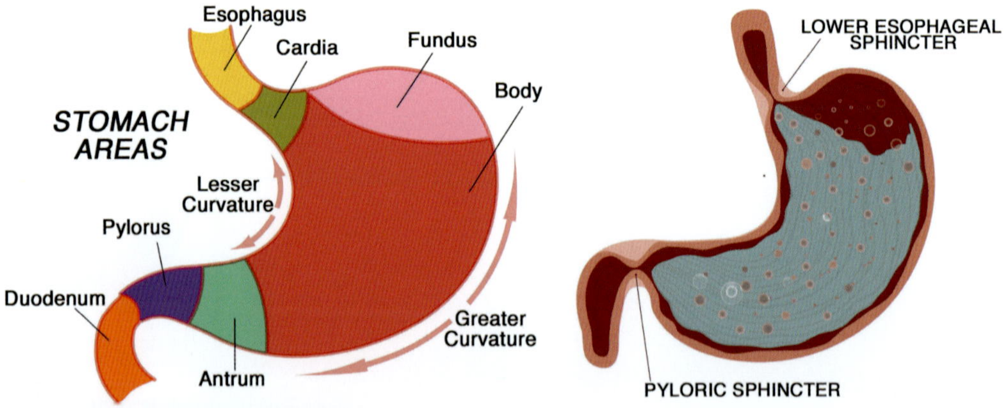

Figure 6-1 Regions of the stomach.

Gastritis and Peptic Ulcer

Gastritis is an acute or chronic inflammation of the stomach lining. It can have different causes, including infection (most commonly *Helicobacter pylori* bacteria), prolonged use of nonsteroidal anti-inflammatory drugs (NSAIDs), alcohol, stress, autoimmunity, and other less common factors. Gastritis can lead to peptic ulcers (ulcers of the stomach or duodenum).

Peptic ulcers usually result from *Helicobacter pylori (H. pylori)* infection. *H. pylori* produces urease, which cleaves urea into CO_2 and ammonia. Ammonia neutralizes the acid, allowing the bacteria to survive in the acidic environment; ammonia also inflames the stomach wall. Peptic ulcers can also be caused by long-term use of nonsteroidal anti-inflammatory drugs (NSAIDs), which irritate the lining of the stomach and small intestine. Corticosteroids inhibit the production of prostaglandins, which protect the stomach lining. Other risk factors include smoking, heavy alcohol use, stress, and some other medications. **Zollinger-Ellison syndrome** is a rare condition in which gastrin-producing tumors cause increased gastric acid production with ensuing ulcers.

Diagnosis of Gastritis and Peptic Ulcer

The patient experiences epigastric pain, nausea, vomiting, bloating, belching, loss of appetite, heartburn, and, in some cases, hematemesis (vomiting of blood) or melena (dark stools from upper GI bleeding). Gastric peptic ulcers cause pain that is often associated with eating, which stimulates acid production and can also irritate the ulcerated area. Duodenal peptic ulcers commonly cause pain that is relieved by eating, as the food triggers the release of hormones and bicarbonate, which reduce the acidity; duodenal ulcer pain typically occurs when the stomach is empty, as in the middle of the night.

Blood Tests:

- CBC to check for anemia (from chronic bleeding)
- Antibodies to *H. pylori* suggests a past infection but this doesn't tell when.

Stool antigen test for *H. pylori*, if positive, indicates current infection. Stool is also tested for occult blood.

Urea breath test for *H. pylori*: The patient drinks a substance containing radiolabeled urea, and the breath is then analyzed for the presence of radiolabeled carbon dioxide, indicating *H. pylori*, which breaks down urea into carbon dioxide and ammonia.)

Endoscopy allows direct visualization of the stomach lining. Biopsy can be taken to check for *H. pylori* infection, atrophy, or malignancy.

Upper GI Series: A barium X-ray is done sometimes to show changes in the lining of the stomach or duodenum, when endoscopy is not available or there is suspicion of other conditions.

Treatment of Gastritis and Peptic Ulcer

Eradication of *H. pylori* is accomplished by a combination of antibiotics (e.g., *clarithromycin, amoxicillin, tetracycline, metronidazole, or rifabutin*) and acid suppressors such as proton pump inhibitors (e.g., *omeprazole, esomeprazole, lansoprazole, pantoprazole,* or *rabeprazole*). Antacids may provide rapid pain relief by neutralizing existing stomach acid. Pepto-Bismol coats the stomach lining and protects it from acid; it also has anti-inflammatory and antibacterial action, mildly reduces acid secretion, and enhances mucus and bicarbonate production, which protect the stomach lining.

Cytoprotective Agents like *sucralfate* (*Carafate*) can coat and protect the stomach or duodenal lining to facilitate healing.

Vitamin B12 may be administered (intramuscular, high-dose oral, sublingual, or nasal) for **autoimmune gastritis**, in which an autoimmune reaction destroys the parietal cells that secrete the intrinsic factor that is necessary for B12 absorption. Here the gastritis is not due to excess acid (since the parietal cells are destroyed) but to the inflammation of the autoimmune reaction.

Bleeding control may be done endoscopically by epinephrine injection, metal clips, cauterization, or hemostatic powders.

Lifestyle and Dietary Modifications:

- Avoid NSAIDs, alcohol, and smoking.
- **Stress Management** (e.g., meditation, relaxation exercises, counseling)
- **Diet:** Avoid spicy, acidic, fried, or other irritating foods. Eat smaller portions and not right before bedtime.

Surgery for duodenal or gastric ulcers may be required in cases of perforation, bleeding, obstruction, or suspicion of cancer. The surgery may aim to excise the ulcer or to reduce acid secretion by vagotomy (the vagus nerve stimulates acid secretion), antrectomy (the antrum of the stomach produces gastrin, which stimulates acid secretion), or pyloroplasty (enlarging the pyloric opening to allow food to pass more quickly).

Gastroenteritis

Gastroenteritis ("stomach flu") is an inflammation of the stomach and small intestine. Symptoms typically include diarrhea, vomiting, abdominal pain, and cramps, sometimes with fever and signs of dehydration (such as dry mouth, decreased urination, and lightheadedness). It can result from certain viruses, bacteria, and parasites, as well as non-infectious causes such as food allergies or medications.

Diagnosis of Gastroenteritis

Physical Exam: Check for signs of dehydration (e.g., decreased skin turgor, orthostatic hypotension), concentrated urine).

Lab Tests:

- **Stool Tests** can identify possible bacterial or parasitic pathogens or detect blood in the stool. Stool tests are often reserved for severe cases, those with blood in the stool, immunocompromised patients, or when symptoms persist. Stool culture or a more specific PCR assay on the stool, can help identify bacterial pathogens. Examination for ova and parasites is of particular importance if there is a history of travel or exposure to contaminated food or water.
- **Electrolytes and Renal Function Tests** may be checked if there is concern about severe dehydration or electrolyte imbalance.

Imaging: Generally imaging studies are not necessary for typical cases of gastroenteritis.

Treatment of Gastroenteritis

Rehydration: Oral or IV if needed
Diet: Include adequate hydration, with initially bland, easily digested food. Dairy products and foods high in fat or sugar may worsen symptoms.

Medications:

- **Anti-diarrheal Medications** such as *loperamide (Imodium)*, can be used in adults, but generally are not recommended for children or for those with bloody diarrhea, as they slow down the removal of bacteria and toxins, mask symptoms, and may have side effects in children.
- **Antiemetics** like *ondansetron* (*Zofran*) can be used to help control vomiting.
- **Antibiotics** or **Antiparasitics** can be useful for a specifically identified bacterial or parasitic pathogen.
- **Probiotics** may be helpful, especially in children. The "good" bacteria in probiotics can help restore the gut bacterial balance.

Prevention:
Hygiene: Frequent handwashing with soap and water is the best defense.
Food Safety: Proper food preparation and storage is important.
Vaccination: Rotavirus vaccination is given in infants, since rotavirus is a common cause of viral gastroenteritis in children.
Clean Water: Ensure safe drinking water, especially when traveling to areas with a higher risk of waterborne illness.

Gastric Cancer

Stomach cancer is often asymptomatic in its early stages and can go undiagnosed until it's at an advanced stage. In the early stages, gastric cancer might cause indigestion, stomach discomfort, a bloated feeling after eating, mild nausea, and loss of appetite. Eventually, symptoms may include stomach pain, weight loss, vomiting (sometimes with blood), and blood in the stool.

Diagnosis of Gastric Cancer

Blood Tests can detect anemia from bleeding or other origins. Tumor markers like CEA (Carcinoembryonic Antigen) can sometimes aid in diagnosis but are not specific. CEA can be useful in monitoring the response to treatment and for early detection of cancer recurrence.

Endoscopy can directly detect and biopsy stomach cancer.

Imaging:

- **Endoscopic Ultrasound** can determine the depth of tumor invasion and involvement of lymph nodes or nearby structures.
- **Computed Tomography (CT) Scan** can assess the extent of the cancer, including metastases. It is also useful for guiding biopsies.
- **Magnetic Resonance Imaging (MRI)** provides better contrast than CT scan for soft tissue imaging and localization. It is better in differentiating between benign and malignant tissues and can provide functional information (e.g., regarding blood flow).
- **Positron Emission Tomography (PET) Scan** provides metabolic information that can locate cancer metastases.

Treatment of Gastric Cancer

Surgery:

- **Endoscopic Resection** is used for very early-stage cancers confined to the stomach lining.
- **Subtotal Gastrectomy** removes part of the stomach when the cancer is still in a limited area.
- **Total Gastrectomy** removes the entire stomach, with nearby lymph nodes and potentially other tissues or organs if the cancer has spread.

Chemotherapy can be used before surgery to shrink the tumor or after surgery to clear up remaining cancer cells.

Radiation Therapy can be used before or after surgery, often together with chemotherapy.

Prevention:

- Reduce the ingestion of smoked, salted, or pickled foods and processed meats, which are associated with an increased risk of gastric cancer.
- Quit smoking.
- Focus on a diet rich in fruits and vegetables. Avoid obesity. Limit alcohol.
- Treat *H. pylori* infection, which can cause stomach ulcers and inflammation, with increased risk of gastric adenocarcinoma.
- Avoid exposure to certain chemicals (e.g., nitrosamines in food products; excess alcohol; asbestos; benzene, polycyclic aromatic hydrocarbons from burning coal, oil, gas, wood, garbage, tobacco, and smoked foods; heavy metals) that can increase the risk of gastric cancer.

Gastroparesis

Gastroparesis is a condition where the muscles in the wall of the stomach work poorly, preventing the stomach from emptying properly. The patient experiences nausea, vomiting, early satiety, bloating, and abdominal pain due to poor gastric emptying.

Diagnosis of Gastroparesis

Tests for Gastroparesis:

Scintigraphy scans the movement of a small amount of radioactive material through the stomach following a small meal.

13C-octanoic Acid Breath Test can be used to measure the rate of gastric emptying, though it's less commonly performed. The patient consumes a meal containing (isotope-labeled) 13C-octanoic acid, which the liver metabolizes to $13CO_2$. The $13CO_2$ is then exhaled in the breath. The rate at which $13CO_2$ appears reflects how fast the stomach is emptying.

Endoscopy can rule out obstruction or other conditions responsible for the symptoms.

Upper GI Series allows the radiologist to observe how the barium moves through the stomach.

Treatment of Gastroparesis

Dietary Modifications: Eat smaller, frequent meals geared more toward liquid or pureed foods, rather than high-fiber or high-fat foods, which can slow down gastric emptying.

Medications:

- **Prokinetic Agents**, e.g., *metoclopramide (Reglan)*, stimulate stomach muscle contractions to help emptying.
- **Anti-Emetics**, e.g., *ondansetron (Zofran)* or *promethazine (Phenergan)* can control nausea and vomiting.
- **Ghrelin Agonist:** *Relamorelin*, an agonist of Ghrelin, the "hunger hormone," stimulates gastric emptying in addition to hunger and food intake.

Gastric Electrical Stimulation uses a gastric pacemaker that sends mild electrical pulses to the stomach muscles to help control nausea and vomiting by coordinating stomach muscle contractions.

Surgery:

- **Stenting of a narrowed pylorus** keeps the pylorus open.
- **Relaxation of the pyloric sphincter** can be done with Botox or incision of the pylorus (**pyloromyotomy**).
- **Jejunostomy** employs a feeding tube placed through the abdominal wall directly into the small intestine in cases that do not respond to less invasive methods.
- **Gastrojejunostomy:** Surgery directly connects the stomach to the jejunum to bypass blockages or facilitate gastric emptying.

Intravenous Nutrition is administered when oral intake is not feasible.

Blood Glucose Control is important in diabetes where gastroparesis is a significant problem.

Gastric Polyps

Most stomach polyps are benign and asymptomatic, but some can become cancerous. They are generally discovered incidentally on endoscopy done for another reason, with biopsy determining the histology. **Hyperplastic Polyps** are the most common and are usually benign and associated with gastric inflammation. **Adenomatous Polyps (adenomas)** have a higher potential to become cancerous, particularly when large. **Fundic Gland Polyps** are generally benign and coincide with prolonged use of proton pump inhibitors.

Treatment of Gastric Polyps

Small asymptomatic benign polyps can simply be observed with periodic endoscopic checks, and with discontinuation of proton pump inhibitors if their chronic use is felt to be a contributing cause. Large or dysplastic polyps can be removed during endoscopy.

Zollinger-Ellison Syndrome

Zollinger-Ellison Syndrome (ZES) results from excess secretion of gastrin hormone by **gastrinomas**, tumors that arise mainly in the pancreas or duodenum. The excess gastrin stimulates the stomach to produce excess acid, which can lead to peptic ulcers. Gastrinomas are often malignant, metastasizing particularly to the liver and lymph nodes. The condition can arise sporadically or be familial, as part of the genetic syndrome **Multiple Endocrine Neoplasia type 1 (MEN1)**.

Diagnosis of Zollinger-Ellison Syndrome

The patient may experience abdominal pain, diarrhea, and GI bleeding, often resistant to standard ulcer treatments. There may also be nausea, vomiting and weight loss.

Blood Tests:

- **Gastrin Levels:** Fasting serum gastrin levels are usually very high, but can also be high in other conditions, e.g., atrophic gastritis, renal failure (decreased gastrin clearance), and use of proton pump inhibitors.
- **Secretin Stimulation Test:** Secretin is a hormone that normally lowers gastrin levels, but in ZES, it paradoxically increases gastrin levels on administration.
- **Chromogranin A**, a protein found in gastrinoma cells, can be elevated in ZES.

Imaging:

- **Endoscopy** can detect the effects of gastrinomas of the pancreas or duodenum (e.g., duodenal ulcers, hypertrophic gastric folds from excess acid production, inflammation, esophagitis).
- **CT** or **MRI scan** can help detect large or metastatic tumors.
- **Somatostatin Receptor Scintigraphy (*Octreotide scan*)** uses radiolabeled octreotide, a chemical similar to somatostatin, to locate tumors that express somatostatin receptors, including gastrinomas.

Esophagogastroduodenoscopy can identify ulcers.
Gastric pH Monitoring can confirm high levels of acid production.

Treatment of Zollinger-Ellison Syndrome

The main treatment for Zollinger-Ellison Syndrome consists of controlling the acid secretion and removing the gastrinomas, whether through surgery or otherwise.

Medications:

- **Proton Pump Inhibitors (PPIs)** to reduce acid
- **Histamine (H2) Blockers:** Less effective than PPIs

Chemotherapy for metastatic disease
Hepatic Artery Embolization blocks the blood supply to liver metastases.
Radiofrequency Ablation destroys liver metastases with heat.
Peptide Receptor Radionuclide Therapy (PRRT) uses a radioactive substance that targets somatostatin receptors, which are often prominent on gastrinomas.

Since Zollinger-Ellison syndrome is often genetic (e.g., MEN1 syndrome; autosomal dominant), genetic counseling may be of value when there is a family history.

Functional Dyspepsia

Functional dyspepsia is a common condition characterized by chronic upper abdominal discomfort or pain without an identifiable medical cause, such as an ulcer or gastroesophageal reflux disease (GERD); it can occur with or without eating. The diagnosis involves ruling out other causes of the discomfort.

Diagnosis of Non-Ulcer Dyspepsia

Blood Tests check for anemia, abnormal liver and pancreas function, and other potential causes.
***Helicobacter Pylori* Testing** is done via breath, blood, or stool test, or endoscopic biopsy.

Imaging and Endoscopy:

- **Endoscopy** is done particularly in patients over the age of 60 or with weight loss, anemia, or GI bleeding, to rule out ulcers, inflammation, or cancer.
- **Ultrasound** can examine the gallbladder and pancreas.

Treatment of Non-Ulcer Dyspepsia

Eating Habits: Eat smaller, more frequent meals, and avoid foods that may trigger the symptoms.

Stress Management

Medications:

- **Proton Pump Inhibitors (PPIs)** or **H2 Blockers** to reduce stomach acid
- **Prokinetics**: E.g., *metoclopramide* to stimulate gastric emptying
- **Antidepressants**: For mood improvement and lessening the perception of pain

- **Antispasmodics:** E.g., *hyoscine butylbromide* or *peppermint oil* to reduce abdominal symptoms
- ***Antibiotics:*** *For H. Pylori* eradication.

Cognitive Behavioral Therapy

Hernia

There are several kinds of abdominal hernia, which may manifest either inside or outside the abdominal wall.

A **hiatal hernia** is a condition where a portion of the stomach pushes up through the diaphragm into the chest cavity. There are two main types: **sliding** and **paraesophageal** (**Fig. 6-2**). The patient may be asymptomatic or experience gastroesophageal reflux (GERD). The symptoms in paraesophageal hernia can be particularly severe if the stomach becomes "strangled" due to its squeezing through the esophageal hiatus and pressing against the esophagus. **Cameron's erosions** are lesions in the stomach where the stomach protrudes through the diaphragm, particularly in paraesophageal hernias.

A **foramen of Bochdalek hernia** is a congenital condition where there is a defect in the posterior diaphragm (usually on the left) in a region called the Bochdalek triangle. Abdominal organs, particularly the intestines can protrude through the defect into the chest cavity of the newborn and can cause respiratory problems. It is diagnosed with an X-ray or CT scan and requires surgical repair of the diaphragmatic defect.

The **treatment** of hiatal hernia often focuses on medical treatment of the GERD symptoms, but surgery may be advised in severe cases, particularly the paraesophageal type. The most common surgery is **fundoplication**, where the fundus of the stomach is wrapped

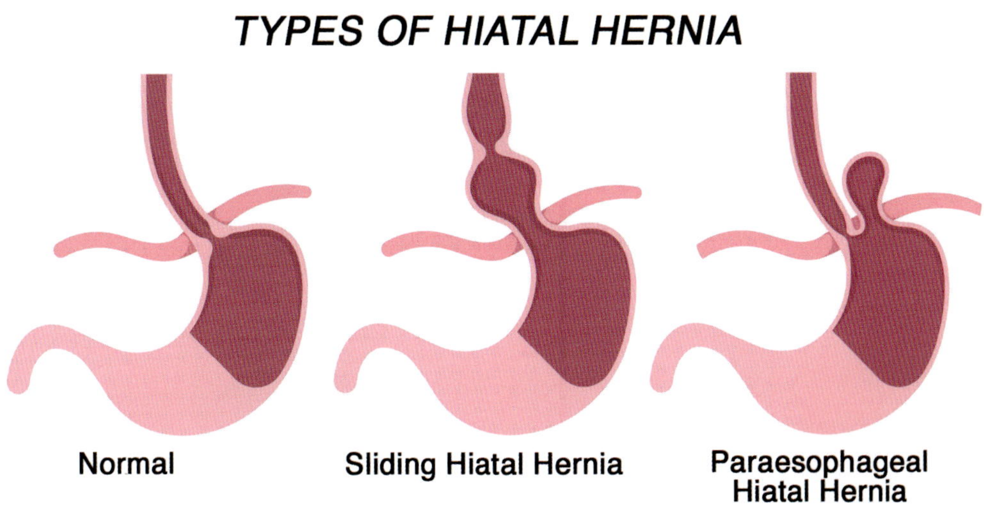

Figure 6-2

around the lower esophagus via surgery to tighten the lower esophageal sphincter muscle and prevent acid reflux (**Fig. 5-1**). If the wrapping procedure is too tight, the patient may experience "**gas-bloat syndrome**," where the patient has bloating, difficulty in belching, and abdominal discomfort due to the prevention by the fundoplication of gas from escaping into the esophagus. In that case, dietary modification may be needed (e.g., eating smaller, more frequent meals, avoiding carbonated beverages or other gas-containing foods, taking medications to reduce gas). In some cases, the fundoplication may need to be surgically revised.

An **umbilical hernia** (**Fig. 6-3**) can involve just fat herniation or may include a portion of bowel as well, which is of greater concern due to the possibility of strangulation of that portion of bowel. Distinguishing the two can be done in several ways. Palpation of bowel may feel more tubular and might gurgle on attempting to push it back. Ultrasound or CT scan is more definitive. Treatment is surgical repair.

Inguinal hernias can be indirect or direct (**Fig. 6-3**). **Indirect inguinal hernias**, which occur particularly in males, occur when fatty or intestinal tissues push into the inguinal canal, the pathway where the spermatic cord and testicles descend into the scrotum in fetal development. The hernia may protrude into the scrotum. **Direct inguinal hernias** are less common than the indirect type. They occur when the abdominal muscles weaken over time (due to aging, physical strain, excess coughing, or obesity. It rarely protrudes into the scrotum. **Femoral hernias** (**Fig. 6-3**) occur more commonly in women. It happens when fatty tissue or a portion of intestine bulges through the wall of the femoral canal, the passage through which the femoral artery, vein, and nerve run from the abdomen into the leg.

Inguinal and femoral hernias, apart from the protrusion itself, can also be painful and may incur a risk of strangulation. Surgical repair is frequently recommended for all three types.

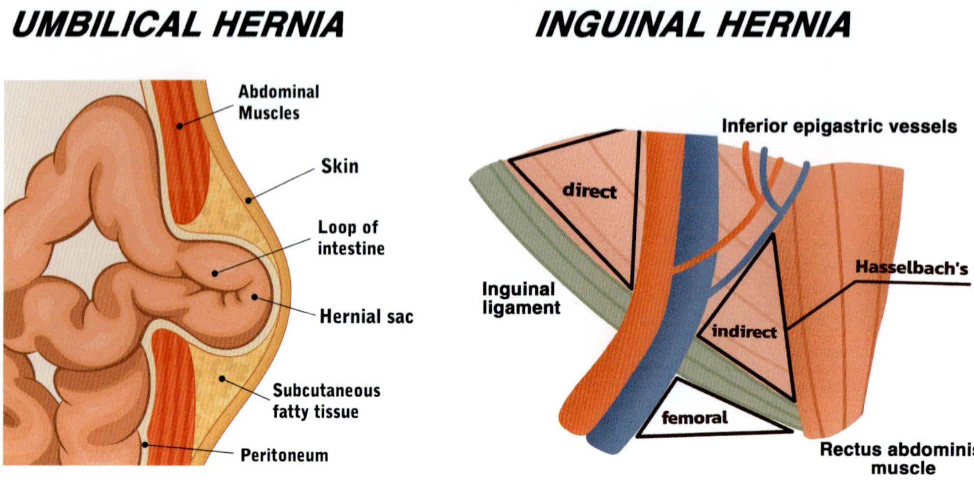

Figure 6-3

Gastric Bleeding

Common causes of gastric bleeding include peptic ulcers, gastritis, GERD, esophageal varices, Mallory-Weiss syndrome, stomach cancer, certain medications, and ingestion of caustic substances or foreign bodies.

Diagnosis of Gastric Bleeding

History and Physical Examination:

Vomiting of blood (hematemesis), whether bright red blood or "coffee grounds" (a sign of partially digested blood), usually suggests an upper GI bleed. Passing dark, tarry stools (melena) also suggests an upper GI bleed. Bright red blood in the stools (hematochezia) suggests a lower GI bleed.

Pallor, low blood pressure, and rapid heart rate can indicate significant blood loss.

Lab Tests:

- **Complete Blood Count (CBC)** can check for anemia and signs of infection.
- **Blood Typing** may be done in case a blood transfusion is needed for significant bleeding.
- **Coagulation Studies** can check for blood-clotting abnormalities, e.g., prothrombin time (PT), INR, partial thromboplastin time (PTT), platelet function tests.

Upper Endoscopy can detect if the bleeding is originating in the esophagus, stomach, or duodenum. It can often assess the cause and severity of the bleeding, enable biopsy for diagnosis, and provide treatment (e.g., cautery, clips or bands, injection, or hemostatic powders to stop bleeding) or remove polyps.

Colonoscopy: If the source isn't found in the upper GI tract, a colonoscopy might be performed to examine the lower GI tract.

Imaging:

CT Scan can identify bleeding and other abnormalities in the abdomen and pelvis.

Capsule Endoscopy: A small, pill-sized camera is swallowed that takes pictures throughout the digestive tract, particularly the small intestine, which is not completely visible by either upper or lower endoscopy.

Treatment of Gastric Bleeding

Stabilize severe bleeds, including IV fluids and blood transfusion as needed.

Medications:

- **Proton Pump Inhibitors**
- **Antibiotics** if there is an infection, e.g., *H. pylori*
- **Anticoagulant Reversal**, e.g., with vitamin K If the bleeding is due to anticoagulants

Endoscopic Treatment:

- **Thermal Coagulation** cauterizes the bleeding vessel.
- **Clipping** bleeding arteries or veins can seal the bleeding vessel. Alternatively, **variceal banding** (ligation of venous varices) or **sclerotherapy** (injection of a sclerosing agent into the dilated veins) can shrink the veins and close off the bleeding.

- **Injection** of chemicals directly into the bleed site can be used to promote clotting.
- Application of hemostatic powders

Angiographic embolization can block the bleeding vessel.

Surgery may be required if the bleeding cannot be controlled with less invasive methods or if there is a perforation or other significant condition.

Dietary changes include avoiding alcohol or NSAIDs.

Treat underlying conditions (e.g., ulcers, gastritis, or esophagitis)

Gastric Antral Vascular Ectasia

Gastric Antral Vascular Ectasia (GAVE) is a rare medical condition characterized by the formation of dilated small blood vessels in the antrum (the lower portion) of the stomach, leading to gastrointestinal bleeding and iron deficiency anemia. Its cause is not known, but it does seem more common in people with certain chronic autoimmune diseases, such as scleroderma, atrophic gastritis, lupus, rheumatoid arthritis, or cirrhosis (often due to autoimmune hepatitis). However, people can have GAVE without these associations.

Diagnosis of Gastric Antral Vascular Ectasia

Endoscopy: On endoscopy, GAVE is characterized by a distinct appearance often described as **"watermelon stomach" (Fig. 6-4)** due to the striped pattern of the blood vessel, which resembles the surface of a watermelon. These differ from **Dieulafoy's lesion**, which is a rare, large caliber arteriole in the stomach wall that can bleed.

Biopsy may be taken during endoscopy to rule out other causes of stomach bleeding and to confirm that it really is GAVE.

Blood Tests assess for anemia and liver disease, which is often associated with GAVE.

Imaging Studies: In some cases, CT scans or MRI may be used to assess the extent of the condition or to look for underlying causes. GAVE is often associated with autoimmune and connective tissue disorders such as scleroderma, as well as with cirrhosis or chronic renal failure.

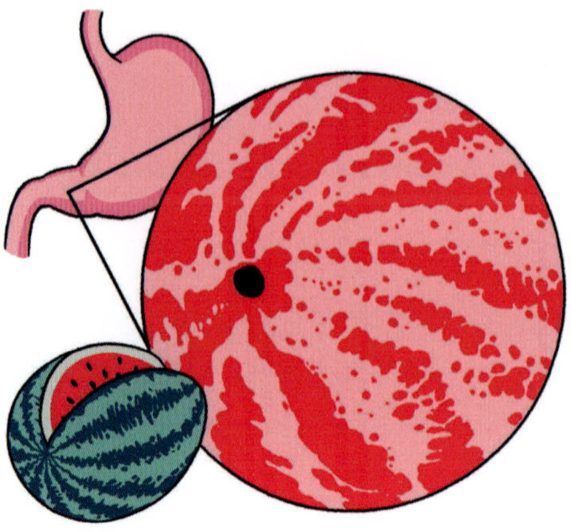

Figure 6-4 *Watermelon stomach in gastric antral vascular ectasia.*

Treatment of Gastric Antral Vascular Ectasia

Endoscopic Treatment uses heat in the form of argon plasma coagulation, electrocoagulation, laser coagulation, or a heat probe to cauterize the bleeding vessels.

Medications: In some cases, drugs might be used to reduce bleeding, e.g., proton pump inhibitors (to increase pH and reduce irritation from stomach acid), or estrogen-progesterone therapy (which might have anti-inflammatory and vasoprotective effects).

Iron Supplements can treat or prevent iron deficiency anemia caused by chronic blood loss.

Blood Transfusions may be used for severe anemia or acute blood loss.

Surgical Intervention might be needed for bleeding if the more conservative treatments are not adequate.

Management of Underlying Conditions: If GAVE is associated with other diseases, such as liver cirrhosis, managing these conditions is also important.

Bile Reflux

Bile can backflow from the small intestine into the stomach or even the esophagus. This can irritate the stomach and esophageal lining, causing gastritis or esophagitis. Reflux may occur after surgery such as gallbladder removal or gastric bypass. Reflux may also result from bile accumulation with duodenal ulcers, delayed gastric emptying, and increased abdominal pressure from obesity. Just as malfunction of the lower esophageal sphincter can cause acid reflux, malfunction of the stomach's pyloric valve can result in bile reflux.

Diagnosis of Bile Reflux

Endoscopy allows direct visualization of the stomach and duodenum. It can detect the dark green to yellowish-brown bile in the stomach as well as inflammation; biopsy can be done if necessary.

A **Gastric Emptying Test** can determine how quickly food leaves the stomach, as delayed gastric emptying can contribute to bile reflux. The test involves mixing a small amount of radioactive material in food and scanning for how long it takes for it to leave the stomach.

The **Bilitec Test** involves placing a probe in the stomach or esophagus to detect bilirubin (a component of bile).

Impedance-pH Monitoring: Can detect both acidic and non-acidic reflux. If the reflux is non-acidic, it may be from the reflux of bile, which is typically alkaline (non-acidic). The esophagus doesn't handle stomach acid or alkaline bile very well.

Treatment of Bile Reflux

Medications:

- **Ursodeoxycholic Acid** interacts with bile, making it less toxic. It also reduces inflammation and protects the mucosal lining of the stomach and esophagus.
- **Proton Pump Inhibitors (PPIs) or H2 Blockers** decrease gastric acid, reducing the damage from reflux.
- **Bile Acid Sequestrants** e.g., *cholestyramine*, bind to bile in the stomach and help reduce symptoms.
- **Prokinetics**, e.g., *metoclopramide,* speed up gastric emptying and reduce reflux.

Lifestyle Changes: Eat smaller, more frequent meals; avoid irritating foods; reduce obesity; avoid alcohol and smoking, elevate the head of the bed.

Surgery may be an option if lesser methods are not effective. **Roux-en-Y gastric bypass (Fig.10-6)**, a procedure used for weight loss, creates a small stomach pouch that bypasses a large part of the stomach and duodenum by connecting directly to the middle of the small intestine (jejunum), reducing the reflux of bile back into the stomach.

Hypertrophic Pyloric Stenosis

Hypertrophic pyloric stenosis, a condition that affects infants, is characterized by a thickened stomach pylorus (**Fig. 6-5**), which blocks food from passing beyond the stomach. The infant, usually between 2-8 weeks old, presents with projectile vomiting, which can cause dehydration and weight loss.

Diagnosis of Hypertrophic Pyloric Stenosis

Physical Examination: The examiner may feel the hypertrophied pylorus as an olive-shaped mass in the right upper quadrant of the abdomen.

Ultrasound visualizes the thickened pylorus.

Blood Tests may show a hypochloremic, hypokalemic metabolic alkalosis due to loss of gastric acid from vomiting.

Treatment of Hypertrophic Pyloric Stenosis

Pyloromyotomy (open or laparoscopic) involves cutting the pyloric muscle to relieve the obstruction. Dehydration or electrolyte imbalance should be corrected before surgery with intravenous fluids. The prognosis is excellent.

Ménétrier's Disease

Ménétrier's disease (Hypertrophic Gastropathy) is a rare condition characterized by the hypertrophy of gastric mucosal folds, leading to excessive mucus production and protein loss. The patient may report pain in the upper/middle abdomen, nausea, vomiting, decreased appetite, weight loss and edema (from protein loss). The symptoms can resemble those of peptic ulcer.

Diagnosis of Ménétrier's Disease

Blood Tests: Hypoalbuminemia is common due to the protein-losing gastropathy. There may also be signs of anemia and inflammation.

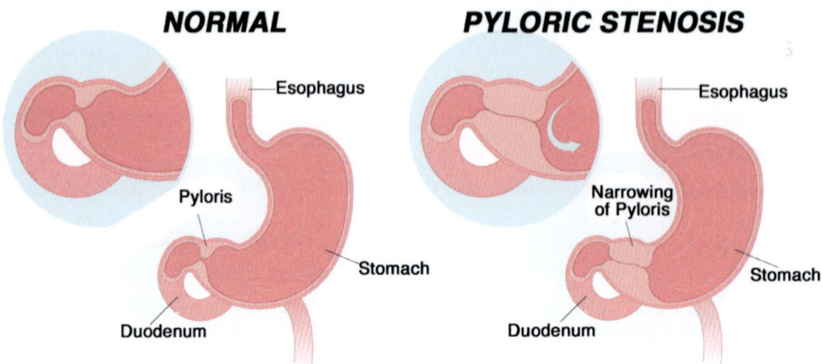

Figure 6-5

Imaging and Endoscopy:

- **Upper GI Series** may show large, tortuous folds in the stomach lining.
- **Endoscopy** can see the thickened gastric folds.
- **Endoscopic Ultrasound** can assess the thickness of the stomach wall.
- **Gastric Biopsy** confirms hyperplasia of the mucus-producing cells of the stomach without evidence of inflammation. A biopsy can also rule out gastric cancer.

Test to rule out *H. pylori* infection.

Treatment for Ménétrier's Disease:

Medications:

- **Proton Pump Inhibitors (PPIs)** or **H2 Receptor Antagonists** to reduce gastric acid secretion
- **Nutritional Support** for protein loss and decreased eating
- **Cytokine Modulators**: *Cetuximab*, a monoclonal antibody against epidermal growth factor (EGFR) may help, since Ménétrier's disease has been associated with increased EGFR signaling.

Gastrectomy may be a consideration in severe, persistent cases.

The prognosis for Ménétrier's disease varies, from spontaneous resolution to gastric cancer.

7

Diseases of the Small Intestine

Celiac Disease

Celiac disease (gluten-sensitive enteropathy; celiac sprue) is an autoimmune genetic disorder where ingesting gluten (a family of proteins – glutenin and gliadin, found in grains like wheat, barley, and rye) damages the small intestine (**Fig. 7-1**). Celiac disease tends to run in families and can develop at any age. The small intestine loses villi along with lymphocyte infiltration from an immune response to gluten. Not everyone who has gluten sensitivity has celiac disease. Some people ("non-celiac gluten sensitivity") do not have the autoimmune or hereditary markers or atrophy of intestinal villi characteristic of celiac disease.

Diagnosis of Celiac Disease

Symptoms may include malabsorptive diarrhea, steatorrhea, bloating, pain, and anemia from iron and B12 deficiency, fatigue, and weight loss. There is an increased risk of developing adenocarcinoma or lymphoma of the small intestine due to chronic untreated irritation of the intestinal lining.

Lab Tests:

- **tTG-IgA Test:** Tissue transglutaminase antibodies (tTG-IgA) are typically elevated in celiac disease. This is the most sensitive test and is usually the first one ordered.
- **EMA Test:** The anti-endomysial antibody (EMA) IgA test is very specific for celiac disease.

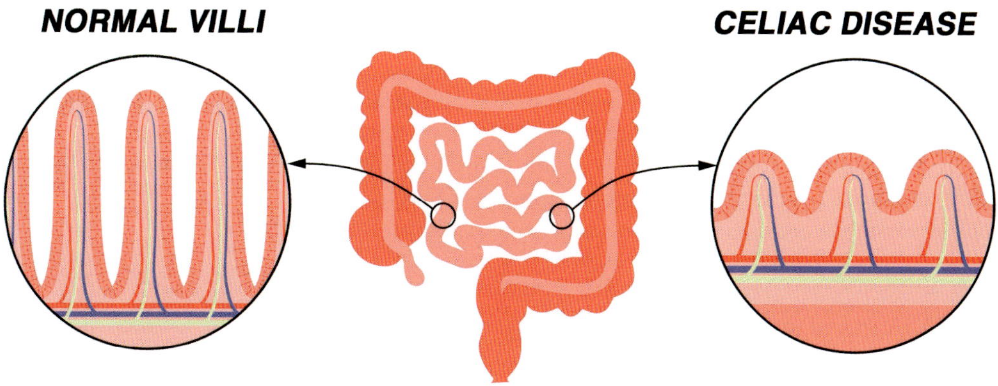

Figure 7-1

- **Total Serum IgA testing** checks for IgA deficiency, which could make tTG-IgA and EMA tests negative despite having the disease.
- The **Deamidated Gliadin Peptide (DGP) Antibodies test** is very specific for celiac disease and is particularly sensitive in detecting these antibodies in children less than the age of 2, who may not always have the other typical celiac antibodies.

Genetic Tests: Tests for HLA-DQ2 and HLA-DQ8 variants, if negative, make celiac disease unlikely.

Endoscopic Biopsy: Upper endoscopy biopsy of the duodenum confirms the diagnosis of celiac disease.

Treatment of Celiac Disease

The treatment for celiac disease is a strict gluten-free diet, particularly avoiding foods that contain wheat, barley, or rye. **Dermatitis herpetiformis**, a blistering skin problem associated with celiac disease may be treated with *dapsone*, an anti-inflammatory medication that helps relieve the itching and blistering experienced with the rash.

The prognosis for celiac disease is generally very good on following the strict gluten-free diet.

Crohn's Disease

Crohn's disease is an inflammatory bowel disease (IBD), as is ulcerative colitis. Crohn's can affect any part of the GI tract from mouth to anus, although it usually affects the terminal ileum (about 2/3 of patients) and the beginning of the colon (**Figs. 8-1** and **8-2**). It is chronic, with periods of inflammation (flares) and remission and affects people to different degrees. The ileum is needed for absorption of bile acids and B12. In the absence of ileum function, the patient may develop B12 deficiency and bile acid diarrhea from lack of reabsorption of bile acids. The cause of Crohn's disease is not clearly established, although it has a strong genetic component and is more common in Ashkenazic Jews.

Diagnosis of Crohn's Disease

Symptoms of Crohn's disease can include diarrhea, abdominal pain, rectal bleeding, weight loss, fever, and fatigue. There may also be extraintestinal manifestations, such as arthritis, skin conditions, eye inflammation, and liver disorders.

Lab Tests: Blood tests may show signs of inflammation (elevated C-reactive protein [CRP], elevated erythrocyte sedimentation rate [ESR]), anemia, or nutrient deficiencies. Stool tests can detect inflammation, infection, or the presence of blood.

Imaging:

- **CT Scan** can identify bowel thickening, obstruction, fistulas, or abscesses.
- **MRI** is particularly helpful for assessing fistulas or abscesses around the anal area and small bowel.

Endoscopic Procedures:

Colonoscopy with Biopsy allows direct visualization of the colon and terminal ileum and biopsy to detect microscopic inflammation, which typically is discontinuous. Follow-up colonoscopy can also be used to confirm whether the disease is in remission.

Capsule Endoscopy is particularly useful in examining the small intestine, which is not easily accessible beyond the duodenum by upper endoscopy or colonoscopy. It uses a capsule, about the size of a large pill, with a camera that takes thousands of pictures while traveling through the GI tract. It is useful not only for diagnosing Crohn's disease but other GI diseases as well, including celiac disease, small intestine tumors, and sources of GI bleeding not detectable with other endoscopic procedures.

Other causes of symptoms, such as infection, ulcerative colitis, or irritable bowel syndrome (IBS) must be ruled out. For instance, bloody diarrhea is more common in ulcerative colitis than in Crohn's or IBS. Stool tests can help rule out infectious causes. Blood tests can check for signs of inflammation (e.g., increased C-reactive protein or ESR, which are more suggestive of an inflammatory bowel disease than IBS). On endoscopy, Crohn's disease can occur anywhere in the GI tract and typically is patchy, while ulcerative colitis is limited to the colon and shows continuous inflammation (**Fig. 8-1**). Biopsy can also differentiate the different causes of colitis. On CT or MRI, fistulas or strictures, which can occur in Crohn's disease, are less likely in ulcerative colitis or IBS. Also, different antibodies are found on blood tests for Crohn's disease than for ulcerative colitis (ASCA antibodies in Crohn's disease, pANCA antibodies in ulcerative colitis). In addition, patients with inflammatory bowel disease often respond to anti-inflammatory medicine, while IBS is managed mainly with dietary changes and medications that target the digestive system.

Treatment of Crohn's Disease

The treatment for Crohn's disease often requires a combination of medication, lifestyle changes, and sometimes surgery. Treatment aims to reduce inflammation, correct nutritional deficiencies, and relieve symptoms.

Medications:

- **Aminosalicylates** (e.g., *sulfazine*), which have an anti-inflammatory effect, can help reduce symptoms of Crohn's disease isolated to the colon (**Crohn's colitis**).

- **Corticosteroids** are anti-inflammatory and can be used orally or intravenously for moderate to severe disease or for flares, but not long-term because of steroid side effects.
- **Immunomodulators** (e.g., *azathioprine* or *methotrexate*) are drugs with a broad effect on the immune system that can be used to maintain remission and reduce the frequency of flare-ups over longer periods.
- **Biologic Therapies: TNF inhibitors** (e.g., *infliximab, certolizumab, adalimumab [Humira]*), **integrin inhibitors** (e.g., *vedolizumab [Entyvio]*), and **interleukin inhibitors** (e.g., *ustekinumab [Stelara]*) are proteins that target specific parts of the immune response and are used in moderate to severe cases.
- **Antibiotics** are used to control bacterial overgrowth or specific complications like fistulas and abscesses.

Nutritional Management: Dietary changes may be needed to manage symptoms and avoid malnutrition.

- Eat smaller, more frequent meals to reduce digestive burden.
- Limit dairy if lactose intolerant.
- Avoid spicy, high fiber, fatty foods if they aggravate symptoms.
- Stay hydrated.

Surgery may be recommended if there is no significant response to medical treatment or there are significant complications, like abscesses, fistulas, strictures or obstructions.

Monitoring: Regular follow-up is important to manage disease activity and adjust treatments. This includes repeat colonoscopies (e.g., every 1-3 years, depending on the state of remission and response to therapy) since there is an increased risk of colorectal cancer in people with chronic Crohn's. Smoking should be discontinued since smoking is a risk factor for Crohn's.

Small Intestinal Bacterial Overgrowth (SIBO)

The small intestine normally carries far fewer bacteria than the large intestine. Bacterial overgrowth in the small intestine may include bacteria not commonly found in the gut. SIBO may arise with intestinal motility disorders, (e.g., diabetes, scleroderma, prior intestinal surgery, anatomical anomalies), chronic use of proton pump inhibitors (reduced gastric acidity predisposes to small intestine bacterial overgrowth), and antibiotic overuse.

Diagnosis of Small Intestinal Bacterial Overgrowth

The patient may have bloating, gas, abdominal pain, diarrhea, and malabsorption, including vitamin B12 and fat-soluble vitamin deficiency, as excess bacteria can interfere with digestion and absorption.

Lab Tests:

Blood tests may suggest a nutritional deficit, as may occur with malabsorption, e.g., a deficiency of vitamins B12, D, E, A, K, folate, or iron.

The **Hydrogen Breath Test** measures hydrogen and methane in the breath after ingestion of a sugar solution that is not normally absorbed (e.g., lactulose). With SIBO, the excess bacteria in the small intestine ferment the lactulose to generate hydrogen and methane, which are absorbed into the bloodstream and can be detected early in the breath. Normally, lactulose is fermented by bacteria in the colon, but if there is an early rise in breath levels of hydrogen or methane, it suggests that an overgrowth of bacteria in the small intestine may be responsible.

Jejunal Aspirate and Culture, taken by endoscopy, is a direct but invasive way of directly analyzing the bacterial overgrowth.

Treatment of Small Intestine Bacterial Overgrowth

Antibiotics (e.g., *rifaximin, neomycin, metronidazole*) may be given, the specific one depending on the organism and its resistance to antibiotics. As the organism is often not known, different antibiotics can be tried in rotating sequence.

Prokinetics (e.g., *metoclopraminde [Reglan], erythromycin, domperidone,*) can increase gut motility, which can help when the SIBO is due to decreased gut motion.

Dietary Changes: A low **FODMAP** (**F**ermentable **O**ligosaccharides, **D**isaccharides, **M**onosaccharides, **A**nd **P**olyols) diet can relieve symptoms by reducing the ingestion of short-chain carbohydrates that are fermented by gut bacteria and produce gas. FODMAP foods include:

- Oligosaccharides (e.g., wheat, rye, onions, garlic, and some other grains; also beans, lentils, and chickpeas)
- Disaccharides, e.g., lactose
- Monosaccharides, e.g., fructose
- Polyols, e.g., sorbitol and mannitol

The FODMAP foods are first eliminated and then reintroduced gradually to determine which ones are most associated with the symptoms.

Treat the Underlying Condition, e.g., diabetes, scleroderma (which can affect the small intestine), prior intestinal surgery, anatomical anomalies, chronic use of proton pump inhibitors (which reduce the acid that normally helps control bacterial growth), or antibiotic overuse.

Ileus

An ileus is a loss of the normal propulsive ability of the intestines. It can be due to various factors, including a postoperative effect, medications, infections, electrolyte imbalance, or bowel obstruction.

Diagnosis of Ileus

The history of ileus may include abdominal distension, pain, nausea, vomiting, inability to pass stool or gas, and lack of bowel sounds on examination.

Imaging:

- **Abdominal X-Rays:** Plain X-rays of the abdomen show dilated loops of bowel with air-fluid levels.
- **CT Scans** provide more detail and are better than plain X-rays for identifying abscesses, tumors, hernias, bowel perforation, ischemia, infection, or other pathology

not seen as well on X-ray. They can also distinguish between ileus and mechanical obstruction, which can present with similar symptoms.

Lab Tests: Blood tests can identify electrolyte imbalances, renal function abnormalities, and signs of inflammation or infection.

Treatment of Ileus

Treatment focuses on the underlying cause and supporting the patient until bowel function returns:

A **Nasogastric (NG) Tube** can remove air and gastric contents that have accumulated from the ileus. It can also prevent vomiting and aspiration, rest the bowels, and be used to administer medication.

Intravenous Fluids maintain hydration and correct electrolyte imbalances.

Medications like *metoclopramide* or *erythromycin* can be used to increase intestinal motility.

Surgery may sometimes be needed, e.g., for a perforation or ischemia.

Intestinal Obstruction

Intestinal obstruction is a serious and potentially life-threatening condition where there is a blockage, whether mechanical (from a physical obstruction, e.g., by fecal impaction or tumor) or functional (from a poorly functioning intestinal wall).

Diagnosis of Intestinal Obstruction

History and Physical may include severe abdominal pain and distension, vomiting, constipation, inability to pass gas, and high-pitched abdominal sounds on auscultation.

Imaging:

- **Abdominal X-rays** may show air-fluid levels and dilated loops of bowel, suggesting obstruction.
- **CT Scan** provides more detailed information as to location and possible cause.
- **Ultrasound**, which does not involve radiation, is sometimes used, especially in children or pregnant women.

Laboratory Tests can show signs of infection, dehydration, electrolyte imbalance, and abnormal kidney function.

Treatment of Intestinal Obstruction

Non-Surgical Treatment:

- A **Nasogastric (NG) Tube** can decompress the stomach and upper intestine from GI secretions or swallowed air and prevent aspiration. Sometimes the contents removed through the tube can be analyzed to help in the diagnosis.
- **Intravenous Fluids**
- **Correction of Electrolyte imbalance** from vomiting or intestinal malfunction

Surgical Treatment: Can relieve the blockage, which might be due to intestinal adhesions, volvulus, stricture, hernia, intussusception, impacted feces in the colon, foreign bodies, gallstones, or tumors.

Constipation with fecal impaction can be a cause or a result of intestinal obstruction. If constipation is the cause, there are a variety of straightforward measures to soften and remove the impacted stool:

Suppositories: *Glycerin* or *bisacodyl* suppositories can be inserted into the rectum for immediate relief, to stimulate a bowel movement and soften the impacted stool.

Enemas: Enemas can be used to soften and break up the impacted stool. These include saline, mineral oil, or soap suds enemas.

Oral Laxatives: Oral laxatives can help soften the stool and stimulate bowel movements. These may include stool softeners (like *docusate*), osmotic laxatives (like *polyethylene glycol* or *lactulose*), or stimulant laxatives (like *senna* or *bisacodyl*).

Manual Disimpaction: In resistant cases, a healthcare provider may need to physically remove the impacted stool using gloved fingers.

Hydration and Diet Modification: Increasing fluid intake and adjusting the diet to include more fiber can help prevent future occurrences of fecal impaction.

Behavioral Changes: Regular toilet habits, such as using the toilet at a set time each day, can help maintain regular bowel movements.

Physical Activity: Regular physical activity can help stimulate bowel movements.

Long-term Management: For chronic constipation, long-term strategies to manage bowel health are important. These might include dietary changes (e.g., high-fiber diet), regular use of laxatives, and exercise.

Intestinal Ischemia

Intestinal ischemia can affect the small intestine, large intestine, or both and can be acute or chronic. It can arise from arterial occlusion of branches of the aorta (e.g., by thrombosis or embolism of the superior mesenteric, inferior mesenteric, or celiac arteries, or the mesenteric arcades and vasa recta, which supply specific segments of the intestines), venous occlusion (e.g., from hypercoagulable states or infections), poor circulation (e.g., from heart failure or certain vasoconstrictors, arterial narrowing from atherosclerosis, strangulated hernia, vasculitis, tumor compressions, fibromuscular dysplasia of the arteries supplying the intestines, or radiation therapy).

Diagnosis of Intestinal Ischemia

Acute ischemia may present with sudden abdominal pain, nausea and vomiting, an urgent need to have a bowel movement, frequent, forceful bowel movements, bloody stools, and abdominal tenderness or distension. Chronic ischemia may present with postprandial pain, weight loss, and fear of eating.

Lab Tests: Blood tests may show an elevated white blood cell count, acidosis (lactic acidosis from a switch to anaerobic metabolism in the ischemic bowel), and elevated lactate levels. D-dimer levels, a reflection of blood clotting and fibrinolysis, can be elevated but are non-specific.

Imaging:

X-rays can show signs of bowel obstruction or perforation.

CT angiography, MRI angiography, and **ultrasound** can show blood flow in the intestinal arteries and veins and may reveal blood vessel blockage or narrowing.

Treatment of Intestinal Ischemia may include surgery to remove the affected portion of the bowel and restore circulation. Other interventions may include stenting, thrombolysis, or anticoagulation (e.g., with heparin) to restore blood flow, and broad-spectrum antibiotics,

Acute mesenteric ischemia has a high mortality rate, especially if treatment is delayed. Chronic Intestinal Ischemia may require surgery, or may improve with dietary changes (e.g., small, frequent meals) or anticoagulants or antiplatelet agents to prevent clotting. Chronic ischemia, if treated before significant complications develop, can have a good prognosis.

Intussusception

Intussusception is a serious condition in which a part of the intestine slides into an adjacent part of the intestine (particularly the ileum into the cecum), like the parts of a telescope (**Fig. 7-2**). It can occur in any part of the intestine, but the most common site is at the ileocecal junction, particularly in children between 6 months and 3 years of age. In adults, intussusception can happen anywhere along the gastrointestinal tract and is more likely to be associated with an identifiable cause, such as a tumor or polyp that serves as a precipitating point for the telescoping of the intestine.

Prompt treatment is important since intussusception can lead to blockage of the intestine, reduced blood flow, and damage to the affected section of bowel.

Diagnosis of Intussusception

Common symptoms include severe, intermittent abdominal pain; vomiting; bloody stools; and, in some cases, a palpable, tender abdominal mass.

Ultrasound is the main diagnostic tool for intussusception. It can visualize the "telescoped" sections of the intestine.

X-rays and **CT scans** can confirm the diagnosis or rule out other conditions.

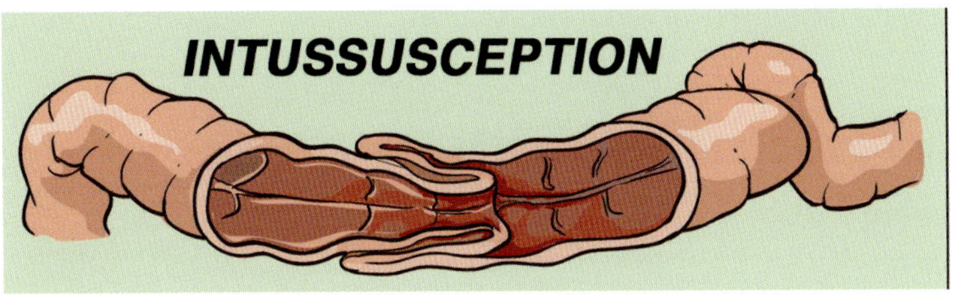

Figure 7-2

Treatment of Intussusception

Non-Surgical Reduction:

- An **air** or **barium enema** can be both diagnostic and therapeutic. Under fluoroscopic guidance, air or barium is introduced into the colon to push the telescoped part of the intestine back into place. This method is successful in many cases, especially in children.
- **Monitoring**: After successful enema reduction, patients are usually monitored for a short time to ensure that intussusception does not recur.

Surgery is necessary if the intussusception cannot be reduced with an enema, if there are signs of bowel perforation, or if there is evidence of compromised blood supply to the intestine. The surgeon manually reduces the intussusception. If part of the intestine is damaged, that section may be removed. If an underlying cause (like a polyp or tumor) is identified as a driving point for the intussusception, it may need to be treated separately.

Recurrence is possible, especially in children, so continued monitoring is important.

Intestinal Perforation

Intestinal perforation is a serious condition that can result from various causes, including trauma, gastrointestinal diseases, obstruction, or surgical complications.

Diagnosis of Intestinal Perforation

The patient has severe abdominal pain, fever, nausea, vomiting, chills, and signs of **acute abdomen**, which can include abdominal rigidity and tenderness.

Physical Examination may show signs of peritonitis (rebound tenderness, guarding, abdominal distention, fever, hypoactive bowel sounds).

Imaging:

- **Abdominal X-ray**: Upright or decubitus X-rays can reveal free air under the diaphragm (**pneumoperitoneum**), suggesting a perforation.
- **CT Scan** can show the location and cause of the perforation (e.g., diverticulitis, Crohn's disease or ulcerative colitis, tumors, foreign bodies), as well as associated free fluid or abscesses.
- **Ultrasound** is less sensitive than CT for detecting pneumoperitoneum.

Lab Tests: Blood tests can show signs of infection such as increased white blood cell count and increased inflammatory markers (e.g., increased C-reactive protein or erythrocyte sedimentation rate).

Treatment of Intestinal Perforation

Surgical Repair:

Laparotomy is an open surgical procedure to repair the perforation. Sometimes, a segment of the intestine may need to be resected and a temporary or permanent stoma created in the abdominal wall. Sometimes, a less invasive repair may be done by laparoscope.

Supportive Care:
Fluid Resuscitation: To treat or prevent shock.

Broad Spectrum Antibiotics
A **Nasogastric Tube** can reduce abdominal distension and prevent further leakage into the abdominal cavity.
Nutritional Support may be given by IV to rest the intestines.

Short Bowel Syndrome

Short bowel syndrome (SBS) is a disorder that typically occurs when a large portion of the small intestine has been removed due to disease or injury, leaving insufficient surface area to absorb nutrients adequately. This malabsorption can lead to a variety of long-term health issues.

Diagnosis of Short Bowel Syndrome

A history of bowel surgery, particularly if large portions of the ileum or jejunum have been removed, is a key indicator. There may be diarrhea, weight loss, and malnutrition.

Lab Tests:

- **Blood tests** may show anemia, electrolyte imbalances, abnormal kidney function, decreased vitamin levels and signs of malnutrition.
- **Stool tests** can confirm decreased fat absorption (**fecal fat test**) and sometimes bacterial overgrowth.

Imaging Studies:
X-ray, CT scan, or **MRI** can evaluate the remaining intestine and rule out other conditions.
Barium studies can provide a different view of the intestinal tract.

Treatment of Short Bowel Syndrome

Treatment focuses on managing symptoms, and ensuring adequate nutrition:

- Frequent small meals low in fat; soluble fiber to help manage diarrhea
- Oral or sometimes parenteral vitamin and mineral supplementation
- IV nutrition or tube feeding, which may be short-term or long-term

Medications:

- **Antidiarrheal Agents**: *Loperamide* or *diphenoxylate* can slow intestinal transit and increase nutrient absorption.
- **Proton Pump Inhibitors or H2 Blockers** can be used to reduce gastric acid secretion, which can be increased in SBS, due in part to reduced inhibitory feedback on acid production.
- **Choleretic Agents**, e.g., *ursodeoxycholic acid* improve bile flow and reduce the chance of gallstones.

- **Growth Factors** e.g., *teduglutide* (a glucagon-like peptide-2 analog) may enhance intestinal absorption and reduce the need for parenteral nutrition.
- **Antibiotics** are given for bacterial overgrowth.
- ***Teduglutide*** (***Gattex***) is a GLP-2 analog that helps promote absorption in the small intestine.

Reconstructive Surgeries: Various procedures can be performed to slow transit time and increase the absorptive surface area of the remaining intestine.

Intestinal Transplant: In severe cases, when parental nutrition is no longer possible, an intestinal transplant may be considered.

Small Intestine Tumors

Tumors of the small intestine are less common than other gastrointestinal tumors. When they occur, they can be benign or malignant (particularly adenocarcinoma). The diagnosis and treatment of small intestine tumors vary, based on their type.

Diagnosis of Small Intestine Tumors

Common symptoms may include abdominal pain, weight loss, nausea, vomiting, or blood in the stool. However, many small intestine tumors are asymptomatic and may be found incidentally.

Imaging:

- **CT** or **MRI Scan** can provide images of masses in the small intestine.
- **Barium X-ray** is less commonly used; it involves swallowing a barium solution that coats the lining of the small intestine to provide clearer X-ray images.

Endoscopic Procedures:

Capsule Endoscopy uses a small, pill-sized camera that is swallowed and can provide images of the length of the small intestine (but cannot take biopsies).

Push Enteroscopy, Double- or **Single-balloon Enteroscopy** and **Spiral Enteroscopy** are special endoscope adaptations that can reach farther into the small intestine than a standard endoscope, and can also take biopsies.

Endoscopic Ultrasound (EUS) combines endoscopy and ultrasound to obtain images and information about the wall of the small intestine and surrounding areas.

Biopsy: The definitive diagnosis of a small intestine tumor is often made through a biopsy.

Treatment of Small Intestine Tumors

Surgery is the most common treatment for tumors in the small intestine, particularly for malignant tumors, and may include removal of the tumor and a portion of the small intestine, as well as lymph node dissection.

Chemotherapy is sometimes used before surgery to shrink the tumor or after surgery to kill any remaining cancer cells.

Radiation Therapy is less commonly used for small intestine tumors unless they cannot be completely removed surgically.

Benign tumors may not need treatment unless they are causing symptoms or have the potential to become malignant.

Lactose Intolerance

Lactose intolerance results from a deficiency of the enzyme *lactase*, which is needed to break down lactose into glucose and galactose for absorption (**Fig. 7-3.**). The undigested lactose is then fermented by bacteria in the large intestine, producing hydrogen, carbon dioxide, and methane. The patient may present with bloating, gas, abdominal pain, and diarrhea (lactose can have an osmotic effect, drawing water into the large intestine).

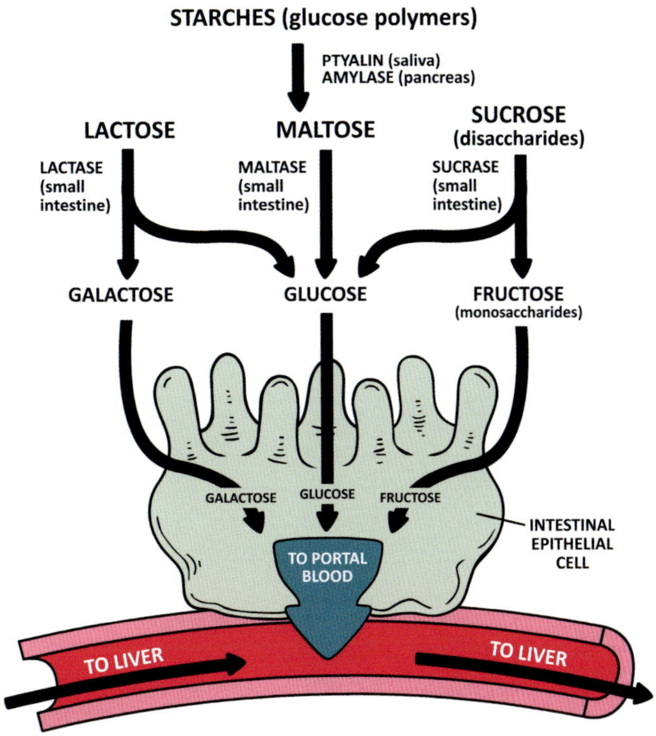

Figure 7-3 Absorption of sugars in the small intestine.

Diagnosis of Lactose Intolerance

Lactose Tolerance Test: After drinking a liquid containing high levels of lactose, blood samples check for a rise in blood glucose, which occurs normally, but not if the patient cannot break down lactose. The patient is also observed during the test for symptoms of lactose intolerance.

Hydrogen Breath Test: After consuming a lactose-rich beverage, the breath is tested at regular intervals to measure hydrogen. Normally hydrogen should not be elevated. If it is, this suggests that the lactose is not being digested but is remaining in the gut, fermenting into hydrogen and other gases. The test is non-invasive and can be used for both adults and children.

Stool Acidity Test: Usually done in infants and children. It measures stool acidity, which increases from lactic acid produced by indigested lactose.

Elimination Diet: Tests whether symptoms disappear on removing lactose from the diet and reappear when reintroducing it

Treatment of Lactose Intolerance

- Limit lactose intake, using alternatives, like lactose-free milk, almond, soy, or rice milk, with calcium and vitamin D supplementation.

- Lactase enzyme supplements
- Probiotics can help some people by altering the gut flora.
- Gradually introducing small amounts of lactose in the diet can help reduce lactose intolerance in some people.

Parasitic Infections of the Small Intestine

Parasitic infections of the small intestine can be caused by various organisms, including protozoa (e.g., *Giardia lamblia, Cryptosporidium*) and helminths (e.g., *hookworms, Ascaris lumbricoides*). These parasites can cause a range of gastrointestinal symptoms, malabsorption, and other systemic problems.

Diagnosis of Parasitic Infection of the Small Intestine

GI symptoms may include diarrhea (constipation sometimes, where there is intestinal obstruction or decreased intestinal motility), abdominal pain, bloating, gas, blood or mucus in the stool, and weight loss, which may involve malabsorption. It is important to obtain a history of travel and possible exposure to contaminated food or water.

Stool Tests:

- **Microscopic Examination** looks for parasite eggs, larvae, or protozoa.
- **Stool Antigen Tests** can detect specific parasitic antigens. A Polymerase Chain Reaction (PCR) test can detect specific genetic material.

Blood Tests:

- Elevated eosinophils are often seen in helminth infections.
- Serology tests can sometimes detect antibodies against specific parasites when they are not detected in the stool (e.g., *Giardia lamblia, Strongyloides stercoralis, Entamoeba histolytica, Cryptosporidium, Toxoplasma gondii,* and *Schistosoma* species).

Imaging Studies: Ultrasound, CT, or MRI can be used to assess the extent of the infection or blockage.

Treatment of Parasitic Infections of the Small Intestine

Medications:

- **Protozoal Infections**: *Metronidazole* or *tinidazole* may be used for Giardia; *nitazoxanide* for *Cryptosporidium*.
- **Helminth Infections**: *Albendazole, mebendazole,* or *ivermectin* can be used for various worm infestations.

Supportive Care: Includes fluid and electrolyte replacement and nutritional support, especially if there is significant diarrhea, weight loss and malabsorption.

Appendicitis

Appendicitis is an inflammation of the appendix. The pain often begins around the umbilicus and over hours or days spreads to the right lower abdomen, becoming sharper.

Other symptoms may include nausea, vomiting, loss of appetite, fever, and an inability to pass gas. It's important to seek immediate medical attention if appendicitis is suspected, as a ruptured appendix can lead to serious complications.

Diagnosis of Appendicitis

Physical Examination:

The abdomen shows tenderness, swelling, or rigidity. Pain commonly is felt at **McBurney's point** (roughly two thirds of the way between the navel and right anterior superior iliac spine) (**Fig. 7-4**). Rebound tenderness (the patient experiences more pain on quick release of pressure on the abdomen) suggests peritoneal inflammation. The **Rovsing's sign** occurs when the examiner presses on the lower left abdomen; the patient experiences pain in the right lower abdomen, due to gas or fecal contents being pushed back toward the cecum and appendix. The **psoas sign** appears when the patient experiences pain in the right lower abdominal quadrant on flexing their right thigh against resistance. The pain occurs because the inflamed appendix contacts the psoas muscle during the flexion.

Lab Tests: Blood tests may detect a high white blood cell count, indicating an infection. Urinalysis is done to rule out a urinary tract infection or kidney stones.

Imaging: An abdominal ultrasound or CT scan can help visualize the appendix, confirm inflammation, and distinguish it from other possible problems.

The **Alvarado Score (MANTRELS score)**, while not definitive, is useful in evaluating if appendicitis is present:

Symptoms:

- **Migratory Right Iliac Fossa Pain**: 1 point
- **Anorexia**: 1 point
- **Nausea/Vomiting**: 1 point

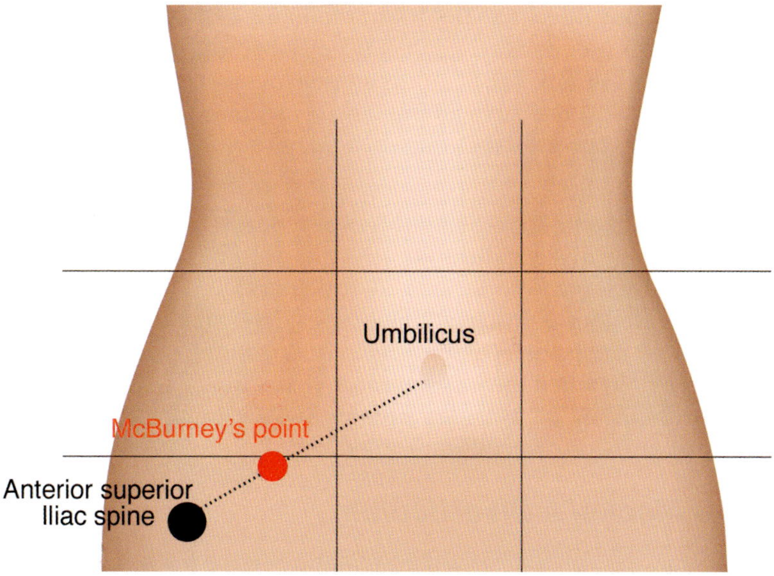

Figure 7-4 *McBurney's point.*

Signs:

- **Tenderness in Right Lower Quadrant**: 2 points
- **Rebound Pain**: 1 point
- **Elevated Temperature (fever)**: 1 point

Laboratory Findings:

- **Leukocytosis (white blood cell count > 10,000 per mm^3)**: 2 points
- **Left Shift (increase in the number of immature neutrophils)**: 1 point

The score is generally interpreted as follows:
Score of 1-4: Low probability of appendicitis
Score of 5-6: Compatible with appendicitis, but more information is needed
Score of 7-8: Probable appendicitis
Score of 9-10: Highly probable appendicitis

Treatment of Appendicitis

Antibiotics may be administered initially for infection.
Surgery (appendectomy) can be done as open surgery or laparoscopically.

Meckel's Diverticulum

Meckel's diverticulum is a congenital condition resulting from the incomplete obliteration of the vitelline duct during embryonic development. It is a small outpouching of the small intestine near the ileocecal valve and is the most common congenital anomaly of the gastrointestinal tract.

Diagnosis of Meckel's Diverticulum

Meckel's diverticulum often remains asymptomatic, but can present with bleeding, inflammation, obstruction, or perforation. It may be discovered incidentally during imaging studies, surgery, or endoscopy for other reasons. However, it can present, particularly in children, with complications such as painless rectal bleeding, or it may present with inflammation (similar to appendicitis), obstruction, or perforation and an acute abdomen.

Imaging:
Technetium-99m Pertechnetate Scan (Meckel's Scan): This diagnostic test is used specifically for Meckel's diverticulum because the isotope is taken up by the gastric mucosa, which can be ectopic in a Meckel's diverticulum.
CT Scan can help diagnose complications such as diverticulitis or obstruction.
Capsule endoscopy can be helpful for direct visualization.
Angiography can help when there is significant bleeding.
Laparoscopy or the more invasive **laparotomy** (which involves a large incision in the abdominal wall) can provide direct visualization.

Treatment of Meckel's Diverticulum

No treatment may be needed for asymptomatic Meckel's diverticulum, but surgery may be required (resection by laparoscopic or open surgery) for symptoms of bleeding, diverticulitis, or obstruction. A segmental resection of the affected intestine may be needed if there is a significant portion of inflamed or necrotic bowel.

Intestinal Tuberculosis

Tuberculosis (*Mycobacterium tuberculosis*) is the great imitator. Intestinal tuberculosis can mimic other gastrointestinal diseases such as Crohn's disease or malignancy and may require several approaches to diagnosis.

Diagnosis of Intestinal Tuberculosis

History and Physical Exam: Is there a history of TB exposure, immunocompromise, or signs of systemic TB, e.g., weight loss, fever, night sweats? Abdominal exam may reveal abdominal pain, distension, and signs of peritonitis (severe diffuse abdominal pain, guarding, rebound tenderness, decreased bowel sounds) along with fever.

Lab Tests:

- **Tuberculin Skin Test (TST)** or **Interferon-Gamma Release Assay (IGRA)** can indicate TB infection but cannot determine if it is active.
- **Complete Blood Count (CBC)** may show signs of chronic infection or anemia.
- **Erythrocyte Sedimentation Rate (ESR)** and **C-Reactive Protein (CRP)** are non-specific inflammatory markers that may be elevated in active TB.

Imaging:

- **Abdominal Ultrasound** or **CT Scan** can detect thickening of the bowel wall, lymphadenopathy, ascites, or other changes suggestive of intestinal TB.
- **Barium Studies** have largely been replaced by CT and MRI but can show strictures, ulcers, and fistulas.

Microbiological and Histological Evaluation:
Stool Cultures can sometimes detect mycobacteria.

Acid-Fast Bacilli (AFB) Staining and Culture: Samples from endoscopic biopsies, ascitic fluid, or tissue can be used for AFB staining, culture, and TB PCR to identify the bacteria.

Colonoscopy or **Upper GI Endoscopy** can identify ulcers, strictures, or mass lesions. Biopsies can be taken for histology, which may show granulomas with caseating necrosis, a hallmark of TB, although not specific for TB.

Treatment of Intestinal TB

The treatment of intestinal TB is like pulmonary TB and typically uses a combination of antituberculous medications, e.g., *isoniazid, rifampicin, pyrazinamide,* and *ethambutol*. Surgery may be required for complications such as obstruction, perforation, fistula formation, or abscesses that do not respond to medical therapy.

Radiation Enteritis

Radiation enteritis is inflammation of the intestines that occurs after radiation therapy, typically for cancers in the abdomen or pelvis. The patient may experience abdominal pain, nausea and vomiting, diarrhea (or constipation with bowel obstruction), intestinal bleeding, weight loss, and fatigue. Radiation enteritis can be acute or chronic, depending on the timing of the symptoms relative to the radiation exposure. Acute radiation enteritis usually occurs during or shortly after radiation therapy and often is self-limiting, resolving with supportive care. Chronic radiation enteritis may arise weeks to years later and can lead to long-term complications.

Diagnosis of Radiation Enteritis

Lab Tests:

- **Complete Blood Count** may show anemia if there is chronic bleeding.
- **Stool Tests** can confirm or exclude infections or inflammatory bowel disease (stool **calprotectin** and **lactoferrin** are markers of inflammation in the GI tract).

Imaging:

- **CT Scan** or **MRI** imaging can help evaluate the extent of bowel inflammation, thickening, or other complications such as fistulas or abscesses.
- **Barium Studies** can demonstrate strictures, dilation, and motility disorders.

Colonoscopy or **Upper GI Endoscopy** allow direct visualization and allow biopsy, which can assess the degree of inflammation and help rule out malignancy.

Treatment of Radiation Enteritis

Dietary Management often includes a low-residue diet to reduce bowel movements. Treatment may include nutritional supplements for malabsorption.

Hydration and Electrolytes

Medications may include anti-diarrheal agents, antispasmodics, analgesics, and sometimes corticosteroids for significant inflammation. Pancreatic enzymes may be administered for pancreatic insufficiency.

Endoscopic or Surgical Intervention: Surgery or endoscopic dilation may be necessary for severe complications like strictures, fistulas, or perforation.

Whipple's Disease

Whipple's disease is a rare bacterial infection that primarily affects the small intestine but can also impact other parts of the body such as the heart, brain, and joints. It interferes with the body's ability to absorb nutrients and is caused by the bacterium *Tropheryma whipplei*.

Diagnosis of Whipple's Disease

There are non-specific signs of abdominal pain, diarrhea, weight loss, and joint pain, which develop slowly over time.

Blood Tests can look for anemia or signs of malnutrition.

Stool Tests: Fatty stool is common, as in other malabsorptive disorders.

Endoscopy: Biopsy often reveals lesions and the presence of periodic acid-Schiff (PAS)-positive macrophages, characteristic of the disease.

Polymerase Chain Reaction (PCR) is a more specific test that can identify *Tropheryma whipplei*.

Treatment of Whipple's Disease

The standard treatment for Whipple's disease is antibiotics, IV at first (e.g., *ceftriaxone* or *meropenem*) for several weeks and then oral (e.g., *doxycycline + hydroxychloroquine*), which may need to be taken for 1-2 years, sometimes lifetime.

The prognosis for Whipple's Disease is good with treatment, but without treatment can be fatal due to malnutrition and systemic effects.

Small Bowel Bleeding

The diagnosis and treatment of small bowel bleeding involve several steps:

Diagnosis of Small Bowel Bleeding

Clinical Evaluation: There may be a history of melena (black, tarry stools), hematochezia (passing fresh blood per rectum), or symptoms of anemia (such as fatigue, shortness of breath, and pallor).

Lab Tests: Blood tests, including a complete blood count (CBC), to check for anemia, and coagulation studies to assess blood clotting.

Imaging:

Computed Tomography (CT) Angiography can help identify bleeding and its origin in the small intestine.

Capsule Endoscopy can identify bleeding sources in the small intestine.

Double-Balloon Enteroscopy allows direct visualization of the small bowel and can also perform biopsies or treat bleeding sites.

Angiography can be used to identify the exact site of active bleeding site and potentially treat it through embolization.

Radionuclide Scanning: A small amount of radioactive material that is taken up by red blood cells is administered intravenously. A special camera can detect the tagged cells where they accumulate from a bleed in the small intestine.

Treatment of Small Bowel Bleeding

Initial treatment may involve IV fluids or blood transfusions for stabilization.

Medical Management: Depending on the cause, treatment may include medications such as proton pump inhibitors (to prevent further small bowel irritation from acid), therapeutic agents for specific conditions like Crohn's disease, or octreotide (which can induce vasoconstriction of blood vessels in the GI tract, inhibit acid secretion, and reduce intestinal motility).

Endoscopic Therapy: If the source of bleeding is identified endoscopically, treatments may include cauterization, clipping, injection sclerotherapy or epinephrine injection.

Angioembolization: If the bleeding site is identified on angiography, embolization can be performed to stop the bleeding by blocking the blood vessel.

Surgery: If other interventions fail or are not possible, surgery may be necessary to remove the bleeding segment of the small intestine.

Treat Underlying Conditions such as inflammatory bowel disease, vascular abnormalities, or tumors.

8

Diseases of the Large Intestine

The main function of the large intestine (colon) is the absorption of water and the concentration of stool, although it does have some role in the absorption of other substances. Abnormal decreases or increases in those functions can result in diarrhea or constipation.

Colon Cancer

The lifetime risk of developing colorectal cancer in the U.S. is about 1 in 23 for men and 1 in 26 for women, with a 5-year survival rate of about 65%, depending on the extent of the cancer and the patient's response to treatment. Regular screening is important, especially for those over the age of 50, who are at higher risk. Apart from age, risk factors include family history of colon cancer, genetic syndromes (e.g., familial adenomatous polyposis), prior colon cancer or polyps, race (Black individuals in the U.S. are at higher risk), and inflammatory bowel disease (Crohn's disease or ulcerative colitis). Modifiable risk factors include a high fat/low fiber diet, inactivity, obesity, smoking and alcohol excess, and diabetes. Currently, colonoscopy is recommended every 10 years for average-risk people age 45-75. The progression from a benign polyp to cancer may take 10–15 years, allowing early successful removal with regular screening.

Diagnosis of Colon Cancer

History and Physical: The patient may at first be asymptomatic, but may present with changes in bowel habits, rectal bleeding, abdominal pain, weight loss, or fatigue. A digital rectal exam may be able to palpate a nearby mass.

Blood Tests:

- CBC can check for anemia.
- Liver function tests can assess the overall health of the liver and potential metastasis.
- Carcinoembryonic antigen (CEA) test may be used to follow patients during and after treatment to look for signs of the cancer returning, but it is not specific or sensitive enough for cancer screening or diagnosis.

Stool Tests: Testing for microscopic traces of blood in the stool, if positive, is relatively sensitive for colon cancer, but is nonspecific, as the presence of blood can mean other things. The **fecal immunochemical test (FIT)** is better than the traditional **guaiac-based fecal occult blood test** in that it specifically targets human hemoglobin protein rather than blood from the diet and is more sensitive in detecting blood than the traditional test. Fecal DNA testing, which detects abnormal DNA sequences as found in cancer cells, is more specific.

Colonoscopy allows direct visualization of the entire colon and rectum, the removal of polyps and biopsy. Colon cancer is believed to develop from an adenomatous polyp.

Imaging:

CT scans of the abdomen and pelvis can determine the extent of the cancer within the colon and check for spread to other organs.

MRI may be used for a more detailed evaluation of cancer spread, particularly if the rectum is involved.

PET scans can sometimes help determine if the cancer has spread.

Biopsy obtained during colonoscopy is the definitive method for diagnosing colon cancer, by providing a sample for histological examination.

Treatment of Colon Cancer

Surgery:

- **Early-stage tumors**: Colonoscopy is used for polypectomy or local excision for very small cancers.
- **Larger tumors**: Partial colectomy may be done to remove the part of the colon that contains the cancer, along with a margin of normal tissue on either side of the cancer.
- **Advanced cancer**: Surgery may involve removing affected adjacent organs if the cancer has spread.
- **Laparoscopic surgery** is a minimally invasive approach for some cancers.

Chemotherapy is used after surgery if the cancer has spread to lymph nodes, to reduce the risk of cancer recurrence. For metastatic cancer, chemotherapy can help to prolong life and improve symptoms.

Radiation Therapy is not typically used in initial treatment of colon cancer but may be used to shrink tumors before surgery or to relieve symptoms of advanced cancer.

Targeted Drug Therapy uses drugs that target specific pathways or genetic mutations within cancer cells. It is used mostly for advanced cancers, especially those that haven't responded to chemotherapy.

Immunotherapy is used for cancers that have specific genetic markers, to help the immune system better attack cancer cells.

Supportive Care: Palliative care can help manage symptoms and improve the quality of life at any stage of cancer.

The prognosis for colon cancer varies significantly with the stage at diagnosis. Early-stage colon cancer has a relatively high survival rate, whereas advanced cancer that has spread to distant organs has a significantly lower survival rate.

Colorectal Polyps

While most colorectal polyps are benign, some can develop into cancer if left untreated.

Types of Colorectal Polyps:

Adenomatous Polyps (adenomas) sometime change into cancer.

Hyperplastic Polyps and **Inflammatory Polyps** are more common and generally do not develop into cancer.

Serrated Types: This category includes hyperplastic polyps and sessile serrated polyps. The latter can become cancerous, especially if they are large (> 10mm) or in the right colon.

Diagnosis of Colorectal Polyps

Colonoscopy is the most accurate test for polyps and allows for their removal during the procedure.

Flexible Sigmoidoscopy allows examination of the lower colon and can detect and remove polyps, but has a limited reach compared to colonoscopy.

CT Colonography (Virtual Colonoscopy) uses CT scanning to find polyps and cancers, but they cannot be removed during the test.

Stool Tests: The **fecal immunochemical test (FIT)** tests for hidden blood in the stool. It is better than the traditional fecal occult blood test in that it specifically targets human hemoglobin protein rather than blood from the diet. The **stool DNA test**, in addition to looking for occult blood, detects specific DNA markers that are often associated with cancer or precancerous colon polyps. While non-invasive, the stool DNA tests is less sensitive in detecting polyps than an actual colonoscopy, where the polyp can be seen, removed and biopsied.

Treatment of Colorectal Polyps

Most polyps can be removed during a colonoscopy with a wire loop or forceps. Larger polyps might require **endoscopic mucosal resection**, where a solution is injected beneath the polyp to lift it and make it easier to remove. For polyps that are too large or too risky to remove during a colonoscopy, laparoscopic or traditional surgery may be required.

A diet high in fruits, vegetables, and fibers with reduced red meat intake, cessation of smoking, regular physical activity, and maintaining a healthy weight are recommended to lower the risk of polyps. Routine colorectal cancer screening is recommended at age 45-75. Removal of a precancerous polyp has an excellent prognosis.

Infectious Colitis

Infectious colitis is inflammation of the colon that is caused by an infection:

Bacteria: E.g, *Campylobacter, Salmonella, Shigella,* and *Escherichia coli*, particularly *E. coli* O157:H7. *Clostridium difficile* (C. diff) can also cause colitis, often after the use of antibiotics.

Viruses: Norovirus, rotavirus, and adenovirus can cause colitis, primarily in children.

Parasites, e.g., *Giardia lamblia* and *Entamoeba histolytica* can cause colitis, usually through contaminated water or food.

The patient may experience diarrhea, which can be bloody or contain mucus, along with abdominal pain, urgency to have a bowel movement, fever, dehydration, or nausea and vomiting. Infectious colitis is often spread through contaminated food or water, or through contact with infected individuals or surfaces. Outbreaks can occur in areas with poor sanitation or contaminated food supply.

Diagnosis of Infectious Colitis

Stool tests may identify the infectious organism.

Blood tests, colonoscopy, or **imaging studies** may provide further information and assess the severity of the condition.

Treatment of Infectious Colitis

Treatment depends on the cause. Bacterial infections may need antibiotics; viral infections typically resolve on their own. Hydration is important to replace lost fluids. More intensive treatment may be needed for severe cases.

Prevention of Infectious Colitis:

Good hygiene practices, including thorough handwashing

Safe food handling and preparation. Drink clean, safe water.

Vaccines (like those for rotavirus) can help prevent some viral causes of colitis.

Microscopic Colitis

Microscopic colitis is a type of colonic inflammation that is only visible under a microscope. Unlike more typical forms of colitis, the inner colon lining doesn't appear inflamed or abnormal during a colonoscopy or sigmoidoscopy. The patient may have a chronic intermittent watery, non-bloody diarrhea, along with abdominal pain, cramps, bloating, and weight loss.

There are two main types of microscopic colitis:

Collagenous Colitis is characterized by a thicker layer of collagen beneath the lining of the colon.

Lymphocytic Colitis has an increased number of lymphocytes in the colon lining.

The exact cause of microscopic colitis is unknown but may be related to an abnormal immune response to bacteria or viruses in the gut. Some medications, like nonsteroidal anti-inflammatory drugs (NSAIDs), proton pump inhibitors, and selective serotonin reuptake inhibitors (SSRIs), have been associated with microscopic colitis. Other potential factors include genetics, autoimmune disorders, and age (it's more common in older adults).

Diagnosis of Microscopic Colitis

While colonoscopy or sigmoidoscopy appear normal, biopsy establishes the diagnosis.

Treatment of microscopic colitis often involves lifestyle changes, such as adjusting the diet (soft, easy-to-digest low-fiber foods) and discontinuing any potentially causative medications. Medications may be prescribed to reduce inflammation (e.g., *budesonide*, a steroid) or reduce diarrhea. Some patients may need immunosuppressive drugs (e.g., *infliximab*, *adalimumab*) if their condition is resistant to other treatments.

Microscopic colitis can be chronic but is generally not life-threatening.

Ulcerative Colitis

Ulcerative colitis (UC) is a chronic inflammatory bowel disease (IBD) that causes inflammation and ulcers in the digestive tract. It mainly affects the large intestine and rectum. It can affect the left colon or the entire colon. Unlike Crohn's disease, its area of gut involvement is continuous, rather than discontinuous. While Crohn's involves inflammation of all layers of the gut wall, UC inflammation typically is confined to the mucosal and submucosal layers (**Figs. 8-1** through **8-3**). The cause of UC is unknown. The treatment goal is to reduce symptoms, achieve and maintain remission, and prevent complications.

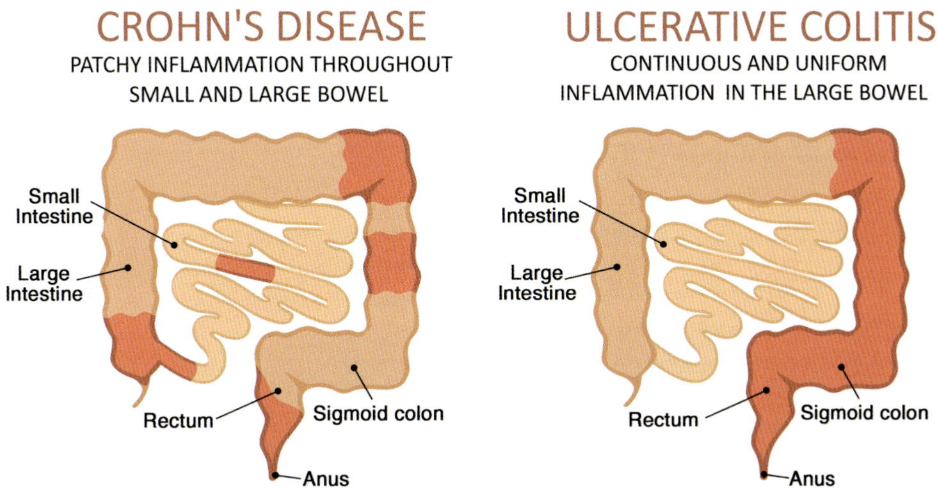

Figure 8-1

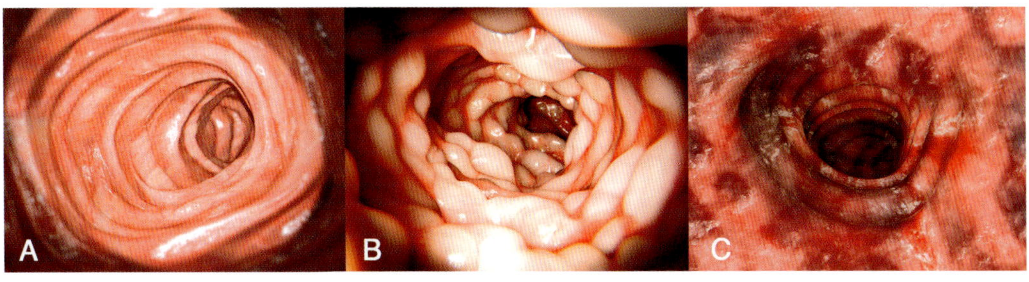

Figure 8-2 *A. Normal colon. B. Crohn's disease. C. Ulcerative colitis.*

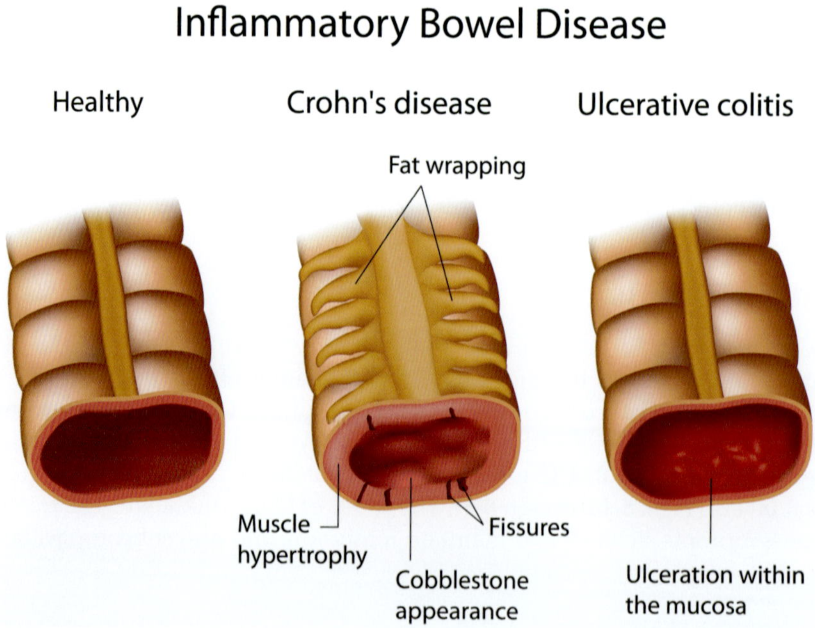

Figure 8-3

Diagnosis of Ulcerative Colitis

The patient may present with abdominal pain, rectal bleeding, diarrhea, and a family history of ulcerative colitis or other irritable bowel disease.

Blood Tests check for anemia, infection, and inflammatory markers, e.g., elevated C-reactive protein (CRP) and erythrocyte sedimentation rate (ESR).

A **Stool Sample** is examined to rule out infections or parasites as the causes of diarrhea and to look for white blood cells (a sign of inflammation).

Colonoscopy allows direct visualization of the colon and the terminal ileum, and enables biopsy to confirm the diagnosis.

Flexible Sigmoidoscopy can only view about 2 feet from the anus, missing the descending colon, transverse colon, ascending colon and cecum, but is less invasive than a colonoscopy and can still be diagnostic of ulcerative colitis and allow biopsy. Flexible sigmoidoscopy is used if a full colonoscopy is not safe or possible.

Imaging Studies such as CT or MRI can be used to evaluate the extent of the disease and complications.

Treatment of Ulcerative Colitis

Medication:

- **Aminosalicylates** (e.g., *sulfasalazine, mesalamine, olsalazine, balsalazide*) are used for their anti-inflammatory effects.
- **Corticosteroids** are used to reduce inflammation for moderate to severe UC during flare-ups, but are not for long-term use.

- **Immunomodulators** (e.g., *azathioprine, 6-mercaptopurine, methotrexate*) reduce inflammation.
- **Biologics** use targeted therapy to block specific pathways of inflammation and include TNF inhibitors (e.g., *adalimumab [Humira]*), integrin inhibitors (e.g., *vedolizumab*), and interleukin inhibitors (e.g., *ustekinumab [Stelara]*).
- **Janus kinase (JAK) inhibitors** (e.g., *tofacitinib*) are a type of oral medication that blocks certain pathways of inflammation.

Diet and Nutrition: While diet does not cause UC, it can trigger symptoms. Patients are often advised to keep a food diary to determine which foods may trigger a flare-up.

Surgery to remove the colon and rectum may be necessary if medication fails or there is perforation or severe inflammation, e.g., **toxic megacolon**, where the colon is very inflamed and dilated. Unlike Crohn's disease, UC can be completely cured by colectomy (although there is still a risk of developing primary sclerosing cholangitis, since the same immune response that causes the colon inflammation may also affect the bile ducts). A common procedure is to perform an ileal pouch-anal anastomosis following removal of the colon. An intermediate stage of the procedure is to first create a temporary ileostomy. This is followed by closing the ileostomy and connecting the terminal ileum to the anus, thereby eliminating the need for the external ostomy bag.

Lifestyle Remedies include managing stress through exercise, relaxation techniques, and quitting smoking.

Diverticulosis

In **diverticulosis**, small, bulging pouches (diverticula) develop in the colon wall. Although diverticula may bleed, diverticulosis is often asymptomatic and discovered incidentally. When one or more of these pouches become inflamed or infected, the condition is known as **diverticulitis**.

Diagnosis of Diverticulosis

The key tools for diagnosing diverticulosis are colonoscopy and CT scan. A barium enema X-ray is less commonly used.

Treatment of Diverticulosis

If diverticulosis is asymptomatic, treatment may not be necessary. Instead, the focus is on prevention of complications like diverticulitis:

- Lifestyle and Dietary Modifications: High-fiber diet, adequate water intake, and exercise; avoid smoking, as it is a risk factor for increased inflammation, which may lead to diverticulitis.
- For symptomatic diverticulosis, OTC pain medication (e.g., *acetaminophen*), probiotics, antispasmodics (e.g., *dicyclomine, hyoscyamine, mebeverine, peppermint oil*) may help reduce symptoms.

Diverticulitis

Diverticulitis is a condition where small, bulging pouches (diverticula) in the digestive tract become inflamed or infected. These pouches are most common in the large intestine.

Diagnosis of Diverticulitis

The patient reports abdominal pain, sometimes accompanied by fever, along with tenderness, bloating, or a mass in the abdomen.

Blood and Urine Tests look for signs of infection (CBC) and / or inflammation (C-Reactive Protein).

A **Pregnancy Test** in women of childbearing age is done to rule out pregnancy as a cause of the abdominal pain.

Liver Function Tests may be done to check for liver or biliary system causes of abdominal pain.

Stool Tests can rule out infection in people who have diarrhea.

A **CT Scan** with contrast can help confirm a diagnosis of diverticulitis and the presence of an abscess.

Ultrasound or **MRI** may be used in cases where the patient cannot undergo a CT scan.

Colonoscopy is not typically used to diagnose diverticulitis due to the risk of possible perforation of the inflamed or infected diverticula.

Treatment of Diverticulitis

- **Mild Diverticulitis** may benefit from antibiotics, a temporary liquid diet to rest the bowel, and over-the-counter pain relievers.
- **Severe Diverticulitis** may require hospitalization and intravenous antibiotics. Surgery may be needed for recurrent diverticulitis or complications such as colon perforation, fistula, or a large abscess. Options may include a bowel resection, removing the affected area of colon. This may be accompanied by a permanent colostomy (**Fig. 8-4**) or a temporary one to allow the distal colon to heal.

Lifestyle Changes: The best way to prevent diverticulosis from progressing to diverticulitis is through diet and lifestyle changes. Future episodes of diverticulitis can be avoided by drinking plenty of water, dietary fiber intake to help stool pass more quickly through the colon, regular exercise, and avoiding smoking.

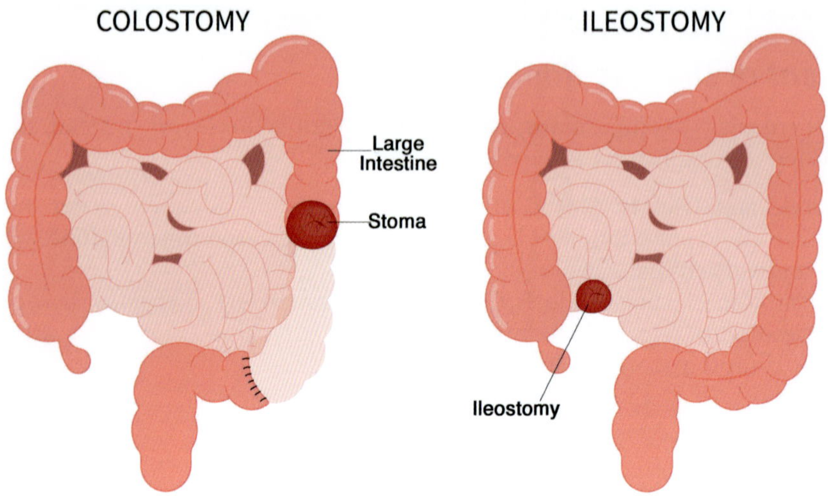

Figure 8-4

Irritable Bowel Syndrome (IBS)

Irritable bowel syndrome (IBS) is a common disorder of the large intestine, characterized by a group of symptoms that include abdominal pain, cramping, bloating, gas, and changes in bowel habits such as diarrhea, constipation, or both. The precise cause of IBS isn't known, but it is believed that it may result from a combination of factors including intestinal muscle contractions, nervous system abnormalities, inflammation in the intestines, changes in gut bacteria, and genetic or psychological factors. There may be a familial predisposition to IBS.

Diagnosis of Irritable Bowel Syndrome

There is no specific test for IBS. Diagnosis is usually made based on symptoms, after ruling out other conditions:

The **Rome Criteria** for IBS include having abdominal pain at least one day per week in the last three months, associated with two or more of the following: pain related to defecation, associated with a change in the frequency of stool, or associated with a change in the form (appearance) of stool.

The Manning Criteria include abdominal pain relieved by defecation, more frequent bowel movements at the onset of pain, looser stools at the onset of pain, visible abdominal bloating, a sensation of incomplete evacuation, and mucus in the stool. The more of these symptoms, the higher the probability of IBS.

The Kruis Criteria consider the presence of abdominal pain, bowel movement frequency (may vary between constipation and diarrhea), consistency of stool (may vary between hard and watery), relief of pain with bowel movements (common), presence of abdominal distention, mucus in stools, and the absence of organic disease. An elevated erythrocyte sedimentation rate (ESR) may suggest an inflammatory or infectious problem rather than IBS, which is a functional disorder without clear biological markers.

Laboratory Tests and Imaging can include blood tests, stool tests, X-rays, CT scan, and colonoscopy, which are often used to rule out other conditions like infections, inflammation, or cancer.

Treatment of Irritable Bowel Syndrome

Treatment of IBS focuses on relieving symptoms and often includes a combination of:

Dietary Changes:

- Identifying and avoiding trigger foods (e.g., dairy, gluten, certain fruits, vegetables, and grains)
- Increasing fiber intake for constipation-predominant IBS, but doing so gradually to avoid gas and bloating
- Following a low FODMAP diet (**F**ermentable **O**ligosaccharides, **D**isaccharides, **M**onosaccharides, **A**nd **P**olyols), which restricts certain carbohydrates that can ferment in the gut

Medications:

- Fiber supplements or laxatives for constipation
- Anti-diarrheal medications for diarrhea
- Anticholinergic medications to relieve painful bowel spasms

- Certain antidepressants can help reduce symptoms.
- Medications like *lubiprostone (Amitiza), linaclotide (Linzess), plecanatide* (*Trulance*), and *tenapanor* (*Ibsrela*) are used for IBS. They can help constipation by increasing fluid secretion in the intestines.

Probiotics can help some people by improving the microbial balance in the gut.

Psychological Counseling can help manage stress and anxiety. Hypnotherapy and mindfulness training can also benefit some people.

Lifestyle Modifications include regular physical exercise, as can stress management (e.g., meditation, deep breathing, yoga).

Prognosis: While IBS can cause discomfort and distress, it does not lead to serious disease, such as cancer. It's a chronic condition, though. Most people with IBS can control their symptoms with diet, stress management, lifestyle modifications, and prescribed medications. Some people, though, may have persistent symptoms that are difficult to treat.

Ischemic Colitis

Ischemic colitis occurs when blood flow to part of the large intestine is reduced, usually due to narrowed or blocked blood vessels, leading to tenderness, inflammation, and injury of the affected tissue. The condition ranges from mild to severe. Severe forms, which are less common, can lead to serious complications and may be life-threatening.

Diagnosis of Ischemic Colitis

Blood Tests can reveal signs of infection or anemia, which might suggest that the colon has been damaged by deficient blood flow.

Stool Tests can rule out infection as a cause of the symptoms.

CT can visualize the colon and check for evidence of ischemic colitis and its severity.

Colonoscopy or **Sigmoidoscopy** allow direct visualization of the inside of the colon and can confirm the diagnosis. Sometimes, a biopsy is taken for closer exam.

Angiography: If other tests are inconclusive and ischemic colitis is still suspected, angiography can be used to view the blood flow in the colon.

Treatment of Ischemic Colitis

Mild Cases:

- **Antibiotics**: To prevent infection
- **IV Fluids**: To prevent dehydration and to rest the bowel
- **Nutrition**: The patient may have to avoid food and drink initially to let the colon rest, followed by a low residue diet.
- **Treatment of Underlying Conditions**: E.g., heart disease or diabetes

Severe Cases:

- **Hospitalization**: For close monitoring and treatment, which may include medications to control pain and other conditions that might be contributing to ischemic colitis

- **Surgery**: If the colon has been damaged significantly or if there is a perforation, dead tissue, or severe infection, like gangrene, surgery may be necessary to remove the affected portion of the colon.

The prognosis for people with ischemic colitis varies. Many people recover completely without surgery, but others may have recurrent episodes. Complications can include chronic colitis, scarring, or stricture of the colon, or, in severe cases, sepsis and death, particularly in cases involving bowel perforation or gangrene. Lifestyle modifications, such as stopping smoking and managing chronic conditions like heart disease and diabetes, are important to reduce the risk of recurrence.

Pseudomembranous Colitis

Pseudomembranous colitis is a form of colon inflammation characterized by the formation of pseudomembranes (layers of inflammatory material, e.g., fibrin, mucus, and inflammatory cells) on the colon lining. It is most associated with the *Clostridioides difficile* bacterium, which typically occurs after the use of antibiotics. This type of colitis can cause significant morbidity if not promptly recognized and treated.

Diagnosis of Pseudomembranous Colitis

Stool Tests can detect toxins produced by *C. difficile* bacteria. PCR tests for the C. *difficile* toxin gene may also be used due to their high sensitivity.

Sigmoidoscopy or **Colonoscopy** can reveal the characteristic pseudomembranes—raised yellow plaques found on the mucosa of the colon—which indicate the disease.

A **CT Scan**, while not diagnostic for *C. difficile*, can show a thickened colon wall, as seen in colitis.

Treatment of Pseudomembranous Colitis

Stop the Implicated Antibiotic, if possible.

Antibiotics: While antibiotics can cause pseudomembranous colitis, appropriate antibiotics are also used to treat it, e.g., *vancomycin* or *fidaxomicin*, which specifically target *C. diff*.

Probiotics: Some evidence suggests that adding probiotics, particularly *Saccharomyces boulardii* and *Lactobacillus* species, may help to restore the normal intestinal flora.

Fluid and Electrolyte Management is helpful for diarrhea and dehydration.

Surgery: In severe cases, particularly those involving complications like **toxic megacolon** (widening and inflammation of the colon) or perforation, surgical intervention may be necessary to remove the affected portion of the colon.

Fecal Transplant: For recurrent *C. diff* infections, fecal transplant is becoming a more common and effective treatment. This involves transplanting stool from a healthy donor into the colon of the affected patient to restore a healthy microbiome.

Constipation

Constipation is a common condition that affects people of all ages. It is characterized by infrequent bowel movements, difficulty passing stools, or the sensation of incomplete evacuation.

Diagnosis of Constipation

The **Rome IV criteria** for constipation (at least two of the symptoms need to be present):

- Fewer than three bowel movements per week
- Hard or lumpy stools
- Straining during bowel movements
- A sense of incomplete evacuation
- The need for manual maneuvers to pass stool
- A feeling of anorectal obstruction/blockage

Diagnostic testing is not usually necessary for most cases of simple constipation. However, if constipation is new, severe, accompanied by blood in the stool, and weight loss, or if it doesn't respond to simple treatments, further diagnostic testing may be warranted to rule out underlying conditions. Tests may include:

Blood Tests: To rule out a systemic condition such as hypothyroidism.

Anorectal Manometry or Transit Studies: To evaluate the muscle function and movement within the intestines.

Colonoscopy: To examine the entire colon and rectum if there is a concern about colorectal cancer, inflammatory bowel disease, or other diseases of the colon.

Treatment of Constipation

Diet and Lifestyle Changes:

- Increase fiber intake through fruits, vegetables, and whole grains.
- Drink plenty of water and other fluids.
- Engage in regular physical exercise.
- Do not unnecessarily delay bowel movements.

Over-the-Counter Remedies:

- **Fiber Supplements**, e.g., *psyllium* husk, *methylcellulose*, or wheat dextrin add bulk to stools.
- **Stool Softeners**, e.g., *docusate sodium*, make stools easier to pass by increasing the amount of water that the stool absorbs in the intestine.
- **Osmotic Agents**, such as *polyethylene glycol* or *lactulose*, draw water into the intestines to soften stools.
- **Stimulant Laxatives**: *Senna* or *bisacodyl [Dulcolax]* can stimulate bowel movements, but should not be used long-term without medical supervision to avoid dependency.
- **Enemas**, whether saline (most common – softens the stool), mineral oil (softens the stool), bisacodyl (stimulates the colonic muscles), phosphate (osmotic, draws fluid into the bowel), or water/soap suds. Enemas are typically recommended for only occasional use, as they can lead to dependence or damage the rectal tissues.

Prescription Medications:

- **Chloride Channel Activators**: *Lubiprostone* (oral) Increases intestinal fluid secretion and motility to help ease the passage of stool.
- **Guanylate Cyclase-C Agonists**: *Linaclotide* and *plecanatide* (both oral) increase fluid secretion and transit in the intestines, thereby softening stools and promoting bowel movements. They also help to reduce abdominal pain.

- **Opioid Receptor Antagonists** (for opioid-induced constipation): *Naloxegol* (oral), *methylnaltrexone* (oral or subcutaneous), and *alvimopan* (oral) block the effects of opioids on the bowel to counteract opioid-induced constipation.
- **5-HT4 Receptor Agonists**: *Prucalopride* (oral) enhances colonic peristalsis.

Biofeedback Therapy can be beneficial for some individuals, particularly those with anorectal dysfunction, by training the pelvic floor muscles how to relax and contract during defecation.

Manual Techniques: Manual removal of stool (**disimpaction**) may be necessary in a healthcare setting.

Diarrhea

Diarrhea is characterized by loose, watery stools that occur more frequently than usual, commonly from increased intestinal motility or decreased absorption of fluids. It can be acute or chronic, with potential causes ranging from infections and inflammation to dietary and medication intolerances, tumor secretions (e.g., serotonin, vasoactive intestinal peptide, gastrin, histamine, calcitonin, prostaglandins, cytokines, substance P), and other intestinal conditions that either decrease fluid absorption (e.g., osmotic-acting laxatives; short bowel syndrome) or increase intestinal motility (e.g., hyperthyroidism). Infections include those due to *E. Coli, Salmonella, Shigella, Campylobacter jejuni, Giardia,* and *Vibrio cholera,* and many other bacteria, viruses, and parasites. Cholera toxins in particular produce a severe, potentially life-threatening, diarrhea from dehydration by causing excess secretion of electrolytes and water into the intestinal lumen.

Diagnosis of Diarrhea

Medical History includes the patient's symptoms, dietary habits, recent travel, medication use, and exposure to illness.

Stool Tests can detect bacteria, parasites, or viruses, and can also assess for the presence of blood or fat.

Blood Tests can check for signs of inflammation or infection and evaluate for conditions like anemia or electrolyte imbalances.

Colonoscopy or **Sigmoidoscopy**: If chronic diarrhea is present, these procedures may be recommended to examine the large intestine.

Imaging: X-ray or CT scan may be used if a structural problem is suspected.

Food Intolerance Tests: If lactose intolerance or celiac disease is suspected, specific tests may be conducted for those conditions.

Treatment of Diarrhea

Rehydration: Oral rehydration solutions are used to replace lost fluids and electrolytes. Severe dehydration may require intravenous fluids.

Dietary Changes: Eat small, frequent meals, avoid high-fiber foods, fatty foods, milk, and caffeine until symptoms improve. Consume **b**ananas, **r**ice, **a**pplesauce, and **t**oast (BRAT diet) to help make stools firmer. Avoid dehydration.

Over-the-Counter Medications:

Antidiarrheal Medications: *Loperamide* (*Imodium*) can reduce the frequency of diarrhea, but it should not be used in cases of bacterial infection or if there is blood in the stool, since slowing the bowel can mask the symptoms and delay the elimination of the pathogen or seeking medical attention.

Bismuth Subsalicylate (e.g., *Pepto-Bismol*) has mild antimicrobial and anti-inflammatory effects; it can bind to bacteria toxins and reduce the secretion of fluids into the intestines in addition to providing a protective coating on the stomach and intestines.

Probiotics may restore a healthy balance of bacteria in the intestines

Prevention of Diarrhea:

Wash hands thoroughly with soap and water, especially after using the bathroom and before eating.

Ensure that food and water are safe by avoiding undercooked meats, raw seafood, and untreated water. When traveling, drink bottled water and avoid ice, raw fruits, and vegetables.

Get vaccinated against rotavirus and cholera where risks are higher.

Bowel Obstruction

Bowel obstruction is a serious and potentially life-threatening condition where there is a blockage that prevents food or liquid from passing through the small intestine or colon.

Diagnosis of Bowel Obstruction

Symptoms of bowel obstruction include abdominal pain, commonly crampy and intermittent, and vomiting, especially in small bowel obstruction. The vomitus may contain bile or, in late stages, feculent material due to backup. Constipation occurs in complete obstruction. In partial obstruction, there may be diarrhea from the liquid that can bypass the obstruction. Abdominal distention and high-pitched tinkling bowel sounds may be present. In late stages, there may be no bowel sounds, indicating ileus. On palpation, there may be abdominal tenderness, guarding, or rebound tenderness, suggesting possible peritonitis secondary to bowel ischemia or perforation. A rectal examination may show absence of stool. There may be signs of dehydration and electrolyte imbalance. A history of abdominal surgery may be relevant and could have led to obstructing adhesions.

Imaging Tests can confirm the presence and location of an obstruction:

- **X-rays** can show areas of obstruction.
- **CT Scan** provides detailed images and can help identify the cause of the obstruction.
- **Ultrasound** is sometimes used in infants and children.

Blood Tests can show signs of dehydration, electrolyte imbalances, or impaired kidney function from bacterial or metabolic toxins that may result from an obstruction.

Treatment of Bowel Obstruction

Non-surgical Treatments:

- **Nasogastric Tube**: Can decompress the intestine by suctioning out air and fluid

- **IV Fluids**: To prevent dehydration and electrolyte imbalance
- **Antibiotics**: If infection is a contributing factor
- **Enemas** or **Oral Laxatives** may be used when the obstruction is not complete and there are no signs of necrosis (fever, tachycardia, peritoneal signs, altered mental status, hypotension and shock, loss of bowel sounds, GI bleeding, or radiologic evidence of bowel wall thickening, gas within the bowel wall, or portal venous gas).

Surgical Treatments:

- **Emergency Surgery** is required if there is a complete obstruction and signs of necrosis or perforation, or if the patient has severe pain or signs of infection. This may involve removing the obstructed section of the intestine and reconnecting the healthy end.
- **Stent Placement**: If the obstruction is due to cancer, sometimes a stent can be placed endoscopically to open up the bowel.

Total Parenteral Nutrition (TPN) may be needed if the obstruction is not resolvable quickly.

Hirschsprung Disease

Hirschsprung disease is a birth defect in which nerve cells are absent in a segment of the large intestine, impairing intestinal motility (**Fig. 8-5**). It typically presents in newborns with symptoms that may include failure to pass meconium, abdominal swelling, and vomiting of green or brown material (bile or fecal matter). The condition can be life-threatening if not treated, due to the risk of serious infection like enterocolitis. It can be familial, although most cases are sporadic.

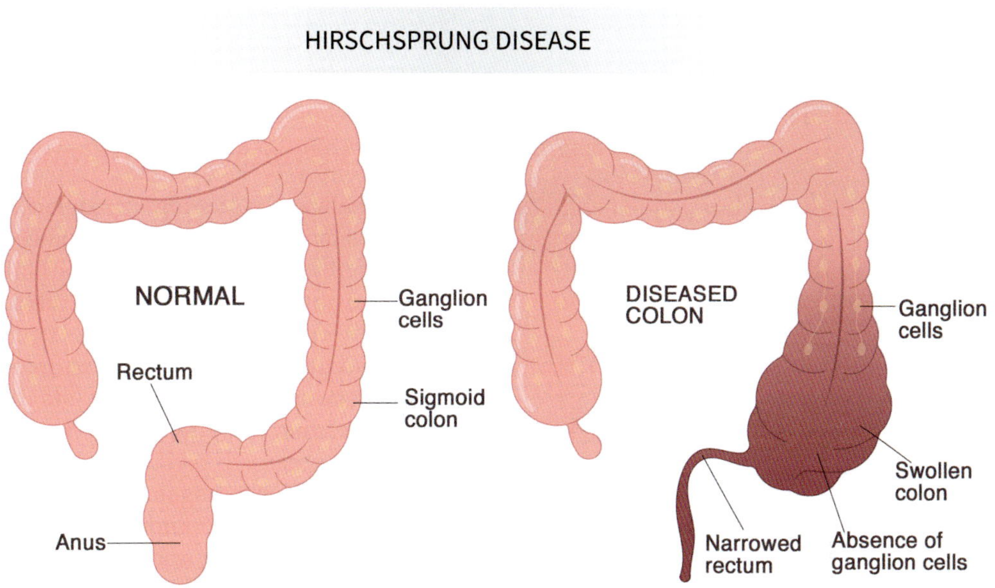

Figure 8-5

Diagnosis of Hirschsprung Disease

Abdominal X-ray can show bowel obstruction and intestinal enlargement.

Anorectal Manometry checks the reflex that normally causes the rectum to relax during a bowel movement. The absence of this reflex suggests Hirschsprung disease.

Rectal Biopsy: A definitive diagnosis is made by biopsy of the wall of the rectum. If nerve cells are absent, this confirms Hirschsprung disease.

Barium Enema provides a clearer image of the large intestine's shape and can highlight any narrowed or blocked areas.

Treatment of Hirschsprung Disease

Surgery: In a **Pull-through procedure**, the diseased segment of the bowel is removed, and the healthy part is pulled down and connected to the anus. In some cases, especially if the child has enterocolitis or significant bowel dilation, an ostomy may be created temporarily to allow the intestine to heal.

Colonic Volvulus

Colonic volvulus is a twisting of the colon that leads to a bowel obstruction. It usually affects the sigmoid colon but can also occur in the cecum. Compromised blood flow to the affected segment of the colon may cause bowel ischemia and gangrene if not treated promptly.

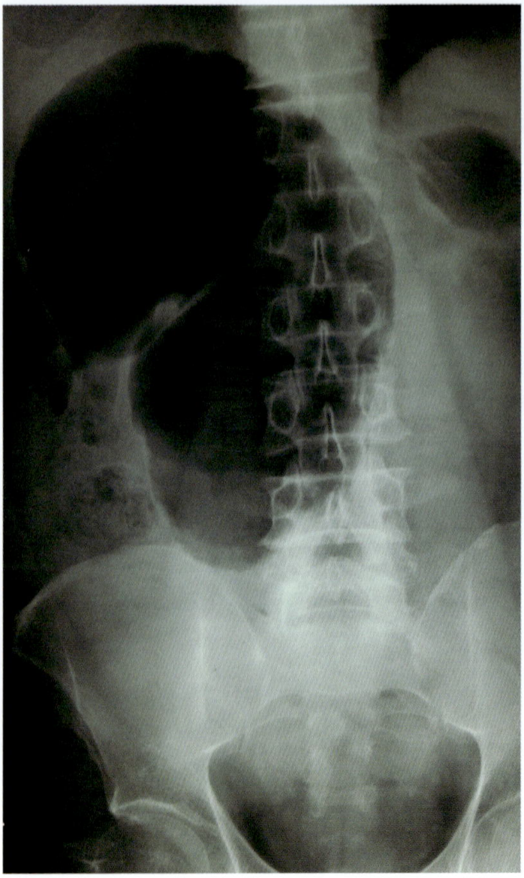

Figure 8-6 Coffee bean sign in sigmoid volvulus.

Diagnosis of Colonic Volvulus

The patient experiences a sudden onset of abdominal pain, distension, and constipation.

Abdominal X-ray may show a characteristic "coffee bean" sign (**Fig. 8-6**) in sigmoid volvulus, indicating the distended loops of bowel.

CT Scan provides detailed images and can confirm the presence of the volvulus, show the extent of bowel distention, and can help identify any complications, such as bowel ischemia or perforation.

Barium Enema has historically been used for diagnosis and can also be therapeutic in reducing a sigmoid volvulus but is less commonly performed now due to the availability of CT scans.

Colonoscopy may be used for both diagnosis and treatment, particularly for sigmoid volvulus.

Treatment of Colonic Volvulus

Non-surgical Treatment:

- **Endoscopic Detorsion**: A sigmoidoscopy or colonoscopy can be used to untwist the volvulus. This is often a temporary solution, and surgery may be needed to prevent recurrence.
- **Rectal Tube Insertion**: After endoscopic reduction, a rectal tube may be placed as a temporary measure to relieve the buildup of pressure and gas in the volvulus and sometimes aid in untwisting the volvulus.

Surgical Treatment: If there is evidence of bowel ischemia or perforation, or if endoscopic reduction is not successful or feasible, emergency surgery is required. The twisted segment of the bowel may be removed and the healthy ends reconnected. In some cases, particularly if the bowel is compromised, an ostomy may be created to allow the bowel to heal.

Colonic Inertia

Colonic inertia is a condition characterized by a slow-moving colon, which can lead to chronic constipation. It's sometimes called "slow-transit constipation." Unlike ordinary constipation, colonic inertia does not respond well to standard laxatives or lifestyle changes.

Diagnosis of Colonic Inertia

Diagnosing colonic inertia usually involves a series of tests to rule out other causes of constipation and to assess the movement of the colon:

- **Colonic Transit Study**: This is often the key diagnostic test, where the patient swallows capsules containing markers visible on X-rays, and subsequent abdominal X-rays are taken over several days to track the progress of the markers through the colon.
- **Anorectal Manometry** evaluates the function of the muscles in the rectum and anus.
- **Defecography** is an imaging test that uses a contrast material to fill the rectum and evaluates with fluoroscopy the efficiency of stool release during a bowel movement. The mechanics of defecation (how the muscles and other structures of pelvis behave during defecation) are analyzed.
- **Colonoscopy** visually inspects the colon and rectum for blockages and to rule out other conditions.
- **Blood Tests** can check for other disorders (e.g., hypothyroidism) that might cause or contribute to the problem.

Treatment of Colonic Inertia

Dietary Changes: High-fiber diets can sometimes help, although patients with colonic inertia may not respond as well as those with ordinary constipation.

Medications:

- **Stool Softeners and Laxatives** are often ineffective for colonic inertia but might be tried initially.
- **Prokinetic Agents**: Medications like *prucalopride,* which stimulates serotonin 5-HT4 receptors in the GI tract to enhance peristalsis, might be helpful to stimulate colonic motility.

Biofeedback: Sensors around the anus show the patient the muscle activity of the pelvic floor. This helps some patients learn how to relax and contract their pelvic floor muscles and coordinate the muscles used to defecate.

Surgery: **Subtotal Colectomy with Ileorectal Anastomosis**, removing the affected portion of the colon, may be considered if there is no response to medical treatment and the condition is severe. However, this is typically a last resort due to potential complications and mixed outcomes.

9

Diseases of the Rectum and Anus

Proctitis

Proctitis is an inflammation of the lining of the rectum. It can cause discomfort, bleeding, and a frequent need to defecate. It can have various causes, including infections, inflammatory bowel diseases (ulcerative colitis or Crohn's disease), radiation therapy, or trauma.

Diagnosis of Proctitis

Anoscopy or **Proctoscopy** can directly visualize the inflamed area.

Sigmoidoscopy or **Colonoscopy** can evaluate the rectum and the lower or entire colon, respectively. These procedures can also involve taking biopsies for further examination.

Lab Tests:

- Stool samples may be tested for bacteria, viruses, parasites, or blood.
- Blood tests may reveal signs of inflammation or anemia.
- Sexually Transmitted Infection (STI) Testing: If the proctitis is believed to be caused by an STI, appropriate tests should be done for gonorrhea, chlamydia, herpes, human papillomavirus (HPV), syphilis, and other STIs.

Imaging: In rare cases, a CT or MRI may be used to assess for complications or to evaluate the extent of disease.

Treatment of Proctitis

Infections: Antibiotics or antiviral medications are prescribed for infection.

Inflammatory Bowel Disease: If proctitis is due to an inflammatory bowel disease, treatment may include aminosalicylates, corticosteroids, immunomodulators, or biologics (made from components of living organisms, often by genetic engineering), all of which have their own mechanisms of reducing inflammation.

Radiation Proctitis: For acute radiation proctitis, treatment is usually supportive, including anti-inflammatory medications, analgesics, and dietary changes. For chronic radiation proctitis, treatments may include formalin application (a chemical cauterization of the affected tissue that can stop bleeding of small blood vessels), endoscopic laser therapy, or hyperbaric oxygen therapy (high oxygen helps tissue healing, stimulates angiogenesis, and reduces inflammation).

Dietary Management: Gradually introduce a high-fiber diet, eliminating foods that can irritate the bowel (e.g., spicy, acidic foods, alcohol and caffeine, fatty and fried foods).

Symptomatic Treatment includes pain relief and anti-inflammatory medications. Topical treatments (suppositories, creams, or enemas) containing anti-inflammatory medications such as steroids or *mesalazine* can be applied directly (suppository or enema) to the inflamed tissue.

STI-Related Proctitis: Treatment is directed towards the specific infection, often with antibiotics or antiviral agents.

Rectal Prolapse

Rectal prolapse is a condition in which the rectum falls from its normal position within the pelvic area and protrudes through the anus (**Fig. 9-1**). It can be uncomfortable and sometimes painful.

Diagnosis of Rectal Prolapse

Clinical History and Physical Examination: Inquire about bowel habits, symptoms, and previous medical or surgical history. The patient may be asked to strain as if having a bowel movement to see if the rectal prolapse occurs.

Proctoscopy or Sigmoidoscopy

Defecography is an imaging test that shows the rectum during a bowel movement following introduction of a contrast material and can demonstrate a prolapse.

Anal Manometry is a test that evaluates the function of the anal sphincter muscles.

Colonoscopy may be performed to rule out other colorectal conditions, particularly in older adults.

Treatment of Rectal Prolapse

Conservative Management: For minor or early-stage prolapses, or for individuals not fit for surgery, treatment may include:

- Dietary changes to manage constipation and straining
- Pelvic floor exercises to strengthen the muscles that support the rectum
- Stool softeners to avoid constipation and straining during bowel movements

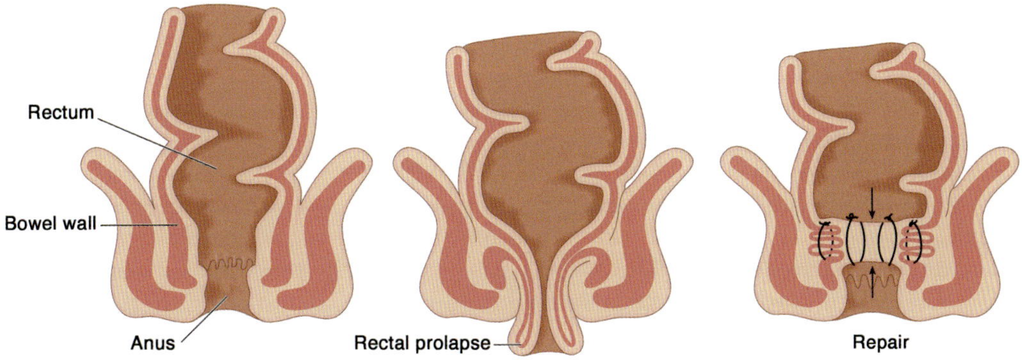

Figure 9-1 *Rectal prolapse.*

Surgical Treatment is the only way to permanently correct rectal prolapse and is usually recommended when symptoms are significant. Surgical approaches include:

- **Abdominal Procedures** such as **rectopexy**, where the rectum is secured back into place, often with the use of mesh, and potentially combined with a resection of part of the colon if constipation is a significant factor.
- **Perineal Procedures:** The *Altemeier procedure* (perineal rectosigmoidectomy) is a resection of the redundant prolapsed rectum and sigmoid colon through the perineum. This is less invasive and may be chosen for patients with a higher surgical risk.

Rectal Ulcers

Rectal ulcers are rare. They can cause rectal bleeding, excessive straining with bowel movements, mucus discharge, and a feeling of incomplete evacuation. They are often associated with rectal prolapse.

Diagnosis of Rectal Ulcers

A thorough medical history to assess symptoms and a physical examination, including a digital rectal exam, are often done first.

Proctoscopy or **Sigmoidoscopy** can directly reveal the ulcer.

Colonoscopy can rule out other conditions, such as inflammatory bowel disease or malignancy, and can inspect the entire colon and rectum. **Biopsy** may be taken during endoscopy to confirm the diagnosis and exclude cancer.

Defecography is a specialized X-ray that examines the mechanics of defecation and can reveal associated rectal prolapse or intussusception.

Anorectal Manometry measures the pressure in the anal canal and rectum. It can detect abnormal function of the anal sphincter and rectal muscles, which can contribute to rectal ulcers through excessive straining.

Treatment of Rectal Ulcers

Conservative Management:

- **Dietary Changes:** A high-fiber diet and increased fluid intake can ease constipation and reduce straining.
- **Stool Softeners**
- **Biofeedback Therapy** teaches patients to gain better control over their pelvic floor muscles.
- **Topical Treatments:** Sucralfate enemas protect the ulcers from irritants present in the feces. Steroid suppositories can be used for their anti-inflammatory effect.

Medications:

- **Aminosalicylates** are given for their anti-inflammatory properties.
- **Sodium Phosphate Enemas** are used to cleanse the lower bowel.

Surgery may be considered for severe cases that don't respond to medical therapy, especially when there's an underlying anatomical problem, such as significant rectal prolapse. Options may include rectopexy to correct prolapse or resection of the affected rectal segment.

Rectal Cancer

Rectal cancer develops from the inner lining of the rectum. Similar to colon cancer, it is often grouped under "colorectal cancer" but has some differences in management.

Diagnosis of Rectal Cancer

The patient may report changes in bowel habits, rectal bleeding, or pain; digital exam may detect an abnormal mass.

Colonoscopy enables exam of the entire colon and rectum, removal of polyps or taking biopsies of suspicious areas.

Imaging:

- **CT** checks for the spread of cancer to other organs.
- **MRI** is particularly useful for evaluating the local extent of rectal cancer and its relationship to surrounding structures.
- **Endorectal Ultrasound** can help assess how deep the cancer has penetrated the rectal wall and if it has spread to nearby lymph nodes.

Blood Tests include CBC and liver enzymes. Carcinoembryonic antigen (CEA) levels, although not diagnostic, can be a marker of the cancer's presence and used to monitor treatment.

Treatment of Rectal Cancer

Surgery:

- **Local Excision** may be done for small, early-stage cancers; the cancer may be removed through the anus without cutting the abdominal wall.

- **Low Anterior Resection (LAR)** involves removal of the rectal cancer and nearby tissue without needing a permanent colostomy.
- **Abdominoperineal Resection (APR)** involves removal of the rectum and anus, with the creation of a permanent colostomy for stool to pass.

Chemotherapy or **Radiation Therapy** may be given before surgery (*neoadjuvant therapy*) to shrink the tumor or after surgery (*adjuvant therapy*) to kill any remaining cancer cells.

Targeted Therapy or **Immunotherapy** may be appropriate for some advanced rectal cancers, especially those that have spread to other parts of the body.

Anal Fistula

An anal fistula is an abnormal connection between the inside of the anus and the skin near the anus. It often results from an infection that starts in an anal gland, leading to an abscess that then drains through the skin. Anal fistulas can cause discomfort, pain, and discharge.

Diagnosis of Anal Fistula

Clinical Examination: The anal area may show an abnormal external opening, swelling, and discharge. The fistula might be felt internally during a digital rectal examination.

Anoscopy can identify any internal openings.

Imaging:

- **Fistulography:** A contrast dye is injected into the fistula tract, and X-rays are taken to delineate the path of the fistula.
- **Ultrasound:** An endoanal or perianal ultrasound can be used to visualize the fistula tract.
- **MRI** provides a detailed view of the fistula tract and is particularly useful in complex or recurrent cases.

Other Diagnostic Procedures:

- **Fistula Probe:** A thin instrument may be used to explore the fistula tract during examination under anesthesia.
- **Colonoscopy** may be done if there is concern about inflammatory bowel disease or other underlying conditions.

Treatment of Anal Fistula

Surgical Repair is the primary treatment for anal fistulas:

Fistulotomy is the most common procedure, where the fistula tract is cut open and flattened out. It's most suitable for simple fistulas with a straightforward tract.

Seton Technique: If the fistula passes through the anal sphincter, a fistulotomy carries a high risk of causing incontinence. In the Seton technique, a surgical thread called a seton is placed in the fistula to help it drain and heal over time, avoiding the need to cut the sphincter muscles.

Advancement Flap Procedures: A piece of tissue (e.g., rectal or anal mucosa) is moved over the internal fistula opening and sewn in place. This is often used for complex fistulas to protect the anal sphincter muscles.

Biologic Tissue Plugs: Bioprosthetic plugs can be used to block the internal opening of the fistula tract and encourage healing.

Fibrin Glue or **Collagen Paste** can be injected into the fistula tract to seal it and promote healing.

Ligation of the Intersphincteric Fistula Tract (LIFT) involves cutting the fistula tract at the intersphincteric space to separate it from the sphincter muscles.

Video-Assisted Anal Fistula Treatment (VAAFT) is a minimally invasive procedure that uses a small camera to help the surgeon see inside the fistula tract and seal it.

Anal Abscess

An anal abscess is a painful condition where a collection of pus develops near the anus. Most anal abscesses are a result of infection from small anal glands.

Diagnosis of Anal Abscess

Symptoms typically include pain around the anus, swelling, redness, fever, and sometimes pus drainage.

Imaging Studies:

- **Ultrasound** can be useful for identifying an abscess, particularly deeper infections that are not palpable on physical examination.
- **CT Scan** can help define the extent of the abscess, especially in the case of complex or recurrent abscesses.
- **MRI** may be indicated in patients with recurrent disease or in whom fistula disease is suspected.

Lab Tests: CBC can indicate infection.

Treatment of Anal Abscess

Surgical Drainage: The primary treatment for an anal abscess is surgical drainage, which can often be performed under local anesthesia. The area is incised to release the pus, and the cavity is cleaned out. A simple abscess may be left open to allow for continuous drainage as it heals.

Antibiotics are not typically required (antibiotics do not penetrate pus well) unless the patient is immunocompromised, or has diabetes, heart valve disease, or other specific conditions, such as cellulitis, sepsis, or an associated fistula.

Pain Management: Pain relievers and warm sitz baths can help ease discomfort after the procedure.

Postoperative Care: Follow-up care is important to ensure proper healing and to check for the development of a fistula. Patients are usually advised to keep the area clean and to perform regular sitz baths to aid in healing and comfort. Since a significant proportion of abscesses can lead to fistulas, follow-up may include an examination or imaging to rule this out.

Lifestyle Adjustments: Dietary changes to avoid constipation may be recommended, as straining during bowel movements can affect healing.

The prognosis for an uncomplicated anal abscess is generally good if treated promptly. However, if left untreated, the infection can progress to a fistula or gangrene.

Hemorrhoids

Hemorrhoids, also known as piles, are swollen veins in the lower part of the anus and rectum. They can cause pain, bleeding, and itching. There are two types of hemorrhoids: internal, located inside the rectum, and external, under the skin around the anus (**Fig. 9-2**).

Diagnosis of Hemorrhoids

Physical Examination: The anal area is examined for external hemorrhoids and felt inside for internal hemorrhoids.

Anoscopy, Sigmoidoscopy, or Colonoscopy can view internal hemorrhoids, and may also be used to rule out other causes of bleeding, such as polyps or colorectal cancer.

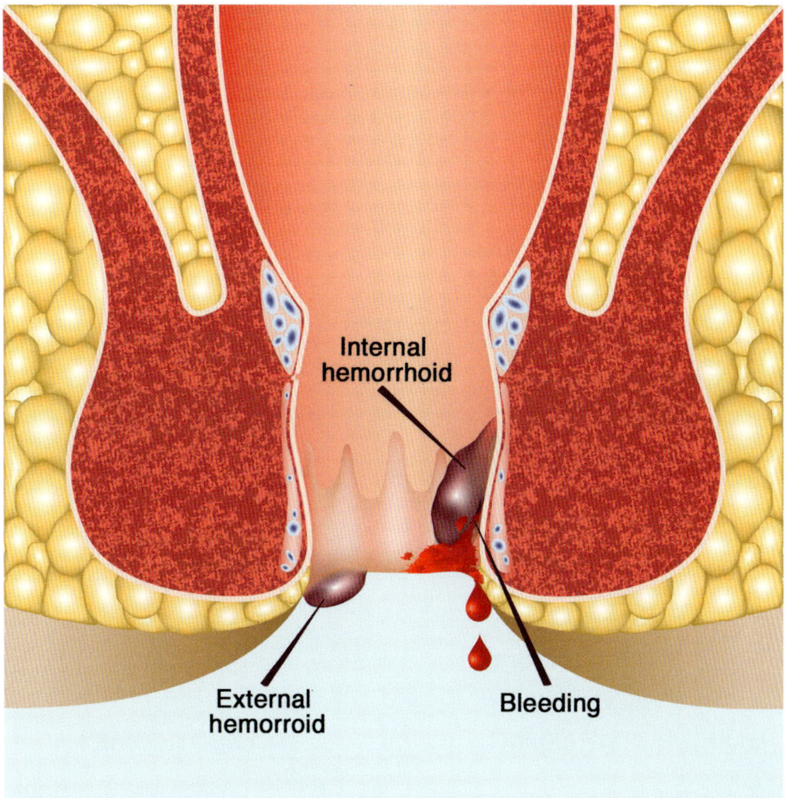

Figure 9-2 *Internal and external hemorrhoids.*

Treatment of Hemorrhoids (Fig. 9-3)

At-Home Treatments of Hemorrhoids:

- **High-Fiber Diet**
- **Topical Treatments**: Over-the-counter creams, ointments, suppositories, or medicated pads designed to treat hemorrhoids can offer relief.
- **Sitz Baths**: Sitting in warm water for 10 to 15 minutes several times a day, especially after bowel movements, can relieve discomfort.
- **Hydration**: Drinking plenty of fluids helps prevent constipation and reduces straining.
- **Pain Relievers**: E.g., acetaminophen, ibuprofen, or aspirin can help relieve discomfort.

Non-Surgical Procedures (For persistent bleeding or painful hemorrhoids):

- **Rubber Band Ligation**: A small band is placed around the base of the hemorrhoid to cut off its blood supply, causing it to wither.

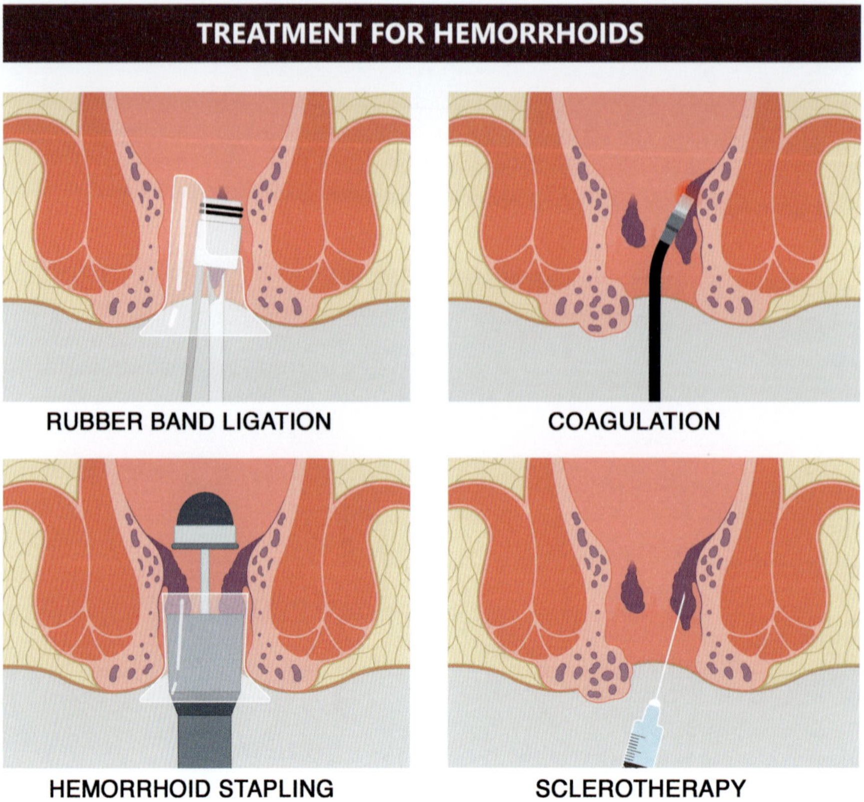

Figure 9-3

- **Sclerotherapy**: A chemical solution is injected around the blood vessel to shrink the hemorrhoid.
- **Infrared** or **Electrocoagulation** uses infrared light or heat to harden and shrivel the hemorrhoid.

Surgical Procedures (or large hemorrhoids or those that do not respond to other treatments):

- **Hemorrhoidectomy**: The excess tissue causing the bleeding is surgically removed under anesthesia. This procedure is effective but can be associated with significant postoperative pain and recovery time.
- **Hemorrhoid Stapling**: This procedure, known as **stapled hemorrhoidopexy**, blocks blood flow to hemorrhoidal tissue. It is typically used only for internal hemorrhoids.

Anal Fissure

An anal fissure is a small tear in the lining of the anus, often causing pain, bleeding, and sometimes spasms of the anal sphincter. Its origin may relate to straining during defecation.

Diagnosis of Anal Fissure

A visual inspection of the anal region usually confirms the presence of a fissure. A digital rectal exam is often avoided if acute fissures are present, as it can cause severe pain.

Anoscopy: If an examination is necessary and tolerable, an anoscope can inspect the anal canal more closely. However, this may not be performed if there is acute pain.

Treatment of Anal Fissure

Conservative Management:

- **High-fiber Diet**: Increasing fiber intake with foods or supplements can soften stool and make passing it easier.
- **Hydration**: Drinking plenty of fluids helps prevent constipation.
- **Sitz Baths**: Sitting in warm water for 10–20 minutes several times a day, especially after bowel movements, can help relax the sphincter and promote healing.

Medications:

- **Topical Anesthetics** can temporarily relieve pain.
- **Topical Nitroglycerin** helps the anal sphincter relax and increases blood flow to promote healing.
- **Topical Calcium Channel Blockers** such as *diltiazem* cream, can also be used to relax the sphincter muscle.
- **Topical Corticosteroids** are not typically recommended for long-term use but may reduce inflammation associated with anal fissures.
- **Botulinum Toxin (Botox)** injection into the anal sphincter can relax the muscles and promote healing.

Surgery: If the fissure does not heal with other treatments, the surgeon may perform a **Lateral Internal Sphincterotomy**, which cuts a small portion of the anal sphincter muscle. This reduces spasms and pain and allows the fissure to heal.

Prevention of Anal Fissure:

Preventive measures focus on maintaining soft stools and regular bowel movements:

- Eat a high-fiber diet.
- Drink plenty of fluids.
- Exercise regularly.
- Respond promptly to the urge to have a bowel movement.
- Use stool softeners if recommended by the physician.

Cryptitis and Papillitis

Cryptitis and papillitis are conditions that affect the anus and rectum, typically presenting as inflammation in these areas. *Cryptitis* involves inflammation of the *anal crypts*, which are small glands located just inside the anus. *Papillitis* is the inflammation of the *anal papillae,* small protrusions that can be found near the anal crypts. Both conditions can be associated with anal discomfort, pain, and sometimes bleeding, and are often seen in conjunction with other anorectal issues like hemorrhoids or fissures.

Diagnosis of Cryptitis and Papillitis

Physical Exam includes inspection of the anal region and a digital rectal examination to feel for tenderness or irregularities.

Anoscopy visualizes the inside of the anal canal and can identify inflammation or other abnormalities.

Proctosigmoidoscopy or **Colonoscopy** may be done if there is concern about more extensive inflammatory bowel disease or other colorectal conditions.

Biopsy is rarely taken; it is used to rule out other conditions if the diagnosis is uncertain.

Treatment of Cryptitis and Papillitis

Conservative Management:

- Warm sitz baths to soothe the area and reduce discomfort
- Dietary modifications, such as increasing fiber intake, to ensure soft stools and reduce straining during bowel movements
- Good anal hygiene, ensuring the area is clean and dry

Medications:

- Topical anesthetics to alleviate pain
- Topical hydrocortisone cream or suppositories can reduce inflammation.

Treatment of Underlying Conditions:

- Address constipation with stool softeners or mild laxatives.
- Treat any associated conditions such as hemorrhoids or fissures.

Surgery may be considered in cases where there is recurrent or persistent inflammation that does not respond to conservative treatment. This might involve excision of the inflamed crypts or papillae.

Pain Management: Over-the-counter pain relievers like ibuprofen or acetaminophen can be recommended for pain control.

Antibiotics may be prescribed If there is evidence of bacterial infection contributing to the inflammation.

Pilonidal Disease

Pilonidal disease is a chronic skin infection in the crease of the buttocks near the coccyx (**Fig. 9-4**). It often begins as a small skin infection but can develop into a chronic problem with the formation of a **pilonidal cyst** that is prone to infection and can become an abscess.

Diagnosis of Pilonidal Disease

Common symptoms include pain at the bottom of the spine, swelling, redness, drainage of pus or blood, and tenderness over the lower sacral or coccygeal area. Physical examination of the area near the coccyx shows a pilonidal cyst, sinus tracts, or active infection, which may be an abscess.

Imaging Studies are typically not required for initial diagnosis but may be necessary in complex or recurrent cases to determine the extent of the disease. Ultrasound, MRI, or CT scans can provide detailed images.

Treatment of Pilonidal Disease

Incision and Drainage: If an abscess is present, it may need to be lanced and drained. This is often done under local anesthesia in an outpatient setting.

Antibiotics are usually prescribed if there is evidence of infection beyond the local abscess area or if the patient is immunocompromised.

Aftercare: Post-drainage care involves keeping the area clean and dry.

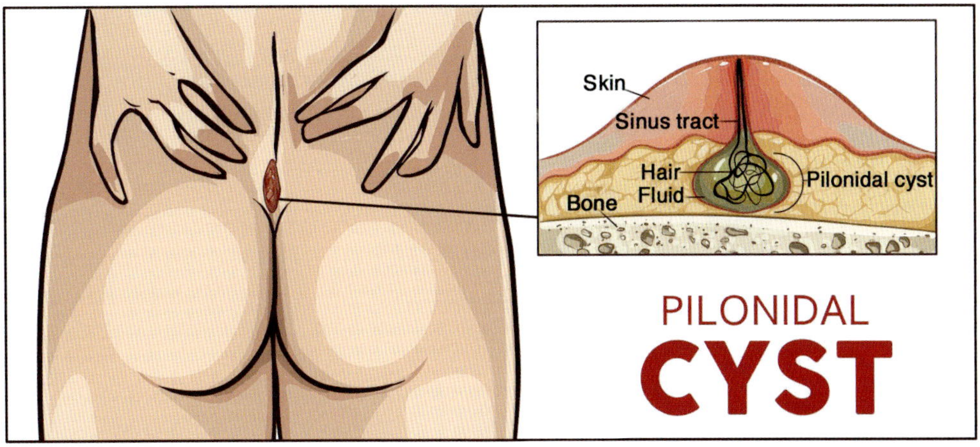

Figure 9-4

Surgical Removal: For recurrent or chronic pilonidal disease, surgery to remove the cyst and sinus tracts may be recommended. Techniques vary, and options include open healing or closure with or without a flap of skin moved to cover the area.

Laser Epilation: Laser hair removal around the area may help prevent recurrence, as pilonidal disease is often associated with ingrown hairs.

Lifestyle Modifications: Keeping the area clean, losing weight if overweight, avoiding prolonged sitting, and removing hair around the area (shaving, laser) can help prevent recurrences.

Wound Care: When the wound is left open to heal, wound care will include regular cleaning, packing the wound, and follow-up to ensure proper healing.

Pain Management: Pain relievers may be needed, especially after surgical procedures.

Fecal Incontinence

Fecal incontinence is the inability to control bowel movements, causing stool to leak unexpectedly from the rectum. It can have various causes, including muscle or nerve damage, and can significantly impact the quality of life.

Diagnosis of Fecal Incontinence

A detailed account of the symptoms, bowel habits, diet, medication use, and past medical or surgical history may be important for diagnosis. Physical exam includes an examination of the anal area for signs of disease, muscle weakness, or structural defects. A digital rectal exam (DRE) assesses muscle tone and sensation.

Anorectal Manometry measures the strength of the anal sphincter muscles, the sensitivity of the rectum, and the neural reflexes that are needed for normal bowel movements. **Endoanal Ultrasound** uses sound waves to create an image of the anal sphincters and can detect damage or defects.

The **Pudendal Nerve Terminal Motor Latency (PNTML) Test** assesses the function of the nerves supplying the anal sphincter. A relatively long delay between the time of electrode stimulation of the pudendal nerve and the muscle response may indicate a problem with nerve function.

Defecography evaluates the shape, position, and function of the rectum and anal sphincter.

MRI can provide detailed images of the muscles and other structures within the pelvis.

Colonoscopy may be performed to rule out other conditions, such as inflammatory bowel disease or tumors.

Treatment of Fecal Incontinence

Dietary Management includes increasing fiber intake to help form stools.

Medications: Anti-diarrheal drugs such as *loperamide* and *diphenoxylate* can help control diarrhea and reduce incontinence. Use stool softeners if constipation contributes to incontinence.

Bowel Training: Scheduled toileting at regular intervals can help some people regain control.

Pelvic Floor Exercises: Kegel exercises strengthen the rectal muscles and can improve anal sphincter control.

Biofeedback can improve bowel control by using special sensors to monitor muscles and provide feedback to the patient to coordinate the proper contraction and relaxation of muscles involved in defecation.

Surgery may be recommended for those who don't respond to conservative treatments and have significant sphincter dysfunction. Surgical options may include sphincter repair, sphincter replacement with an artificial sphincter (a doughnut-shaped inflatable cuff implanted around the anal canal), or colostomy in severe cases.

Nerve Stimulation: Sacral nerve stimulation (SNS) involves using electrical impulses to stimulate the nerves that control the rectum and anus. This can improve the strength and function of the muscles in the bowel and pelvic floor.

Injectable Bulking Agents: Materials are injected into the tissue around the anus to narrow the anal canal and reduce incontinence.

Supportive Devices: Anal plugs or barriers can be used to prevent leakage.

Management of Underlying Conditions: Treat conditions that may contribute to fecal incontinence, such as diabetes (which can affect nerve function and gastrointestinal motility) or neurological diseases.

Anal Itching (Pruritus Ani)

Diagnosis of Pruritus Ani

Causes of anal itching may include dietary factors, hygiene habits, topical agents, and systemic diseases.

An inspection of the anal region is performed to check for signs of infection, worms (pinworms often come out at night), skin conditions (eczema, psoriasis, dermatitis), or anatomical abnormalities that might cause or contribute to the itching.

A digital rectal exam and anoscopy may be performed to rule out internal hemorrhoids, fissures, or other rectal pathologies.

If contact dermatitis is suspected, patch testing may be used to identify allergens.

Stool cultures and examination for pinworm eggs or worms are used to rule out infections.

Blood glucose tests are done for diabetes mellitus, which can be associated with pruritus.

Biopsy can be done rarely, if there is an unusual lesion or if skin cancer is suspected.

Treatment of Pruritus Ani

General Measures: Keep the anal area clean and dry. Avoid the use of soap on the anal area, which can remove protective oils. Instead, clean with water alone and then dry thoroughly. Avoid scratching, as this can exacerbate the condition.

Dietary Modifications: Limit or avoid potential irritants like caffeine, citrus fruits, spicy foods, and dairy products.

Topical Treatments: Zinc oxide ointment can protect the skin and reduce irritation. Hydrocortisone cream may be used for a short time to reduce inflammation, but prolonged use can thin the skin and worsen symptoms. Antifungal or antibacterial medications may be prescribed if an infection is present. Antihistamines can reduce severe itching.

Treat Underlying Causes, e.g., hemorrhoids, fungal infections, or STIs if they are diagnosed.

Management of Systemic Diseases: Control diabetes or other systemic conditions that may contribute to pruritus ani.

Surgical Intervention may be suggested, e.g., for hemorrhoids, fissures, or skin tags.

Anal Cancer

Anal cancer, which occurs in the anal canal, is relatively rare. It differs from colorectal cancer. Most anal cancers are squamous cell carcinomas, although some can be adenocarcinomas, small cell carcinomas, or melanomas. Colorectal cancers are mainly adenocarcinomas. Anal cancers can be associated with human papillomavirus (HPV) infection and are more commonly seen in patients with some degree of immunosuppression, as in HIV, or in chronic anal inflammation.

Diagnosis of Anal Cancer

The patient may report rectal bleeding, anal itching, a lump at the anal opening, pain or fullness in the anal region, abnormal discharge from the anus, diarrhea, or constipation. Inquire about risk factors (e.g., HPV infection, multiple sex partners, anal intercourse, HIV, smoking, chronic anal irritation, or a history of cervical, vaginal, or vulvar cancer). A digital rectal exam may be performed. There may be swollen lymph nodes in the anal or groin area.

Anoscopy can detect abnormal growths.

Biopsy is the definitive diagnostic test.

Imaging:

- **Anal Ultrasound** can help determine how deep the tumor has grown into the tissues around the anus.
- **CT Scan** provides detailed cross-sectional images of the body and can show if cancer has spread.
- **MRI** offers detailed images and is useful for looking at soft tissues.
- **Positron Emission Tomography (PET) Scans** can detect areas of increased metabolic activity, such as cancer cells, and can reveal distant metastases.

Treatment of Anal Cancer

Chemoradiation: The primary treatment for most anal cancers is a combination of chemotherapy and radiation therapy (chemoradiation), which often can cure the cancer without surgery.

Surgery: Local resection may suffice for very small, early-stage anal cancers. **Abdominoperineal Resection (APR)** is used for larger cancers or cancers that have not responded to chemoradiation. Surgery to remove the anal canal and surrounding tissue may be necessary, resulting in a permanent colostomy.

Chemotherapy: Drugs may be used to help shrink the tumor before surgery or to treat cancer that has spread.

Targeted Therapy: For some advanced anal cancers, targeted drugs might be used when standard chemotherapy is no longer effective.

Immunotherapy uses the body's immune system to fight cancer. It may be an option for advanced anal cancer that has not responded to other treatments that have a proven track record.

HPV Vaccination: While not a treatment for existing cancer, vaccination against HPV can prevent anal infections with HPV and may reduce the risk of anal cancer.

Sexually Transmitted Infections

Sexually transmitted infections (STIs) affecting the anal and rectal areas can include a variety of pathogens, including herpes simplex virus (HSV), human papillomavirus (HPV), gonorrhea, chlamydia, syphilis, and human immunodeficiency virus (HIV).

Diagnosis of STIs of the Anal Area

A history of sexual practices is taken to assess risk factors for STIs. Inspection of the anal area is done for lesions, discharge, or other signs of infection. Digital rectal exam (DRE) may be performed with caution, especially if there is pain or lesions suggestive of herpes. Diagnosis of **genital warts (condyloma acuminatum)** is usually made by visual inspection of the warts. Condyloma acuminatum is a sexually transmitted infection caused by certain types of human papillomavirus (HPV). These warts are typically flesh-colored, can be smooth or rough, and may appear as small bumps or larger, cauliflower-like growths in the genital or anal area.

Lab Tests:

- **Swabs:** Rectal swabs can be taken for gonorrhea and chlamydia NAAT (Nucleic Acid Amplification Test).
- **Blood Tests:** Syphilis can be diagnosed with specific blood tests like RPR or VDRL, confirmed with FTA-ABS or TPPA. Blood tests can also be used to diagnose HIV and HSV.
- **HPV Testing:** Human papillomavirus (HPV) is often diagnosed based on clinical presentation, such as the presence of warts or through high-resolution anoscopy to examine the anal tissue more closely for dysplasia in individuals at higher risk (men who have sex with men, HIV-positive individuals, and those with a compromised immune system). Anal HPV testing, while not routine, can be done on cells collected from the anal canal in higher-risk individuals.

Visual Diagnosis: For genital warts caused by the human papilloma virus, a visual diagnosis is often sufficient. Herpes lesions are typically diagnosed based on their appearance but can be confirmed with a swab for PCR or culture.

Anoscopy: In some cases, especially if symptoms like rectal discharge or bleeding are present, anoscopy can visualize lesions inside the rectum.

For genital warts, acetic acid application to the skin can sometimes cause genital warts to whiten, which can make them more visible, but this method is not specific and may lead to false positives. If there is doubt about the diagnosis or if the warts do not respond to standard treatments, a biopsy may be performed to examine the tissue for signs of HPV. **HPV Typing,** although not commonly done on warts, can be used to confirm the diagnosis and determine if the specific type of HPV is one that is associated with the development of cancer.

Treatment of STIs of the Anal Area

Antibiotics: Bacterial infections like gonorrhea, chlamydia, and syphilis are treated with specific systemic antibiotics according to current guidelines.

Antivirals: Herpes infections are treated with antiviral medications such as *acyclovir, valacyclovir*, or *famciclovir*. HIV is treated with antiretroviral therapy (ART), a combination of medicines to treat HIV. The HPV vaccine protects against various strains of human papillomavirus.

Topical Treatments: Genital warts may be treated with topical agents like *imiquimod, podofilox*, or *trichloroacetic acid (TCA)*.

Cryotherapy or **Surgical Removal:** Larger warts may require physical removal methods such as cryotherapy, electrosurgery, or excision.

Vaccination: While not a treatment for existing warts, the HPV vaccine can prevent future infections with certain types of HPV, including some that cause genital warts.

It's important to note that while treatment can remove genital warts, none of these therapies can completely eradicate the virus. HPV may remain in the body in a latent state, and warts may recur, particularly in the first three months after treatment. Regular follow-up is often necessary to monitor for recurrence of warts.

Patients with genital warts and other STIs should be screened for other STIs; sexual partners should be informed and may also need examination and treatment. Most common STIs (e.g., chlamydia, gonorrhea, HPV, HSV, HIV, syphilis, hepatitis B and C) can be transmitted even when the infected person is asymptomatic.

10

Diseases of the Liver

The liver has many functions, including detoxification; storage of glycogen, iron, copper, and vitamins A, D, and B12; synthesis of important proteins, cholesterol, triglycerides, and the bile necessary for digestion. It can be affected by a wide range of diseases, including those that affect GI functioning.

The liver has two vascular inputs – the **hepatic portal vein**, which brings absorbed nutrients from the gastrointestinal tract to the liver, and the **hepatic artery**, which brings oxygen. Blood leaves the liver via the **hepatic veins**, which connect with the **inferior vena cava** (**Fig. 10-1**).

Bile produced by the liver leaves the liver by the right and left hepatic ducts, which connect with the common bile duct (**Fig. 10-1**).

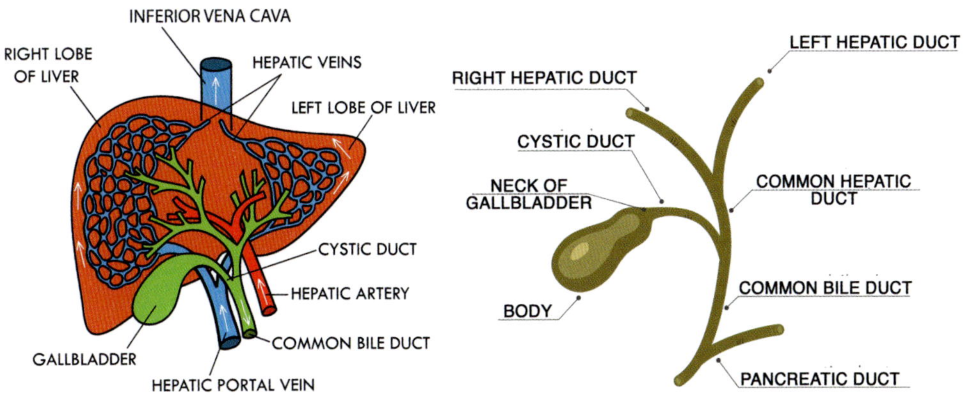

Figure 10-1 *Liver and bile duct anatomy.*

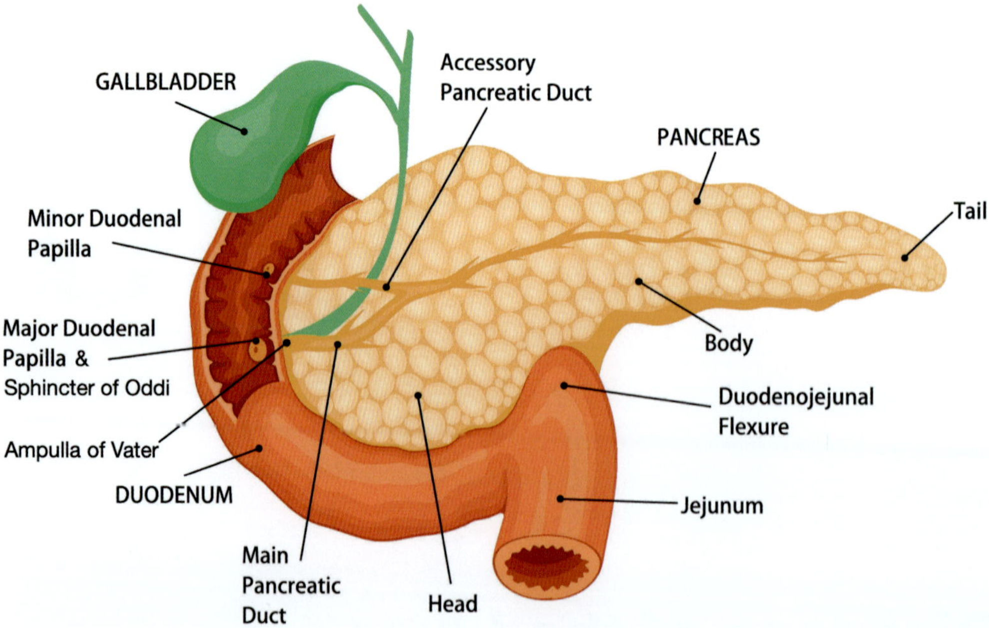

Figure 10-2 *Pancreatic ducts.*

The **main pancreatic duct** converges with the **common bile duct** to form the **ampulla of Vater**, a small bulb-like structure that protrudes slightly into the second (descending) part of the duodenum and empties there via the major duodenal papilla. About 10% of individuals have an **accessory pancreatic duct**, which empties through a **minor duodenal papilla**, an alternate pathway for digestive juices to flow from the pancreas to the duodenum (**Fig. 10-2**).

Hepatitis

Hepatitis is an inflammation of the liver, often caused by viral infections, but also by other things such as excess alcohol use, toxins, medications, and certain medical conditions, such as hemochromatosis, Wilson's disease, and alpha-antitrypsin deficiency.

In a nutshell:

- There are different types of viral hepatitis, including hepatitis A, B, C, D, and E, each caused by a different virus.
- The ends, A and E, of the letter sequence "ABCDE," correspond to hepatitis A and E being spread by the oral/fecal route, the ends of the GI tract. The others, BCD, are spread by blood-to-blood contact (e.g., needles) or exchange of bodily fluids (e.g., unprotected sexual contact).
- While A, B, C, D, and E can all cause acute hepatitis. B, C, and D can also cause chronic hepatitis and are risk factors for the development of cirrhosis and hepatocellular carcinoma. (Hepatitis D can only infect people who are also infected with hepatitis B.)

- Hepatitis C is the leading cause of chronic hepatitis in the U.S. and the leading cause of liver transplantation. Fortunately, hepatitis C can be cured with newer antivirals.
- Hepatitis B can be treated with interferons, nucleoside analogs (e.g., lamivudine, adefovir, entecavir, telbivudine, tenofovir), but there is still a possibility of relapse.
- There are vaccines effective for preventing hepatitis A and B.
- In general: The presence of viral antigens, viral antibodies, and viral genetic material in the blood quantified by PCR (polymerase chain-reaction) helps determine whether an individual has been exposed to virus, immunized against virus, or whether there is dormant or active infections. The presence of viral antigens or viral genetic material in the blood indicates active infection and potential infectivity. The patient who has viral antigens for hepatitis A or B, or antibodies in hepatitis C is considered potentially infectious. The presence of antibodies only (no viral antigens or viral genetic material) indicates past exposure or immunity and lack of infectivity in hepatitis A or B. In the case of hepatitis C (HCV) the antigen test is not very sensitive; the patient may still be infectious with HCV even if HCV antigen is not detected. The HCV **RNA** test by PCR (polymerase chain reaction) can detect lower levels of the virus than the antigen test. A test positive for anti-HCV antibodies and negative for HCV RNA indicates that the patient has been exposed to HCV but is not infectious. If both are positive, it indicates active infection, even if the antigen test for HCV is negative (see **Figures 10-3A**, **10-3B**, and **10-3C** for more details).

FIGURE 10-3A HEPATITIS A VIRUS TESTING

Test	Result	Interpretation
Anti-HAV IgM	Positive	Acute or recent Hepatitis A infection.
Anti-HAV IgM	Negative	No acute Hepatitis A infection.
Anti-HAV Total (IgG)	Positive	Past infection or immunity due to vaccination.
Anti-HAV Total (IgG)	Negative	No prior exposure or immunity to Hepatitis A.

FIGURE 10-3B HEPATITIS B VIRUS TESTING

Test	Result	Interpretation
HBsAg (Surface Antigen)	Positive	Active infection (acute or chronic).
HBsAg	Negative	No active Hepatitis B infection.
Anti-HBs (Surface Antibody)	Positive	Immunity due to vaccination or recovery from past infection.
Anti-HBs	Negative	No immunity to Hepatitis B.
Anti-HBc (Core Antibody)	Positive	Past or ongoing Hepatitis B infection.
Anti-HBc IgM	Positive	Acute Hepatitis B infection.
HBV DNA (Viral Load)	Detectable	Active viral replication.
HBV DNA (Viral Load)	Undetectable	No active viral replication.

FIGURE 10-3C HEPATITIS C VIRUS TESTING		
Test	**Result**	**Interpretation**
Anti-HCV (Antibody)	Positive	Current or past Hepatitis C infection.
Anti-HCV	Negative	No evidence of Hepatitis C exposure.
HCV RNA (Viral Load)	Detectable	Active Hepatitis C infection (confirmatory test).
HCV RNA (Viral Load)	Undetectable	No active Hepatitis C infection.
HCV Genotype	Genotype 1-6	Determines the strain of HCV for treatment planning.

Diagnosis of Hepatitis

The symptoms of hepatitis may include fatigue, jaundice, abdominal pain, nausea and vomiting, decreased appetite, dark urine (excess bilirubin excreted by the kidneys), pale stools (reduced bilirubin secreted into the intestines), joint pain, fever, and itching. The medical and travel history, vaccination status, lifestyle (including alcohol consumption), and any possible exposures to hepatitis viruses are all relevant to the diagnosis.

Blood Tests:

- **Liver Function Tests** assess levels of liver enzymes (ALT, AST, GGT, alkaline phosphatase), bilirubin, and proteins, which can indicate liver inflammation or damage.

ALT and AST are most prominent in liver hepatocytes, while GGT and alkaline phosphatase are most prominent in the walls of the bile ducts (**Fig. 10-4**). Viral hepatitis, which damages the hepatocytes, initially causes high ALT and AST levels, while GGT, alkaline phosphatase, and bilirubin are only mildly elevated. With worsening of the hepatitis, liver swelling narrows the intrahepatic bile canals; bilirubin backs up and there is damage to the bile duct walls, resulting in rising levels of bilirubin, GGT, and alkaline phosphatase. Serum albumin levels can decrease due to impaired liver function, as the liver normally synthesizes albumin.

In contrast, a stone blocking the *bile ducts* results in high levels of alkaline phosphatase, GGT, and bilirubin, while AST and ALT rise only a small amount. Simplistically, this may relate to the different presence of these molecules in the liver versus the bile ducts. (**Fig. 10-4**). Serum albumin levels may initially remain normal but decrease with prolonged obstruction and liver damage.

- **Hepatitis Virus Serology**: Specific blood tests can identify antigens and antibodies related to different hepatitis viruses, indicating acute or past infections or immunity.
- **PCR Tests** can detect viral RNA or DNA for hepatitis to determine the presence of active viral replication, especially for hepatitis C.

Imaging: Ultrasound, CT scan, or MRI can be used to visualize the liver and assess the extent of liver damage.

Liver Biopsy may be performed in some cases to determine the severity of liver inflammation and fibrosis.

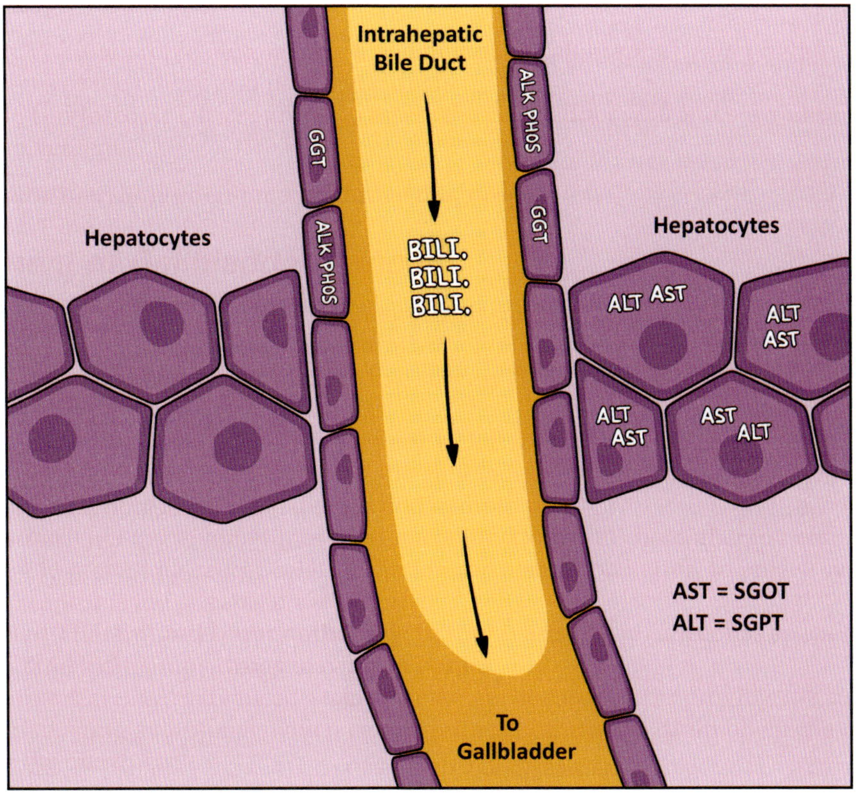

Figure 10-4 *Liver and bile duct enzymes. (From Gladwin, M.T., Trattler, W, and Mahan, C.S. Clinical Microbiology Made Ridiculously Simple, Medmaster)*

Treatment of Hepatitis

Hepatitis A:

Supportive Care: Hepatitis A is usually self-limiting and doesn't require specific antiviral treatment. Support includes adequate hydration, rest, and avoiding alcohol and liver-toxic medications.

Vaccination: Post-exposure prophylaxis with the hepatitis A vaccine or immune globulin may be recommended for close contacts of infected individuals.

Hepatitis B:

Acute Hepatitis B: Most adults clear the infection spontaneously, and treatment is supportive.

Chronic Hepatitis B: Antiviral medications such as *tenofovir* and *entecavir* can be used to reduce viral replication and liver damage.

Regular Monitoring: Chronic hepatitis B requires monitoring for liver function and signs of liver cancer.

Vaccination: A vaccine is available and recommended to prevent hepatitis B.

Hepatitis C:

Hepatitis C is a major reason for liver transplantation. Direct-acting antivirals (DAAs), which target specific steps in the hepatitis C life cycle, have revolutionized the treatment of hepatitis C, offering cure rates of over 90%. These include NS3/4 protease inhibitors, NS5A inhibitors, and NS5B inhibitors. *Pegylated interferon-alpha*, a stable form of interferon, is sometimes used to boost the immune system's antiviral response. Those with chronic hepatitis C, especially those who have developed cirrhosis, need regular surveillance for liver cancer.

Hepatitis D:

Coinfection with Hepatitis B: Treatment may involve medications used for hepatitis B, as hepatitis D requires the hepatitis B virus to replicate.

Hepatitis E is generally self-resolving; treatment is supportive, with rest and hydration. Antivirals like *ribavirin* may be used in chronic cases, primarily in immunocompromised patients.

Other Considerations:

Avoid Alcohol: Alcohol can exacerbate liver inflammation and should be avoided in hepatitis.

Medication Review: Some medications can be hepatotoxic, and their use should be assessed and modified as needed.

Preventative measures include vaccinations for hepatitis A and B, practicing safe hygiene and food handling, safe sex practices, and avoiding the sharing of needles or personal items that could be contaminated with blood.

The prognosis for hepatitis varies widely depending on the type, severity, the individual's overall health, and how early the disease is diagnosed and treated.

Fatty Liver Disease

Fatty liver disease (**hepatic steatosis**) occurs when fat accumulates in the liver. This has the potential to cause serious liver damage through inflammation and fibrosis, including cirrhosis. It can be broadly categorized into two types: **nonalcoholic fatty liver disease (NAFLD)** and **alcoholic liver disease (ALD)**. NAFLD includes a spectrum from simple fatty liver (steatosis) to **Metabolic Associated Steatohepatitis (MASH** – replaces the older term **NASH** for nonalcoholic steatohepatitis), which can progress to cirrhosis and liver failure. ALD is due to excessive alcohol consumption.

Diagnosis of Fatty Liver Disease

History and Physical Exam: inquire about alcohol intake and look for signs on exam suggesting liver involvement, e.g., jaundice or hepatomegaly.

Blood Tests:

- **Liver Function Tests (LFTs)**: Elevated liver enzymes may suggest liver inflammation.
- **Lipid Profile**: To evaluate dyslipidemia
- **Fasting Blood Glucose** and **HbA1c** are done to check for diabetes. Insulin resistance in type 2 diabetes can lead to fat accumulation in the liver.

Other Tests: Additional tests check for thyroid function (hypothyroidism can lead to metabolic disturbances and fatty liver), metabolic syndrome indicators (abdominal obesity, high triglycerides, low HDL, high blood pressure, high fasting blood sugar), and screen for viral hepatitis.

Imaging:

- **Ultrasound** can show fat in the liver. CT and MRI can provide more detail.
- **FibroScan** is a special ultrasound that can estimate the degree of liver fibrosis.

Liver Biopsy is invasive but can assess the severity of inflammation and fibrosis in pronounced cases where the results may significantly impact management.

Treatment of Fatty Liver Disease

Lifestyle Modifications:

- **Weight Loss**
- **Diet**: Low in saturated fats, trans fats, and simple sugars. The Mediterranean diet (rich in fruits, vegetables, whole grains, legumes, lean proteins such as fish and poultry), and healthy fats (like olive oil and nuts) is often recommended.
- **Exercise**: Regular physical activity can improve liver enzymes and reduce liver fat even without weight loss.

Medications and Supplements:

- *Vitamin E,* by reducing inflammation and fibrosis, may improve liver histology in some non-diabetic patients with non-alcoholic fatty liver disease.
- *Pioglitazone* makes the body more responsive to insulin and may help in some patients with non-alcoholic steatohepatitis.
- *Omega-3 Fatty Acids* reduce liver fat.

Manage Comorbidities such as diabetes, dyslipidemia (e.g., statins), and hypertension.

Alcohol abstinence is advised in alcoholic liver disease and moderation in non-alcoholic liver disease.

Avoid or adjust medications that can worsen liver health.

Bariatric (weight loss) Surgery may improve non-alcoholic steatohepatitis and other metabolic conditions in cases of morbid obesity.

Simple fatty liver has a better prognosis than non-alcoholic steatohepatitis, which can progress to cirrhosis and liver cancer.

Cirrhosis

Cirrhosis is a late stage of fibrosis (scarring) of the liver caused by many forms of liver diseases, such as hepatitis and chronic alcoholism (**Fig. 10-5**). A liver with cirrhosis can't function properly, leading to long-term liver failure. Associated portal vein hypertension may be accompanied by GI bleeding, ascites, peritonitis, hepatic encephalopathy, and kidney dysfunction (**hepatorenal syndrome**) due to portal hypertension changes in blood pressure and renal blood flow.

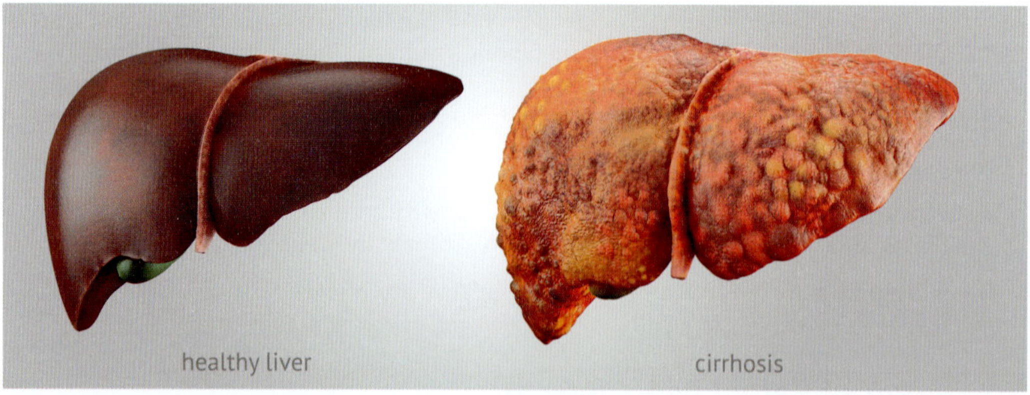

Figure 10-5 Normal and cirrhotic liver.

Diagnosis of Cirrhosis

The diagnosis of cirrhosis involves several steps:

History and Physical: What is the degree of alcohol intake? Is there a personal or family history of liver disease? Are there physical signs such as jaundice, spider angiomas, palmar erythema, ascites (from low serum albumin and portal hypertension), or splenomegaly? There may be signs of easy bruising from deficiency of clotting factor synthesis in the liver. Peritonitis may occur from infected ascites fluid.

Blood Tests:

- **Liver Function Tests** assess the function of the liver (e.g., albumin, which decreases in cirrhosis) and the extent of liver damage (ALT, AST, alkaline phosphatase, GGT, and bilirubin, all of which rise in cirrhosis).
- **Complete Blood Count** may show thrombocytopenia, anemia, or leukopenia. These can arise from sequestration of platelets and red blood cells by an enlarged spleen from portal hypertension along with hepatic and nutritional insufficiency.
- **Clotting Tests**: INR may be elevated due to insufficient liver production of clotting factors.
- **Serologies** include tests for hepatitis B and C.

Imaging:

- **Ultrasound** can detect signs of cirrhosis and portal hypertension, and screen for liver cancer.
- **CT Scan** and **MRI** provide more detail and can be used to evaluate the liver's structure.
- **Transient Elastography (FibroScan)** is a non-invasive test that measures liver stiffness to estimate fibrosis. It is an ultrasound-based test that evaluates liver stiffness by emitting a pulse of energy and calculating the speed of its return, which correlates with the amount of fibrosis in the liver.

Endoscopy may be performed to look for esophageal varices, which can develop as a complication of cirrhosis.

Liver Biopsy confirms the diagnosis by showing the extent of liver damage and fibrosis, though biopsy is not always necessary with all the other evidence.

Treatment of Cirrhosis

Treat Underlying Causes: For hepatitis, antiviral drugs may be used. For alcoholic liver disease, cessation of alcohol intake is critical.

Medications:

- **Beta-blockers** reduce the risk of variceal bleeding by lowering portal blood pressure.
- **Diuretics** can help manage ascites and edema.
- ***Lactulose*** and ***Rifaximin*** can reduce the risk of hepatic encephalopathy by targeting the gut bacteria that produce ammonia.
- **Vitamin K** or **fresh frozen plasma** can be used to replace clotting factors.
- **Vaccination against hepatitis B** and **safe behavior to prevent hepatitis C** (spread through blood contact, needles, sexual contact, and infected mother-to-baby).

Paracentesis of ascites fluid can alleviate the discomfort of abdominal distension.

Transjugular intrahepatic portosystemic shunt (TIPS) is used for severe ascites. It shunts the inflowing portal vein to the outflowing hepatic vein with a stent. This lowers portal venous pressure, lowering the risk of variceal bleeding, lessens ascites, and improves renal blood flow.

Variceal banding or **sclerotherapy** can control esophageal variceal bleeding.

Lifestyle Modifications:

- **Alcohol**: Complete cessation in cases of alcoholic liver disease
- **Nutrition**: Dietary changes, including a low-sodium diet for ascites and a balanced diet for malnutrition
- **Avoidance of Liver Toxins**: E.g., acetaminophen, NSAIDs, certain antibiotics, and cholesterol medication that may have hepatotoxic effects

Liver Transplant may be recommended for eligible patients with end-stage liver disease.

Liver Cancer

Liver cancer is one of the most common types of cancer worldwide and is especially linked to liver cirrhosis and chronic hepatitis.

Diagnosis of Liver Cancer

Ask about a history of cirrhosis, hepatitis, alcohol use, and a family history of liver cancer. While liver cancer is not typically inherited per se, there are some familial conditions that predispose to it, such as hereditary hemochromatosis, alpha-1 antitrypsin deficiency, Wilson's disease, autoimmune hepatitis, a family history of hepatitis B or C, and other rare genetic conditions.

Blood Tests:

- **Alpha-fetoprotein (AFP)**: An elevated level can be a sign of liver cancer, although not all liver cancers raise AFP levels, and not all increased AFP is due to liver cancer.
- **Liver Function Tests** assess the general health of the liver.

Imaging:

- **Ultrasound** is often used as a screening tool, especially in patients with cirrhosis.
- **CT Scan** and **MRI** can provide detailed images and help in staging the cancer by showing the size and number of the tumors and whether the cancer has spread.

Biopsy: A needle biopsy of the liver can confirm the diagnosis, but in cases where imaging is conclusive, a biopsy might not be needed to start treatment.

Other Tests: If the cancer is suspected to have spread, additional tests like a bone scan or chest X-ray might be performed.

Treatment of Liver Cancer

Surgery:

Resection of the tumor and surrounding tissue may be feasible if the cancer is in an early stage, liver function is good, and the tumor is not too large.

Liver Transplant is suitable for small tumors when resection isn't possible due to poor liver function or other reasons. The most common reason for liver transplant is cirrhosis.

Local Non-Surgical Therapies:

Radiofrequency Ablation (RFA)/Microwave Ablation (MWA) uses heat to destroy cancer cells via a probe inserted through the skin into the tumor, with ultrasound, CT, or MRI guidance.

Percutaneous Ethanol Injection of alcohol into the tumor kills cancer cells.

Cryotherapy freezes and destroys cancer cells.

Transarterial Chemoembolization (TACE) delivers chemotherapy directly to the liver followed by a substance that blocks the artery feeding the cancer cells.

Radioembolization (Y90) delivers radiation in the form of tiny beads to the liver tumor via blood vessels.

Radiation Therapy uses external beam radiation to target specific areas of the liver.

Chemotherapy, delivered systemically, isn't typically very effective against liver cancer but may be used in some cases.

Targeted Therapy uses drugs like *sorafenib*, *lenvatinib*, and others to target specific aspects of cancer cells.

Immunotherapy helps the immune system to recognize and attack cancer cells by targeting specific proteins that cancer cells use to protect themselves from the immune system. These drugs (**checkpoint inhibitors**) include drugs such as *nivolumab* (*Opdivo*), *pembrolizumab* (*Keytruda*), *atezolizumab* (*Tecentriq*), *ipilimumab* (*Yervoy*), *and durvalumab* (*Imfinzi*).

The prognosis for liver cancer depends heavily on the stage at diagnosis and the underlying liver function. Early diagnosis often leads to a better prognosis. Follow-up care is critical to monitor for recurrence or progression of the disease.

Prevention of Liver Cancer:

- Vaccinate against hepatitis B.
- Treat and regularly monitor for chronic hepatitis B and C infections.
- Limit alcohol and tobacco use.
- Maintain a healthy weight and diet. Obesity is a risk factor for liver cancer.

Liver Abscess

Liver abscesses often result from infection in the bile ducts, the gastrointestinal tract, or the bloodstream. There are several types of infection:

- **Bacterial** infections are the most common, e.g., *E. coli, Klebsiella pneumoniae, Streptococcus* species.
- **Parasitic**, e.g., *Entamoeba histolytica*
- **Fungal**, e.g., *Candida, Aspergillus* species
- **Mixed**, i.e., caused by multiple organisms

Diagnosis of Liver Abscess

The patient may present with fever, chills, upper abdominal pain, jaundice, and general malaise. Physical exam may reveal tenderness in the right upper quadrant of the abdomen.

Lab Tests:

Blood tests may show an elevated white blood cell count, abnormal liver function tests (e.g., elevated AST, ALT, alkaline phosphatase, or bilirubin), and inflammatory markers (like C-reactive protein).

Blood cultures may identify a bacterial pathogen.

Serology tests can check for antibodies against specific parasitic infections, e.g., amoebic or *Echinococcus* tapeworm. They can also test for antibodies against specific viruses (e.g., hepatitis A, B, C, D, or E, cytomegalovirus, Epstein-Barr, or herpes simplex), indicating a past or current infection.

Imaging:

- **Ultrasound** can identify fluid collections in the liver.
- **CT Scan** provides a more detailed view and can help determine the size, number, and location of abscesses, as well as guide drainage procedures.
- **MRI** may be used for further delineation if needed.

Aspiration and Culture: In many cases, percutaneous needle aspiration under imaging guidance is performed not only to confirm the diagnosis of infection but also for microbiological culture to identify the specific pathogen.

Treatment of Liver Abscess

Antibiotics: Broad-spectrum antibiotics are started empirically as soon as the diagnosis is suspected, and they are later adjusted based on culture and sensitivity results. Therapy is often prolonged, typically lasting 4-6 weeks.

Percutaneous Drainage is the standard treatment for large or multiple abscesses. It is done by inserting a needle or catheter through the skin with ultrasound or CT guidance. This procedure removes pus from the liver and can provide significant symptomatic relief.

Surgical Drainage may be required if percutaneous drainage is not possible or effective, or if there are complicating factors, such as rupture or hemorrhage within the abscess.

Management of the Underlying Cause: If the abscess is secondary to conditions like biliary tract disease, these must also be addressed to prevent recurrence.

Hemochromatosis

Hemochromatosis is a genetic disorder causing the body to absorb too much dietary iron. The excess iron is then deposited in various organs, especially the liver, heart, and pancreas, which can lead to conditions such as liver cirrhosis and liver cancer, heart disease, and diabetes. The most common type is caused by a mutation in the HFE gene.

Diagnosis of Hemochromatosis

The patient may have symptoms of fatigue, joint and abdominal pain, skin darkening (bronze or grey color from iron deposits in the skin), diabetes (from pancreatic damage), liver problems (e.g., hepatomegaly, cirrhosis, liver failure, liver cancer), weight loss, and sexual dysfunction. There may be a family history.

Blood Tests:

- **Serum Transferrin Saturation** measures the amount of iron bound to transferrin protein, which carries iron in the blood. Saturation above 45% is considered high.
- **Serum Ferritin** indicates the amount of iron stored in the body. Elevated levels may suggest hemochromatosis.
- **Liver Function Tests** help establish if the liver is involved.

Imaging Studies: **MRI** can estimate the degree of iron overload in the liver by measuring its magnetic properties.

Liver Biopsy can be used to assess the degree of liver damage (cirrhosis) if other tests are inconclusive.

Genetic Testing can confirm the diagnosis by identifying mutations in the HFE gene (most commonly C282Y and H63D mutations).

Treatment of Hemochromatosis

Phlebotomy is the main treatment for hereditary hemochromatosis; the body does not have a good way of otherwise eliminating excess iron.

Chelation Therapy uses a chelating (binding) chemical (e.g., *deferoxamine*), which is administered by intramuscular injection or IV; the bound iron is excreted mainly in the urine.

Dietary Changes: Avoid iron supplements and multivitamins containing iron; limit excess intake of vitamin C, which can increase iron absorption. Limit alcohol, which can increase liver damage in patients with iron overload. Avoid eating raw shellfish, which have a high iron content. Also, people with hemochromatosis are at higher risk of bacterial infections from shellfish, because a bacterium found in shellfish (*Vibrio vulnificus*) likes to eat iron and can more easily infect persons with hemochromatosis.

Wilson's Disease

Wilson's disease is a rare autosomal recessive disorder characterized by excess copper storage in various body tissues, particularly the liver, brain, and eyes. This accumulation can lead to hepatic, neurological, and psychiatric symptoms.

Diagnosis of Wilson's Disease

Physical Exam may show signs of:

- Liver disease, ranging from asymptomatic liver function abnormalities to fulminant hepatic failure (jaundice, altered mental status, bleeding or clotting problems, hypoglycemia, ascites, malaise, nausea and vomiting, abdominal pain, and even multiorgan failure)
- Neurological symptoms (tremors, slurred speech, ataxia, dystonia, parkinsonism)
- Psychiatric disturbances (depression, neurotic behaviors, personality changes)
- **Kayser-Fleischer rings** (copper deposits in the cornea, visible via slit-lamp examination)
- Hematological signs (hemolytic anemia from copper damage to red blood cells)

Lab Tests:

- **Serum ceruloplasmin levels** are usually low in Wilson's disease. Ceruloplasmin is a copper-carrying protein synthesized in the liver. In Wilson's disease, the liver cannot incorporate copper into ceruloplasmin. The unbound copper deposits particularly in the liver and brain, while the level of serum ceruloplasmin is reduced.
- **Serum copper** is typically low (due to decreased ceruloplasmin), but can be normal.
- **Urinary copper** is elevated in a 24-hour urine copper excretion test.
- **Liver biopsy** shows increased hepatic copper content.

Genetic Testing: ATP7B gene mutation analysis confirms the diagnosis.

Imaging: MRI of the brain can show characteristic changes in the basal ganglia related to copper deposition.

Treatment of Wilson's Disease

Chelating Agents: *D-penicillamine* or *trientine* binds copper and increases its excretion. *Tetrathiomolybdate* (mainly given orally) chelates copper and reduces copper absorption from the GI tract.

Zinc: Zinc acetate or sulfate works by blocking the absorption of copper in the intestinal tract.

Antioxidants: Some patients might benefit from vitamin E and other antioxidants to mitigate the oxidative stress caused by copper.

Liver Transplantation may be considered in patient's unresponsive to medical therapy or in end-stage liver disease.

Dietary Management: Reduce the intake of copper-rich foods (e.g., shellfish, nuts, chocolate, mushrooms, and organ meats). Avoid copper-containing supplements and water from copper pipes.

Genetic counseling for family members may be advised, since Wilson's disease is an autosomal recessive disorder.

Primary Sclerosing Cholangitis

Primary Sclerosing Cholangitis (PSC) is a chronic liver disease characterized by inflammation and fibrosis of the bile ducts both inside and outside the liver. This leads to bile duct strictures, cholestasis, and progressive liver damage; PSC can ultimately lead to cirrhosis, liver failure, or cholangiocarcinoma (bile duct cancer). It may require liver transplantation. PSC is often associated with inflammatory bowel disease (IBD), particularly ulcerative colitis.

PSC is believed to arise from a combination of genetic, autoimmune, and environmental factors and is often suspected in patients with known Inflammatory Bowel Disease (IBD) who develop abnormal liver function tests, particularly an elevated alkaline phosphatase. Alkaline phosphatase is normally found in the liver, bile ducts, and bone. Elevated levels suggest cholestasis (e.g., from bile duct blockage), liver damage, or bone turnover.

PSC can also occur in patients without IBD. Some drugs can cause chronic bile duct inflammation, e.g., *Adriamycin*. IgG4-associated cholangiopathy may result when there are high levels of IgG4 antibody (which may respond to immunosuppressive agents).

Diagnosis of Primary Sclerosing Cholangitis

The patient may present with fatigue, itching, jaundice, and right upper quadrant abdominal pain. However, many patients are asymptomatic, especially in the early stages.

Tests and Procedures:

Blood tests check for elevated liver enzymes (alkaline phosphatase, GGT, AST, ALT) and bilirubin.

MRCP (Magnetic Resonance Cholangiopancreatography) is a type of MRI that visualizes the biliary tree and can show characteristic changes without the need for invasive procedures. PSC typically shows a beaded appearance of the bile ducts due to alternating strictures and dilations.

ERCP (Endoscopic Retrograde Cholangiopancreatography): A contrast material is injected by endoscope into the bile duct where the duct enters the duodenum. This enables X-ray images to be taken of the ducts. In addition, tools can be passed through the endoscope to remove gallstones, relieve obstructions, take biopsies, and insert stents to keep the ducts open, or perform other procedures.

Liver biopsy may be performed to assess the degree of liver inflammation and fibrosis. Biopsy of the ampulla of Vater can confirm the diagnosis of IgG4-associated cholangiopathy by showing infiltration of IgG4-positive plasma cells.

PSC should be distinguished from **Secondary Sclerosing Cholangitis**, which has other causes (e.g., chronic biliary inflammation due to chronic choledocholithiasis or injury during cholecystectomy; HIV cholangiopathy or cholangiopathy resulting from *cryptosporidiosis*, *giardia* or other infections that can be detected in a stool test).

Treatment of Primary Sclerosing Cholangitis

Treatment is primarily aimed at managing symptoms or complications such as portal hypertension, varices, or ascites. ERCP may be performed, such as endoscopic dilation or stent insertion, for bile duct stricture. Surgery may be performed for resecting a cholangiocarcinoma. Liver transplantation may be considered for severe cases of advanced cirrhosis. There are other options for SSC, which is caused by identifiable and often treatable external factors.

Medications for Primary Sclerosing Cholangitis:

Ursodeoxycholic acid (UDCA), a bile acid, may help bile flow and has an anti-inflammatory and protective effect on liver cells. However, its effectiveness in PSC is not well-established.

Antibiotics may be used for bacterial cholangitis.

Vitamin supplementation with fat-soluble vitamins (A, D, E, and K) may be prescribed for malabsorption caused by cholestasis.

Medications for itching (from backup of bile acids) include *cholestyramine* (to bind bile acids), *rifampicin* (to stimulate the metabolism and excretion of bile acids), or *naltrexone* (blocks opioid receptors involved in itch sensation).

Patients with PSC are at higher risk for colorectal cancer, particularly those with ulcerative colitis. Regular colonoscopy screening is recommended.

Autoimmune Hepatitis

Autoimmune hepatitis (AIH) is a chronic inflammatory liver disease characterized by immune-mediated destruction of hepatic cells, which can lead to cirrhosis and liver failure if untreated. It is believed to result from a combination of genetic and environmental factors that trigger an inappropriate immune response against liver cells.

Diagnosis of Autoimmune Hepatitis

Patients may present with symptoms of fatigue, abdominal discomfort, jaundice, itching, joint pains, and amenorrhea. However, some patients may be asymptomatic and are discovered incidentally due to abnormal liver function tests.

Lab Tests:

Autoantibodies: Antinuclear antibodies (ANA), smooth muscle antibodies (SMA), liver/kidney microsomal type 1 antibodies (LKM-1), and soluble liver antigen/liver pancreas antibodies (SLA/LP) are typically tested for confirmation.

Hypergammaglobulinemia: Elevated levels of immunoglobulin G (IgG) are common.

Liver function tests: Transaminases (ALT and AST) and bilirubin are elevated; alkaline phosphatase levels tend to be relatively low because autoimmune hepatitis mainly affects the liver cells (hepatocytes) rather than the bile ducts, which have the most alkaline phosphatase.

Liver Biopsy: Histology shows **interface hepatitis** (characteristic inflammation and damage at the boundary between the liver parenchyma and portal tracts), infiltration of lymphocytes and plasma cells, and hepatic rosette pattern formation.

Imaging: Although not diagnostic for AIH, ultrasound, CT scan, or MRI might be used to rule out other liver diseases.

Other Tests like viral serologies, serum ceruloplasmin, and iron studies may be performed to rule out viral hepatitis, Wilson's disease, hemochromatosis and other liver diseases.

Treatment of Autoimmune Hepatitis

Corticosteroids can be used to reduce inflammation.

Azathioprine (an immunosuppressant) or other immunosuppressants (e.g., *mycophenolate mofetil, cyclosporine,* or *tacrolimus*) can be used to decrease the autoimmune inflammation.

Liver Transplant is considered in cases of severe liver damage.

Alcoholic Hepatitis

Alcoholic hepatitis is an inflammatory condition of the liver resulting from excess alcohol consumption. It's part of a spectrum of alcohol-related liver disease which also includes fatty liver disease and cirrhosis.

Diagnosis of Alcoholic Hepatitis

History: Heavy and prolonged alcohol use. Some patients may not be forthcoming about their alcohol intake, making history-taking challenging.

Physical: Signs may include jaundice, hepatomegaly, ascites, and other features of chronic liver disease, such as **spider angiomas** (small, spider-like blood vessels seen under the skin), **gynecomastia**, and **caput medusae** (enlarged veins around the navel). Spider angiomas and gynecomastia may result from increased estrogen due to the liver's deficit in metabolizing hormones. Caput medusae result from portal hypertension. There may be hepatic encephalopathy in advanced cases with **asterixis** (wrist flapping), and confusion.

Lab Tests:

Liver Function Tests:

- There may be elevated **AST** and **ALT** levels, with AST typically higher than ALT, usually in a 2:1 ratio, although this is not specific to alcoholic hepatitis.
- **Gamma-glutamyl transferase (GGT)** is often elevated. Alcohol increases the production of GGT in the liver and biliary epithelium.
- **Bilirubin** levels may be significantly elevated.
- **Complete Blood Count (CBC)** may show anemia, elevated white blood cell count, decreased platelets and, occasionally, eosinophilia (possibly an allergic reaction triggered by alcohol or medication used to treat the hepatitis).
- **Prothrombin Time (PT)** may be prolonged due to liver impairment in producing clotting factors, including prothrombin.
- **Albumin** levels may be low because the liver is not producing enough.
- **Inflammatory markers** such as C-reactive protein (CRP) may be elevated.

Imaging: Ultrasound, CT scan, or MRI can assess for liver damage, including fatty infiltration and cirrhosis, and exclude other causes of liver disease.

Liver biopsy can confirm the diagnosis by showing characteristic histological features, such as ballooning degeneration (swelling of hepatocytes), neutrophil infiltration, Mallory bodies (abnormal clumps of protein in hepatocytes), and fibrosis. However, biopsy is not always necessary for diagnosis, especially if the clinical picture is clear.

Exclusion of Other Causes: Other causes of hepatitis should be excluded, such as viral hepatitis, autoimmune hepatitis, and medication-induced hepatitis.

Treatment of Alcoholic Hepatitis

The primary treatment for alcoholic hepatitis is abstinence from alcohol, nutritional support, and management of liver complications. Total cessation of alcohol intake is crucial. Counseling, support groups such as Alcoholics Anonymous (AA), and treatment for alcohol withdrawal may be necessary.

Corticosteroids may be prescribed to reduce inflammation in severe cases, particularly those with a high **Maddrey's Discriminant Function (DF) score**:

$$(DF = 4.6 \times (\text{prothrombin time in seconds} - \text{control time}) + \text{serum bilirubin level in mg/dL})$$

Pentoxifylline is a phosphodiesterase inhibitor that has been used to treat severe alcoholic hepatitis due to its anti-inflammatory effects.

Liver Transplant can be considered for patients with severe alcoholic hepatitis who don't respond to medical therapy and have stopped drinking.

Management of Complications: Ascites, variceal bleeding, hepatic encephalopathy, and infections should be treated as per standard guidelines for liver disease.

Metabolic Associated Steatohepatitis (MASH)

Metabolic Associated Steatohepatitis (MASH) is a type of nonalcoholic fatty liver disease (NAFLD)(a newer name for NAFLD is "Metabolic Dysfunction-associated Steatotic Liver Disease", or MASLD). MASH is a more serious stage of MASLD, characterized by fatty liver (steatosis), inflammation, and liver cell injury. While MASLD is mostly a benign fat accumulation in the liver, MASH can progress to fibrosis and cirrhosis. Risks include insulin resistance, metabolic syndrome, obesity, and a family history of diabetes, particularly type 2.

Diagnosis of MASH

Patients might be asymptomatic or have nonspecific symptoms like fatigue or right upper quadrant discomfort.

Blood Tests: Liver enzymes may be elevated, although they can also be normal. Other tests may indicate insulin resistance or dyslipidemia.

Imaging: Ultrasound, CT, or MRI can detect fatty liver.

Elastography (e.g., **FibroScan**) assesses liver stiffness as an indirect sign of fibrosis.

Liver Biopsy is the only definitive way to diagnose MASH and assess the degree of inflammation and fibrosis.

Treatment of MASH

There is no specific medication approved for MASH, so treatment focuses on managing underlying conditions and lifestyle modifications.

Lifestyle Changes: Weight loss through diet and exercise is the primary treatment. A weight loss of 7-10% can improve liver enzymes, steatosis, inflammation, and fibrosis. A healthy diet, such as the Mediterranean diet, is often recommended. Regular physical activity, even without weight loss, can improve metabolic parameters. Alcohol should be consumed in moderation or not at all, and patients should avoid medications that can worsen liver health.

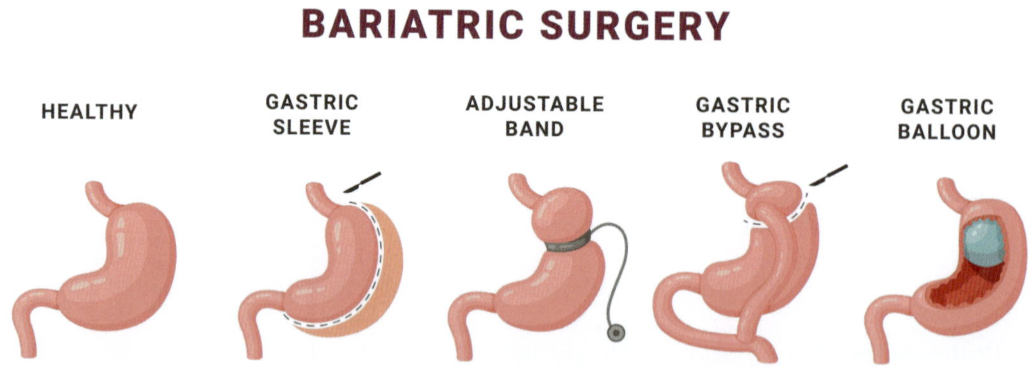

Figure 10-6 Bariatric Surgery

Tight control of diabetes, management of dyslipidemia, and treatment of hypertension are important.

Medications:

- *Vitamin E* at specific doses has been shown to improve liver histology in non-diabetic patients with MASH.
- *Pioglitazone*, a medication for type 2 diabetes that increases sensitivity to insulin, can improve MASH in some patients but is associated with weight gain and potential long-term risks.
- *Resmetirom* (*Rezdiffra*) is a selective thyroid hormone receptor beta agonist that reduces liver fat and inflammation in adults with noncirrhotic MASH and moderate to advanced fibrosis.

Potential for Bariatric Surgery: In selected patients, particularly those with obesity and who are not able to achieve weight loss through lifestyle changes alone, bariatric (weight loss) surgery may be considered (**Fig. 10-6**).

Liver Transplantation may be an option for patients who develop cirrhosis and liver failure or hepatocellular carcinoma.

Drug-Induced Liver Injury

Drug-induced liver injury (DILI) is a condition where liver damage is caused by medications, herbal or dietary supplements, or other toxins. DILI can range from mild elevations in liver enzymes to severe liver damage, including acute liver failure. Symptoms may include jaundice, dark urine, abdominal pain, or pruritus.

Diagnosis of Drug-induced Liver Injury

History: Identify the intake of any prescription drugs, over-the-counter medications, herbal products, supplements, or toxins that could cause liver damage. DILI can occur days to months after drug initiation.

Lab Tests may show elevated liver enzymes, particularly alanine aminotransferase (ALT) for hepatocellular injury and alkaline phosphatase (ALP) for cholestatic or mixed injury. Bilirubin levels and coagulation profile (INR) can also provide insight into the severity of liver injury.

Imaging: Ultrasound, CT, or MRI can help rule out obstructive causes of liver injury, such as gallstones.

Liver Biopsy may be necessary to confirm the diagnosis and to assess the extent and cause of liver damage, especially if the clinical picture is unclear.

Roussel Uclaf Causality Assessment Method (RUCAM) is a way to help determine the likelihood that a drug caused the liver injury. It takes into consideration:

- **Time to onset** after starting the drug
- **Course of the reaction** after stopping the drug
- **Risk factors** such as age, alcohol use, and pregnancy
- **Concomitant use of drugs** that may also be hepatotoxic
- **Exclusion of alternative causes** like viral hepatitis, biliary obstruction, etc.
- **Previous information on the hepatotoxicity** of the drug
- **Response to unintentional or deliberate re-exposure** to the drug

Treatment of Drug-Induced Liver Injury

Immediate cessation of the drug suspected of causing liver injury is the most important step. In cases where the suspected drug is necessary for treating a critical condition, a risk-benefit analysis must be performed. Treatment is mostly supportive, addressing symptoms and managing complications.

For cases of acute liver failure, management in an intensive care setting might be required.

Corticosteroids may be administered in certain cases, such as those with autoimmune features or hypersensitivity reactions. **N-acetylcysteine** replenishes hepatic glutathione stores, which are important for the detoxification of harmful substances (e.g., in acetaminophen overdose).

Gilbert's Syndrome

Gilbert's syndrome is a common, mild liver disorder in which the liver doesn't properly process bilirubin. It doesn't require treatment, but it can cause jaundice with no other signs of liver disease, due to increased blood levels of unconjugated bilirubin, which the liver won't conjugate (**Fig. 10-7**). Patients often report episodes of jaundice that appear during times of exertion, stress, fasting, or infections.

Diagnosis of Gilbert's Syndrome

Blood Tests:

Unconjugated bilirubin levels are elevated, without other abnormalities in liver function tests (LFTs). CBC is normal. A fasting challenge test may be conducted, which can cause bilirubin levels to rise in someone with Gilbert's syndrome.

Genetic Testing: Gilbert's syndrome is caused by a genetic mutation in the UGT1A1 gene, which leads to reduced activity of the enzyme UDP-glucuronosyltransferase that is

BILE METABOLISM AND CAUSES OF JAUNDICE

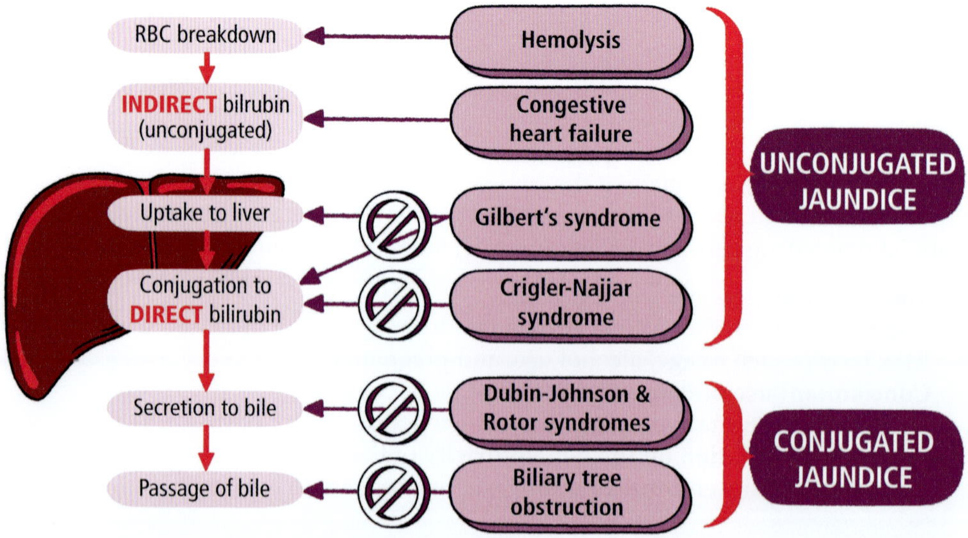

Figure 10-7 *(From Berkowitz, A., Clinical Pathophysiology Made Ridiculously Simple, Medmaster)*

responsible for bilirubin processing. Genetic testing can confirm the diagnosis, although it's not commonly performed since the condition is harmless.

Treatment of Gilbert's Syndrome

- Avoid fasting or diets that cause rapid weight loss, as these may trigger jaundice.
- Stress management can be beneficial since stress may exacerbate symptoms.
- Moderate exercise is advised; however, intense exertion should be approached with caution as it may increase bilirubin levels.

Crigler-Najjar Syndrome

Crigler-Najjar Syndrome is a rare genetic disorder in which the liver cannot conjugate bilirubin (**Fig. 10-7**). The unconjugated (indirect) bilirubin, which, unlike conjugated bilirubin, cannot be excreted by the kidneys, accumulates and can cause neonatal jaundice with **kernicterus** (brain damage from bile accumulation in the brain).

Diagnosis of Crigler-Najjar Syndrome

Blood tests show elevated levels of unconjugated bilirubin, without signs of liver damage or hemolysis.

Genetic testing can confirm mutations in the UBT1A1 gene, the activity of which is more severely reduced than in Gilbert's syndrome.

Treatment of Crigler-Najjar Syndrome

Phototherapy can be used to convert the bilirubin into a form that the body can excrete without having to be conjugated. Milder cases can be treated with **phenobarbital**, which stimulates bilirubin conjugation.

Plasmapheresis can temporarily reduce bilirubin.

A liver transplant may provide a cure for refractory cases.

Dubin-Johnson and Rotor Syndromes

Dubin-Johnson Syndrome is a rare genetic liver disorder in which the liver ***can*** conjugate bilirubin but cannot secrete it into the biliary tract (**Fig. 10-7**). Conjugated bilirubin accumulates, causing jaundice.

Diagnosis of Dubin-Johnson Syndrome

Blood tests show a conjugated hyperbilirubinemia, with otherwise normal liver enzymes and no evidence of hemolysis. **Liver biopsy** shows a diagnostic dark brown pigment in liver hepatocytes.

Treatment is usually not needed for Dubin-Johnson since the condition is generally benign, although phototherapy may be used in newborns.

Rotor Syndrome, like Dubin-Johnson, is a condition in which the liver can conjugate bilirubin but cannot secrete it into the biliary tract (**Fig. 10-7**). It is due to mutations in the SLCO1B1 and SLCO1B3 genes. Since it is benign, no specific treatment is usually necessary.

Budd-Chiari Syndrome

Budd-Chiari syndrome (BCS) is a rare condition that occurs when there is obstruction of the hepatic veins (**Fig. 10-1**), which drain the liver; it can lead to liver damage. The severity of the condition can vary from mild to life-threatening.

Diagnosis of Budd-Chiari Syndrome

The physical exam may reveal features of liver congestion, e.g., abdominal pain, hepatomegaly, ascites, and jaundice.

Blood Tests: Liver function tests may show elevated liver enzymes, bilirubin, and INR (elevated INR indicates decreased clotting ability, which may be attributed to liver damage and using up the clotting factors during clotting of the hepatic veins).

Imaging:

- Ultrasound with Doppler can assess blood flow in the hepatic veins and inferior vena cava (IVC).
- CT or MRI can provide detailed images of the liver and hepatic vasculature and may show hepatic vein thrombosis or webs (thin, membrane-like structures that can form in the hepatic veins and cause obstruction).
- Angiography may can confirm the diagnosis and guide therapeutic interventions.

- Liver biopsy may be performed if the diagnosis is unclear, although it may be risky if there is significant portal hypertension, due to the risk of bleeding.
- Tests for clotting disorders may be part of the workup.

Treatment of Budd-Chiari Syndrome

Medical Management:
Anticoagulation: Lifelong anticoagulation is often required to prevent further clotting.
Diuretics reduce ascites and edema.
Sodium restriction is recommended to manage ascites.

Endovascular Procedures:

- **Stenting** can widen narrowed or blocked veins.
- **TIPS (Transjugular Intrahepatic Portosystemic Shunt):** If the response to medical treatment is poor, TIPS can be used to redirect blood flow from the portal vein to the inferior vena cava or partially functioning hepatic vein, bypassing the liver and helping relieve portal hypertension and liver congestion.

Surgery:

- **Thrombectomy**: Surgical removal of the clot might be considered in acute cases.
- **Paracentesis** may be required for ascites.
- **Endoscopic treatment** may be needed to stop bleeding esophageal varices.
- **Liver transplantation** may be the only option in severe cases.

Alpha-1 Antitrypsin Deficiency

Alpha-1 antitrypsin deficiency (AATD) is a genetic condition that can lead to lung and liver disease. It is caused by mutations in the SERPINA1 gene; this leads to a deficiency or dysfunction of the alpha-1 antitrypsin (AAT) protein, which is important in protecting the lungs from enzyme damage. In the liver, misfolded alpha-1 antitrypsin can damage hepatocytes. The patient presents with pulmonary symptoms that may include shortness of breath, wheezing, recurrent respiratory infections, asthma, and reduced exercise tolerance. Liver-related symptoms may include elevated liver function tests, jaundice, ascites, and pedal edema from fluid accumulation.

Diagnosis of Alpha-1 Antitrypsin Deficiency

Blood Test: A simple blood test can measure the level of AAT protein in the blood, which will be reduced. **Genetic Testing:** DNA testing can confirm the specific genetic mutations (e.g., the Z or S allele) responsible for AATD.

Pulmonary Function Tests are used to assess lung function.

Imaging: Chest X-ray or CT scans can show evidence of emphysema, which is often associated with AATD.

Liver Function Tests can detect liver damage associated with AATD, particularly in children and infants.

Liver Biopsy may be done to assess the degree of liver damage, especially in cases where the diagnosis is unclear.

Treatment of Alpha-1 Antitrypsin Deficiency

There is no cure for AATD, but treatments can help manage the symptoms and slow the progression of the disease:

Augmentation Therapy: For individuals with lung involvement, augmentation therapy with intravenous infusions of AAT derived from donated human plasma can help to increase AAT levels and reduce the rate of decline in lung function.

Lifestyle Changes: Avoiding smoking is critical as smoking accelerates lung damage in AATD. Alcohol should be consumed in moderation, if at all, due to the risk of liver disease.

Management of Lung Diseases:

- Inhaled bronchodilators and corticosteroids may be used to treat COPD symptoms.
- Vaccinations, such as influenza and pneumococcal vaccines, are important to prevent infections.
- In severe cases of liver disease, a liver transplant may be necessary.

Genetic Counseling: Since AATD is an autosomal recessive genetic condition, genetic counseling may be considered for the patient and family.

Hepatic Encephalopathy

Hepatic encephalopathy (HE) is characterized by a spectrum of neurological manifestations ranging from mild confusion to deep coma and is a serious complication of liver cirrhosis or acute liver failure. It results from the liver's impaired ability to detoxify the blood, with the accumulation in the blood of ammonia particularly.

Diagnosis of Hepatic Encephalopathy

The diagnosis of hepatic encephalopathy is primarily clinical, based on the patient's history, symptoms, and neurological examination, in the context of liver disease:

Clinical Assessment involves evaluation of mental status changes, including levels of consciousness, personality changes, intellectual function, and motor coordination. The **West Haven Criteria** is a commonly used grading scale for the severity of HE, ranging from Grade 0 (mild confusion) to Grade 4 (coma).

Lab Tests: Blood tests include liver function tests, ammonia levels, electrolytes, complete blood count, and renal function tests to assess overall health and function of the liver and kidneys, as these can influence HE. Arterial blood gases may be checked to rule out hypoxia and metabolic disturbances.

Imaging: Brain imaging such as CT scan or MRI can exclude other causes of altered mental function such as stroke or brain lesions.

Electroencephalogram (EEG) may show characteristic changes in brain activity in HE but is not specific or necessary for the diagnosis.

It's important to rule out other potential causes of altered mental status, such as infection, bleeding, or drug intoxication.

Treatment of Hepatic Encephalopathy

The treatment of hepatic encephalopathy focuses on reducing the production and absorption of toxins, particularly ammonia, that affect brain function:

Lactulose is a synthetic sugar that is not absorbed from the digestive tract. Its administration helps trap ammonia in the gut where the ammonia is expelled in the stool.

Antibiotics: *Rifaximin* may be used to reduce the number of ammonia-producing bacteria in the gut.

Dietary Changes: Protein intake may need to be adjusted. While proteins are essential, excessive protein can increase ammonia production.

Primary Biliary Cholangitis

Primary biliary cholangitis (PBC), formerly known as **primary biliary cirrhosis**, is a chronic autoimmune liver disease characterized by progressive destruction of the small bile ducts within the liver, leading to bile accumulation and liver damage. Symptoms of fatigue and itching (pruritis) are common but nonspecific. Physical findings may include hepatomegaly or signs of advanced liver disease, such as jaundice.

PBC (Primary Biliary Cholangitis) is not the same as PSC (Primary Sclerosing Cholangitis). While both are chronic liver diseases with progressive inflammation of the bile ducts, there are differences:

- PSC involves both the intra-and extrahepatic bile ducts, affects younger males, can lead to cholangiocarcinoma and liver transplantation, and is often associated with inflammatory bowel disease.
- PBC mainly affects the small intrahepatic bile ducts, is autoimmune (associated with antimitochondrial antibodies), is more commonly seen in middle-aged women, and has a more favorable prognosis, due to the availability of effective treatments, such as ursodeoxycholic acid, which promotes bile flow, reduces bile acid toxicity, and protects liver cells from damage.

Diagnosis of Primary Biliary Cholangitis

Blood Tests:

- **Antimitochondrial Antibodies (AMA)** are present in approximately 95% of patients with PBC and are considered a hallmark of the disease.
- **Liver Function Tests** commonly show elevations in alkaline phosphatase (ALP) and gamma-glutamyl transferase (GGT).
- **Cholesterol Levels**, including total cholesterol and HDL, may be elevated due to the backup of cholesterol excretion.

Imaging Studies: Ultrasound, CT, or MRI may be used to assess the liver and bile ducts' structure and to rule out other causes of bile duct obstruction.

Liver Biopsy can confirm the presence of lymphocytic infiltration surrounding and destroying the bile ducts and can assess the stage of liver damage.

Treatment of Primary Biliary Cholangitis

There is no cure, but treatment can help manage symptoms and slow disease progression:

Ursodeoxycholic Acid (UDCA) Is a non-toxic bile acid that helps move bile out of the liver and can decrease inflammation and scarring.

Obeticholic Acid (OCA) is a second-line treatment for patients who do not respond adequately to UDCA. It reduces bile acid synthesis and the accumulation of inflammatory bile acids.

Fibrates: Medications like *fenofibrate* may be used in some cases. It can improve lipid levels, reduce inflammation, and improve the flow of bile through the liver.

Symptom Management:

Pruritus: *Cholestyramine, rifampicin, naltrexone,* or *sertraline* may be used to relieve itching.

Dry Eyes and Mouth (as may be present in coinciding **Sjogren's syndrome**, another autoimmune syndrome) may be treated with artificial tears and saliva substitutes; *pilocarpine* or *cevimeline,* two parasympathomimetic agents, can be used if symptoms are severe, to stimulate tear and saliva production.

Liver Transplant: In cases of liver failure or complications from advanced cirrhosis, a liver transplant may be considered.

Lifestyle Measures: Patients should avoid alcohol and medications that can further damage the liver. Smoking cessation is particularly important since smoking can accelerate the fibrosis in PBC.

Liver Cysts

Liver cysts are fluid-filled cavities in the liver that are typically benign and often discovered incidentally during imaging studies done for other reasons. They can be solitary or multiple and are usually asymptomatic. However, some patients may experience discomfort or pain if the cysts are large or if there is bleeding into the cysts.

Diagnosis of Liver Cysts

Imaging:

- **Ultrasound:** Cysts appear as round, clearly defined areas.
- **CT Scan** and **MRI** can provide more detailed information about the size, number, and relation of cysts to other liver structures.

Blood Tests: Routine liver function tests may be conducted to assess liver function and look for any signs of associated liver disease. These are usually normal in cases of simple cysts.

In some cases, especially if there is suspicion of a more complex cyst (like a hydatid cyst caused by *Echinococcus* infection), serologic tests or additional imaging may be needed to rule out parasitic infections.

Treatment of Liver Cysts

Usually, no treatment is necessary for simple asymptomatic liver cysts. Routine follow-up imaging may be recommended to monitor for any changes in their size. For symptomatic liver cysts, aspiration of the fluid from the cyst can be done using a needle under ultrasound or CT guidance. After aspiration, a sclerosant can be injected into the cyst to reduce the chance of fluid reaccumulating. Surgery may be considered for large symptomatic cysts that do not respond to other measures or are suspicious for malignancy. Options include laparoscopic **deroofing** (removing of a significant part of the cyst wall) or **fenestration** (creating a window in the cyst), both of which aim to promote cyst drainage.

Cysts that are suspected to be malignant or parasitic may need more extensive surgical intervention or medical treatment. **Hydatid cysts** (from larval *Echinococcus* tapeworm) require antiparasitic medication (e.g., *albendazole*) in addition to surgical removal. **Cystadenomas** or **cystadenocarcinomas** may require surgical resection due to the risk of cancer.

Polycystic Liver Disease

Polycystic liver disease (PLD) is characterized by *multiple* cysts scattered throughout the liver (**Fig. 10-8**). It is often seen in association with polycystic kidney disease, but it can also occur alone. The patient may be asymptomatic or present with abdominal distension and abdominal discomfort. In some cases, the cysts may cause a mass effect on adjacent organs. The cysts cause symptoms by compressing the stomach, bile ducts, gallbladder, intestines, or blood vessels, or press up against the diaphragm and cause difficulty breathing. If they press on the heart, they may cause palpitations or other discomfort.

Diagnosis of Polycystic Liver Disease

Imaging:

- **Ultrasound** is commonly used initially to visualize cysts within the liver.
- **CT Scan** and **MRI** provide a more detailed view of the liver and can help assess the number, size, and distribution of cysts.

Genetic Testing: If there is a family history, genetic testing may be used to diagnose Autosomal Dominant Polycystic *Liver* Disease or Autosomal Dominant Polycystic *Kidney* Disease.

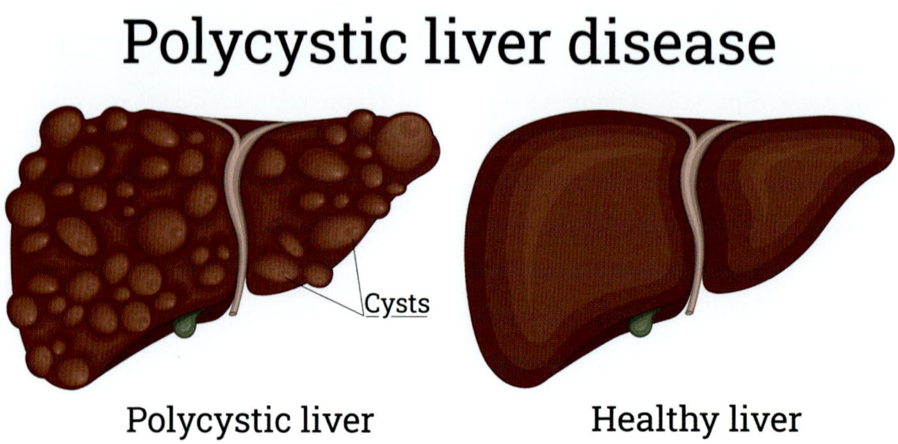

Figure 10-8

Blood Tests: Liver function tests may be conducted to assess the impact of the cysts on liver function, though they are often normal in PLD unless there is significant liver obstruction or compression.

Treatment of Polycystic Liver Disease

The treatment for PLD is usually aimed at managing symptoms, as the condition is not curable.

Aspiration and Sclerotherapy: The cysts can be aspirated under imaging guidance, and a sclerosing agent can be injected to prevent refilling.

Cyst Fenestration: Surgical removal or opening of large cysts can relieve symptoms.

Liver Transplantation may be considered in rare cases where the liver function is compromised, or symptoms are unmanageable.

Liver Hemorrhage

Liver hemorrhage can cause abdominal pain, swelling and signs of shock (e.g., low blood pressure and tachycardia). It can result from trauma, abdominal surgery, other liver problems, or systemic problems that involve disorders of blood coagulation or that affect liver blood flow, such as portal hypertension.

Diagnosis of Liver Hemorrhage

There may be a recent history of trauma, abdominal surgery, other liver problems, or coagulopathy.

Blood tests can check for anemia, liver function, and coagulation disorders.

Ultrasound, apart from assessing the liver, can detect fluid in the abdomen.

CT scan may identify the source of the bleeding and help assess the degree of liver damage.

MRI can provide more detailed information.

Treatment of Liver Hemorrhage

The patient must be initially stabilized, including IV fluid replacement or blood transfusion if needed.

Medication might be used to control bleeding. This includes treatment for any known coagulopathies or to reduce portal hypertension. Otherwise, the condition might be dealt with by arterial embolization to block the bleeding vessel or surgery to repair the damaged liver.

Treatment includes management of any underlying liver disease or other condition that might have contributed to the bleed.

Ascites

Ascites is the accumulation of fluid in the peritoneal cavity. It commonly arises from liver disease, e.g., cirrhosis, where there is increased pressure in the portal venous system as well as decreased albumin and other protein production by the liver; albumin is important in maintaining the oncotic pressure in blood vessels. Ascites can also result from other causes of decreased plasma protein, such as malnutrition, protein-losing enteropathy, kidney diseases like nephrotic syndrome, where protein is lost in the urine, and certain chronic diseases where inflammation breaks down protein. Also, heart failure can cause ascites if there is liver congestion from the backup of pressure into the hepatic veins.

Diagnosis of Ascites

The patient may present with abdominal swelling and discomfort, weight gain and changes in bowel habits. There may be a history of liver disease, heart failure, kidney disease, or cancer.

The **physical exam** may show a **fluid wave** (a wave-like motion felt through the abdominal fluid on tapping one side of the abdomen) or **shifting dullness** on percussion (a change in dullness on percussing the abdomen when the patient shifts from side to side. There may also be jaundice, edema from heart or kidney failure, or signs of malignancy.

Imaging Studies:

- **Ultrasound** can detect ascites while also evaluating the liver, kidneys and other abdominal organs.
- **CT** and **MRI** can provide more detailed information.

Blood Tests:

- Liver function tests, kidney function tests, and CBC can evaluate the liver and kidneys as well as check for signs of infection or inflammation.
- **Serum-ascites albumin gradient (SAAG)** (serum albumin concentration minus ascitic fluid albumin concentration) can help determining the cause of ascites, whether is due to portal hypertension (e.g., from cirrhosis, heart failure, or Budd-Chiari syndrome) or from another cause, such as malignancy, tuberculosis, nephrotic syndrome, or pancreatic injury. A high SAAG indicates low albumin in an ascitic *transudate* due to portal hypertension. A low SAAG suggests high albumin in an ascitic *exudate* from other causes than portal hypertension.
- Analysis of the ascitic fluid (cell count, protein content, SAAG, culture) by paracentesis can help tell if the source of the ascites is transudative (e.g., cirrhosis, heart failure) or exudative (e.g., cancer, infection, pancreatitis).
- ECG and other cardiology tests can be done to assess if there is a cardiac cause.

Laparoscopy can directly visualize the abdominal organs for signs of tumor or TB.

Endoscopy can check for varices in the esophagus or stomach that might implicate portal hypertension.

Treatment of Ascites

Treatment may include:

- Sodium and water restriction
- Medications: Diuretics, and albumin infusions; antibiotics for infection; beta-blockers to reduce portal hypertension

- Paracentesis to remove fluid from the abdomen for symptomatic relief and for diagnosis
- Treating the underlying cause
- Palliative care when the condition is end-stage

Acute Intermittent Porphyria

Acute intermittent porphyria is a rare disease that is mentioned here because it can present as attacks of severe diffuse abdominal pain that are easily misdiagnosed and may even lead to unnecessary surgery. It is caused by a deficiency of the enzyme *porphobilinogen deaminase*, which is important for heme synthesis. The enzyme deficiency can lead to a buildup of toxic heme precursors in the body, leading to abdominal pain (possibly from neurotoxic effects of the heme precursors), and, in some cases, peripheral neuropathy, ascending paralysis, central nervous system involvement (e.g., confusion, hallucinations, seizures, or coma). Flareups can be triggered by certain medications, alcohol consumption, fasting, infections, hormonal changes, and stress.

Diagnosis of Acute Intermittent Porphyria

A clue to the diagnosis is the darkening of standing urine, which frequently occurs. Family history is also important since the disease is inherited as an autosomal dominant, and there may be close relatives with the same condition. A urine sample can be tested for elevated levels of porphobilinogen and aminolevulinic acid during an acute attack. Plasma porphyrins may be elevated. Genetic testing can help identify mutations and may be useful for family screening and counseling.

Treatment of Acute intermittent Porphyria

- Hospitalization may be necessary, with adequate pain management, hydration, high-carbohydrate intake and hemin therapy (both of which reduce the synthesis of toxic heme precursors).
- Long term, it is important for the patient to avoid triggers, e.g. certain medications, alcohol, smoking, and fasting.

11

Diseases of the Gallbladder and Biliary Ducts

Bile is made of bile acids, bilirubin, cholesterol, phospholipids, and electrolytes. It is produced in the liver, stored in the gallbladder, and released into the small intestine via the bile duct. The main function of bile acids is to aid the digestion and absorption of dietary fats and fat-soluble vitamins in the small intestine by emulsifying fats so that they can be broken down more easily by pancreatic lipase. Bile also helps in the excretion of excess cholesterol and bilirubin, a breakdown product of red blood cells. Bile acids are recycled by absorption in the small intestine, transported back to the liver via the portal system (the **enterohepatic circulation)**, and reincorporated into liver hepatocytes for reuse (**Fig. 11-1**).

Bile is absorbed mainly in the ileum of the small intestine. Glucose, amino acids, and fat are absorbed mainly in the duodenum and jejunum. Bile, glucose, and amino acids get to the liver by the portal venous system; fats are first absorbed into the lymphatic system as chylomicrons and eventually reach the liver by the bloodstream (**Fig. 11-1**).

Gallstones and Cholecystitis

Diseases of the gallbladder and biliary ducts often involve the formation of gallstones and inflammation.

Gallstones (cholelithiasis) are hardened deposits, generally made of cholesterol or bilirubin. They may be symptomatic or asymptomatic. Complications of gallstones include acute **cholecystitis** (inflammation of the gallbladder), **cholangitis** (inflammation of the

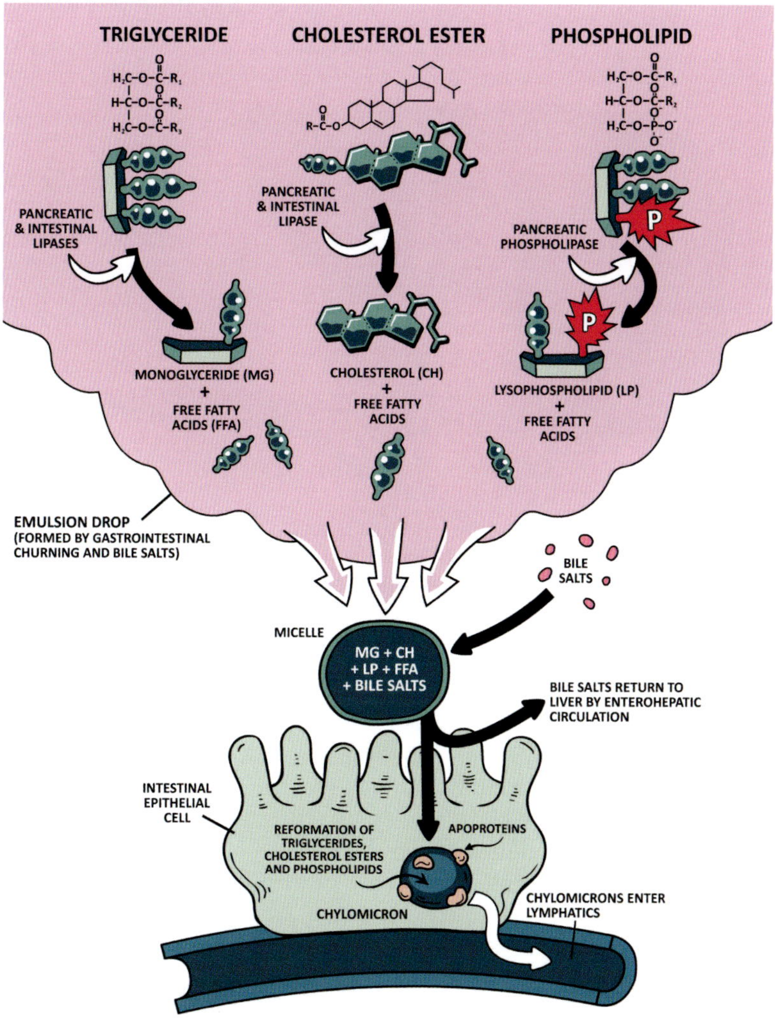

Figure 11-1 *Lipid absorption in the small intestine.*

bile ducts), and **pancreatitis**, which may occur if a gallstone blocks the common bile duct (**Fig. 11-2**). Pancreatic stones tend to be made of calcium carbonate that crystallizes out of pancreatic secretions and deposits in the pancreatic duct.

Diagnosis of Gallstones and Cholecystitis

The patient may experience **biliary colic**, a sharp, cramping pain in the upper right part of the abdomen. The pain may radiate to the back or right shoulder and often occurs after eating a fatty meal.

Tenderness occurs on pressing in the right upper quadrant of the abdomen; it may cause the patient to involuntarily stop a deep inhalation due to pain during palpation of the gallbladder (**Murphy's sign**).

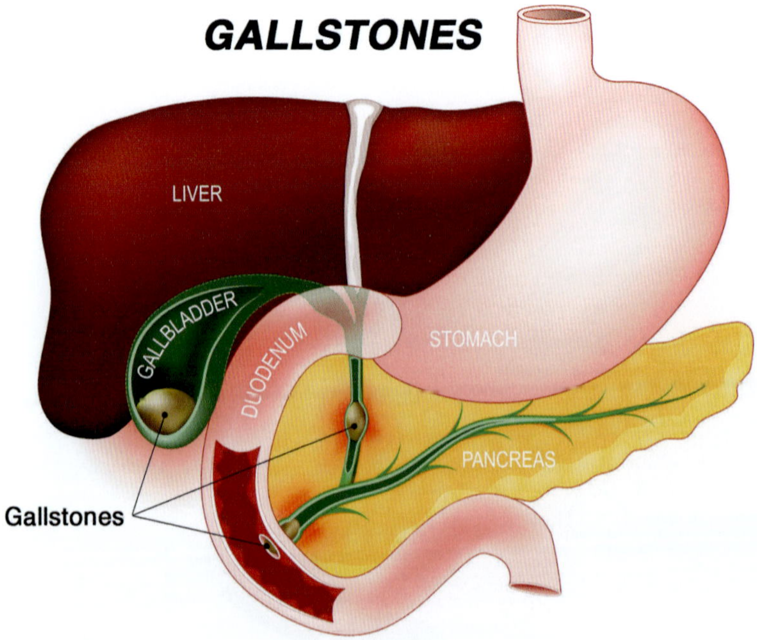

Figure 11-2

Blood Tests: While not diagnostic for gallstones, **liver function tests** can show abnormalities if gallstones are causing a blockage of the bile ducts. **CBC** may show leukocytosis, suggesting infection or inflammation. Elevated **amylase** and **lipase** suggest pancreatitis, which may accompany gallbladder disease. Elevated **C-reactive protein** suggests inflammation.

Imaging:

Ultrasound, the main diagnostic tool for detecting gallstones, is non-invasive and highly sensitive. It may show gallstones, a thickened gallbladder wall, and pericholecystic fluid, which are suggestive of cholecystitis.

CT scan may be used to detect gallstones but is less sensitive than ultrasound for this purpose. It can be used when ultrasound is inconclusive and to rule out other causes of abdominal pain.

Common bile duct stones can also be seen with an intraoperative cholangiogram done during laparoscopic cholecystectomy or by MRI.

HIDA scan (Hepatobiliary Iminodiacetic Acid Scan): While not directly visualizing gallstones like ultrasound does, HIDA can assess gallbladder function and diseases related to gallstones. It involves injecting a radioactive tracer which is processed by the liver and excreted into the bile. The scan can measure how well the gallbladder empties over several hours or if there is biliary dyskinesia, where the gallbladder does not empty properly.

Treatment of Gallstones

Typically, no treatment is required for asymptomatic gallstones. For severe symptoms, the patient may be hospitalized on IV fluids while fasting, with pain medication and antibiotics for infection. Surgery can be done laparoscopically for symptomatic gallstones and is one of the most common surgical procedures. Alternatively, *ursodeoxycholic acid*, an oral medication, may be used to dissolve cholesterol gallstones in certain patients who cannot undergo surgery, but it is less effective than surgery and may take months or even years to completely dissolve gallstones.

Endoscopic Retrograde Cholangiopancreatography (ERCP) may be done to remove stones in the common bile duct, before or after gallbladder removal. In this procedure, an endoscopic catheter cannulates the common bile duct or pancreatic duct and injects a contrast material that can be seen with fluoroscopy. This can visualize stones in the biliary or pancreatic ducts, which can be removed endoscopically during the same procedure.

Percutaneous Cholecystostomy may be done in very ill patients who cannot undergo surgery. An interventional radiologist inserts a tube through the skin into the gallbladder to drain the infection. The gallbladder can also be drained using ERCP: A guidewire is passed through the cystic duct and a stent is passed over the wire to allow drainage of the gallbladder. A stent can also be made that connects the gallbladder to the stomach or small intestine.

Choledocholithiasis

Choledocholithiasis (common bile duct stones), occurs when one or more gallstones are present in the common bile duct. These stones can originate in the gallbladder and migrate into the bile duct or form in the duct itself.

Diagnosis of Choledocholithiasis

Patients may have a history of gallstones or cholecystectomy and present with symptoms such as jaundice, dark urine (from conjugated bilirubin), light-colored stools (from not passing bile into the intestines), and upper abdominal pain. Fever and chills may indicate the development of cholangitis, which is an emergency.

Blood Tests:

- **Liver Function Tests (LFTs)** may show elevated bilirubin, alkaline phosphatase, and liver enzymes (AST and ALT).
- **Complete Blood Count (CBC)** may show an elevated white blood cell count, particularly if infection is present.

Imaging:

- **Transabdominal Ultrasound** is often the initial test; it can show dilated bile ducts and may identify stones.
- **Endoscopic Ultrasound (EUS)** is highly sensitive for detecting smaller stones and bile duct dilation.
- **Magnetic Resonance Cholangiopancreatography (MRCP)** is a non-invasive method to visualize the biliary and pancreatic ducts and is often used to confirm the diagnosis.
- **Endoscopic Retrograde Cholangiopancreatography (ERCP)** is both a diagnostic and therapeutic procedure used to identify and remove bile duct stones.

METHODS OF GALLBLADDER DRAINAGE

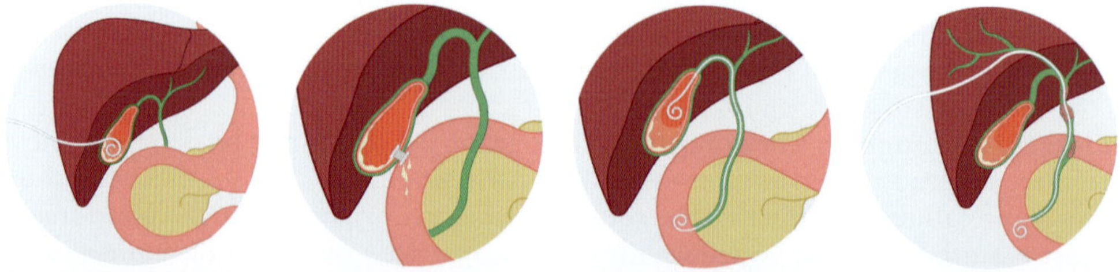

Figure 11-3

Treatment of Choledocholithiasis

Endoscopic Retrograde Cholangiopancreatography (ERCP) removes bile duct stones via an endoscope with instruments to extract stones or to place stents to bypass obstructions.

Lithotripsy, breaking up stones using shock waves, may be needed In cases where stones are too large to be removed by ERCP.

Cholecystectomy is typically done following successful ERCP to prevent recurrence.

Medical Therapy: While not typically a primary treatment for choledocholithiasis, medications may be used sometimes. *Ursodeoxycholic acid,* administered orally, can help dissolve small stones or fragments left after ERCP.

Surgical Intervention: If ERCP is not successful or not possible, a surgical bile duct exploration may be necessary.

Antibiotics are administered if there is evidence of infection of the bile ducts or if the patient is at high risk of developing an infection after procedures like ERCP.

Biliary Drainage (Fig. 11-3) is done if immediate stone removal is not possible, particularly in the setting of cholangitis. **Percutaneous transhepatic cholangiography (PTC)** may be used to better visualize the biliary tree so that a blockage can be decompressed by placing a catheter to drain bile externally. A stent can also be placed to keep a narrowed duct open (**Fig. 11-3**).

Cholangitis

Cholangitis is an inflammation of the bile duct system, usually caused by bacteria ascending from the duodenum. This condition often arises due to an obstruction, such as a bile duct stone, stricture, or tumor, which causes bile to stagnate and become infected.

The classic presentation of cholangitis is **Charcot's triad**, which consists of jaundice, right upper quadrant abdominal pain, and fever. If the patient also has hypotension and altered mental status, this is known as **Reynold's pentad** and indicates a more severe form of the disease, called **acute suppurative cholangitis.**

Diagnosis of Cholangitis

Blood Tests:

- **Liver Function Tests (LFTs)** typically reveal conjugated hyperbilirubinemia and elevated alkaline phosphatase, an enzyme found in the bile duct wall. Transaminases may be elevated but often to a lesser extent.
- **Inflammatory markers** include an elevated white blood cell count, C-reactive protein (CRP), and erythrocyte sedimentation rate (ESR).
- **Blood** cultures should be taken to identify the causative organism, although the culture may not always be positive.

Imaging:
Ultrasound is commonly the first imaging modality used; it can show biliary dilation and potential causes such as gallstones.

CT Scan can provide detailed images of the biliary tree and surrounding structures and identify the level and cause of obstruction.

Magnetic Resonance Cholangiopancreatography (MRCP) is non-invasive and shows highly detailed imaging of the biliary and pancreatic ducts.

Endoscopic Retrograde Cholangiopancreatography (ERCP) has both diagnostic and therapeutic roles. It can visualize the biliary tree and can remove stones or place stents.

Treatment of Cholangitis

Antibiotics: Immediate broad-spectrum antibiotics are required to cover gram-negative enteric organisms and anaerobes, which are common causes. The choice of antibiotic may later be refined based on culture results.

Biliary Drainage:
Endoscopic Retrograde Cholangiopancreatography (ERCP) is the preferred method for both diagnosing and managing the cause of obstruction.

Percutaneous Transhepatic Cholangiography (PTC): If ERCP is not possible or unsuccessful, PTC may be used for drainage.

Surgical Decompression is rarely used but may be necessary if less invasive methods fail or are not feasible.

Without prompt treatment, cholangitis can lead to sepsis, liver abscess, and multiple organ failure, which are serious and potentially life-threatening.

Gallbladder Polyps

Gallbladder polyps are growths that protrude from the inside lining of the gallbladder. They are usually benign. Most are asymptomatic, but large ones may be painful.

Diagnosis of Gallbladder Polyps

Ultrasound Examination is the most common and reliable method for detecting gallbladder polyps. Polyps are typically seen as immobile structures projecting from the gallbladder wall. The size of the polyp is an important factor in management. Polyps larger than 10 mm are at risk for future malignancy and often warrant closer investigation or cholecystectomy.

Endoscopic Ultrasound (EUS) can be used for more detailed imaging and assessment.

MRI or **MRCP (Magnetic Resonance Cholangiopancreatography)** may provide additional detail about the gallbladder and bile ducts.

Treatment of Gallbladder Polyps

Observation: Small polyps (< 10 mm) without suspicious features may be monitored with periodic ultrasounds.

Cholecystectomy is generally recommended for:

- Polyps larger than 10 mm due to the increased risk of gallbladder cancer
- Polyps that are symptomatic
- Polyps that show rapid growth on follow-up ultrasounds
- Patients with primary sclerosing cholangitis, as they have a higher risk of gallbladder cancer
- Patients with polyps and gallstones, especially if they have symptoms

Laparoscopic Cholecystectomy is the most common procedure for removing the gallbladder. It is minimally invasive and has a shorter recovery time compared to open surgery.

Open Cholecystectomy may be necessary in more complex cases or if unexpected complications arise during laparoscopic surgery.

Post-cholecystectomy, patients may need to adjust their diet, such as reducing fat intake to help manage digestion since the gallbladder's bile storage function is lost.

Gallbladder Cancer

Gallbladder cancer is relatively rare and often hard to diagnose early because the gallbladder is tucked beneath the liver, and early-stage cancer typically doesn't cause many specific symptoms. Symptoms may include jaundice, abdominal pain, nausea, vomiting, and weight loss. Physical examination may reveal gallbladder enlargement or signs of jaundice.

Diagnosis of Gallbladder Cancer

Blood Tests:

- Liver function tests check for signs of liver disease or biliary obstruction.
- Tumor markers (e.g., CA 19-9) may be elevated in some cases but are not specific for gallbladder cancer.

Imaging:

- **Ultrasound** is often the first test to image the gallbladder.
- **CT** (and **MRI**) provide more detailed images and can help assess the extent of the disease and whether it has spread.
- **MRCP** (Magnetic Resonance Cholangiopancreatography) is useful to visualize the bile ducts.

Endoscopic Examinations:

- **ERCP** (Endoscopic Retrograde Cholangiopancreatography) can provide detailed images of the biliary and pancreatic ducts.
- **EUS** (Endoscopic Ultrasound) can assess the gallbladder wall and surrounding tissue involvement.

Biopsy usually is needed for a definitive diagnosis.

Treatment of Gallbladder Cancer

Surgery: If diagnosed early, the main treatment is surgical removal of the gallbladder, often with some surrounding liver tissue and nearby lymph nodes (**radical cholecystectomy**). For more advanced disease, more extensive surgery may be required to remove additional liver tissue and other affected structures.

Chemotherapy can be used after surgery to kill any remaining cancer cells (adjuvant chemotherapy). For advanced or metastatic gallbladder cancer, chemotherapy may be the primary treatment to control the disease and symptoms.

Radiation Therapy is sometimes used in conjunction with chemotherapy after surgery to target any remaining cancer cells. Radiation can also be palliative, to relieve symptoms when the cancer is too advanced for surgery.

Targeted Therapy and Immunotherapy: In some cases, if the cancer has specific genetic changes, targeted therapy drugs may be an option.

Palliative Care: For advanced stages, treatment focuses on improving the quality of life and managing symptoms, which can include procedures to drain bile if the cancer is blocking the bile ducts.

Biliary Dyskinesia

Biliary dyskinesia is a functional gallbladder disorder characterized by biliary colic in the absence of gallstones, due to abnormal gallbladder motility. It's a diagnosis of exclusion, meaning it is typically diagnosed after other conditions have been ruled out.

Diagnosis of Biliary Dyskinesia

The patient experiences pain in the right upper quadrant of the abdomen, particularly related to fatty meals.

Blood Tests: Liver function tests are normal, which helps exclude other liver or bile duct diseases.

Imaging: Ultrasound is often performed to exclude gallstones or other gallbladder pathology.

Hepatobiliary iminodiacetic acid (HIDA) scan is a key diagnostic test for biliary dyskinesia. It measures gallbladder ejection fraction after administering a stimulant to gallbladder contraction, e.g., IV cholecystokinin, with a low ejection fraction (< 35-40%) suggesting biliary dyskinesia.

Endoscopy may be done to rule out other sources of abdominal pain, like peptic ulcer disease or gastroesophageal reflux disease.

Exclusion of Other Causes: Conditions like irritable bowel syndrome, pancreatitis, and chronic cholecystitis need to be excluded.

Treatment of Biliary Dyskinesia

Surgical: Cholecystectomy is the most common treatment if the patient's symptoms correlate with the results of the HIDA scan, and other causes have been ruled out. Laparoscopic cholecystectomy is the standard approach, offering a minimally invasive option with quicker recovery.

Dietary Modifications: Some patients might benefit from changes in diet, such as reducing fat intake to minimize symptoms.

Medications: While not typically used to treat biliary dyskinesia, some medications that improve bile flow, like *ursodeoxycholic acid*, or antispasmodic medications, might provide symptomatic relief in some cases. Pain management with appropriate analgesics may be administered while preparing for surgery.

Bile Duct Stricture

Bile duct stricture can obstruct bile flow from the liver into the intestine. Strictures can be benign or malignant and may be caused by a variety of conditions, including chronic pancreatitis, cholangitis, trauma, surgical complications, or cancer.

Diagnosis of Bile Duct Stricture

Symptoms may include jaundice, pruritus (itching), dark urine, pale stools, and abdominal pain.

Blood Tests: Liver function tests may show elevated bilirubin and alkaline phosphatase levels indicative of cholestasis.

Imaging:

- **Ultrasound** is often the initial imaging modality to detect bile duct dilation with the backup of bile from the stricture.
- **Magnetic Resonance Cholangiopancreatography (MRCP**) is a non-invasive method to delineate the biliary tree and identify strictures. An IV contrast material may be given to enhance visibility.
- **Endoscopic Retrograde Cholangiopancreatography (ERCP)** can provide detailed images and the opportunity to take biopsies, place stents, or perform balloon dilation.
- **CT** can provide more information about the surrounding structures and help in staging if cancer is a concern.
- **Percutaneous Transhepatic Cholangiography (PTC)** can be used to visualize the biliary tree, especially in cases where ERCP is not successful or contraindicated. A thin needle is inserted through the skin and liver directly into the bile ducts, where a contrast dye is injected that is identified by X-ray. This outlines the bile ducts within the liver and allows for the detection of obstructions, strictures, stones, or tumors in the bile ducts.

Biopsy may be necessary to determine if the stricture is benign or malignant.

Treatment of Bile Duct Strictures

Stent placement using ERCP can be used to relieve obstruction.

Balloon dilation of the stricture may also be performed during ERCP. In cases where ERCP is not feasible, percutaneous approaches can be used for stenting or dilation.

Surgical resection may be necessary, especially if the stricture is due to cancer. Biliary enteric bypass is an option for benign strictures not amenable to endoscopic or percutaneous interventions.

Liver transplantation might be an option in selected cases, especially if the stricture is part of a more diffuse liver disease, like primary sclerosing cholangitis.

Gallbladder Empyema

Gallbladder empyema is the accumulation of pus within the gallbladder. It is typically the result of an untreated or severe case of acute cholecystitis. The condition is serious and can be life-threatening if not treated quickly.

Diagnosis of Gallbladder Empyema

Patients often present with signs and symptoms of acute cholecystitis, which include severe right upper quadrant abdominal pain, fever, and leukocytosis. In the case of empyema, symptoms may be more pronounced, including chills and a toxic appearance.

Lab Tests: A complete blood count (CBC) often shows elevated white blood cells. Liver function tests (LFTs) may show abnormal liver enzymes and bilirubin levels.

Imaging: Ultrasound is typically the first-line imaging modality. Findings may include gallbladder wall thickening, distended gallbladder, and the presence of bright material within the gallbladder suggestive of pus. There may not be any stones, but bile flow may be reduced or absent. **CT scan** can be more sensitive in identifying the extent of inflammation, the presence of gallbladder wall thickening, pericholecystic fluid, and any complications like perforation.

Treatment of Gallbladder Empyema

Broad-spectrum antibiotics are initially given intravenously.

Surgical Intervention: Cholecystectomy is the definitive treatment for gallbladder empyema. This may be performed by laparoscope or by open surgery. A percutaneous cholecystostomy can also be performed. This procedure involves the placement of a drainage catheter into the gallbladder to drain the pus, which can help to stabilize the patient before surgery.

Biliary Fistula

A biliary fistula is an abnormal connection between the biliary system and another organ or the outside body.

Diagnosis of Biliary Fistula

Symptoms depend on the location and type of the fistula. Patients may experience jaundice, cholangitis, abdominal pain, or fecal changes. External fistulas may be evident due to the presence of bile drainage through the skin.

Lab Tests: Blood tests, including liver function tests, may show elevated bilirubin levels, elevated alkaline phosphatase, and signs of inflammation or infection.

Imaging:

Ultrasound can identify dilated bile ducts.

CT can provide details about the anatomy and the presence of complications such as abscesses.

Magnetic Resonance Cholangiopancreatography (MRCP) is a non-invasive way to visualize the biliary tree.

Endoscopic Retrograde Cholangiopancreatography (ERCP) is both diagnostic and therapeutic, allowing direct visualization of the biliary tree and the fistula as well as the ability to remove stones, insert stents, drain bile, or close off the fistula.

Hepatobiliary Iminodiacetic Acid (HIDA) Scan can sometimes identify biliary leaks by following the movement of IV injected radioactive material through the liver into the bile ducts, gallbladder, and intestine.

Treatment of Biliary Fistula

Conservative Management: Some biliary fistulas can close spontaneously, especially if they are small and there is no distal obstruction. This approach requires careful monitoring.

Endoscopic Therapy: For certain fistulas, ERCP can be used to place stents to redirect bile flow directly into the intestine rather than through the fistula, allowing the fistula to heal naturally. Sphincterotomy of the sphincter of Oddi or the placement of a nasobiliary drain can also be performed during ERCP. This is to increase the drainage of bile and relieve elevated pressure from blockage in the bile duct which may be causing the fistula.

Surgical: Surgery may be required to close the fistula and repair the bile ducts if the fistula does not heal with conservative management.

Biliary Atresia

Biliary atresia is a serious condition in infants where the bile ducts inside or outside the liver are scarred and blocked. Since bile can't flow into the intestine, bile builds up in the liver and can lead to liver damage.

Diagnosis of Biliary Atresia

The child typically presents within the first few weeks of life. Progressive jaundice, pale stools, and dark urine are common. Hepatomegaly and eventually splenomegaly due to portal hypertension may appear.

Blood Tests: Liver function tests typically show conjugated hyperbilirubinemia and elevated liver enzymes. Coagulation studies are important because the liver's ability to produce clotting factors may be deficient. Also, vitamin K absorption may be compromised due to a lack of bile in the intestines.

Abdominal Ultrasound is used to assess the liver and bile ducts and to rule out other causes of jaundice.

Hepatobiliary Iminodiacetic Acid (HIDA) Scan uses a radioactive tracer to see if bile is able to flow from the liver into the small intestine. In biliary atresia, there is little or no excretion of the tracer into the intestine.

Liver Biopsy shows characteristic bile duct proliferation, as the liver attempts to compensate for the obstruction; portal tract edema; and fibrosis.

Cholangiogram: An X-ray views contrast that has been directly placed into the bile ducts, either via endoscope or percutaneously injected into the liver and bile ducts to see if they are open or closed.

Treatment of Biliary Atresia

Kasai Procedure (Hepatoportoenterostomy): This surgery involves removing the damaged bile ducts outside the liver and attaching a loop of the small intestine directly to the liver to restore bile flow. It is ideally performed before the infant is 8 weeks old for the best outcomes. It is not a cure, and many children eventually need a liver transplant, which has a good success rate.

Gallstone Ileus

Gallstone ileus is a rare form of small bowel obstruction caused by a gallstone that has entered the gastrointestinal tract. This condition is most common in the elderly and can be life-threatening if not treated.

Diagnosis of Gallstone ileus

The patient has abdominal pain, vomiting, and sometimes a history of gallbladder disease. Physical examination may reveal signs of bowel obstruction, such as distention and hyperactive bowel sounds.

Imaging:

- **Abdominal X-ray** may show air in the biliary tree (**pneumobilia**), indicating a biliary-enteric fistula, along with evidence of intestinal obstruction.
- **CT** is the most sensitive imaging study for gallstone ileus; it can show the gallstone, the site of the obstruction, and air in the biliary tree.
- **Ultrasound** or **MRI** might be useful, but less so than CT for this condition.

Blood Tests typically include a CBC, serum electrolytes, renal function tests, liver function tests, and inflammatory markers.

Treatment of Gallstone ileus

Initial Management involves stabilization of the patient, which includes fluid resuscitation, correction of electrolyte imbalances, nasogastric decompression, and the administration of antibiotics if infection is suspected.

Surgical Intervention is the definitive treatment for gallstone ileus. The approach can vary based on the patient's condition, the location of the obstruction, and the surgeon's preference.

Enterolithotomy is the most common procedure, where the bowel is opened at the site of the obstruction and the stone is removed.

Fistula Repair: In some cases, the biliary-enteric fistula may also be repaired during the initial surgery, but in many cases, it may be managed conservatively due to the high surgical risk in these often elderly and frail patients.

Cholecystectomy is typically not performed during the initial surgery unless there are other indications, as it poses additional risks. It might be considered later once the patient has recovered from the acute illness.

Mirizzi's Syndrome

Mirizzi's syndrome is a rare condition characterized by compression of the common hepatic duct by a gallstone that is impacted in the cystic duct or neck of the gallbladder, leading to obstructive jaundice. It is classified into different types depending on the presence and extent of any associated cholecystobiliary fistula.

Diagnosis of Mirizzi's Syndrome

Symptoms may include jaundice, right upper quadrant abdominal pain, and sometimes fever or chills if cholangitis is present. Physical examination can show jaundice, and there is tenderness in the right upper quadrant.

Lab Tests: Liver function tests typically show elevated bilirubin and alkaline phosphatase levels. CBC may show leukocytosis if infection is present.

Imaging:

Ultrasound is usually the first imaging modality used, which can show dilation of the biliary tree and the presence of gallstones.

MRCP (Magnetic Resonance Cholangiopancreatography) is highly useful for defining the anatomy and identifying the level and cause of obstruction.

ERCP (Endoscopic Retrograde Cholangiopancreatography) can be both diagnostic and therapeutic. It provides detailed images of the biliary tree and can also be used to relieve obstruction.

CT is useful to evaluate the extent of the disease, especially if malignancy needs to be ruled out.

Treatment of Mirizzi's Syndrome

Endoscopic Treatment: ERCP may be used to remove the stone or place a stent to bypass the obstruction and treat jaundice. This is often temporary before definitive surgery.

Surgical Treatment: Surgery is the definitive treatment and can vary depending on the type of Mirizzi's syndrome and whether a cholecystobiliary fistula (a direct connection between the gallbladder and bile ducts) is present, which would make the surgery more complicated than just removing the stone.

Cholecystectomy may be done in cases without fistula and with a relatively intact gallbladder, often laparoscopically.

Bilioenteric anastomosis may be done if there is a fistula or the cystic duct is not identifiable. A more complex surgery such as a hepaticojejunostomy may be required to bypass the obstructed duct.

Open vs. Laparoscopic Surgery: Open surgery may be required in complex cases or if there is extensive inflammation and scarring. Laparoscopic surgery may be attempted in less severe cases.

Bile Duct Cancer

Symptoms of bile duct cancer (**cholangiocarcinoma**) can include jaundice, itching, dark urine, pale stools, abdominal pain, loss of appetite, weight loss, and fever. These symptoms often present late, making early diagnosis difficult.

Diagnosis of Bile Duct Cancer

Lab Tests:

Liver function tests may show elevated bilirubin levels, alkaline phosphatase, and gamma-glutamyl transferase (GGT).

Tumor markers such as CA 19-9 and CEA may be elevated but are not specific for bile duct cancer.

Imaging:

Ultrasound is often the first imaging test done to evaluate jaundice.

CT and **MRI** provide more detailed information about the location and extent of the cancer, and whether it has spread.

MRCP (Magnetic Resonance Cholangiopancreatography) is a non-invasive method to visualize the biliary and pancreatic ducts.

ERCP (Endoscopic Retrograde Cholangiopancreatography) can provide images and allow for biopsy and stent placement if needed.

Percutaneous Transhepatic Cholangiography (PTC) may be used if ERCP is not possible.

Biopsy confirms the diagnosis through cytology or histology, often obtained during ERCP or PTC.

Treatment of Bile Duct Cancer

Surgical Resection: The only potential cure for cholangiocarcinoma is complete surgical removal of the tumor. Depending on the tumor location, surgery may involve removing part of the bile duct, liver resection, or even a Whipple procedure (pancreatoduodenectomy) (**Fig. 11-4**).

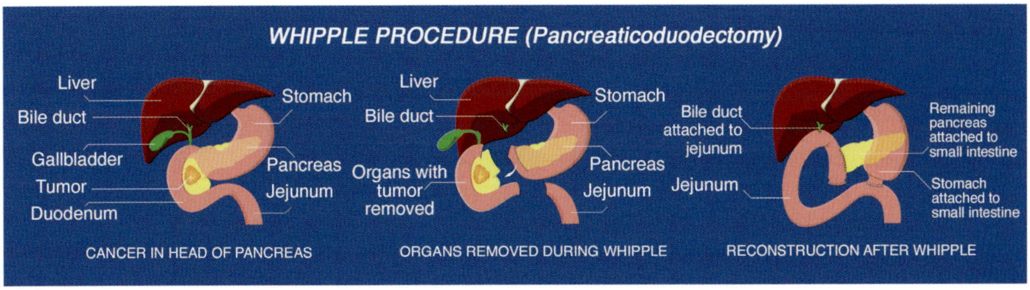

Figure 11-4

Liver Transplantation: In selected cases, particularly for perihilar cholangiocarcinomas (near the hepatic duct bifurcation – **Fig. 10-1**), liver transplantation may be an option following preoperative chemo- or radiotherapy to shrink the cancer.

Adjuvant Therapy: After surgery, adjuvant chemotherapy or chemoradiation may be recommended to reduce the risk of recurrence.

Palliative Treatments: For unresectable or metastatic cancers, palliative treatments aim to relieve symptoms and improve the quality of life. Endoscopic or percutaneous stenting can relieve bile duct obstruction and jaundice. Chemotherapy, targeted therapy, and radiation therapy can also be used to manage symptoms and control the spread of the disease. Some tumors may have specific mutations that can be targeted with newer drugs.

The prognosis for bile duct cancer is generally better if it is diagnosed early and surgically removed. Unfortunately, many patients are diagnosed at a later stage when the tumors are not resectable.

Bile Duct Cysts

Bile duct cysts (choledochal cysts) can be found anywhere in the bile duct pathways. They may be multiple. The patient can present with abdominal pain, jaundice, or a mass in the abdomen. There may be a history of pancreatitis or cholangitis.

Diagnosis of Bile Duct Cysts

Lab Tests: Liver function tests check for signs of jaundice or liver dysfunction. The CA 19-9 tumor marker may be elevated in some cases, as such cysts have the potential for malignant transformation.

Imaging:

- **Ultrasound** can detect the cysts.
- **CT**, **MRI**, **Magnetic Resonance Cholangiopancreatography (MRCP)**, or **Endoscopic Retrograde Cholangiopancreatography (ERCP)**, can provide more anatomical detail.

Histological Examination: If a surgical excision is performed, the cyst can be examined histologically to confirm the diagnosis and to check for malignancy.

Treatment of Bile Duct Cysts

Treatment often involves surgical intervention, especially due to the potential for malignancy. The specific treatment depends on the type of cyst and related symptoms:

Surgical Resection is the definitive treatment, whether by open surgery or laparoscopy. Surgical resection may include excision of the cyst and reconstruction of the biliary tract, often with a hepaticojejunostomy (anastomosis of the hepatic duct to the jejunum).

Drainage Procedures: In some cases, cysts may be drained internally or externally, but this is not a definitive treatment and is more palliative or temporary.

Endoscopic Treatments: ERCP can be used for stent placement or sphincterotomy to relieve obstruction in certain types of biliary dilation.

Management of Complications includes treatment of cholangitis, pancreatitis, or any malignancy that may arise in association with the cysts.

In rare cases with severe biliary disease, liver transplantation may be considered. The potential for malignant transformation in some biliary cysts necessitates careful long-term follow-up.

Ampullary Disease

"Ampullary disease" generally refer to conditions affecting the ampulla of Vater (**Fig. 10-2**), which is located where the bile duct and pancreatic duct join and empty into the duodenum. These diseases can impact both the gallbladder and the pancreas due to their shared pathway to the duodenum.

- **Ampullary Stones (Choledocholithiasis)** arise when gallstones, formed in the gallbladder, pass into the bile duct, and become lodged near the ampulla of Vater. This can block the flow of bile and pancreatic juice, leading to pain, jaundice, and pancreatitis.
- **Ampullary Stenosis** is the stricture of the ampulla of Vater, which can obstruct bile flow. This may result from chronic inflammation, post-surgical scarring, or other conditions.
- **Ampullary Tumors,** either benign or malignant, can develop in the ampulla of Vater. Ampullary cancer, although rare, can obstruct bile flow and is often associated with jaundice.
- **Cholangitis**, inflammation of the bile duct system, can involve the ampulla and often occurs due to bacterial infection that ascends from the duodenum.
- **Pancreatitis**: While pancreatitis is primarily a disease of the pancreas, blockage of the ampulla (such as by gallstones) can cause backflow of pancreatic enzymes, leading to inflammation of the pancreas.

Diagnosis of ampullary diseases often involves imaging studies like ultrasound, CT scans, MRI, or more specifically MRCP (Magnetic Resonance Cholangiopancreatography). Endoscopic procedures, such as ERCP (Endoscopic Retrograde Cholangiopancreatography), are not only diagnostic but can also be therapeutic, allowing for the removal of stones, biopsy of tumors, or dilation of strictures. Depending on the condition, ***treatment*** may include endoscopic procedures, medication, or surgery.

12

Diseases of the Pancreas

The pancreas produces digestive enzymes to help break down food in the small intestine but also produces hormones, such as insulin and glucagon, to regulate blood sugar levels. Diseases and conditions affecting the pancreas can have significant impacts on digestion and metabolism. Normally, digestive enzymes are secreted in an inactive state so that they don't digest the pancreas.

The main pancreatic duct usually joins with the common bile duct to form the **ampulla of Vater**, a small enlargement that opens into the duodenum at the **major duodenal papilla** (**Fig. 10-2**). An accessory pancreatic duct (**Duct of Santorini**), which is not always present, connects the pancreas to the duodenum through a **minor duodenal papilla (papilla of Santorini)** (**Fig. 10-2**) The **sphincter of Oddi** is a muscular valve that surrounds the ampulla of Vater and helps control the flow of bile and pancreatic juice into the intestine. It also prevents the contents of the duodenum from backflowing into the bile and pancreatic ducts.

Pancreatitis

Pancreatitis can be acute, occurring suddenly and lasting days, or chronic, occurring over many years, and may have many causes, apart from alcohol. Stones in the common bile duct or pancreatic duct can block flow from the pancreatic duct, as can pancreatic cancer and sticky mucus from cystic fibrosis, causing pancreatitis. Pancreatitis can result from premature activation of pancreatic digestive enzymes, which then autodigest the pancreas; this can occur in trauma and other conditions, such as hypercalcemia (the mechanism in hypercalcemia may in part relate to calcium depositing as stones in the pancreatic duct). There are also some medications that can cause pancreatitis, e.g., certain diuretics, antibiotics, and chemotherapy drugs. Sometimes, the cause is not found.

Diagnosis of Pancreatitis

Acute pancreatitis typically presents with a sudden onset of severe, constant upper abdominal pain, not relieved by a change in position, and often radiating to the back. The pain may be associated with nausea and vomiting, fever, and jaundice. There may be a **Grey Turner's sign** (bruising of the flank on one or both sides from retroperitoneal hemorrhage) or **Cullen's sign** (bruising around the navel from intraperitoneal hemorrhage). There may also be dehydration, decreased urine output, increased hematocrit, hypotension, respiratory distress, metabolic acidosis, and kidney failure.

Chronic pancreatitis may present similarly but also may include weight loss and diabetes due to the loss of endocrine function of the pancreas, as well as steatorrhea (fatty stools) from lipase deficiency and malabsorption of fat. Chronic pancreatitis is considered a risk factor for development of pancreatic adenocarcinoma.

Lab Tests: Blood tests in acute pancreatitis show elevated levels of pancreatic enzymes - amylase and lipase. Liver function tests may also be affected, especially if the bile duct is involved. In chronic pancreatitis, amylase and lipase are less likely to be elevated due to damage to the pancreas that decreases its ability to synthesize these enzymes; fecal tests may show fat malabsorption due to deficits in digestive enzymes, particularly lipase.

Imaging:

Plain abdominal X-ray may show calcifications suggestive of chronic pancreatitis. Plain films may also show a "sentinel loop," i.e., a dilated portion of small intestine suggesting an ileus (an area of poor intestinal contraction). Sometimes, calcified stones may be seen in the gallbladder or common bile duct,

CT Scan is often used to diagnose acute pancreatitis and its complications.

MRI/MRCP (magnetic resonance cholangiopancreatography) can provide detailed images of the gallbladder, bile duct, pancreas and pancreatic duct.

Endoscopic Ultrasound (EUS) is used for detailed imaging and sometimes for biopsy of the pancreas, where a fine needle is passed from the endoscope through the wall of the duodenum or stomach into the pancreas for biopsy samples.

ERCP (Endoscopic Retrograde Cholangiopancreatography): Can be diagnostic and therapeutic if there is an associated bile duct obstruction.

Treatment of Pancreatitis

Acute Pancreatitis: Initial treatment is supportive and includes pain management and fasting to rest the pancreas. Intravenous fluids prevent dehydration. Nutritional support is often with a nasogastric feeding tube if the pancreatitis is severe or prolonged and the patient cannot tolerate oral food.

Chronic Pancreatitis: Treatment includes pain management by nerve block or medication, pancreatic enzyme supplements to aid digestion, dietary changes, and management of diabetes if present. Other measures include abstinence from alcohol and smoking and alteration of medication if drug-induced pancreatitis is suspected. Treatment may include removal of pancreatic duct stones, correction of strictures by endoscopy or surgery, relief of pressure on an obstructed pancreatic duct, removal of selected areas of chronic pancreatitis, or total pancreatectomy. If the pancreas is removed, a pancreatic islet cell autotransplant may be done to ensure a continuing supply of insulin.

Endoscopic Treatments: ERCP may be used to remove bile duct stones, dilate narrowed ducts, or stent strictures.

Surgical Treatment: Sometimes it is necessary to drain fluid collections or remove damaged tissue. In chronic pancreatitis, surgery might also be required to relieve a blocked pancreatic duct or to resect part of the pancreas.

Antibiotics may be used that penetrate the pancreas wall (e.g., *imipenem, meropenem, fluoroquinolones*) to deal with potential infection in a necrotic pancreas.

Management of Complications: Acute complications such as pseudocysts (a fluid-filled sac in the abdomen containing pancreatic enzymes, blood, and necrotic tissue) or abscesses, may require drainage. Chronic measures might include the treatment of chronic pain or surgical management of pancreatic duct strictures.

Diet and Lifestyle Modifications: Dietary changes include low-fat meals to reduce the workload on the pancreas. In chronic cases, cessation of alcohol and smoking is essential. Small, frequent meals may be recommended for chronic pancreatitis.

Pancreatic Cancer

Pancreatic cancer is one of the most difficult cancers to treat, partly because it often goes undetected until it is advanced. Risk factors include age > 45 (most over 65), smoking, chronic pancreatitis, type 2 diabetes, family history, genetic syndromes, e.g., Lynch syndrome (colonic polyposis), ataxia telangiectasia (unsteady coordination + red spider veins on the skin), heavy alcohol use, exposure to toxic chemicals, chronic infections in the area, race, and gender (African Americans have a slightly higher incidence; males are affected somewhat more than females).

Diagnosis of Pancreatic Cancer

Symptoms may include pain in the upper abdomen that radiates to the back, loss of appetite, weight loss, jaundice, light-colored stools, dark urine, and new-onset diabetes. A tumor of the head of the pancreas can compress and obstruct the distal common bile duct.

Blood Tests: While there are no specific blood tests to diagnose pancreatic cancer, certain markers like CA 19-9 can be elevated. Liver function tests can also be abnormal if the cancer blocks the bile ducts.

Imaging:

- **CT Scan** is often the first imaging test done, providing detailed cross-sectional images of the pancreas.
- **MRI/MRCP (Magnetic Resonance Cholangiopancreatography)**. The latter is a specialized type of magnetic resonance imaging (MRI) that can show detailed images of the pancreas and surrounding structures.
- **Endoscopic Ultrasound (EUS)** can provide images inside the abdomen and is often used to guide needle biopsies.
- **Positron Emission Tomography (PET) Scan** can help show if cancer has spread to other parts of the body.

- **ERCP (Endoscopic Retrograde Cholangiopancreatography)** is used to take images of the bile and pancreatic ducts and can help in diagnosing and relieving obstructions.

Biopsy: The definitive diagnosis is usually made by a biopsy, which can be done during EUS, ERCP, or through a needle inserted into the tumor during a CT or ultrasound-guided procedure.

Treatment of Pancreatic Cancer

Surgery is the only potentially curative treatment, but only a small percentage of patients are candidates due to the advanced stage at diagnosis. Types of surgery may include a Whipple procedure (pancreaticoduodenectomy, **Fig. 11-4**), distal pancreatectomy, or total pancreatectomy, depending on the tumor's location and size.

Chemotherapy: Chemotherapy may be given before surgery (**neoadjuvant therapy**) to shrink the tumor, after surgery (**adjuvant therapy**) to eliminate microscopic disease, or as the main treatment if the cancer is advanced.

Radiation Therapy may be used in combination with chemotherapy either before surgery to shrink the tumor or after to kill any remaining cancer cells.

Targeted Therapy: For certain genetic mutations in pancreatic cancer, targeted therapies can be used that specifically attack those cancer cells.

Immunotherapy: Currently, immunotherapy is not widely used for pancreatic cancer but may be an option for some patients, especially those with certain genetic changes that may make tumors more responsive to immunomodulatory therapies.

Palliative Care is critical for managing symptoms and maintaining quality of life, including pain management, nutritional support, and managing jaundice with stenting or bypass surgery if the bile duct is blocked.

Pancreatic Cysts

Some pancreatic cysts are benign, while others can become cancerous. The diagnosis and treatment of pancreatic cysts often depend on the type of cyst and the risk of it becoming malignant.

Diagnosis of Pancreatic Cysts

Many pancreatic cysts are asymptomatic and are found incidentally on imaging for other reasons. When symptoms do occur, they may include abdominal pain, nausea, vomiting, or jaundice.

Imaging:

- **CT Scan** provides detailed cross-sectional images and can identify cysts.
- **Magnetic Resonance Imaging (MRI)**, including MRCP (Magnetic Resonance Cholangiopancreatography), can provide detailed images of ducts.
- **Endoscopic Ultrasound (EUS)** allows for close examination of the cyst and is often used to guide fine-needle aspiration (FNA) for fluid and tissue sampling.

Lab Tests: Analysis of cyst fluid obtained through EUS-FNA can check for cancer cells, infection, and chemical markers, like amylase or CEA (carcinoembryonic antigen). The finding of amylase would suggest a connection between the cyst and the pancreatic ductal system, often the result of (non-neoplastic) pancreatitis. The finding of CEA raises suspicion of a neoplasm. CEA level in the fluid can help differentiate between mucinous cysts (which can be precancerous and have elevated CEA levels) and serous cysts (which are usually benign). DNA analysis of cyst fluid can detect mutations associated with malignancy.

Treatment of Pancreatic Cysts

Many cysts, especially small and asymptomatic ones, can be monitored with periodic imaging to check for changes in size or characteristics.

Surgical removal is considered if the cyst is large, causes symptoms, or has characteristics suggestive of cancer or a high risk of becoming cancerous. Types of surgery include:

- **Cystectomy:** Removal of the cyst
- **Partial Pancreatectomy:** Removal of part of the pancreas
- **Whipple Procedure (Fig. 11-4)** if the cyst is in the head of the pancreas

Endoscopic Treatment may include endoscopic drainage or stenting for certain cysts. In some cases, cysts may be treated with ethanol or other sclerosing agents to reduce the size and symptoms.

Pancreatic Insufficiency

Pancreatic insufficiency is a condition where the pancreas does not produce enough of the enzymes necessary to digest food properly, leading to malabsorption and a range of digestive symptoms. It often occurs with chronic pancreatitis, cystic fibrosis, pancreatic cancer, or surgery that affects the pancreas.

Diagnosis of Pancreatic Insufficiency

Symptoms may include weight loss, steatorrhea, abdominal pain, and diarrhea.

The **Fecal Elastase Test** is a stool test that measures the amount of elastase, an enzyme produced by the pancreas. Low levels indicate pancreatic insufficiency.

The **Fecal Fat Test** determines the amount of fat in the stool. Excessive fat can indicate malabsorption of fat due to pancreatic enzyme insufficiency.

Blood tests can check for nutritional deficiencies that may result from malabsorption (such as fat-soluble vitamins A, D, E, and K).

Imaging tests such as CT, MRI, or endoscopic ultrasound can look for structural abnormalities of the pancreas.

Pancreatic Function tests that measure bicarbonate and enzyme production can be performed during endoscopy, but are rarely used today.

Treatment of Pancreatic Insufficiency

Pancreatic Enzyme Replacement Therapy (PERT): Oral pancreatic enzymes are taken with meals and snacks to aid in the digestion and absorption of nutrients.

Dietary Changes may include a high-calorie, high nutrient diet that is low in fiber, for easier digestion.

Fat-Soluble Vitamin Supplementation: Vitamins A, D, E, and K may need to be supplemented due to malabsorption.

Management of Diabetes: Pancreatic insufficiency can lead to diabetes due to the loss of insulin-producing cells. Blood sugar monitoring and insulin therapy may be necessary.

Pain Management is important, particularly if chronic pancreatitis is the underlying cause.

Avoidance of Alcohol and Smoking: These can exacerbate pancreatic damage.

Treatment of Underlying Causes: Addressing conditions like chronic pancreatitis, cystic fibrosis, or obstruction may improve pancreatic function.

Pancreatic Stones

Pancreatic stones (pancreatic calculi) are often associated with chronic pancreatitis. They can block the flow of pancreatic digestive enzymes and cause abdominal pain or exacerbate the symptoms of pancreatitis.

Diagnosis of Pancreatic Stones

Imaging:

- **Abdominal Ultrasound** can detect larger stones within the pancreatic duct.
- **CT** can provide detailed images and help to determine the exact location and size of the stones.
- **Magnetic Resonance Cholangiopancreatography (MRCP)** can visualize the pancreatic ducts and detect stones non-invasively.
- **Endoscopic Ultrasound (EUS)** is highly sensitive for detecting pancreatic stones and can also be used to guide therapeutic procedures.
- **Endoscopic Retrograde Cholangiopancreatography (ERCP)** can provide diagnostic information and is used to remove stones.

Lab Tests:

- **Blood Tests** check for signs of infection, inflammation, or elevated pancreatic enzymes.
- **Stool Tests** measure the levels of fat and could indicate the pancreas isn't releasing enough digestive enzymes.

Treatment of Pancreatic Stones

Conservative Management:

- **Pain management** is often necessary to manage the abdominal pain associated with pancreatic stones.
- **Dietary change** to a low-fat diet can help reduce symptoms.
- **Pancreatic enzyme supplements** can aid digestion if the stones are inhibiting enzyme flow.
- **ERCP with sphincterotomy** can help remove stones and debris from the pancreatic duct.
- **Extracorporeal Shock Wave Lithotripsy (ESWL)** uses high-energy sound waves to break up stones into smaller pieces that can pass through the duct more easily.

Surgical Treatment:

- **Pancreaticojejunostomy (Puestow Procedure):** Surgery drains the dilated pancreatic duct into the small intestine
- **Pancreatectomy:** Partial or total removal of the pancreas may be necessary in severe cases.
- **Stenting:** Placing a stent in the pancreatic duct can help keep it open and allow stones to pass.

Pancreatic Neuroendocrine Tumors (PNETS)

Pancreatic neuroendocrine tumors (PNETs) arise from pancreatic endocrine cells. They can be hormone-producing or non-functional and can be benign or malignant.

Diagnosis of Pancreatic Neuroendocrine Tumors

Symptoms depend on whether the tumor is functional (causing hormone-related symptoms) or non-functional (often asymptomatic until they grow large and cause pain or jaundice).

Hormone Level Measurement includes blood and urine tests for hormone levels, such as gastrin, insulin, glucagon, VIP (vasoactive intestinal peptide), and chromogranin A (a marker for neuroendocrine tumors).

Imaging Tests include CT scan, MRI, or ultrasound to visualize the tumor.

- **Endoscopic Ultrasound (EUS)** is particularly useful for smaller tumors.
- **Somatostatin Receptor Scintigraphy (Octreoscan)** or **PET** scans with Gallium-68 DOTATATE can detect PNETs based on their expression of somatostatin receptors.

Biopsy can confirm the diagnosis.

Genetic Testing may be recommended for hereditary syndromes associated with PNETs (like Multiple Endocrine Neoplasia type 1).

Treatment of Pancreatic Neuroendocrine Tumors

Surgery is the main treatment for PNETs, aiming to remove the tumor completely. This can be a Whipple procedure, distal pancreatectomy, or local removal, depending on the tumor's location and size.

Medical Therapy: For functional tumors, somatostatin analogs like *octreotide* or *lanreotide* can control hormone overproduction and symptoms. Targeted therapies such as *sunitinib* or *everolimus* are used for advanced PNETs.

Peptide Receptor Radionuclide Therapy (PRRT) is a targeted therapy using radioactive somatostatin analogs to deliver radiation directly to the tumor cells.

Chemotherapy may be recommended for more aggressive or advanced PNETs, although these tumors are often less responsive to traditional chemotherapy.

Hormone Management might be necessary to manage hormone-induced symptoms.

Embolization or **Ablation** techniques may be employed for liver metastases. These procedures involve cutting off the blood supply to the tumor (embolization) or directly destroying tumor cells by radiofrequency ablation (RFA) or cryoablation, where a cryoprobe or RFA probe is passed through the skin into the liver tumors under CT or ultrasound guidance.

Pancreatic Pseudocysts

Pancreatic pseudocysts are fluid collections that can occur inside or outside the pancreas after an episode of acute pancreatitis, chronic pancreatitis, or abdominal trauma. They are not true cysts as they lack an epithelial lining.

Diagnosis of Pancreatic Pseudocysts

Patients may be asymptomatic or present with abdominal pain, bloating, nausea, vomiting, or even jaundice if the cyst is compressing the common bile duct.

Blood tests may show elevated amylase and lipase levels, indicative of pancreatitis.

Imaging:

- Abdominal ultrasound can help detect fluid collections.
- CT scan is more sensitive and can assess the size and location of the cysts.
- Magnetic resonance imaging (MRI) or magnetic resonance cholangiopancreatography (MRCP) may be used for further evaluation.

Aspiration: Fluid aspiration under imaging guidance can help rule out infection or malignant cysts by analyzing the fluid's chemical makeup, cytology, and amylase content.

Treatment of Pancreatic Pseudocysts

Small, asymptomatic pseudocysts without any complications can be managed conservatively with observation, as they often resolve on their own.

Endoscopic Management: Endoscopic ultrasound-guided fine-needle aspiration (EUS-FNA) for drainage is preferred for pseudocysts that are causing symptoms or complications.

Stenting: Endoscopic placement of a stent allows continuous drainage of the pseudocyst into the stomach or small intestine.

Percutaneous Catheter Drainage: A drainage catheter that drains to the skin may be placed into the pseudocyst from outside the body, guided by imaging.

Surgical Drainage is indicated if the pseudocyst is not amenable to less invasive treatments or if there are complications like infection, hemorrhage, or rupture. Options for drainage include cystogastrostomy (connecting the cyst to the stomach), cystoduodenostomy (connecting the cyst to the duodenum), or cystojejunostomy (connecting the cyst to the jejunum).

Laparoscopic Surgery is a less invasive option than open surgery for drainage or cyst removal.

Antibiotics are given if needed.

Cystic Fibrosis

Cystic fibrosis (CF) is a genetic disorder that primarily affects the lungs and pancreas due to the production of abnormally thick and sticky mucus. It is caused by mutations in the cystic fibrosis **transmembrane conductance regulator (CFTR)** gene, of which there are over 2,000 known mutations, resulting in variations on the severity of the disease.

Diagnosis of Cystic Fibrosis

Newborn Screening: Most developed countries include CF in their newborn screening programs, where a blood test is used to check for elevated levels of immunoreactive trypsinogen (IRT), which can indicate CF.

Sweat Chloride Test is the gold standard for CF diagnosis. It measures the amount of chloride in sweat. A high level (greater than 60 millimoles per liter) typically confirms the diagnosis.

Genetic Testing: DNA tests can identify mutations in the CFTR gene.

Prenatal Testing can be done on the parents, placenta or amniotic fluid for families with a known history of CF.

Additional Tests: Chest X-rays, lung function tests, sputum cultures, fecal fat tests, and measurements of pancreatic function may be used to evaluate organ involvement and disease progression.

Treatment of Cystic Fibrosis

Airway Clearance: Techniques to clear mucus from the lungs are fundamental, including chest physiotherapy, exercise, and devices that help with mucus clearance.

Medications:

- **CFTR Modulators** are drugs that target the defective CFTR protein to improve its function. The use of these drugs depends on the specific mutation that a patient has.
- **Bronchodilators**
- **Mucolytics** such as *dornase alfa* thin the mucus.
- **Antibiotics** are used to treat and prevent lung infections.
- **Anti-inflammatory drugs** can reduce lung inflammation.

Pulmonary Rehabilitation: A structured exercise and education program is designed to improve the well-being of people with chronic respiratory diseases.

Nutritional Support includes a high-calorie diet, pancreatic enzyme replacement therapy to aid digestion, fat-soluble vitamin supplements, and nutritional supplements.

Hereditary Pancreatitis

Hereditary pancreatitis is a genetic, usually autosomal dominant, condition characterized by recurrent episodes of pancreatitis. It is often associated with mutations in the PRSS1 gene, which encodes for trypsinogen, an inactive form of the enzyme trypsin that can become prematurely activated with the mutation. This can result in autodigestion of the pancreas. There is increased risk of developing pancreatic cancer later in life.

Diagnosis of Hereditary Pancreatitis

Recurrent episodes of acute pancreatitis without obvious precipitating factors (e.g., alcohol, smoking, certain medications) can suggest hereditary pancreatitis, especially if they begin in childhood.

There may be a family history. Since the condition is autosomal dominant, the child has a 50% chance of inheriting it. Family counseling is often recommended.

Genetic Testing can identify mutations in genes such as PRSS1, SPINK1, CFTR, or CTRC that are associated with hereditary pancreatitis.

Imaging: CT, MRI, or endoscopic ultrasound (EUS) are used to assess the structure of the pancreas.

Functional Tests like fecal elastase (low) or serum trypsinogen (often elevated due to gene mutations) can evaluate the exocrine function of the pancreas.

Treatment of Hereditary Pancreatitis

Hospitalization may be necessary for severe cases of acute pancreatitis, with intravenous fluids, pain management, and nutritional support. Chronic pain may be managed with analgesics, nerve blocks, or endoscopic therapies to remove any blockages.

Pancreatic Enzyme Replacement Therapy (PERT) can be used to treat malabsorption due to exocrine pancreatic insufficiency.

Diet: A low-fat diet is often recommended, along with small, frequent meals to reduce the metabolic load on the pancreas.

Pancreas Divisum

Pancreas divisum is a common congenital anomaly of the pancreatic ducts where the dorsal and ventral pancreatic ducts fail to fuse during embryological development (**Fig. 12-1**). This condition can lead to pancreatic fluid outflow obstruction when the

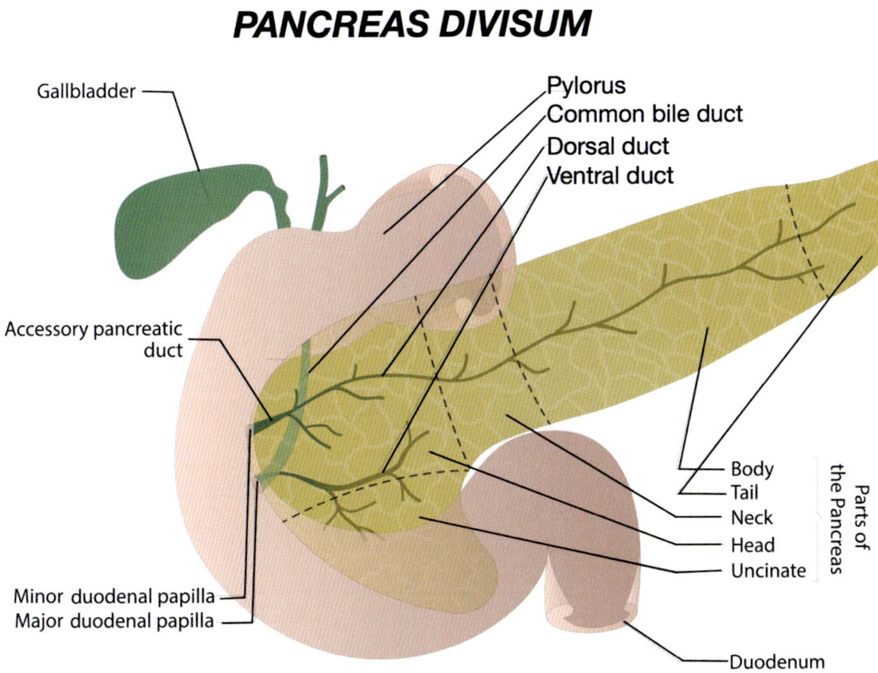

Figure 12-1

majority of pancreatic secretions drain through the smaller and less efficient minor papilla, which can sometimes be associated with pancreatitis.

Diagnosis of Pancreas Divisum

Many individuals with pancreas divisum are asymptomatic. However, it can be associated with recurrent episodes of pancreatitis.

Imaging: Magnetic Resonance Cholangiopancreatography (MRCP) can show the separate pancreatic duct systems. **Endoscopic ultrasound** can provide detailed images of the pancreas and can be used if MRCP is inconclusive. **Endoscopic Retrograde Cholangiopancreatography (ERCP)**, although more invasive, is considered the gold standard for diagnosing pancreas divisum since it can directly visualize the ductal anatomy and allow for therapeutic intervention.

Secretin Stimulation Test: During MRCP or ERCP, secretin, which stimulates pancreatic secretion, can be administered to enhance the visualization of pancreatic fluid secretion and ductal anatomy. The secretin stimulation results in a disproportionately large amount of pancreatic juice coming out of the minor papilla into the duodenum.

Treatment of Pancreas Divisum

Treatment for pancreas divisum is generally only recommended if the patient is symptomatic, typically with recurrent pancreatitis.

Endoscopic Therapy:

- **Minor papillotomy**: Cutting of the minor papilla (the accessory pancreatic duct entrance to the duodenum) eliminates blockage and improves ductal drainage.
- **Stenting** of the dorsal pancreatic duct can facilitate drainage if the duct is too narrow.

Surgical Intervention: If endoscopic therapy fails, surgical minor papillotomy or pancreaticojejunostomy may be considered to improve pancreatic fluid flow.

Pain Management: Analgesics may be used to manage abdominal pain associated with pancreatitis.

Annular Pancreas

Annular pancreas is a rare congenital anomaly where a ring of pancreatic tissue surrounds the second part of the duodenum. This can cause duodenal obstruction.

Diagnosis of Annular Pancreas

In infants, it can present with feeding intolerance, vomiting (often with bile), and failure to thrive. In adults, symptoms may include abdominal pain, nausea, vomiting, and signs of intestinal obstruction or pancreatitis.

Abdominal Ultrasound may suggest the diagnosis in neonates with duodenal obstruction.

CT Scan can show the ring of pancreatic tissue surrounding the duodenum.

Magnetic Resonance Imaging (MRI)/Magnetic Resonance Cholangiopancreatography (MRCP) can provide detailed images.

Upper Gastrointestinal Series: An X-ray examination with contrast may show a characteristic "windsock" deformity caused by the annular pancreas.

Endoscopy can directly visualize the narrowing of the duodenal lumen and may also be useful for ruling out other causes of obstruction.

Treatment of Annular Pancreas

The treatment depends on the severity of the symptoms and the presence of complications, such as obstruction. Without symptoms, some cases of annular pancreas may be discovered incidentally and may not require treatment.

Surgical Intervention: The mainstay of treatment for symptomatic annular pancreas is surgery. The specific procedure depends on the patient's anatomy and symptoms.

- **Duodenoduodenostomy** or **Duodenojejunostomy** bypasses the obstructed segment of the duodenum by creating a new connection to a downstream part of the intestine.
- **Web Excision:** If there is a duodenal web, excision may relieve obstruction-

Pancreatoduodenectomy (Whipple Procedure, Fig. 11-4): In very rare cases with complicated or malignancy-associated annular pancreas, more extensive surgery might be required.

Since annular pancreas can be associated with other congenital anomalies, a thorough evaluation is often necessary.

Pancreatic Trauma

Pancreatic trauma is a rare but potentially life-threatening injury, often resulting from blunt abdominal trauma or penetrating wounds. The pancreas is a deep-seated organ, so it is less commonly injured compared to other abdominal organs. However, its location near major blood vessels and other vital structures can make pancreatic injuries serious.

Diagnosis of Pancreatic Trauma

Patients may present with abdominal pain, tenderness, or signs of peritonitis. Back pain is also a potential symptom due to the retroperitoneal location of the pancreas. Elevated serum amylase and lipase levels may indicate pancreatic injury but are not definitive.

Imaging:

CT is the gold standard for diagnosing pancreatic trauma. It can reveal the extent of the injury, including lacerations, contusions, injuries of the pancreatic duct, and the presence of fluid collections.

MRI or **Magnetic Resonance Cholangiopancreatography (MRCP)** can be used to assess ductal injuries if not clearly seen on CT.

Focused Assessment with Sonography for Trauma (FAST): This rapid bedside ultrasound examination is used to detect free intraperitoneal fluid but is not specific for pancreatic injury.

Diagnostic Peritoneal Lavage (DPL) is rarely used, but it can detect blood in the abdominal cavity.

Endoscopic Retrograde Cholangiopancreatography (ERCP) is both a diagnostic procedure and a potentially therapeutic one that can place stents in a damaged pancreatic duct to prevent pancreatic juice leakage.

Treatment of Pancreatic Trauma

Non-operative Management is usually reserved for minor injuries without ductal involvement. It Includes bowel rest, nutritional support (often with total parenteral nutrition or enteral feeding distal to the injury), and close monitoring for complications.

Surgical Intervention is indicated for major injuries, especially those with ductal involvement or if the patient has other injuries requiring surgery. Surgery may involve drainage through placement of drains near the injury, or distal pancreatectomy if the injury is to the body or tail of the pancreas. **Pancreaticoduodenectomy (Whipple Procedure) (Fig. 11-4)** may be suggested for complex injuries involving the head of the pancreas, although this procedure is rarely done for pancreatic trauma, due to high morbidity.

ERCP with Stent Placement across the injury can allow it to heal without the need for surgery.

Pancreatic Ascariasis

Pancreatic ascariasis is an infection of the pancreas by the roundworm *Ascaris lumbricoides*. This condition can occur when the parasitic larvae or adult worms migrate from the small intestine to the pancreatic duct. It can cause acute pancreatitis and is more common in tropical and subtropical areas where ascaris infection is endemic.

Diagnosis of Pancreatic Ascariasis

Symptoms may include abdominal pain, nausea, vomiting, and signs of acute pancreatitis. There may be a history of passage of worms in the stool or vomit.

Lab Tests:

- Elevated serum amylase and lipase levels may indicate pancreatitis.
- CBC may show eosinophilia, which is common in parasitic infections.
- Stool examination may reveal ascaris eggs.

Imaging:

Ultrasonography (USG) can visualize worms in the bile duct or pancreatic duct as echogenic, non-shadowing (like a cyst), linear or curved structures with or without associated dilation of the ducts.

CT or **MRI** may show dilated pancreatic ducts and can occasionally visualize the worm itself.

Treatment of Pancreatic Ascariasis

Endoscopic Retrograde Cholangiopancreatography (ERCP): While primarily therapeutic in relieving obstruction, ERCP can also be diagnostic as it may visualize worms within the ducts. It may also be used to extract an obstructing worm.

Anthelmintic medication, e.g., *albendazole* or *mebendazole*, is administered to kill the worms.

Autoimmune Pancreatitis

Autoimmune pancreatitis (AIP) is a form of chronic dysfunctional pancreatitis that is thought to be caused by an autoimmune response. It is characterized by the swelling and inflammation of the pancreas. There are two types of AIP: Type 1, which is more common and is part of a disease called IgG4-related disease, and Type 2, which is less common and not associated with IgG4.

Diagnosis of Autoimmune Pancreatitis

Patients may present with jaundice, abdominal pain, weight loss, and new-onset diabetes. Some may have no symptoms and AIP is discovered incidentally through imaging.

Lab Tests: Elevated serum IgG4 levels are often found in Type 1 AIP but are not specific and can be elevated in other conditions. Elevated levels of IgG, as well as the presence of autoantibodies (such as ANA, RF), can be indicative. Type 2 AIP is not associated with IgG4 and does not have a specific serologic test.

Imaging:

- **CT** and **MRI** may show a diffusely enlarged pancreas with a "sausage-like" appearance, a delayed and gradual enhancement, and a rim-like capsule.
- **Endoscopic Ultrasound (EUS)** is useful for imaging and for obtaining tissue for biopsy.
- **Endoscopic Retrograde Cholangiopancreatography (ERCP)** may show diffuse or segmental narrowing of the pancreatic duct in a "sausage-like" appearance due to alternating strictures and dilatations.

Histology: A biopsy showing lymphoplasmacytic sclerosing pancreatitis with obliterative phlebitis and storiform (whorled) fibrosis suggests Type 1 AIP. Type 2 AIP is characterized by granulocytic epithelial lesions (GELs).

Other Diagnostic Criteria: The **HISORt** criteria (**H**istology, **I**maging, **S**erology, **O**ther organ involvement, **R**esponse to therapy) can be used for diagnosis. AIP responds to corticosteroids; pancreatic cancer does not.

Treatment of Autoimmune Pancreatitis

Corticosteroids (*prednisone* or *prednisolone*) are the first-line treatment for AIP, which often results in rapid improvement of symptoms and imaging abnormalities.

Immunomodulators: For those who relapse upon tapering steroids, immunomodulators such as *azathioprine*, *6-mercaptopurine*, or *mycophenolate mofetil* may be used.

Biologic Agents: *Rituximab*, an anti-CD20 monoclonal antibody, has been used in cases resistant to steroids and immunomodulators, particularly in Type 1 AIP.

Biliary stents may be needed if there is concurrent biliary obstruction. Pancreatic enzyme supplements may be used in case of exocrine insufficiency.

Glossary

Achalasia: Loss of coordinated muscle contractions in the esophagus and failure of the lower esophageal sphincter to relax due to degeneration of nerves supplying the esophagus, resulting in difficulty swallowing (dysphagia)
ALP: Alkaline phosphatase
ALT: Alanine aminotransferase
Anorexia: Loss of appetite
Ascites: Fluid collection in the abdominal cavity
Bariatric surgery: Weight loss surgery
Biliary atresia: Congenital absence or closure of the bile ducts
Biologics: Drugs manufactured from biological sources
Bulimia: Episodes of binge eating followed by compensatory behaviors like self-induced vomiting, excess exercise, or laxative abuse to prevent weight gain
Capsule endoscopy: Endoscopy using a small wireless camera that travels through and views the GI tract, particularly the small intestine
Cholangiocarcinoma: Cancer of the bile duct
Cholangiogram: Imaging of the bile ducts with X-ray and contrast
Cholangitis: Inflammation of the bile ducts
Cholecystectomy: Removal of the gallbladder
Cholecystitis: Inflammation of the gallbladder
Cholecystotomy: Opening the gallbladder, e.g., to remove stones or remove pus
Choledocholithiasis: Stones in the common bile duct
Cholelithiasis: Gallstones
Cholestasis: Decreased bile flow
Colon: Large intestine
CPK: Creatine phosphokinase
CRP: C-Reactive Protein
CT: Computerized Tomography
Diverticulitis: Inflammation of one or more diverticula in the lining of the digestive system, particularly the colon
Diverticulosis: Small bulging pouches (diverticula), particularly in the colon, without inflammation
Dyspepsia: Indigestion. Burning, over-fullness and bloating after eating
Dysphagia: Difficulty swallowing
Endoscope: An instrument that can be introduced into the body to view its internal parts
Endoscopic Retrograde Cholangiopancreatography (ERCP): A technique that combines endoscopy and fluoroscopy to diagnose and treat certain problems of the biliary or pancreatic ductal systems
Endoscopic Ultrasound (EUS): A technique combining endoscopy with ultrasound to obtain images of internal organs or their adjacent structures
Endoscopy: Use of an endoscope to examine the interior surfaces of an organ or tissue.
Enteroscopy: A form of endoscopy that examines the small intestine
ERCP: Endoscopic retrograde cholangiopancreatography

ESR: Erythrocyte Sedimentation Rate
EUS: Endoscopic Ultrasound
Exudates: Cells or other cellular substances with relatively high protein content in often cloudy fluid that leaks from blood vessels, usually from inflamed tissues (as opposed to transudates).
Functional disorder: One where no structural of biochemical abnormalities are found to account for the symptoms
Gastric: Related to the stomach
Gastritis: Inflammation of the stomach lining
Gastroenteritis: Inflammation of the stomach and intestines
Gastroparesis: Delayed gastric emptying, often seen in diabetes
GERD: gastroesophageal reflux disease
GGT: Gamma-glutamyl transferase
GI: Gastrointestinal
Hematochezia: Bright red blood in the stools from lower GI bleeding
Hepatitis: Inflammation of the liver
Hepatobiliary Iminodiacetic Acid (HIDA) Scan: A scan that follows the movement of IV injected radioactive material through the liver into the bile ducts, gallbladder, and intestine
HIDA Scan: Hepatobiliary Iminodiacetic Acid Scan
IBD: Inflammatory Bowel Disease (Crohn's disease or ulcerative colitis)
IBS: Irritable Bowel Syndrome
Ileostomy: An opening on the abdomen to divert waste from the ileum into an ostomy bag
Ileus: Inability of the bowel to contract
Immunotherapy: Cancer treatment that enhances the body's immune response to cancer cells
Inflammatory Bowel Disease (IBD): Crohn's disease or ulcerative colitis
INR: International Normalized Ratio, a standardized way of measuring how long it takes for blood to clot, used to monitor patients on anticoagulants
Intussusception: Telescoping of part of the intestine (usually small intestine) into itself
Irritable Bowel Syndrome (IBS): A condition marked by abdominal pain, bloating, and altered bowel habits, without an identifiable underlying organic cause
Laparoscopy: A surgical procedure where a fiber-optic instrument is inserted through the abdominal wall to view or operate inside the abdominal cavity
Laparotomy: Surgical incision through the abdominal wall to access the abdominal cavity
Leukocytosis: High white blood cell count
LFTs: Liver Function Tests
Lithotripsy: A technique for breaking up kidney, gallbladder, or other stones using ultrasound shock waves
Magnetic Resonance Cholangiopancreatography (MRCP): An imaging technique that uses magnetic resonance imaging to visualize the biliary and pancreatic ducts non-invasively
Melena: Black, tarry stools from upper GI bleeding
Mesenteric ischemia: Inadequate blood supply to the small intestine
Microbiome: The collective genomes of microorganisms that live inside the body
MRCP: Magnetic resonance cholangiopancreatography
Necrosis: Tissue death from disease or injury

Pancreatitis: Inflammation of the pancreas

Paracentesis: Withdrawal of ascitic fluid via needle or catheter passed through the abdominal wall into the peritoneal cavity

PCR: Polymerase Chain Reaction

Percutaneous transhepatic cholangiography (PTC): A contrast dye is injected through the skin into the bile ducts inside the liver, and X-rays are taken for better visualization of the biliary duct tree.

Peristalsis: Muscular wave-like movement that propels food through the digestive tract

Peritoneal cavity: The space between the inner lining of the abdominal wall and the outer lining of the abdominal viscera

Phlebitis: Inflammation of a vein

Porphyria: A group of rare hereditary disorders resulting from abnormal heme production, leading to the accumulation of porphyrins or porphyrin precursors, which may cause various symptoms, including diffuse abdominal pain

PSC: Primary Sclerosing Cholangitis

Pyelonephritis: Infection (typically bacterial) and inflammation of the kidney

Sclerosing: Hardening and thickening of tissue, often from chronic inflammation or disease

Sphincterotomy: Cutting of a sphincter muscle

Steatohepatitis: Inflammation of the liver with fat accumulation in liver cells

Steatorrhea: Fatty stools

Steatosis: Fatty liver

Stoma: Surgical exteriorization of the small bowel (ileostomy) or large bowel (colostomy) through the anterior abdominal wall

Targeted therapy: Cancer treatment that targets specific molecules in cancer cells

Toxic megacolon: Rapid swelling of the colon often associated with inflammatory bowel disease or infection

Transudates: Thin, clear, watery fluids with usually low protein content that leak through blood vessels, often cause by increased hydrostatic pressure or decreased oncotic pressure (e.g., heart failure, cirrhosis, hypoalbuminemia), as opposed to exudates.

Volvulus: Obstruction of the small or large intestine from abnormal twisting on itself

Index

Bayesian Machine Learning in Quantitative Finance

Wilson Tsakane Mongwe · Rendani Mbuvha ·
Tshilidzi Marwala

Bayesian Machine Learning in Quantitative Finance

Theory and Practical Applications

palgrave
macmillan

Wilson Tsakane Mongwe
Department of Electrical
and Electronic Engineering
University of Johannesburg
Johannesburg, South Africa

Rendani Mbuvha
School of Statistics and Actuarial
Science
University of Witwatersrand
Johannesburg, South Africa

Tshilidzi Marwala
United Nations University
Tokyo, Japan

ISBN 978-3-031-88430-6 ISBN 978-3-031-88431-3 (eBook)
https://doi.org/10.1007/978-3-031-88431-3

This Palgrave Macmillan imprint is published by the registered company Springer Nature Switzerland AG
The registered company address is: Gewerbestrasse 11, 6330 Cham, Switzerland

Wilson Tsakane Mongwe dedicates this book in loving memory of his mother
Monica Mmanyedi Mongwe

Preface

The finance landscape has undergone a transformative evolution, marked by the integration of sophisticated mathematical models and advanced computational techniques. Among these, Bayesian machine learning has emerged as a powerful tool, enabling practitioners to navigate the complexities of financial markets with enhanced precision and insight. This book, *Bayesian Machine Learning in Quantitative Finance: Theory and Practical Applications*, is a comprehensive guide designed to bridge the gap between theoretical foundations and practical implementations in the dynamic field of quantitative finance.

The application of Bayesian methods in finance is not new. Bayesian inference, emphasizing probability and uncertainty, naturally aligns with the stochastic nature of financial markets. However, recent advancements in machine learning have propelled Bayesian techniques to new heights, allowing for more nuanced and adaptive models that can respond to the ever-changing financial landscape. This book aims to elucidate these advancements, providing a robust framework for understanding and applying Bayesian machine learning in various financial contexts.

This book firstly delves into the theoretical underpinnings of Bayesian statistics and machine learning. We begin with a detailed exploration of Bayesian inference, discussing its principles, advantages, and how it differs from traditional frequentist approaches. This section also covers critical concepts such as prior and posterior distributions, likelihood functions, variational inference, and Markov Chain Monte Carlo methods, including advanced techniques like Hamiltonian Monte Carlo and Shadow Hybrid Monte Carlo, providing readers with a solid foundation in Bayesian theory. The Bayesian framework allows us to naturally answer questions, such as: (1) How can we explain the prediction or output of the models?, (2) What is the distribution of the parameters of the model?, (3) How do we select between the different models in a statistically principled manner?, and (4) Which inputs are most relevant for the task at hand?

The book secondly focuses on the practical applications of Bayesian machine learning in quantitative finance. Here, we explore how Bayesian methods can be applied to analyze sell-side investment analyst reports, volatility surface analysis, recovery rate modeling on defaulted loans, credit rating models for corporations, municipal financial management, option pricing, yield curve modeling, and motor insurance claim modeling. Each chapter presents real-world examples and case studies demonstrating the effectiveness of Bayesian approaches in addressing complex financial problems. We also provide detailed code implementations, allowing readers to experiment with and extend the models discussed.

We also look toward the future, examining emerging trends and potential developments in Bayesian machine learning and their implications for quantitative finance. Topics such as Bayesian deep learning, normalizing flows, and distributed Gaussian processes are discussed, offering a glimpse into the cutting-edge research and innovations that will shape the field's future.

This book is intended for a diverse audience, including finance professionals, quantitative analysts, researchers, and students. A background in statistics and machine learning will be helpful, but we have endeavored to make the material accessible to those with varying levels of expertise. Each chapter builds progressively, with clear explanations and practical insights designed to facilitate a deep understanding of Bayesian machine learning and its applications in finance.

In writing this book, our goal has been to create a resource that is both informative and inspiring. We hope to equip our readers with the knowledge and tools necessary to leverage Bayesian machine learning in their own work, driving innovation and excellence in quantitative finance. As you embark on this journey through the following pages, we invite you to explore the fascinating intersection of Bayesian methods and financial theory and discover the immense potential within.

Johannesburg, South Africa	Wilson Tsakane Mongwe
London, UK	Rendani Mbuvha
Tokyo, Japan	Tshilidzi Marwala
June 2025	

Acknowledgements Wilson Tsakane Mongwe thanks his wife, Gavaza, and his children, Vuthlari, Vutivi, and Vumbhoni, who have been very supportive and patient through the highs and lows of producing this book. Last but not the least, he would like to thank the all-mighty God who has ordered his steps throughout this journey. All the glory be to God. It is all by the grace of God!

All the authors want to acknowledge the Center for High-Performance Computing (CHPC) at the Council of Scientific and Industrial Research (CSIR) South Africa for providing them with the resources that they used to perform the computations in this book.

Competing Interests The authors have no competing interests to declare that are relevant to the content of this manuscript.

Contents

About the Authors

Wilson Tsakane Mongwe was born in Tembisa (Gauteng, South Africa) and matriculated from Bankuna High School in 2008, where he was the overall second-best-performing learner in the Limpopo Province. He holds a B.Sc. in Computing from the University of South Africa (cum laude), B.Bus.Sci. in Actuarial Science from the University of Cape Town (with a distinction in Statistics and class medals for 2nd and 3rd-year Statistics modules), a Masters in Mathematical Finance from the University of Cape Town (the degree and dissertation with distinction) and a Ph.D. in Artificial Intelligence (specializing in Bayesian machine learning) from the University of Johannesburg. He received a Google Ph.D. fellowship in machine learning, which supported his Ph.D. research. He received the Mail and Guardian Top 200 Young South Africans for 2020 and was recognized as one of 30 Young Mandela's in 2022 by News24. Wilson is passionate about human capacity development and supervises honors, master's, and Ph.D. research projects at the intersection of machine learning and quantitative finance. He has authored over twenty intentional conference and journal machine learning research papers. He is the author of a Bayesian machine learning book entitled "Hamiltonian Monte Carlo Methods In Machine Learning" published by Academic Press (Elsevier) in March 2023. He is a leader in financial services and has experience in the banking and insurance sectors. Wilson is currently an Associate Director and the Head Quantitative Analyst at a Big Four audit firm's Financial Services Advisory business unit and was previously the Head Of Market Risk And Capital Analytics at a tier 1 South African bank's Global Markets division. His research interests include computational finance, Bayesian machine learning, and Markov Chain Monte Carlo algorithms.

Rendani Mbuvha born in Venda (Limpopo, South Africa), is an Associate Professor of Actuarial Science at the University of Manchester. He was the DeepMind Academic Fellow in Machine Learning at Queen Mary University of London. He is a Fellow of the Institute of Faculty of Actuaries and a holder of the Chartered Enterprise Risk Actuary designation. He holds a B.Sc. with Honours in Actuarial Science and Statistics from the University of Cape Town and an M.Sc. in Machine Learning from KTH, Royal Institute of Technology in Sweden. He is a recipient of the Google Ph.D. fellowship in machine learning which supported his Ph.D. research at the University of Johannesburg. Rendani is an Honorary Senior Research Associate in Computer Science at University College London and a visiting associate professor at the University of Witwatersrand.

Tshilidzi Marwala who was born in Venda, South Africa, is a distinguished artificial intelligence (AI) engineer, academic leader, and author, currently serving as the Rector of the United Nations University and a UN Under-Secretary-General. Known for his contributions to AI applications in engineering, economics, and education. Marwala has consistently championed the integration of advanced technologies to address pressing global challenges. As the Principal of the University of Johannesburg, he spearheaded initiatives that positioned AI at the core of academia and innovation, fostering its use for societal benefit. He has written over 25 books on AI, leadership, and the Fourth Industrial Revolution, advancing discourse on the transformative potential of technology. Marwala earned a Ph.D. in AI from the University of Cambridge, a Master's in Mechanical Engineering from the University of Pretoria, and a Bachelor of Science in Mechanical Engineering with magna cum laude from Case Western Reserve University. An advocate for responsible AI development, his expertise and impact have earned him fellowships in the American Academy of Arts and Sciences, the Chinese Academy of Sciences, and the African Academy of Sciences.

Abbreviations

AGSA	Auditor General South Africa
AI	Artificial Intelligence
ANN	Artificial Neural Network
ARD	Automatic Relevance Determination
ARD-NS	Automatic Relevance Determination Nelson and Siegel
ATM	At The Money
AUC	Area Under The Receiver Operating Curve
BNN	Bayesian Neural Network
EAD	Exposure AT Default
ECB	European Central Bank
ESS	Effective Sample Size
GLM	Generalized Linear Model
GP	Gaussian Processes
HMC	Hamiltonian Monte Carlo
JDP	Jump-Diffusion Process
JSE	Johannesburg Stock Exchange
LA	Laplace Approximation
LGD	Loss Given Default
MALA	Metropolis Adjusted Langevin Algorithm
MCMC	Markov Chain Monte Carlo
MH	Metropolis-Hastings
MHMC	Magnetic Hamiltonian Monte Carlo
MLR	Multinomial Logistic Regression
MSE	Mean Square Error
NPL	Non-Performing Loans
NS	Nelson and Siegel

NUTS	No-U-Turn Sampler
PD	Probability of Default
PoE	Product of Experts
RMHMC	Riemannian Manifold Hamiltonian Monte Carlo
ROC	Receiver Operating Curve
S2HMC	Separable Shadow Hamiltonian Hybrid Monte Carlo
SABR	Stochastic Alpha Beta Rho
SVM	Support Vector Machine
VI	Variational Inference

List of Figures

List of Tables

List of Algorithms

CHAPTER 1

Introduction to Bayesian Machine Learning in Quantitative Finance

1.1 Introduction

The fourth industrial revolution is driven by a confluence of technologies such as artificial intelligence and cyber-physical systems (Xing & Marwala, 2017). A subset of artificial intelligence known as machine learning has been instrumental in driving breakthroughs in the fourth industrial revolution. These machine learning methods are based on learning input-output mappings using data, with the most popular machine learning techniques being those based on neural networks. Machine learning has impacted all fields, such as autonomous driving, energy, climate, and vision, and finance is no exception (Marwala et al., 2023). A subset of finance known as quantitative finance has successfully used machine learning technologies.

Quantitative finance is a cross-discipline field that integrates finance with tools from computer science, physics, statistics, and mathematics (Sidogi, 2023). Quantitative methods are used to solve real-world finance problems in this quantitative finance domain. These quantitative methods are typically founded in economic theory, with many models being parsimonious and readily interpretable to practitioners (Heston, 1993). Quantitative finance methods have applications that range from asset management to banking, insurance, derivative modeling, and general risk

W. T. Mongwe et al., *Bayesian Machine Learning in Quantitative Finance*, https://doi.org/10.1007/978-3-031-88431-3_1

and financial management. Broadly, these fields can be split into sell-side (where product structures are constructed) as well as the buy-side (where the constructed product structures are consumed). This book explores each of these domains.

In the derivative modeling domain, quantitative methods were introduced by Louis Bachelier in his PhD thesis—which became the foundation of modern-day mathematical finance (Bachelier, 1900; Choi et al., 2022). In his work, Bachelier modeled changes in asset prices with Brownian motions and preceded the work of Albert Einstein (Bachelier, 1900; Choi et al., 2022). The main disadvantage of the Bachelier model was that it allowed for negative values for the variable being modeled, but it has recently become popular since the low interest-rate environment has introduced the possibility of negative interest rates (Choi et al., 2022). The breakthrough in quantitative finance came through the Black and Scholes (1973) model, which has become the standard for pricing and risk management of options—a consequence of which is that the Bachelier model has been forgotten as a part of history until recently (Choi et al., 2022). The Black and Scholes (1973) framework has numerous assumptions, the key of which is that volatility is constant throughout the life of the option. It assumes that there is no market skew or term structure of volatility. The crises of 1989 resulted in a volatility skew forming in the market, rendering the assumptions of Black and Scholes (1973) invalid. This has resulted in an explosion of models that aim to capture the skew, such as the Heston stochastic volatility model and jump-diffusion processes, among others (Kou, 2007; Heston, 1993; Mongwe et al., 2022). In recent times, there has also been an increase in the exploration of using data-driven approaches in derivative pricing and risk management within the literature (Buehler et al., 2019; Mikkilä & Kanniainen, 2023; Wiese et al., 2020). A key result has been the deep hedging work of Buehler et al. (2019), which showed that deep learning could be utilized to hedge options successfully. Other studies that use machine learning include those that utilize machine learning in the pricing of instruments, calibrating more exotic models such as rough stochastic volatility models, and synthetic data generation through generative adversarial networks (Horvath et al. 2021; Ruf & Wang 2019; Sidogi et al. 2022a; Wiese et al. 2020). However, most of the approaches in the literature produce point estimates with little exploration of Bayesian methods, which naturally encapsulate uncertainties in estimates and the calibrated model parameters.

A critical decision that individuals and institutions must make is the optimal capital allocation between various assets. This is commonly referred to as portfolio theory, with one of the founding fathers being Markowitz (1991). Furthermore, Sharpe (1964) and Lintner (1975) introduced the capital asset pricing model (CAPM), which can be used for the estimation of the cost of capital for firms and for evaluating the performance of managed portfolios. Fama and French (2004) later introduced their factor models, which have become the cornerstone of fundamental investing. Machine learning has also been used within portfolio theory. Wang and Chen (2023) utilize a dynamic CAPM model incorporating machine learning to measure systematic risk in the Chinese market with success, with various authors exploring portfolio optimization using machine learning. Sidogi et al. (2022b) use machine learning to combine analysts' sell-side forecasts to improve the bidirectional accuracy of sell-side forecasts. Rough path theory combined with traditional machine learning techniques has also enhanced the directional accuracy of forecasting stock prices using limit order book data (Sidogi et al., 2023). These results show that data-driven approaches can enhance and transform portfolio and risk management.

Banks have often utilized traditional statistical techniques to understand the risk involved in granting loans and to model the amounts recoverable from loan accounts that have already defaulted (Hlongwane et al., 2024, 2024a). Loan default modeling in retail credit is traditionally tackled using logistic regression in practice (Hlongwane et al., 2024). This is mainly driven by regulations requiring that the models used in the granting of credit should be easy to explain to customers as to why they were not granted credit, for example (Hlongwane et al., 2024, 2024a). Recently, machine learning techniques have been explored for this task, including tree-based methods such as random forests and boosted methods such as XGBoost (Hlongwane et al., 2024, 2024a). However, the uptake of more complex models, such as neural networks within banking, has been low due to the black-box nature of these models. Furthermore, once loans have defaulted, banks have traditionally used Beta regression and zero-inflated versions to model the recoveries on defaulted loans (Bellotti & Crook, 2012; Hoechstoetter et al., 2012; Loang et al., 2023; Ye & Bellotti, 2019). Credit risk assessment is not limited to retail credit but also incorporates ratings of corporations—and this amounts to modeling the credit ratings of these corporations. Rating agencies like Moodys and S&P have pioneered techniques for rating sovereigns and corporations (Wallis et al., 2019). However, alternative approaches have been explored, given the costs of obtaining these ratings—which involve experts working through company records. Various machine learning techniques, such as trees and neural networks, have been successfully explored for this task (Hajek & Michalak, 2013; Huang et al., 2004; Muñoz Izquierdo et al., 2022; Wallis et al., 2019).

Sound financial management within organizations is crucial for the organization's sustainable future. Lapses in economic management are entrenched in public institutions in South Africa, with the Auditor General of South Africa uncovering these year after year (Auditor-General South Africa, 2011, 2023). In addition, manipulations of the financial accounts of listed entities have led to millions of dollars being lost at local and international stock exchanges (Bratton, 2001; Moepya et al., 2014a). Prominent examples include the scandals of Enron, Wirecard, Steinhoff, and Tongaard-Hullet, which have brought to the fore the rampant management fraud that is being perpetrated across the world (Bratton, 2001; Cotterill, 2018; Donnelly, 2018; Mongwe & Malan, 2020a; O'Donnel, 2020). The ability of stakeholders to model and detect fraud or poor audit outcomes is crucial. Furthermore, being able to detect the presence of irregular, unauthorized, or overlapping unlawful expenditures in public entities would provide further insight into the sources of these acts and how to prevent them best. Accurately modeling audit outcomes and unlawful expenditures would allow auditors to perform better risk ratings and deploy resources more efficiently (Mabelane et al., 2023; Marwala et al., 2023; Mongwe & Malan, 2020a, 2020b; Mongwe et al., 2021). Given the increase in financial and alternative data, machine learning techniques are prime to be used for these tasks. Within the context of modeling audit opinions, various studies have successfully utilized logistic regression, support vector machines, Naïve Bayes classifiers, and neural networks in multiple jurisdictions worldwide (Kim et al., 2020; Kirkos et al., 2007; Moepya et al., 2014a, 2014b). On the other hand, very few studies have been conducted on using machine learning to model unlawful expenditures (Sikhosana, 2021). This is still an open area of research.

Insurance is an effective risk transfer mechanism. The policyholder transfers the risk from exposure to an insurable risk factor to the insurer for a fee. Various types of insurance coverage exist, including life and non-life insurance. Machine learning techniques have been utilized in this insurance domain to address limitations of data (Ngwenduna & Mbuvha,

2021), to model mortality (Bjerre, 2022), to enhance motor claim predictions (Poufinas et al., 2023), and to reduce risk in weather index insurance (Eltazarov et al., 2023), among others. These studies show the inherent potential of utilizing machine learning methods to understand better and mitigate the impact of various risk factors covered by insurance.

Advancements in artificial intelligence, led by increased data and computing power, have led to the growth of data-driven pricing and risk management models in finance. The explosion of machine learning in quantitative finance has raised several questions, such as: How can we explain the prediction or output of the models? What is the distribution of the parameters of the model? How do we select between the different models in a statistically principled manner? Which inputs are most relevant to the task at hand? This book aims to provide a potential framework that can be used to answer these questions within quantitative finance. The framework that we explore in this book to answer these questions is the Bayesian inference framework. The Bayesian framework is based on Bayes theorem, which describes how our prior beliefs are updated by new information through the likelihood, with the product of the prior distribution and the likelihood being normalized by the Bayesian evidence. These components of the Bayes theorem provide a mechanism to answer the questions highlighted above in this way: The posterior

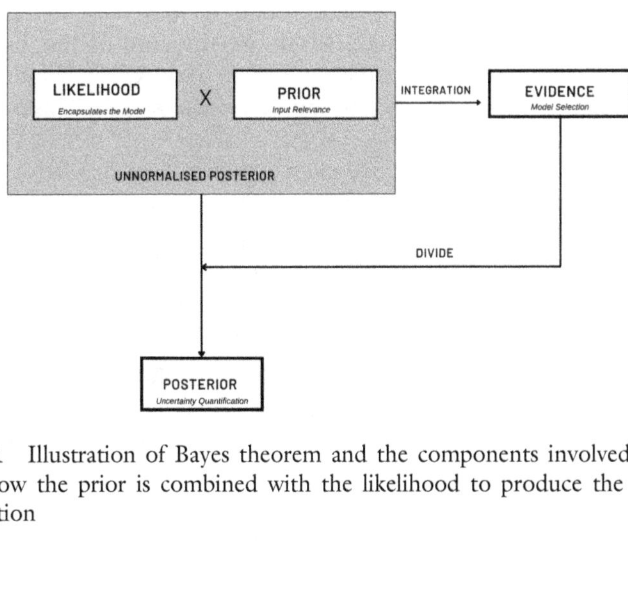

Fig. 1.1 Illustration of Bayes theorem and the components involved. It illustrates how the prior is combined with the likelihood to produce the posterior distribution

captures the distribution of the parameters and the distribution of the predictions/outputs. The likelihood encapsulates the model and considers new data as it becomes available. The prior provides a means of automatically determining which input variables are essential for the task at hand, making the results more accessible to stakeholders and non-experts. Finally, the Bayesian evidence metric can be used to compare and select between different models, which is very important as there is a proliferation of data-driven models within the quantitative finance space. The components of the Bayes theorem are illustrated in Fig. 1.1, where we also show how these components can assist us in answering the questions highlighted above.

This book covers the theory and related applications of this Bayesian framework to various quantitative finance problems. The aim is to highlight its utility in solving multiple quantitative finance tasks while indicating its potential benefits and drawbacks.

1.2 Themes of the Book

This book covers the theory and applications of the Bayesian framework in quantitative finance. The themes covered in this book are shown in Fig. 1.2 and are discussed in more detail below:

1. We start by providing a background to Bayesian inference and Bayesian machine learning , which are the core of this book. We discuss the variational inference and Markov Chain Monte Carlo techniques that can be used to train Bayesian models. This is covered in **Chapter** 2.
2. We explore utilizing the Bayesian framework in derivative pricing, model calibration, and volatility surface modeling. This has the benefit of providing confidence bands, distribution of the calibrated parameters, and no requirements for external arbitrage conditions to be added to the loss for option pricing. This ***derivative modeling*** theme is covered in the following chapters:
    - **Chapter** 3: On the Stochastic Alpha Beta Rho Model and Hamiltonian Monte Carlo Techniques.
    - **Chapter** 4: Learning Equity Volatility Surfaces Using Sparse Gaussian Processes.

   - **Chapter** 5: Analyzing South African Equity Option Prices Using Normalizing Flows.

3. We utilize the Bayesian framework for financial management. We consider topics important for banks, such as predicting a corporation's credit rating and modeling recoveries on defaulted loans. We then consider municipal financial management and provide a framework for selecting models for audit outcome prediction and for detecting unauthorized expenditure in South African municipalities. This *financial management* theme is covered in the following chapters:
   - **Chapter** 6: Sparse and Distributed Gaussian Processes for Modeling Corporate Credit Ratings.
   - **Chapter** 7: Bayesian Detection of Recovery on Charged-Off Loan Accounts.
   - **Chapter** 8: Bayesian Audit Outcome Model Selection Using Normalizing Flows.
   - **Chapter** 9: Bayesian Detection Of Unauthorized Expenditure Using Langevin and Hamiltonian Monte Carlo.
4. We then consider applications of the Bayesian framework in the insurance and investments space. We use Bayesian inference to infer motor insurance claims, calibrate yield curve models, and introduce the Bayesian sell-side investment analyst. This *insurance and investments* theme is covered in the following chapters:
   - **Chapter** 10: Bayesian Neural Network Inference of Motor Insurance Claims.
   - **Chapter** 11: Shadow and Adaptive Hamiltonian Monte Carlo Methods For Calibrating the Nelson and Siegel Model.
   - **Chapter** 12: Static and Dynamic Nested Sampling for Yield Curve Model Selection.
   - **Chapter** 13: A Bayesian Investment Analyst on the Johannesburg Stock Exchange.

As each theme is tackled, we emphasize the theoretical and practical elements to be considered—with the associated samples of the code used

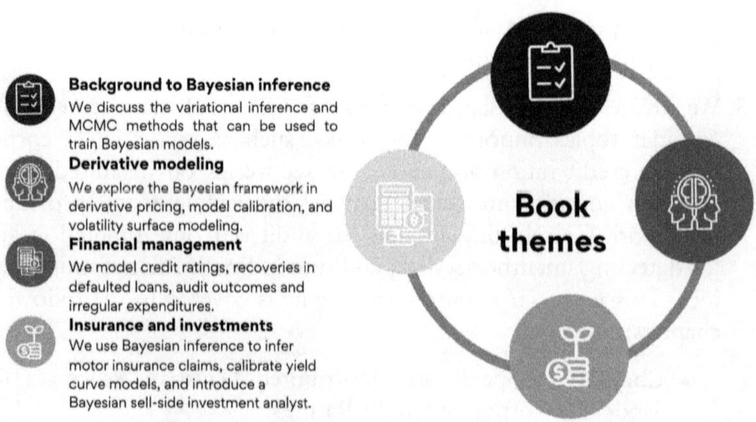

Fig. 1.2 Summary of the main themes covered in this book being the (1) background to Bayesian inference, (2) derivative modeling, (3) financial management, and (4) insurance and investments

to generate the results for each chapter also provided. The book is carefully structured, allowing each chapter to be read in isolation. This design feature allows readers to focus on specific topics of interest, while the main dependencies are on the background chapters, which lay the foundation for the book.

1.3 Conclusion

This chapter laid the foundation for the remainder of the book. We explored the various fields of quantitative finance that this book covers. Furthermore, we introduced the Bayesian framework, which is used in this book to answer questions such as: How can we explain the prediction or output of the models? What is the distribution of the parameters of the model? How do we select between the different models in a statistically principled manner? Which inputs are most relevant to the task at hand? This book aims to utilize the Bayesian inference framework to answer these questions within the quantitative finance domain.

The next chapter provides an overview of Bayesian methods used to train machine learning models, such as variational inference and Markov Chain Monte Carlo. We also discuss the associated performance metrics for these inference techniques and the metrics we use to assess the performance of the models and algorithms used in later chapters of the book.

References

Auditor-General South Africa (2011). *Background to the three aspects we audit.* https://www.agsa.co.za/portals/0/AGSA_Terminology.pdf. Last Retrieved: 16 August 2020.

Auditor-General South Africa (2023). *Consololidated general report on local government audit outcomes - mfma 2021-22.* https://mfma-2022.agsareports.co.za/report/mfma_report_2021_22_final_31_may_2023.pdf. Last Retrieved: 16 November 2023.

Bachelier, L (1900). *Th é orie de la Sp é culation Annales Scientifiques de l'Ecole Normale Sup é rieure S é r.*

Bellotti, T., & Crook, J. (2012). Loss given default models incorporating macroeconomic variables for credit cards. *International Journal of Forecasting, 28*(1), 171–182.

Bjerre, D. S. (2022). Tree-based machine learning methods for modeling and forecasting mortality. *ASTIN Bulletin: The Journal of the IAA, 52*(3), 765–787.

Black, F., & Scholes, M. (1973). The pricing of options and corporate liabilities. *Journal of Political Economy, 81*(3), 637–654. ISSN: 00223808.

Bratton, W. W. (2001). Enron and the dark side of shareholder value. *Tulane Law Review, 76*, 1275.

Buehler, H., Gonon, L., Teichmann, J., & Wood, B. (2019). Deep hedging. *Quantitative Finance, 19*(8), 1271–1291.

Choi, J., Kwak, M., Tee, C. W., & Wang, Y. (2022). A Black-Scholes user's guide to the Bachelier model. *Journal of Futures Markets, 42*(5), 959–980.

Cotterill, J. (June 2018). *Steinhoff shareholders sue Deloitte for damages.* https://www.ft.com/content/4f4d591a-6f0f-11e8-92d3-6c13e5c92914. Last Retrieved: 15 November 2019.

Donnelly, L. (June 2018). *PIC still limping from Steinhoff blow.* https://mg.co.za/article/2018-06-08-00-pic-still-limping-from-steinhoff-blow. Last Retrieved: 18 August 2020.

Eltazarov, S., Bobojonov, I., Kuhn, L., & Glauben, T. (2023). Improving risk reduction potential of weather index insurance by spatially downscaling gridded climate data-a machine learning approach. *Big Earth Data, 7*(4), 937–960.

Fama, E. F., & French, K. R. (2004). The capital asset pricing model: Theory and evidence. *Journal of Economic Perspectives, 18*(3), 25–46.

Hajek, P., & Michalak, K. (2013). Feature selection in corporate credit rating prediction. *Knowledge-Based Systems, 51*, 72–84.

Heston, S. L. (1993b). A closed-form solution for options with stochastic volatility with applications to bond and currency options. *The Review of Financial Studies, 6*(2), 327–343. ISSN: 08939454.

Hlongwane, R., Ramabao, K., & Mongwe, W. (2024). A novel framework for enhancing transparency in credit scoring: Leveraging Shapley values for interpretable credit scorecards. *Plos One, 19*(8), Article e0308718.

Hlongwane, R., Ramaboa, K. K. K. M., & Mongwe, W. (2024). Enhancing credit scoring accuracy with a comprehensive evaluation of alternative data. *Plos One, 19*(5), Article e0303566.

Hoechstoetter, M., Nazemi, A., Rachev, S. T., & Bozic, C. (2012). Recovery rate modelling of non-performing consumer credit using data mining algorithms. *Review of*.

Horvath, B., Muguruza, A., & Tomas, M. (2021). Deep learning volatility: a deep neural network perspective on pricing and calibration in (rough) volatility models. *Quantitative Finance, 21*(1), 11–27.

Huang, Z., Chen, H., Hsu, C.-J., Chen, W.-H., & Wu, S. (2004). Credit rating analysis with support vector machines and neural networks: a market comparative study. *Decision Support Systems, 37*(4), 543–558.

Kim, A. W., Nyengerai, T., & Mendenhall, F. (2020). Evaluating the mental health impacts of the COVID-19 pandemic: Perceived risk of COVID-19 infection and childhood trauma predict adult depressive symptoms in urban South Africa. *Psychological Medicine*, 1–13.

Kirkos, E., Spathis, C., Nanopoulos, A., & Manolopoulos, Y. (Dec. 2007). Identifying qualified auditors' opinions: A data mining approach. *Journal of Emerging Technologies in Accounting, 4*(1), 183–197. https://doi.org/10.2308/jeta.2007.4.1.183

Kou, S. G. (2007). Jump-diffusion models for asset pricing in financial engineering. *Handbooks in operations research and management science, 15*, 73–116.

Lintner, J. (1975). The valuation of risk assets and the selection of risky investments in stock portfolios and capital budgets. In *Stochastic optimization models in finance* (pp. 131–155). Elsevier.

Loang, O. K., Ahmad, Z., & Naveenan, R. V. (2023). Non-performing loans, macroeconomic and bank-specific variables in Southeast Asia during COVID-19 pandemic. *The Singapore Economic Review, 68*(03), 941–961.

Mabelane, K., Mongwe, W. T., Mbuvha, R., & Marwala, T. (2023). An analysis of local government financial statement audit outcomes in a developing economy using machine learning. *Sustainability, 15*(1), 12.

Markowitz, H. M. (1991). Foundations of portfolio theory. *The Journal of Finance, 46*(2), 469–477.

Marwala, T., Mbuvha, R., & Mongwe, W. T. (2023). *Hamiltonian Monte Carlo methods in machine learning*. Elsevier.

Mikkilä, O., & Kanniainen, J. (2023). Empirical deep hedging. *Quantitative Finance, 23*(1), 111–122.

Moepya, S. O., Akhoury, S. S., & Nelwamondo, F. V. (Dec. 2014a). Applying Cost-Sensitive Classification for Financial Fraud Detection under High Class-Imbalance. In *2014 IEEE international conference on data mining workshop* (pp. 183–192). https://doi.org/10.1109/icdmw.2014.141

Moepya, S. O., Nelwamondo, F. V., & Van Der Walt, C. (2014b). A support vector machine approach to detect financial statement fraud in South Africa: A first look. In *Intelligent information and database systems* (pp. 42–51). Springer International Publishing. https://doi.org/10.1007/978-3-319-05458-2_5

Mongwe, W. T., & Malan, K. M. (2020a). A survey of automated financial statement fraud detection with relevance to the South African context. *South African Computer Journal, 32*(1).https://doi.org/10.18489/sacj.v32i1.777

Mongwe, W. T., & Malan, K. M. (2020b). The efficacy of financial ratios for fraud detection using self organising maps. In *2020 IEEE symposium series on computational intelligence (SSCI)* (pp. 1100–1106). IEEE.

Mongwe, W. T., Mbuvha, R., & Marwala, T. (2021). Bayesian inference of local government audit outcomes. *Plos One*. https://doi.org/10.1371/journal.pone.0261245

Mongwe, W. T., Sidogi, T, Mbuvha, R., & Marwala, T. (2022). Probabilistic inference of south african equity option prices under jump-diffusion processes. In *2022 IEEE symposium on computational intelligence for financial engineering and economics (CIFEr)* (pp. 1–8). IEEE.

Muñoz-Izquierdo, N., Segovia-Vargas, M. J., Camacho-Miñano, M., & Pérez-Pérez, Y. (2022). Machine learning in corporate credit rating assessment using the expanded audit report. *Machine Learning, 111*(11), 4183–4215.

Ngwenduna, K. S., & Mbuvha, R. (2021). Alleviating class imbalance in actuarial applications using generative adversarial networks. *Risks, 9*(3), 49.

O'Donnel, J. (July 2020). *Who's to blame for Wirecard? Germany passes the buck.* https://www.reuters.com/article/us-wirecard-accounts-responsibility/whos-to-blame-for-wirecard-germany-passes-the-buck-idUSKBN24320O. Last Retrieved: 18 August 2020.

Poufinas, T., Gogas, P., Papadimitriou, T., & Zaganidis, E. (2023). Machine learning in forecasting motor insurance claims. *Risks, 11*(9), 164.

Ruf, J., & Wang, W. (2019). Neural networks for option pricing and hedging: a literature review. arXiv preprint arXiv:1911.05620

Sharpe, W. F. (1964). Capital asset prices: A theory of market equilibrium under conditions of risk. *The Journal of Finance, 19*(3), 425–442.

Sidogi, T., Mongwe, W. T., Mbuvha, R., & Marwala, T. (2022a). Creating synthetic volatility surfaces using generative adversarial networks with static arbitrage loss conditions. In *2022 IEEE symposium series on computational intelligence (SSCI)* (pp. 1423–1429). IEEE.

Sidogi, T., Mongwe, W. T., Mbuvha, R., & Marwala, T. (2022b). Fusing sell-side analyst bidirectional forecasts using machine learning. *IEEE Access, 10*, 76966–76974.

Sidogi, T. (2023). Machine learning methods for financial data challenges in quatitative finance. PhD thesis. University of Johannesburg.

Sidogi, T., Mongwe, W. T., Mbuvha, R., Olukanmi, P., & Marwala, T. (2023). A signature transform of limit order book data for stock price prediction. *IEEE Access*.

Sikhosana, M. J. (2021). The relationship between unlawful expenditure and municipal financial performance in a South African context. PhD thesis.

Wallis, M., Kumar, K., & Gepp, A., (2019). Credit rating forecasting using machine learning techniques. In *Managerial perspectives on intelligent big data analytics* (pp. 180–198). IGI Global.

Wang, J., & Chen, Z. (2023). Exploring low-risk anomalies: A dynamic CAPM utilizing a machine learning approach. *Mathematics, 1114*, 3220.

Wiese, M., Knobloch, R., Korn, R., & Kretschmer, P. (2020). Quant GANs: deep generation of financial time series. *Quantitative Finance, 20*(9), 1419–1440.

Xing, B., & Marwala, T (2017). Implications of the fourth industrial age on higher education. arXiv preprint arXiv:1703.09643

Ye, H., & Bellotti, A. (2019). Modelling recovery rates for non-performing loans. *Risks, 7*(1), 19.

CHAPTER 2

Background to Bayesian Machine Learning in Quantitative Finance

2.1 Introduction

Statistical inference is approached either through the Bayesian or frequentist paradigms. In Bayesian inference, parameters are random variables with their own distribution, while frequentist inference is based on the idea that probability is a limiting frequency (Wagenmakers et al., 2008). Bayesian inference is older than the frequentist paradigm but was initially neglected (Hackenberger, 2019). The primary cause for Bayesian inference being neglected was that Bayesian statistics could only be applied in a limited number of situations where conjugate priors were known and could not be employed in situations where a closed form of the posterior was unavailable (Hackenberger, 2019). The resurgence of Bayesian statistics in recent years can be attributed to the rapid growth of computational power and data volume and the development of novel mathematical algorithms (Hackenberger, 2019). The development of Markov Chain Monte Carlo (MCMC) techniques in the 1950s, including the Hastings (1970) algorithm, was particularly noteworthy because it made it possible to create random sampling algorithms from a probability distribution and compute Bayesian hierarchical models (Marwala et al., 2023). A few years later, statisticians started using MCMC, which marked the beginning of the contemporary Bayesian statistics period (Hackenberger, 2019).

W. T. Mongwe et al., *Bayesian Machine Learning in Quantitative Finance*, https://doi.org/10.1007/978-3-031-88431-3_2

Unlike the frequentist paradigm, which relies on other unobserved quantities, Bayesian inference uses the observed data that contain all relevant information needed to draw an inference (Hackenberger, 2019; Wagenmakers et al., 2008). Regardless of the predetermined experimental design, validity is preserved if the prior distribution is appropriately specified. The use of p-values in frequentist hypothesis testing is frequently criticized because these values are partially based on data that have never been observed. Although Bayesian methods do not employ null and alternative hypotheses, the primary criticism directed toward them is the subjectivity of the chosen prior distribution (Hackenberger, 2019; Wagenmakers et al., 2008). Furthermore, selecting a prior cannot be done in a single, well-defined, and recommended way. As a result, different studies may choose different priors for the same experiment, resulting in different posteriors and, hence, conclusions. However, Bayesian techniques merely ascertain an event's likelihood. Additionally, using various priors makes it possible to measure the experiment findings' sensitivity to different prior distribution assumptions (Hackenberger, 2019; Wagenmakers et al., 2008).

Given the benefits and drawbacks of the Bayesian paradigm, we chose to use it in this book as it allows us to naturally answer questions such as: How can we explain the prediction or output of the models? What is the distribution of the parameters of the model? How do we select between the different models in a statistically principled manner? Which inputs are most relevant to the task at hand? As highlighted in the previous chapter, the Bayesian framework is founded on the Bayes theorem, allowing one to update prior beliefs through new observations encapsulated through the assumed underlying model. The following section discusses Bayesian machine learning and its relation to the Bayesian inference paradigm.

2.1.1 *Bayesian Machine Learning*

To produce predictions and their associated uncertainties, Bayesian machine learning blends computational models with the ideas of Bayesian inference (Bharadiya, 2023; Tipping, 2003). Bayesian machine learning's foundation is the Bayesian framework, which enables modeling uncertainty and updating beliefs in light of observed data and past knowledge (Bharadiya, 2023; Tipping, 2003). Bayesian machine learning combines probability distributions over model parameters and predictions, offering a more thorough account of uncertainty than classic machine learning techniques, which produce point estimates (Bharadiya, 2023; Marwala et al., 2023; Tipping, 2003). They provide benefits, including flexible modeling, the capacity to incorporate prior information, and the systematic treatment of uncertainty (Bharadiya, 2023; Tipping, 2003). Nevertheless, they also pose difficulties with scalability and computing complexity (Tipping, 2003). Future research in Bayesian machine learning aims to develop scalable algorithms, increase computational efficiency, bridge the gap between Bayesian approaches and deep learning, and address interpretability difficulties (Marwala et al., 2023; Tipping, 2003). In general, Bayesian machine learning offers a practical paradigm for describing uncertainty and producing well-informed predictions in machine learning tasks. The advantages and disadvantages of Bayesian machine learning compared to frequentist machine learning are presented in Table 2.1 (Bharadiya, 2023).

2.1.2 Bayesian Machine Learning Models

Bayesian machine learning approaches contain an assortment of methodologies that apply Bayesian principles to draw inferences and make predictions (Bharadiya, 2023). Examples of Bayesian machine learning models as outlined in Bharadiya (2023) are as follows:

- **Bayesian Logistic Regression:** Through adding prior distributions across the model parameters, Bayesian logistic regression expands on the concepts of classical logistic regression. In light of the observed data, it offers a posterior distribution across the parameters and quantifies uncertainty in the parameter estimations (Bharadiya, 2023).
- **Bayesian Mixture Models:** Probabilistic models known as Bayesian mixture models assume that the data is derived from a combination of underlying distributions. Bayesian mixture models handle uncertainty in the model parameters and enable density estimation and clustering by imposing priors on the mixture proportions and the parameters of each component distribution (Bharadiya, 2023).
- **Gaussian Processes:** Gaussian processes (GPs) are non-parametric models that are flexible and describe a prior distribution over functions. GPs can identify intricate patterns in the data and offer estimations of prediction uncertainty. Regression, classification, and time series analysis are among their common uses (Bharadiya, 2023).

Table 2.1 Summary of the comparison between the Frequentist and Bayesian paradigms in machine learning

Metric	*Frequentist*	*Bayesian*
Uncertainty Quantification	Frequentist approaches do not naturally incorporate uncertainties as the predictions produced by the models are point estimates	Bayesian techniques capture uncertainty in the model parameters and predictions through probability distributions (Bharadiya, 2023; Tipping, 2003)
Prior Beliefs	Frequentist approaches have no notion of a prior. Thus, a user cannot naturally impose prior beliefs into the inference process.	The prior distribution captures the prior beliefs about model parameters. The prior is then updated through new observations using Bayes' theorem (Bharadiya, 2023)
Regularization and Over-fitting	Frequentist approaches don't naturally impose regularization, and the practitioner must select the most suitable penalty to apply so as to regularize the model	Bayesian techniques naturally incorporate regularization techniques through prior distributions over model parameters—which prevents chances of overfitting and leads to more generalizable models (Bharadiya, 2023)
Model Selection	Model selection is often performed using a K-fold cross-validation or leave-on-out procedure. In general, there is currently no agreed-upon state-of-art metric used to select between models (Guyon et al., 2010)	The Bayesian evidence metric, which is the normalizing constant for the posterior distribution, provides a principled way to select and compare models (Bharadiya, 2023)
Scalability	Unlike Bayesian approaches, frequentist methods scale considerably more easily to huge dimensions and datasets (Bharadiya, 2023; Marwala et al., 2023)	Frequently involving intricate calculations, Bayesian approaches can be computationally demanding and difficult to scale to large datasets (Bharadiya, 2023)

- **Bayesian Neural Networks:** Through adding prior distributions over the network weights, Bayesian neural networks (BNNs) expand on the architecture of classical frequentist neural networks. BNNs can estimate posterior distributions over the weights using methods like variational inference or Markov chain Monte Carlo (MCMC) sampling, allowing for Bayesian model averaging and uncertainty quantification (Bharadiya, 2023).
- **Bayesian formulation of economic models**: This is when a traditional model, for example, the Heston stochastic volatility model, is framed within the Bayesian framework. These models are explored in more detail in each relevant chapter in this book.

In the relevant chapters of this book, we expand on the details of each utilized model. The parameters of the models discussed above need to be estimated. In the following section, we discuss how one can estimate or calibrate the parameters of Bayesian models.

2.1.3 Training Bayesian Machine Learning Models

The Bayesian framework, and hence Bayesian machine learning , is founded on Bayes theorem , which states that for a given model M with parameters $\mathbf{w}$ and data D, we have:

$$\underbrace{\mathbb{P}(\mathbf{w}|D, M)}_{\text{posterior}} = \frac{\overbrace{\mathbb{P}(D|\mathbf{w}, M)}^{\text{likelihood}} \overbrace{\mathbb{P}(\mathbf{w}|M)}^{\text{prior}}}{\underbrace{\mathbb{P}(D|M)}_{\text{evidence}}} \tag{2.1}$$

where $\mathbb{P}(\mathbf{w}|D, M)$ is the posterior of the parameters given the model M and data D, $\mathbb{P}(D|\mathbf{w}, M)$ is the likelihood of the data D, $\mathbb{P}(\mathbf{w}|M)$ is the prior distribution for the parameters and $\mathbb{P}(D|M)$ is the Bayesian evidence for model M and can be utilized for model selection (Mobiny et al., 2021; Marwala et al., 2023). A Bayesian model is fully specified when the prior distribution $\mathbb{P}(\mathbf{w}|M)$ and the likelihood function $\mathbb{P}(D|\mathbf{w}, M)$ have been specified. The prior is typically chosen to be a Gaussian distribution, with the standard deviation sometimes allowed to be different for each parameter. Furthermore, the likelihood is typically chosen as the equivalent loss function that would have been utilized on the frequentist inference. For example, for a regression problem, the likelihood would be the least squares error.

The aim of training Bayesian machine learning models is to infer the posterior distribution of the parameters $\mathbb{P}(\mathbf{w}|D, M)$. The posterior distribution $\mathbb{P}(\mathbf{w}|D, M)$ is typically not available in closed form due to the Bayesian evidence $\mathbb{P}(D|M)$ not being available in closed form, and thus, numerical techniques are often required to determine the posterior (MacKay, 1992). The common approaches for training models, which amounts to determining the posterior distribution within the Bayesian framework, are variational inference techniques (Hinton & Van Camp, 1993; Hoffman et al., 2013) and Markov Chain Monte Carlo (MCMC) algorithms. MCMC algorithms are preferable to variational techniques as they can converge to the correct target distribution if the sample size is sufficiently large (Ruiz & Titsias, 2019; Salimans et al., 2015), with MCMCs main disadvantage being its slow execution compared to variational methods. Typically, the variational and MCMC methods do not simultaneously estimate the Bayesian evidence and the posterior during inference—with the Bayesian evidence only being computed as a post-processing step. However, some probabilistic methods aim to estimate the Bayesian evidence directly (for example, the nested sampling algorithm of Skilling (2006) and produce the posterior distribution of the parameters $\mathbb{P}(\mathbf{w}|D, M)$ as a by-product. The following sections discuss these various approaches to training Bayesian models.

2.1.3.1 Variational Inference

When performing Bayesian inference, one is interested in obtaining the posterior distribution of the model parameters. An approximate inference technique that has found favour in the literature is variational inference (VI). VI is a Bayesian inference approach that aims to obtain an approximation to the true posterior , with the approximation coming from a simpler family of distributions. The Gaussian distribution is a commonly used family of distributions, as it is easy to work with mathematically (Ghosh et al., 2021). Through approximating using simpler distributions, the sampling problem can be transformed into an optimization problem in which the Kullback-Leibler divergence between the target posterior and the approximating distribution is minimized (Ghosh et al., 2021). Due to this property, variational methods are generally much

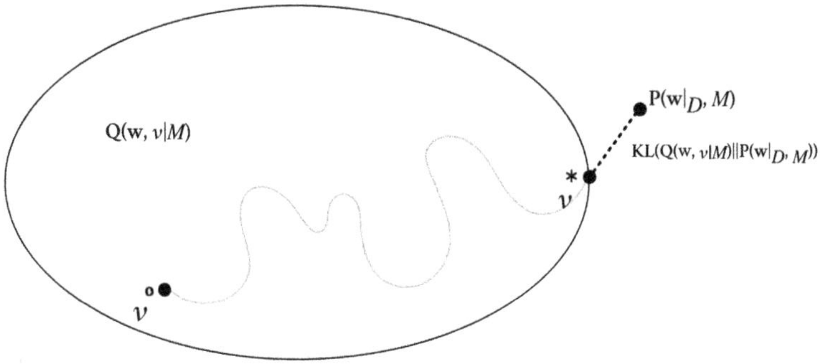

Fig. 2.1 Illustration of variational inference showing how the variational parameters ν of the variational distribution $\mathrm{Q}(\mathbf{w}, \nu|M)$ are obtained from the initial parameters ν^0 to the solution at ν^* which minimizes the Kullback-Leibler divergence

faster than MCMC approaches (Hinton & Van Camp, 1993; Ghosh et al., 2021).

Variational inference works by first positing a variational family of distributions $\mathrm{Q}(\mathbf{w}, \nu|M)$ over the parameters $\mathbf{w}$ for model M, and then fitting the variational parameters ν to be close to the posterior (in terms of some measure of distance from the exact posterior). This process is illustrated in Fig. 2.1 where the variation parameters are initialized at ν^0, and through optimization, we end up with the optimal variational parameters at ν^*. The typical approach when undertaking variational inference is to minimize the Kullback-Leibler divergence between variational distribution $\mathrm{Q}(\mathbf{w}, \nu|M)$ and the target posterior $\mathbb{P}(\mathbf{w}|D, M)$:

$$KL(\mathrm{Q}(\mathbf{w}, \nu|M)||\mathbb{P}(\mathbf{w}|D, M)) = \int \mathrm{Q}(\mathbf{w}, \nu|M) \log\left[\frac{\mathrm{Q}(\mathbf{w}, \nu|M)}{\mathbb{P}(\mathbf{w}|D, M)}\right] d\mathbf{w} \tag{2.2}$$

Note that we introduced VI as a way of avoiding estimating $\mathbb{P}(\mathbf{w}|D, M)$ directly as the Bayesian evidence $\mathbb{P}(D|M)$ is not tractable, but Eq. 2.2 has the evidence $\mathbb{P}(D|M)$ in the equation, which makes computing the *KL* also not tractable. This is seen as follows:

$$
\begin{aligned}
KL &= \int \mathbb{Q}(\mathbf{w}, \nu|M) \log\left[\frac{\mathbb{Q}(\mathbf{w}, \nu|M)}{\mathbb{P}(\mathbf{w}|D, M)}\right] d\mathbf{w} \\
&= \int \mathbb{Q}(\mathbf{w}, \nu|M)\big[\log \mathbb{Q}(\mathbf{w}, \nu|M) - \log \mathbb{P}(\mathbf{w}|D, M)\big] d\mathbf{w} \\
&= \int \mathbb{Q}(\mathbf{w}, \nu|M) \log \mathbb{Q}(\mathbf{w}, \nu|M) - \mathbb{Q}(\mathbf{w}, \nu|M) \log \mathbb{P}(\mathbf{w}|D, M) d\mathbf{w} \\
&= \int \mathbb{Q}(\mathbf{w}, \nu|M) \log \mathbb{Q}(\mathbf{w}, \nu|M) d\mathbf{w} - \int \mathbb{Q}(\mathbf{w}, \nu|M) \log \mathbb{P}(\mathbf{w}|D, M) d\mathbf{w} \\
&= \mathbb{E}_{\mathbb{Q}}[\log \mathbb{Q}(\mathbf{w}, \nu|M)] - \mathbb{E}_{\mathbb{Q}}[\log \mathbb{P}(\mathbf{w}|D, M)] \\
&= \mathbb{E}_{\mathbb{Q}}[\log \mathbb{Q}(\mathbf{w}, \nu|M)] - \mathbb{E}_{\mathbb{Q}}\left[\log \frac{\mathbb{P}(\mathbf{w}, D|M)}{\mathbb{P}(D|M)}\right] \\
&= \mathbb{E}_{\mathbb{Q}}[\log \mathbb{Q}(\mathbf{w}, \nu|M)] - \mathbb{E}_{\mathbb{Q}}[\log \mathbb{P}(\mathbf{w}, D|M)] + \mathbb{E}_{\mathbb{Q}}[\log \mathbb{P}(D|M)] \\
&= \mathbb{E}_{\mathbb{Q}}[\log \mathbb{Q}(\mathbf{w}, \nu|M)] - \mathbb{E}_{\mathbb{Q}}[\log \mathbb{P}(\mathbf{w}, D|M)] + \log \mathbb{P}(D|M) \\
&= \mathbb{E}_{\mathbb{Q}}[\log \mathbb{Q}(\mathbf{w}, \nu|M)] - [\log \mathbb{P}(\mathbf{w}, D|M)] + \log \mathbb{P}(D|M) \\
&= \mathbb{L}(D, \nu|M) + \underbrace{\log \mathbb{P}(D|M)}_{\text{intractable}}
\end{aligned}
\tag{2.3}
$$

where $\mathbb{L}(D, \nu|M)$ is the evidence lower bound (ELBO) as $KL \geq \mathbb{L}(D, \nu|M)$. As can be seen from Eq. 2.3, the KL is not tractable due to the evidence term. However, in practice, it is often convenient to consider the equivalent task of maximizing the ELBO $\mathbb{L}(D, \nu|M)$ (which only has tractable terms), which is equivalent to maximizing the KL as well as the Bayesian evidence simultaneously. In effect, we have converted the sampling problem into an optimization problem wherein we are finding the optimal parameters ν^* for the variational distribution $\mathbb{Q}(\mathbf{w}, \nu|M)$ that is close to the true posterior distribution $\mathbb{P}(\mathbf{w}|D, M)$. The optimal ν^* can be found by obtaining the gradient of $\mathbb{L}(D, \nu|M)$ with respect to the parameters ν of the variational distribution $\mathbb{Q}$ and then update ν in the direction of the steepest gradient. The optimization problem formulation will depend on the model M and the family of variational distributions $\mathbb{Q}$ being considered. More details on this can be found in Blei et al. (2017).

In contrast to MCMC , which we address in the following section, variational inference has the following benefits: It scales more quickly to high dimensions, enables us to leverage complexity and accuracy, and facilitates effective mini-batch optimization that handles large amounts of data. Among its drawbacks is that because we only consider a family of parametric distributions, bias is introduced by construction. It implies that, generally speaking, we cannot get an exact approximation of the posterior distribution.

2.1.3.2 Markov Chain Monte Carlo

The foundation of contemporary Bayesian inference is using models with difficult-to-compute posteriors and the accompanying approximation procedures (Blei et al., 2017). MCMC has been the predominant paradigm for approximation inference for more than 50 years (Blei et al., 2017). It was first created in the 1940s by scientists including Ulam, Von Neumann, Fermi, and Metropolis, among others (Robert & Casella, 2011). As highlighted previously, the main drawback of MCMC is its inability to scale to higher dimensions. In the MCMC approach, we initially build a Markov chain on the parameters, with the posterior serving as its stationary distribution (Blei et al., 2017; Neal, 1993). After that, we take long-term samples from the chain in the hopes of gathering independent samples from the stationary distribution (Blei et al., 2017; Mongwe et al., 2021e). These MCMC methods have been successfully applied to train Bayesian models in various domains such as cosmology, finance, and energy (Marwala et al., 2023; Mbuvha & Marwala, 2020; Mbuvha et al., 2021; Mongwe et al., 2021e.

The seminal Metropolis-Hastings (MH) algorithm is a gradient-free foundational MCMC algorithm that also forms the core of more advanced MCMC methods, with the Gibbs sampler being an indispensable tool for Bayesian statisticians (Geman, 2002; Hastings, 1970). Our goal in Bayesian inference is to determine the posterior distribution of the parameters $\mathbf{w}$ from some model M. Through the use of some proposal distribution $T(\mathbf{w}^*|\mathbf{w})$, the MH technique generates recommended samples (Marwala et al., 2023; Mongwe et al., 2021c, 2021e, 2021f). The ratio of likelihoods is used to determine whether to accept or reject the following state, $\mathbf{w}^*$ as follows (Brooks et al., 2011; Marwala et al., 2023; Mbuvha et al., 2021):

$$\mathbb{P}(\text{accept } \mathbf{w}^*) = \min\left(1, \frac{\pi(\mathbf{w}^*)T(\mathbf{w}|\mathbf{w}^*)}{\pi(\mathbf{w})T(\mathbf{w}^*|\mathbf{w})}\right) \quad (2.4)$$

where, for each given $\mathbf{w}$, $\pi(\mathbf{w})$ is the stationary target density evaluated at $\mathbf{w}$.

When we use the Gaussian distribution with the mean being the current state as the proposal, we end up with the commonly utilized version of MH known as random walk Metropolis algorithm (Marwala et al., 2023; Mbuvha et al., 2021). The transition density for this algorithm is given as $\mathcal{N}(\mathbf{w}, \epsilon\Sigma)$, where $\epsilon\Sigma$ is the covariance matrix of the proposal distribution (Marwala et al., 2023; Mbuvha et al., 2021). Note that Σ is typically set to be the identity matrix in practice, leaving only ϵ to be specified and tuned by the user. When the proposal distribution is symmetric, for example when it is Gaussian, it results in $T(\mathbf{w}|\mathbf{w}^*) = T(\mathbf{w}^*|\mathbf{w})$ and leads to Eq. (2.4) becoming (Mbuvha et al., 2021):

$$\mathbb{P}(\text{accept } \mathbf{w}^*) = \min\left(1, \frac{\pi(\mathbf{w}^*)}{\pi(\mathbf{w})}\right) \tag{2.5}$$

The proposal density in random walk Metropolis-Hastings often induces random walk behavior, resulting in elevated autocorrelations among the produced samples and slow convergence (Marwala et al., 2023; Mbuvha et al., 2021).

One major drawback of the MH seminal approach is the relatively high autocorrelations between the generated samples (Marwala et al., 2023). Large sample sizes are required because high autocorrelations cause the Monte Carlo estimates to converge slowly. To lessen the random walk behavior seen in MH, strategies that enhance the conventional MH method usually utilize the structure of the target posterior distributions, such as the gradient (which encapsulates the first-order gradient information) and the Hessian (which captures the second-order gradient information and the local curvature) of the target (Girolami and Calderhead, 2011; Marwala et al., 2023). First-order gradient information techniques include those based on Hamiltonian and Langevin dynamics on a Euclidean manifold, while the methods that utilize second-order gradient information focus on Riemannian and other manifolds (Brofos and Lederman, 2020a; Duane et al., 1987; Girolami and Calderhead, 2011; Marwala et al., 2023; Tripuraneni et al., 2017).

The most widely used MCMC algorithm in the literature on machine learning is HMC (Marwala et al., 2023). It has been applied in various fields such as finance, cosmology, and health (Heide et al., 2021; Marwala et al., 2023; Mbuvha and Marwala, 2020; Mongwe et al., 2021c, 2021d, 2021e; Radivojevic and Akhmatskaya, 2017; Tsaih et al., 2009). Its popularity stems mainly from its ability to suppress the random walk behavior seen with the random walk MH algorithm (Betancourt, 2017; Neal, 2012) by using first-order gradient information of the posterior distribution to direct its exploration. Samples from any differentiable target on Euclidean spaces can be easily sampled using this method (Brofos and Lederman, 2020a; Neal, 2012). The geometrical underpinnings of HMC and the circumstances in which HMC is geometrically ergodic—that is, the algorithm will ultimately traverse every region of the parameter space—are outlined in Betancourt (2017). It can also be shown that the Metropolis-Adjusted Langevin Algorithm (MALA) is a special case of HMC with the path length being equal to one, but typically generates highly correlated samples compared to the more advanced HMC method. Numerous studies have attempted to improve HMC. These have led to advanced algorithms such as the No-U-Turn Sampler (NUTS), Magnetic Hamiltonian Monte Carlo (MHMC), and the Separable Shadow Hamiltonian Hybrid Monte Carlo, among others.

The step size and trajectory length parameters for HMC can be automatically adjusted with Hoffman and Gelman's NUTS technique (Hoffman and Gelman, 2014). By aiming for a user-specified acceptance rate in the generated samples, the step size parameter is modified during the burn-in phase using the primal-dual averaging technique (Afshar et al., 2021; Andrieu & Thoms, 2008; Hoffman and Gelman, 2014; Marwala et al., 2023; Mongwe et al., 2021a, 2021b). Until specific requirements are met, the trajectory length is determined by gradually doubling it (Afshar et al., 2021; Hoffman & Gelman, 2014; Mongwe et al., 2021a, 2021b). Without requiring costly tuning iterations or human intervention, empirical results show that NUTS performs at least as well as, and occasionally better than, a properly calibrated standard HMC approach (Hoffman and Gelman, 2014; Marwala et al., 2023). Additionally, NUTS has been extended to Riemannian manifolds (Betancourt, 2013), enabling the automatic adjustment of Riemannian Manifold Hamiltonian Monte Carlo (RMHMC) parameters. A Bayesian optimization framework for adjusting the parameters of HMC and RMHMC samplers is presented by Wang et al. (2013), Wang and Freitas (2011), Marwala et al. (2023). The authors demonstrate how their method is ergodic and occasionally eliminates the need for more intricate samplers.

The practical findings demonstrate that compared to NUTS, this method has more suitable samples per calculation unit. Compared to NUTS, Hoffman et al. (2021) demonstrate that their adaptive MCMC scheme for adjusting the trajectory length parameter in HMC usually produces larger effective sample sizes normalized by the number of gradient evaluations. This method may also be effectively used with GPUs and operated in parallel, unlike NUTS (Marwala et al., 2023).

Non-canonical dynamics are used by MHMC to improve posterior exploration when compared to HMC (Brofos & Lederman, 2020b; Mongwe et al., 2021c; Tripuraneni et al., 2017). In addition to the force field already in HMC, MHMC adds a magnetic field to HMC. The magnetic field accelerates convergence to the target distribution and decreases autocorrelations in the generated samples (Gu & Sun, 2020; Mongwe & Malan, 2020b; Tripuraneni et al., 2017). When the magnetic component is removed, MHMC performs similarly to HMC. This suggests that the magnetic component provides more flexibility to improve HMC's performance. Mongwe et al. (2021f) introduce the Quantum Inspired Magnetic Hamiltonian Monte Carlo (QIMHMC) and Adaptive Magnetic Hamiltonian Monte Carlo (A-MHMC) algorithms, which rely on using a random mass matrix instead of a fixed mass in MHMC and in tuning the path length parameter in MHMC, respectively. The authors show that these versions of MHMC result in improved sampling compared to the classical MHMC algorithm. Brofos and Lederman (2020a) have extended MHMC to manifolds, showing that it is superior to MHMC. However, MHMC's drawback is that the user must specify the magnetic component. There are currently no canonical methods for tuning the magnetic component in the literature on MHMC (Brofos & Lederman, 2020b; Marwala, 2010; Mongwe et al., 2021c, 2022; Tripuraneni et al., 2017.

Following the foundational research of Izaguirre and Hampton (2004) on integrator-dependent shadow Hamiltonians, there has been a proliferation of shadow HMC techniques in the literature. The shadow Hamiltonian techniques are based on the fact that shadow Hamiltonians are conserved better when compared to the true Hamiltonians (Izaguirre & Hampton, 2004). This facilitates one to use larger step sizes or perform sampling on problems with larger dimensions without a significant decrease in the acceptance rates when compared to HMC methods (Akhmatskaya & Reich, 2006; Radivojevic & Akhmatskaya, 2017; Heide et al., 2021). However, this method introduces an additional parameter to control the momentum generation that the user has to specify. Through applying a canonical transformation to the parameters and momentum, Sweet et al. (2009) enhances the work of Izaguirre and Hampton (2004). The non-separable Hamiltonian proposed by Izaguirre and Hampton (2004) is made separable by substituting this canonical transformation. Izaguirre and Hampton's original shadow HMC approach (Izaguirre & Hampton, 2004) is less computationally efficient than the processed leapfrog integration scheme that is produced by the canonical transformation. This is due to eliminating the necessity for computationally costly momentum generation for the non-separable Hamiltonian. Additionally, the technique uses the same parameters as classical HMC and does not introduce new hyperparameters. This novel method is called the Separable Shadow Hamiltonian Hybrid Monte Carlo (S2HMC) algorithm. Mongwe et al. (2021b) introduce an adaptive version of S2HMC based on automatically tuning the path length parameter of S2HMC. This enhancement makes the S2HMC algorithm accessible to non-expert users.

For a detailed exposition of MCMC methods, we refer the reader to Marwala et al. (2023). In this book, we will present the details of each Bayesian inference algorithm used in each application chapter and the various problems that may be amenable to the Bayesian methods discussed in this chapter.

2.2 Performance Metrics

The performance metrics that we have employed throughout this book to assess the effectiveness of the models and algorithms are now presented. For both MCMC and variational techniques, we evaluate the predictive performance on unseen data, while for the MCMC methods, we take into account the multivariate Effective Sample Size (ESS), the multivariate ESS normalized by the execution time.

The ESS measure is often used to assess the sampling efficiency of MCMC algorithms. The number of uncorrelated samples among all the generated samples is captured by this performance metric (Marwala et al., 2023; Radivojevic & Akhmatskaya, 2017). The higher the ESS, the more efficient is the MCMC technique at generating quality samples. The ESS normalized by execution time measure takes into account the computational resources needed to generate the samples in order to penalize MCMC algorithms that use greater computer resources to produce the same number of uncorrelated samples (Marwala et al., 2023). The larger this metric is, the more efficient the algorithm is. This book employs the multivariate ESS metric developed by Vats et al. (2019) in place of the minimum univariate ESS metric often employed for analyzing MCMC findings (Mongwe et al., 2021b; Marwala et al., 2023). The multivariate ESS metric can take into account correlations between the dimensions, whereas the minimum univariate ESS measure is unable to capture the relationships between the various parameter dimensions (Girolami & Calderhead, 2011; Mongwe et al., 2021c, 2021d; Vats et al., 2019). The estimate of the ESS produced by minimum univariate ESS metric is dominated by the parameter dimensions that mix the slowest and disregard all other dimensions, according to the minimal univariate ESS computation (Marwala et al., 2023; Mongwe et al., 2021c; Vats et al., 2019). We also normalize this ESS metric with the execution time of the methods to account for the fact that different MCMC methods have different execution times.

The performance metrics we consider for classification are the same as those in Marwala et al. (2023) and include the accuracy, sensitivity, precision, recall, and F-measure. The other classification performance measurements used in this book are the Receiver Operating Curve (ROC) and the Area Under the Receiver Operating Curve (AUC). The y-axis of ROC plots the true positives from the model against the x-axis of false positives (Marwala et al., 2016; Mongwe & Malan, 2020a). The Area Under the ROC, or AUC , indicates the average miss-classification rate. On the other hand, the coefficient of determination (R^2), Mean Absolute Error (MAE), and the Mean Squared Error (MSE) are the performance metrics that are utilized in regression problems in this book—which are the same as those in Marwala et al. (2023). While R^2 indicates the percentage of the target variable's variability that the model explains, MSE and MAE are similar in quantifying the difference between the observations and the forecasts. Low levels of MSE and MAE and high R^2 are associated with a good model (Marwala et al., 2016).

2.3 Conclusion

This chapter introduced the Bayesian framework, some typical Bayesian models, and how to train these models in this framework, focusing on the variational and MCMC approaches. In the following chapter, we calibrate the Stochastic Alpha Beta Rho (SABR) stochastic volatility model using Bayesian models and show the benefits of this in terms of uncertainty quantification without loss of model accuracy.

References

Afshar, H. M., Oliveira, R., & Cripps, S. (2021). Non-volume preserving Hamiltonian Monte Carlo and No-U-TurnSamplers. In *International conference on artificial intelligence and statistics*. PMLR (pp. 1675–1683).

Akhmatskaya, E., & Reich, S. (2006). The targeted shadowing hybrid Monte Carlo (TSHMC) method. In *New algorithms for macromolecular simulation* (pp. 145–158). Springer.

Andrieu, C., & Thoms, J. (2008). A tutorial on adaptive MCMC. *Statistics and Computing, 18*(4), 343–373.

Betancourt, M. (2013). Generalizing the No-U-Turn Sampler to Riemannian manifolds. arXiv preprint arXiv:1304.1920

Betancourt, M. (2017). A conceptual introduction to Hamiltonian Monte Carlo. arXiv preprint arXiv:1701.02434

Bharadiya, J. P. (2023). A review of Bayesian machine learning principles, methods, and applications. *International Journal of Innovative Science and Research Technology, 8*(5), 2033–2038.

Blei, D. M., Kucukelbir, A., & McAuliffe, J. D. (2017). Variational inference: A review for statisticians. *Journal of the American statistical Association, 112*(518), 859–877.

Brofos, J. A., & Lederman, R. R (2020a). Magnetic Manifold Hamiltonian Monte Carlo. arXiv preprint arXiv:2010.07753

Brofos, J. A., & Lederman, R. R. (2020b). Non-canonical Hamiltonian Monte Carlo. arXiv preprint arXiv:2008.08191

Brooks, S., Gelman, A., Jones, G., & Meng, X.-L. (2011). *Handbook of Markov chain Monte Carlo*. CRC Press.

Duane, S., Kennedy, A. D., Pendleton, B. J., & Roweth, D. (1987). Hybrid Monte Carlo. *Physics Letters B, 195*(2), 216–222.

Geman, H. (2002). Pure jump Levy processes for asset price modelling. *Journal of Banking Finance, 26*(7), 1297.

Ghosh, S., Birrell, P., & De Angelis, D. (2021). Variational inference for nonlinear ordinary differential equations. In *International conference on artificial intelligence and statistics*. PMLR (pp. 2719–2727).

Girolami, M., & Calderhead, B. (2011). Riemann manifold langevin and hamiltonian monte carlo methods. *Journal of the Royal Statistical Society: Series B (Statistical Methodology), 73*(2), 123–214.

Gu, M., & Sun, S. (2020). Neural langevin dynamical sampling. *IEEE Access, 8*, 31595–31605.

Guyon, I., Saffari, A., Dror, G., & Cawley, G. (2010). Model selection: Beyond the bayesian/frequentist divide. *Journal of Machine Learning Research, 11*(1).

Hackenberger, B. K. (2019). Bayes or not Bayes, is this the question? *Croatian Medical Journal, 60*(1), 50.

Hastings, W. K. (1970). Monte Carlo sampling methods using Markov chains and their applications. *Biometrica, 57*(1), 97–109.

Heide, C., Roosta, F., Hodgkinson, L., & Kroese, D. (2021). Shadow manifold Hamiltonian Monte Carlo. In *International conference on artificial intelligence and statistics*. PMLR (pp. 1477–1485).

Hinton, G. E., & Van Camp, D. (1993). Keeping the neural networks simple by minimizing the description length of the weights. In *Proceedings of the sixth annual conference on Computational learning theory* (pp. 5–13). ACM.

Hoffman, M. D., Blei, D. M., Wang, C., & Paisley, J. (2013). Stochastic variational inference. *Journal of Machine Learning Research, 14*(5).

Hoffman, M., Radul, A., & Sountsov, P. (2021). An adaptive-MCMC scheme for setting trajectory lengths in Hamiltonian Monte Carlo. In *International conference on artificial intelligence and statistics*. PMLR (pp. 3907–3915).

Hoffman, M. D., & Gelman, A. (2014). The No-U-turn sampler: Adaptively setting path lengths in Hamiltonian Monte Carlo. *Journal of Machine Learning Research, 15*(1), 1593–1623.

Izaguirre, J. A., & Hampton, S. S. (Nov. 2004). Shadow hybrid Monte Carlo: An efficient propagator in phase space of macromolecules. *Journal of Computational Physics, 200*(2), 581–604. ISSN: 0021-9991. https://doi.org/10.1016/j.jcp.2004.04.016

MacKay, D. J. C. (1992). A practical Bayesian framework for backpropagation networks. *Neural Computation, 4*(3), 448–472.

Marwala, T. (2010). Finite-element-model updating using a Bayesian approach. In *Finite-element-model updating using computional intelligence techniques: Applications to structural dynamics* (pp. 183–201).

Marwala, T., Boulkaibet, I., & Adhikari, S. (2016). *Probabilistic finite element model updating using Bayesian statistics: Applications to aeronautical and mechanical engineering*. Wiley.

Marwala, T., Mbuvha, R., & Mongwe, W. T. (2023). *Hamiltonian Monte Carlo methods in machine learning*. Elsevier.

Mbuvha, R., & Marwala, T. (2020). Bayesian inference of COVID-19 spreading rates in South Africa. *PloS One, 15*(8), Article e0237126.

Mbuvha, R., Mongwe, W. T., & Marwala, T. (2021). Separable Shadow Hamiltonian hybrid Monte Carlo for Bayesian neural network inference in wind speed forecasting. *Energy and A, 1*, Article 100108.

Mobiny, A., Yuan, P., Moulik, S. K., Garg, N., Wu, C. C., & Van Nguyen, H. (2021). Dropconnect is effective in modeling uncertainty of Bayesian deep networks. *Scientific Reports, 11*(1), 1–14.

Mongwe, W. T., & Malan, K. M. (2020a). A survey of automated financial statement fraud detection with relevance to the South African context. *South African Computer Journal, 32*(1). https://doi.org/10.18489/sacj.v32i1.777

Mongwe, W. T., & Malan, K. M. (2020b). The efficacy of financial ratios for fraud detection using self organising maps. In *2020 IEEE symposium series on computational intelligence (SSCI)* (pp. 1100–1106). IEEE.

Mongwe, W. T., Mbuvha, R., & Marwala, T. (2021a). Adaptive magnetic Hamiltonian Monte Carlo. *IEEE Access, 9*, 152993–153003. https://doi.org/10.1109/ACCESS.2021.3127931

Mongwe, W. T., Mbuvha, R., & Marwala, T. (2021b). Adaptively setting the path length for separable shadow Hamiltonian hybrid Monte Carlo. *IEEE Access, 9*, 138598–138607.

Mongwe, W. T., Mbuvha, R., & Marwala, T. (2021c). Antithetic magnetic and Shadow Hamiltonian Monte Carlo. *IEEE Access, 9*, 49857–49867.

Mongwe, W. T., Mbuvha, R., & Marwala, T. (2021d). Antithetic Riemannian manifold and quantum-inspired Hamiltonian Monte Carlo. arXiv preprint arXiv:2107.02070

Mongwe, W. T., Mbuvha, R., & Marwala, T. (2021e). Bayesian inference of local government audit outcomes. *Plos One*. https://doi.org/10.1371/journal.pone.0261245

Mongwe, W. T., Mbuvha, R., & Marwala, T. (2021f). Quantum-inspired magnetic Hamiltonian Monte Carlo. *Plos One, 16*(10), Article e0258277.

Mongwe, W. T., Mbuvha, R., & Marwala, T. (2022). Shadow magnetic Hamiltonian Monte Carlo. *IEEE Access, 10*, 34340–34351. https://doi.org/10.1109/ACCESS.2022.3161443

Neal, R. M. (1993). Bayesian learning via stochastic dynamics. In *Advances in neural information processing systems* (Vol. 5). Morgan Kaufmann Publishers Inc. (pp. 475–482). ISBN: 1-55860-274-7. http://dl.acm.org/citation.cfm?id=645753.667903

Neal, R. M. (2012). *Bayesian learning for neural networks* (Vol. 118). Springer Science & Business Media.

Radivojević, T., & Akhmatskaya, E. (2017). Mix & Match Hamiltonian Monte Carlo. arXiv preprint arXiv:1706.04032

Robert, C., & Casella, G. (2011). *A short history of MCMC: Subjective recollections from incomplete data* (pp. 49–61). Chapman and Hall/CRC.

Ruiz, F., & Titsias, M. (2019). A contrastive divergence for combining variational inference and mcmc. In *International conference on machine learning*. PMLR (pp. 5537–5545).

Salimans, T., Kingma, D., & Welling, M. (2015). Markov chain monte carlo and variational inference: Bridging the gap. In *International conference on machine learning*. PMLR (pp. 1218–1226).

Skilling, J. (2006). Nested sampling for general Bayesian computation. *Bayesian Analysis, 1*(4), 833–859.

Sweet, C. R., Hampton, S. S., Skeel, R. D., & Izaguirre, J. A. (2009). A separable shadow Hamiltonian hybrid Monte Carlo method. *The Journal of Chemical Physics, 131*(17), Article 174106.

Tipping, M. E. (2003). Bayesian inference: An introduction to principles and practice in machine learning. In *Summer school on machine learning* (pp. 41–62). Springer.

Tripuraneni, N., Rowland, M., Ghahramani, Z., & Turner, R. (2017). Magnetic Hamiltonian Monte Carlo. In *International conference on machine learning*. PMLR (pp. 3453–3461).

Tsaih, R.-H., Lin, W.-Y., & Huang, S.-Y. (2009). Exploring fraudulent financial reporting with GHSOM. In *Intelligence and security informatics* (pp. 31–41). Springer. https://doi.org/10.1007/978-3-642-01393-5_5

Vats, D., Flegal, J. M., & Jones, G. L. (Apr. 2019). Multivariate output analysis for Markov chain Monte Carlo. *Biometrika, 106*(2), 321–337. ISSN: 0006-3444. eprint: https://academic.oup.com/biomet/article-pdf/106/2/321/28575440/asz002.pdf

Wagenmakers, E.-J., Lee, M., Lodewyckx, T., & Iverson, G. J. (2008). Bayesian versus frequentist inference. In *Bayesian evaluation of informative hypotheses* (pp. 181–207).

Wang, Z., & de Freitas, N. (2011). Predictive adaptation of hybrid Monte Carlo with Bayesian parametric bandits. In *NIPS deep learning and unsupervised feature learning workshop* (Vol. 30).

Wang, Z., Mohamed, S., & Freitas, N. (2013). Adaptive Hamiltonian and Riemann manifold Monte Carlo. In *International conference on machine learning*. PMLR (pp. 1462–1470).

CHAPTER 3

On the Stochastic Alpha Beta Rho Model and Hamiltonian Monte Carlo Techniques

3.1 Introduction

The two most popular models for vanilla options pricing are the Black and Scholes (1973) model and the Black (1976) model. One critique aimed at these two pricing models is their presumption of constant volatility during the option's duration, which is not corroborated by actual market volatility (Marwala et al., 2023; Mongwe, 2015; Mongwe et al., 2022b; Yang et al., 2015). Implied volatility has a distinct value for every combination of strike price and time to maturity, which is now a well-established and stylized fact. The volatility smile shows the variation in volatility, for a given maturity, for each strike price. The volatility's time-to-maturity variation for a given strike price is described by its term structure (Mongwe et al., 2022b). Using a constant volatility model to hedge an extensive portfolio of options is not feasible given these market findings, as options with varying maturities and strikes are typically pooled together for hedging purposes (Yang et al., 2015).

Dupire et al. (1994) proposed a local volatility model, which implies that the underlying volatility is a local function of the strike price and

Supplementary Information The online version contains supplementary material available at https://doi.org/10.1007/978-3-031-88431-3_3.

W. T. Mongwe et al., *Bayesian Machine Learning in Quantitative Finance*, https://doi.org/10.1007/978-3-031-88431-3_3

maturity, as an alternative to the Black and Scholes (1973) and Black (1976) models, for hedging and pricing exotic options. The implied volatility curve from the local volatility model predicts that the market volatility skew moves in the opposite direction of the underlying asset's price, as shown mathematically by Hagan et al. (2002). This behavior deviates from how option prices typically behave in the market. Accordingly, using a local volatility model for delta hedging is likewise erroneous since the delta formula contains a correction term: the model-predicted change in implied volatility due to the underlying asset change (Hagan et al., 2002). In contrast to what is seen in the actual market, this correction term suggests that the implied volatility curve changes to the right when the forward price falls and to the left when the forward price rises (Hagan et al., 2002).

To resolve these short-falls of the Dupire local volatility formulation, Hagan et al. (2002) developed the Stochastic Alpha Beta Rho (SABR) model, a stochastic volatility model in which the asset price and volatility are correlated. The authors use single perturbation methods to create a closed-form algebraic formula for implied volatility based on today's forward price and strike when pricing European options using their SABR model (Hagan et al., 2002; Yang et al., 2015). Black's formula may then be used to quickly determine the market price and sensitivities, such as Volga and Vanna risks, thanks to its closed-form implied volatility formula. Additionally, the SABR model offers decent and occasionally outstanding fits to the inferred volatility curves seen in the market (Hagan et al., 2002). The SABR model has been widely adopted in the financial industry for European options' pricing and risk management, owing to its intuitive and parsimonious parameterization (Choi & Seo, 2023). The Hagan et al. (2002) SABR model has since been extended to allow for negative interest rates, including the shifted, free boundary, and the mixture SABR models with promising results (Antonov et al., 2015).

This chapter calibrates the SABR model using simulated and market-observed ZAR swaption prices. We intend to produce a distribution of the calibrated model parameters and naturally incorporate confidence intervals for the model's predictions. To this end, we calibrate the SABR model by employing the Bayesian inference framework. The Bayesian inference framework relies on Bayes theorem, which asserts that for a given model, the posterior distribution equals the likelihood multiplied by the prior over the parameters divided by the Bayesian evidence. In this chapter, we aim to determine the posterior distribution of parameters for the original formulation of the SABR model. This will allow us to use the SABR model to produce predictions and determine how well it matches the volatility skew. To get the posterior, one must frequently use numerical approaches as the posterior distribution is usually not accessible in closed form (MacKay, 1992). Within the Bayesian framework, variational inference techniques (Hinton & Van Camp, 1993; Hoffman et al., 2013) and Markov Chain Monte Carlo (MCMC) algorithms are commonly used for training models and thus producing the posterior distribution. If the sample size is large enough, MCMC methods are guaranteed to converge to the right target distribution (Marwala et al., 2023; Ruiz & Titsias, 2019; Salimans et al., 2015), thus presenting themselves as a better option compared to variational inference approaches. A discussion of variational inference and MCMC can be found in Chapter 2 of this book.

We introduce a first-in-literature use of the Separable Shadow Hamiltonian Hybrid Monte Carlo (S2HMC) (Izaguirre & Hampton, 2004; Mongwe et al., 2021b, 2021c, 2021f, 2022a, 2022b), Hamiltonian Monte Carlo (Duane et al., 1987; Mongwe et al., 2022b) (HMC), and Metropolis-Adjusted Langevin Algorithm (Girolami & Calderhead, 2011; Mongwe et al., 2022b) (MALA) methods in the calibration of the SABR model to simulated and ZAR observed market swaption data as at 28 June 2024. Our analysis reveals that the Bayesian framework can reproduce the true parameters for the simulated data and can further fit the volatility skew on ZAR observed swaption data. In addition, we obtain confidence bands on the predicted volatility skew, with the results showing that the bands are wider at the wings of the skew and narrow around the at-the-money point.

The remainder of this chapter is structured as follows: We first describe the Stochastic Alpha Beta Rho model used to fit the volatility skew for each expiry in Sect. 3.2; we then detail the Markov Chain Monte Carlo methods used to train the model in Sect. 3.3; we then present the experiment setup, after which we present the results, discuss them, and provide the conclusion in Sects. 3.4–3.6 respectively.

3.2 Stochastic Alpha Beta Rho Model

The Stochastic Alpha Beta Rho Model (SABR) model is a stochastic volatility model specified by the following system of stochastic differential equations (Hagan et al., 2002):

$$dF_t = \sigma_t F_t^{\beta} dW_t \tag{3.1}$$

$$d\sigma_t = \sigma_t \nu dZ_t \tag{3.2}$$

where F_t, and σ_t (where $\sigma_0 = \alpha$) are the processes for the forward price and volatility respectively, ν is the volatility of volatility, $\beta \in [0, 1]$ is the elasticity parameter, and W_t and Z_t are standard Brownian motions correlated through ρ as $dW_t dZ_t = \rho dt$ with $\rho \in [-1, 1]$ (Hagan et al., 2002). The model assumes that the underlying process is already a (local) martingale under some equivalent martingale measure (Kennedy et al., 2012).

In the original Hagan et al. (2002) model, the price of European options, assuming log-normal volatilities, is given by Black's formula:

$$V_{call} = D(t)(fN(d_1) - kN(d_2))) \tag{3.3}$$

$$d_{1/2} = \frac{\ln(f/k) \pm \sigma_B^2 t}{\sigma_B \sqrt{t}} \tag{3.4}$$

where the implied volatility $\sigma_B(f, k)$ is given by:

$$\sigma_B(f,k) = \frac{\alpha}{(fk)^{\frac{1-\beta}{2}}\left\{1 + \frac{(1-\beta)^2}{24}(\ln(f/k))^2 + \frac{(1-\beta)^4}{1920}(\ln(f/k))^4 + \ldots\right\}} \times \frac{z}{x(z)} \times \left\{1 + \left[\frac{(1-\beta)^2}{24}\frac{\sigma^2}{(fk)^{1-\beta}} + \frac{1}{4}\frac{\rho\beta\nu\alpha}{(fk)^{(1-\beta)/2}} + \frac{2-3\rho^2}{24}\nu^2\right]t + \ldots \tag{3.5}$$

where

$$z = \frac{\nu}{\alpha}(fk)^{(1-\beta)^2/2}\ln(f/k) \tag{3.6}$$

and

$$x(z) = \ln\left(\frac{\sqrt{1 - 2\rho z + z^2} + z - \rho}{1 - \rho}\right) \tag{3.7}$$

For the special case of at-the-money options, options struck at $f = k$, this formula reduces to:

$$\sigma_{ATM} = \sigma_B(f, f) = \frac{\alpha}{f^{1-\beta}}\left\{1 + \left[\frac{(1-\beta)^2}{24}\frac{\alpha^2}{f^{2-2\beta}} + \frac{1}{4}\frac{\rho\beta\nu\alpha}{f^{1-\beta}} + \frac{2-3\rho^2}{24}\nu^2\right]t + \ldots\right. \tag{3.8}$$

The parameters we want to perform inference on are $\{\alpha, \beta, \rho, \nu\}$. It is worth noting the following constraints on the parameters: $\alpha \in [0, \infty]$, $\beta \in [0, 1]$, $\rho \in [-1, 1]$, and $\nu \in [0, \infty]$. The forms of the skews and smiles are determined in part by each parameter in the SABR model. The key influence on the skew is the parameter β. Specifically, when $\beta = 1$ and $\rho > 0$, decreasing β from 1 to 0 results in an implied volatility curve with a more significant negative (downward) slope (Hagan et al., 2002).

Similar effects are seen on the volatility skew by the SABR model's ρ parameter; a larger negative ρ allows for a curve that slopes further downward (Hagan et al., 2002). As a result, ρ is frequently used to match the skew. In addition, varied degrees of curvature are seen in the implied volatility curves in practice. When choosing a less sophisticated choice for the parameter, a large curvature typically appears, and with an increase in expiry, the smile tends to flatten out (Hagan et al., 2002). Because of this, the market-given parameter T (maturity) is always considered together with ν, also known as Volvol (volatility of volatility). Lastly, the initial volatility α plays a role in matching the implied volatility of the at-the-money point, which in each market correlates to the option with the highest level of liquidity. The correlation ρ and exponent β have comparable effects on the volatility smile (Hagan et al., 2002). As the strike k fluctuates, they both result in a downward-sloping skew in $\sigma_B(f, k)$ (Hagan et al., 2002). It is challenging to discern the two parameters from a single market snapshot of $\sigma_B(f, k)$ as a function of f at a given k (Hagan et al., 2002). The remaining parameters, $\{\alpha, \rho, \nu\}$, are calibrated to market data, and the β parameter is usually fixed. This is also the approach taken in this chapter.

In this chapter, we utilize the Bayesian inference framework to calibrate the parameters by minimizing the squared error between the implied normal volatility from the SABR model and what we observe from the swaption market. Hagan et al. (2002) normal implied volatility expansion is given in formula (B.67a) in Hagan et al. (2002). The implied normal volatility $\sigma_B(f, k)$ expansion is given as:

$$\sigma_B(f, k) = \alpha \times \frac{z}{x(z)} \times A(1 + (B + C + D)t) \tag{3.9}$$

where

$$A = \frac{(1-\beta)(f-k)}{f^{(1-\beta)} - k^{(1-\beta)}} \tag{3.10}$$

$$B = \frac{-\beta(2-\beta)\alpha^2}{24(\sqrt{fk})^{(2-2\beta)}} \tag{3.11}$$

$$C = \frac{\rho\alpha\nu\beta}{4(\sqrt{fk})^{(1-\beta)}} \tag{3.12}$$

$$D = \frac{2-3\rho^2}{6}\frac{\nu^2}{4} \tag{3.13}$$

$$z = \frac{\nu}{\alpha}(k-f) \tag{3.14}$$

and

$$x(z) = \ln\left(\frac{\sqrt{1+2\rho z+z^2}+z+\rho}{1+\rho}\right) \tag{3.15}$$

It is worth noting that when $\beta = 0$, this implied normal volatility simplifies to (Choi and Seo, 2023):

$$\sigma_B(f, k) = \alpha\frac{z}{x(z)}\left(1 + \frac{2-3\rho^2}{6}\frac{\nu^2}{4}t\right) \tag{3.16}$$

In this chapter, we utilize the *full* (i.e., when β is not zero) implied normal volatility expansion in Eq. 3.9. However, in all our experiments, we set $\beta = 0.5$, which aligns with what is typically done in practice.

In the following section, we explore the Markov Chain Monte Carlo techniques that we use to calibrate the SABR model.

3.3 Markov Chain Monte Carlo Methods

We now describe the MALA, HMC, and S2HMC Markov Chain Monte Carlo (MCMC) methods for calibrating the SABR model to simulated and ZAR market-observed swaption price data. We implemented all the MCMC methods using the PyTorch framework in Python.

3.3.1 Metropolis-Adjusted Langevin Algorithm

The Metropolis-Adjusted Langevin Algorithm (MALA) enhances the Metropolis-Hastings (MH) method through the use of first-order gradient information of the target posterior. MALA reduces the random walk behavior of MH via the use of Langevin dynamics where the drift component is the derivative of the log of the target posterior, and the diffusive component is Brownian motion which is represented as follows (Gu & Sun, 2020; Marwala et al., 2023; Mongwe et al., 2021e, 2022b):

$$d\mathbf{w}_t = \frac{1}{2} f'(\mathbf{w})dt + dZ_t \tag{3.17}$$

where $\mathbf{w}$ are the parameters, $f'(\mathbf{w})$ is the first derivative of the target $f(\mathbf{w})$ with respect to the parameters, and Z_t is a Brownian motion process at a fictitious time t. The Langevin dynamics in Eq. 3.17 typically cannot be solved analytically, and numerical methods such as the Euler-Maruyama integration scheme are typically used (Marwala et al., 2023). This, however, introduces errors that can break the detailed balance condition, which would not guarantee that the method would converge to the correct target distribution (Marwala et al., 2023). To rectify this, a Metropolis acceptance step is incorporated into the algorithm to ensure detailed balance (Marwala et al., 2023). The MALA algorithm converges to the stationary distribution at a faster pace than the MH algorithm because it takes into account the density's first-order gradient data, which is represented by $f'(\mathbf{w})$ (Girolami & Calderhead, 2011; Gu & Sun, 2020; Marwala et al., 2023). The samples produced using the MALA method are still highly correlated. Girolami and Calderhead (2011) incorporate second-order gradient information of the target by extending MALA from being on a Euclidean manifold to a Riemannian manifold (Marwala et al., 2023). Despite a corresponding increase in compute time, this approach demonstrated significant gains in the sampling performance of the MALA method (Marwala et al., 2023).

3.3.2 *Hamiltonian Monte Carlo*

Hamiltonian Monte Carlo (HMC) is a popular MCMC method for performing Bayesian inference and has been utilized in various disciplines such as finance, health, and energy (Duane et al., 1987; Mbuvha & Marwala, 2020; Mbuvha et al., 2021; Mongwe et al., 2021d, 2022b). The method is premised on using Hamiltonian dynamics, which naturally considers the first-order gradient information of the target posterior. The dynamics that underpin HMC are as follows (Marwala et al., 2023; Neal, 1993):

$$\frac{d\mathbf{w}}{\partial t} = \frac{\partial \mathrm{H}(\mathbf{w}, \mathbf{p})}{\partial \mathbf{p}}; \quad \frac{d\mathbf{p}}{\partial t} = -\frac{\partial \mathrm{H}(\mathbf{w}, \mathbf{p})}{\partial \mathbf{w}} \tag{3.18}$$

where $\mathbf{w}$ are the parameters, $\mathbf{p}$ is the auxiliary momentum variable with the same dimensionality as $\mathbf{w}$, and $\mathrm{H}(\mathbf{w}, \mathbf{p})$ is the Hamiltonian—which represents the total energy (i.e., potential energy defined by the target posterior and kinetic energy which is typically captured through a multivariate Gaussian distribution) from this system (Mongwe et al., 2021b, 2022a). This HMC method allows distant proposals, which results in a significant reduction in the autocorrelations of the generated samples (Marwala et al., 2023). The pseudo-code for HMC is shown in Algorithm 3.1.

The HMC technique is composed of two steps. The first step integrates Hamiltonian dynamics in Eq. 3.18 typically using the leapfrog integrator (Duane et al., 1987; Marwala et al., 2023; Neal, 1993), and the second step utilizes a Metropolis-Hastings correction to account for the numerical integration errors arising from the first step (Duane et al., 1987; Hastings, 1970; Neal et al., 2011). The parameter and momentum update equations for the leapfrog integration scheme (corresponding to the first step of HMC) are given as follows:

$$\begin{aligned}
\mathbf{p}_{t+\frac{\epsilon}{2}} &= \mathbf{p}_t + \frac{\epsilon}{2}\frac{\partial H\left(\mathbf{w}_t, \mathbf{p}_t\right)}{\partial \mathbf{w}} \\
\mathbf{w}_{t+\epsilon} &= \mathbf{w}_t + \epsilon \mathbf{M}^{-1}\mathbf{p}_{t+\frac{\epsilon}{2}} \\
\mathbf{p}_{t+\epsilon} &= \mathbf{p}_{t+\frac{\epsilon}{2}} + \frac{\epsilon}{2}\frac{\partial H\left(\mathbf{w}_{t+\epsilon}, \mathbf{p}_{t+\frac{\epsilon}{2}}\right)}{\partial \mathbf{w}}
\end{aligned} \tag{3.19}$$

where ϵ is the discretization step size and $\mathbf{M}$ is a covariance matrix emanating from the kinetic energy component in $\mathrm{H}(\mathbf{w}, \mathbf{p})$. If the integration of the Hamiltonian dynamics in the first step were solved precisely, the second step would not be required. However, due to the discretization errors, a Metropolis-Hastings acceptance step is typically required where the $\mathbf{w}^*$ proposed by the first step are accepted with probability:

$$\mathrm{P}(\text{accept } \mathbf{w}^*) = \min\left(1, \frac{\exp(-\mathrm{H}(\mathbf{w}^*, \mathbf{p}^*))}{\exp(-\mathrm{H}(\mathbf{w}, \mathbf{p}))}\right). \tag{3.20}$$

Algorithm 3.1: Hamiltonian Monte Carlo

Input: $N, \epsilon, L, w_{\text{init}}, H(w, p)$
Output: $(w)_{m=0}^{N}$
$w_0 \leftarrow w_{\text{init}}$
for $m \rightarrow 1$ **to** N **do**
  $p_{m-1} \sim \mathcal{N}(0, \mathbf{M})$
  $p_m, w_m =$ **Leapfrog**$(p_{m-1}, w_{m-1}, \epsilon, L, H)$ in equation (3.19)
  $\delta H = H(w_{m-1}, p_{m-1}) - H(w_m, p_m)$
  $\alpha_m = \min(1, \exp(\delta H))$
  $u_m \sim \text{Unif}(0, 1)$
  $w_m =$ **Metropolis**$(\alpha_m, u_m, w_m, w_{m-1})$ in equation (3.20)
end for

The parameters of HMC are the discretization step size ϵ, which is required for the first step in HMC, and the trajectory length, which determines the number of times the integration is performed. The step size parameter is typically set to obtain a user-specified target acceptance rate using the dual averaging method (Hoffman & Gelman, 2014; Marwala et al., 2023) while tuning the trajectory length parameter is a more complex problem (Hoffman & Gelman, 2014). It can further be shown that when the trajectory length parameter is set to 1, the HMC method becomes the MALA method. The overall HMC sampling process follows a Gibbs sampling scheme, where we sample $\mathbf{p}$ auxiliary momentum variable and then sample a new set of parameters $\mathbf{w}$ given the drawn momentum $\mathbf{p}$. As can be seen from Algorithm 3.1, this procedure is repeated until the required number of samples N are generated (Marwala et al., 2023; Mongwe et al., 2021a, 2021b).

3.3.3 *Separable Shadow Hamiltonian Hybrid Monte Carlo*

Although significantly better than MALA, the HMC method still produces auto-correlated samples (Heide et al., 2021; Marwala et al., 2023). This is mainly driven by the fact that the leapfrog integration scheme in Eq. 3.19 only preserves the Hamiltonian up to second order $\mathcal{O}(\epsilon^2)$. This causes the change in the Hamiltonian in step 5 of Algorithm 3.1 to become large, thus leading to more rejections in step 8 of Algorithm 3.1 (Heide et al., 2021; Marwala et al., 2023). There are two possibilities to address this issue; one can either create more accurate (i.e., better than $\mathcal{O}(\epsilon^2)$) integration schemes to integrate the Hamiltonian dynamics, or only run the integration scheme for small step sizes ϵ and short path lengths L—or a combination of these two approaches. However, all these approaches attract longer execution times (Marwala et al., 2023).

It can be shown that when one runs a backward error analysis through the leapfrog integrator in Eq. 3.19, we can derive a modified Hamiltonian (which is called the shadow Hamiltonian) whose energy is better preserved by the leapfrog integrator than the true Hamiltonian (Marwala et al., 2023). By design, the numerical integrator precisely conserves the perturbations of the Hamiltonian of the shadow Hamiltonians . However, as this Hamiltonian is not the true Hamiltonian, we would effectively be sampling from an importance distribution, which we would need to correct so as not to introduce bias in the generated samples (Heide et al., 2021).

At its core, the shadow or modified Hamiltonian is an asymptotic expansion in the powers of the discretization step size ϵ around the Hamiltonian:

$$\tilde{\mathrm{H}} = \mathrm{H} + \epsilon \mathrm{H}_2 + \epsilon^2 \mathrm{H}_3 + \epsilon^3 \mathrm{H}_4 + \dots \tag{3.21}$$

However, to ensure that this expansion does not diverge, a kth order truncation of the expansion is utilized in practice:

$$\begin{aligned} \tilde{\mathrm{H}}^{[k]} &= \mathrm{H} + \epsilon \mathrm{H}_2 + \epsilon^2 \mathrm{H}_3 + \epsilon^3 \mathrm{H}_4 + \dots \\ &= \tilde{\mathrm{H}} + \mathcal{O}(\epsilon^k) \end{aligned} \tag{3.22}$$

Through comparing the associated elements of the Taylor series in terms of ϵ and the extended precise flow of the modified differential equation of the Hamiltonian, the H_k terms can be found. For symplectic integrators like the leapfrog integrator, these altered equations can be regarded as being Hamiltonian (Marwala et al., 2023). This chapter considers a fourth-order truncation of the shadow Hamiltonian under the leapfrog integrator. The fourth-order truncation is conserved with more accuracy ($\mathcal{O}^4$) than the true Hamiltonian since the leapfrog is second-order accurate ($\mathcal{O}^2$). The fourth-order shadow Hamiltonian for the leapfrog integrator after matching coefficients from the flow and the asymptotic expansion is expressed as:

$$\tilde{H}^{[4]} = U(\mathbf{w}) + K(\mathbf{p}) + \frac{\epsilon^2}{12} K_{\mathbf{p}}^T U_{\mathbf{ww}} K_{\mathbf{p}} - \frac{\epsilon^2}{24} U_{\mathbf{w}}^T K_{\mathbf{pp}} U_{\mathbf{w}} + \mathcal{O}(\epsilon^4) \quad (3.23)$$

where $U_{\mathbf{w}}$, $U_{\mathbf{ww}}$, $K_{\mathbf{p}}$ and $K_{\mathbf{pp}}$ are Jacobians and Hessians of the potential and kinetic energies respectively. It can be noted that the modified Hamiltonian in Eq. 3.23 is non-separable in terms of the parameter and momentum vectors. This is problematic as it requires potential tuning of additional parameters and momentum acceptance criterion that is computationally expensive (Izaguirre & Hampton, 2004; Marwala et al., 2023; Sweet et al., 2009).

Separable Shadow Hamiltonian Hybrid Monte Carlo (S2HMC) utilizes a processed leapfrog integrator to create a separable Hamiltonian (Sweet et al., 2009). Before passing through the leapfrog integrator, the parameter vector and momenta are pre-processed to minimize computational overhead. The resultant separable Hamiltonian in S2HMC is

$$\tilde{H}(\mathbf{w}, \mathbf{p}) = U(\mathbf{w}) + K(\mathbf{p}) + \frac{\epsilon^2}{24} U_{\mathbf{w}}^T M^{-1} U_{\mathbf{w}} + \mathcal{O}(\epsilon^4) \quad (3.24)$$

The positions and momenta are propagated on the shadow Hamiltonian after performing the reversible mapping $(\hat{\mathbf{w}}, \hat{\mathbf{p}}) = \mathcal{X}(\mathbf{w}, \mathbf{p})$, where $(\hat{\mathbf{w}}, \hat{\mathbf{p}})$ is found through fixed point iterations as:

$$\hat{\mathbf{p}} = \mathbf{p} - \frac{\epsilon}{24}\left[U_{\mathbf{w}}(\mathbf{w} + \epsilon\, \mathbf{M}^{-1}\hat{\mathbf{p}}) - U_{\mathbf{w}}(\mathbf{w} - \epsilon\, \mathbf{M}^{-1}\hat{\mathbf{p}})\right] \quad (3.25)$$

$$\hat{\mathbf{w}} = \mathbf{w} + \frac{\epsilon^2\, \mathbf{M}^{-1}}{24}\left[U_{\mathbf{w}}(\mathbf{w} + \epsilon\, \mathbf{M}^{-1}\hat{\mathbf{p}}) + U_{\mathbf{w}}(\mathbf{w} - \epsilon\, \mathbf{M}^{-1}\hat{\mathbf{p}})\right] \quad (3.26)$$

After the leapfrog is performed, this mapping is reversed using post-processing of the following fixed point iterations:

$$\mathbf{w} = \hat{\mathbf{w}} - \frac{\epsilon^2 \mathbf{M}^{-1}}{24}\left[\mathrm{U}_{\mathbf{w}}(\mathbf{w} + \epsilon \mathbf{M}^{-1}\hat{\mathbf{p}}) + \mathrm{U}_{\mathbf{w}}(\mathbf{w} - \epsilon \mathbf{M}^{-1}\hat{\mathbf{p}})\right] \tag{3.27}$$

$$\mathbf{p} = \hat{\mathbf{p}} + \frac{\epsilon}{24}\left[\mathrm{U}_{\mathbf{w}}(\mathbf{w} + \epsilon \mathbf{M}^{-1}\hat{\mathbf{p}}) - \mathrm{U}_{\mathbf{w}}(\mathbf{w} - \epsilon \mathbf{M}^{-1}\hat{\mathbf{p}})\right] \tag{3.28}$$

Importance weights are computed after the samples are obtained using the S2HMC (Marwala et al., 2023; Mongwe et al., 2021d) to guarantee that the shadow canonical density is used rather than the true density. The differences between the true and shadow Hamiltonians are the basis for determining the importance weights. It is worth noting that S2HMC degenerates to HMC when the shadow Hamiltonian is set to equal the true Hamiltonian. A detailed exposition on S2HMC, HMC, and MALA can be found in Marwala et al. (2023).

3.4 Numerical Experiments

In this section, we describe the experimental setup used in this chapter. We present a description of the dataset utilized and the performance metrics used to compare against the different methods.

3.4.1 *Data Description*

The performance of the MALA, HMC, and S2HMC methods in calibrating the SABR model is compared to real-world and simulated datasets. The simulated data is from the SABR model with known parameters being $\{\alpha = 0.0130, \rho = -0.23, \nu = 1.21\}$ for the 1W into 1Y swaption. In contrast, the real-world data is from the South African (ZAR) swaption data as observed in the market for the 6M into 1Y swaption as at 28 June 2024, extracted from a calibrated model from a market data provider.

3.4.2 *Performance Metrics*

The performance metrics used in this chapter are predictive performance on unseen data. The predictive performance metrics used are the Mean Square Error (MSE), Mean Absolute Error (MAE), coefficient of determination (R^2), and Mean Percentage Error (MAPE). For all the MCMC algorithms, we set the pre-conditioning matrix $\mathbf{M} = \mathbf{I}$, which is the typical approach in practice (Marwala et al., 2023).

We generated five chains with 2000 samples for all the datasets with a burn-in period of 1000. This was adequate for all of the methods to converge across all datasets. The number of steps required to create each sample was set at 25 for HMC and S2HMC. The step sizes were chosen by targeting an acceptance rate of 60% for MALA and 80% for HMC and S2HMC methods through the dual averaging methodology (Hoffman & Gelman, 2011; Mongwe et al., 2021a).

3.5 Results and Discussions

In this section, we present the results and the discussions from the numerical experiments. Table 3.1 shows the calibrated parameters and standard deviations on simulated data using the MALA, HMC, and S2HMC methods, while Table 3.2 shows the calibration results on the ZAR market-observed swaption data using all the MCMC methods. Tables 3.3 and 3.4 show the performance on unseen data using various performance metrics on the simulated and ZAR market-observed swaption data, respectively, across all the MCMC algorithms.

Figures 3.1 to 3.2 show the inference results for the Bayesian framework across all the MCMC algorithms on the simulated and ZAR market observed volatility skew. Figures 3.3 to 3.11 show the posterior distribution inference results for the α, ρ and ν parameters in the SABR model using the MALA, HMC, and S2HMC algorithms on both the simulated and the ZAR market swaption data.

Table 3.1 shows that the MALA, HMC, and S2HMC algorithms can reproduce the parameters that produced the simulated data. We note that the S2HMC algorithm produces the highest standard deviations for each parameter, while MALA has the lowest standard deviations. Table 3.2 shows that the methods agree on the parameters, with S2HMC producing the largest standard deviations across all the parameters, while MALA produces the lowest. This is consistent with what was observed on the simulated data, thus suggesting that MALA can generally produce the lowest standard deviations on the parameters. Tables 3.3 and 3.4 show that the methods produce similar performance on unseen data, with the HMC and S2HMC algorithms displaying the best performance across the various performance metrics.

Table 3.1 Results of the MCMC calibration on the simulated swaption data for the 1W into 1Y swaption. The true and calibrated parameters are displayed. The results show that the MALA, HMC, and S2HMC algorithms can reproduce the true parameters. The HMC and S2HMC methods both use a path length of 25. The values in the parenthesis are the standard deviations from the posterior distribution. The entries in **bold** indicate the MCMC method that outperforms

Parameter	*True parameters*	MALA	HMC_{25}	$S2HMC_{25}$
α	0.0130	0.0129 (**0.0191**)	0.0129 (0.0264)	0.0130 (0.0277)
ρ	–0.23	–0.2301 (**0.0092**)	–0.2302 (0.0106)	–0.2303 (0.0104)
ν	1.21	1.2147 (**0.0098**)	1.2116 (0.0131)	1.2106 (0.0136)

Table 3.2 Results of the MCMC calibration on the ZAR market-observed swaption data for the 6M into 1Y swaption as at 28 June 2024. The results show that the MALA, HMC, and S2HMC algorithms agree on the calibrated parameters. The HMC and S2HMC methods both use a path length of 25. The values in the parenthesis are the standard deviations from the posterior distribution. The entries in **bold** indicate the MCMC method that outperforms

Parameter	MALA	HMC_{25}	$S2HMC_{25}$
α	0.0347 (**0.0027**)	0.0347 (0.0029)	0.0347 (0.0031)
ρ	0.6004 (**0.0043**)	0.6001 (0.0044)	0.6004 (0.0045)
ν	0.9176 (**0.0044**)	0.9182 (0.0051)	0.9183 (0.0053)

Table 3.3 Results of the MCMC calibration on the simulated unseen swaption data for the 1W into 1Y swaption. The entries in **bold** indicate the MCMC method that outperforms for the given metric. The results show that the MALA and S2HMC algorithms perform best across the various performance metrics. The HMC and S2HMC methods both use a path length of 25

Metric	MALA	HMC_{25}	$S2HMC_{25}$
R2	0.9999992851	0.999999230	**0.999999659**
MSE	0.0007668415	0.000825566	**0.000365645**
MAPE	0.0004271379	0.00046407	**0.0003041687**
MAE	0.0220524944	0.023652592	**0.015996114**

Table 3.4 Results of the MCMC calibration on the ZAR unseen observed market swaption data as at 28 June 2024 for the 6M into 1Y swaption. The entries in **bold** indicate the MCMC method that outperforms for the given metric. The results show that the HMC and S2HMC algorithms perform best across the various performance metrics. The HMC and S2HMC methods both use a path length of 25

Metric	MALA	HMC_{25}	$S2HMC_{25}$
R2	0.9999933461	0.9999932867	**0.9999934771**
MSE	0.0124373011	0.0125490858	**0.0121925901**
MAPE	0.0007746001	**0.0007267914**	0.0007388930
MAE	0.0882670898	**0.0854889729**	0.0856298624

Figure 3.1a shows that all the methods can fit the skew on the simulated data, with the fit being more certain around the at-the-money (ATM) point and less confident as we move further away from the ATM point. We note that the methods are less confident on the skew's right wing than the skew's left wing. Similar observations are also noted on the ZAR market-observed swaption data in Fig. 3.2a, except that all the methods are confident in the predictions on the left wing of the skew. We also note in Fig. 3.1b and Fig. 3.2b that all the methods have converged on both the simulated and market-observed data.

On both the simulated and ZAR market swaption data, the three MCMC approaches agree on the shape of the posterior distribution for the α, ρ, and ν parameters in the SABR model, as shown in Figs. 3.3, 3.4, 3.5, 3.6, 3.7, 3.8, 3.9, 3.10 and 3.11. Practitioners may use these probability distributions to learn more about the likely values of the parameters, information not provided by more conventional calibration techniques like maximum-likelihood fitting techniques. Creating realistic stress scenarios for the parameters is also easier, which may be important in determining how the skew affects the institution's economic capital, among other metrics.

3.6 Conclusions

Fitting the volatility skew is of utmost importance for practitioners dealing in non-linear derivatives, with the Stochastic Alpha Beta Rho (SABR) model being the commonly used model in the interest-rate market. This

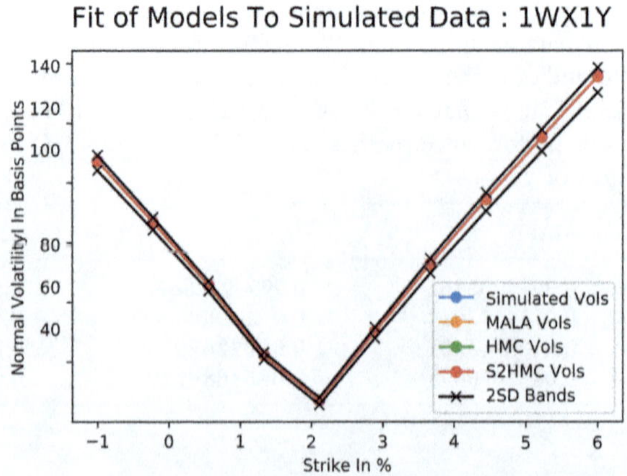

(**a**) Fit over the the simulated volatility skew for the 1W into 1Y swaption using the MALA, HMC, and S2HCM algorithms. We also show the two standard deviation confidence bands using the S2HMC algorithm.

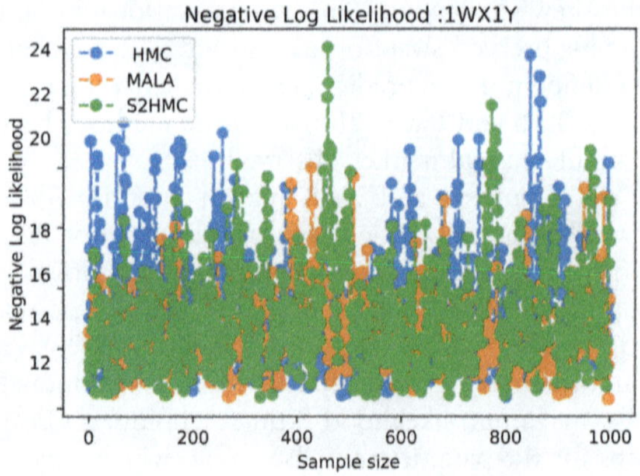

(**b**) Convergence profile based on the negative likelihood for the MALA, HMC, and S2HMC on the simulated volatility skew for 1W into 1Y swaption.

Fig. 3.1 Inference results for the Bayesian framework across all the MCMC algorithms on the simulated swaption market data

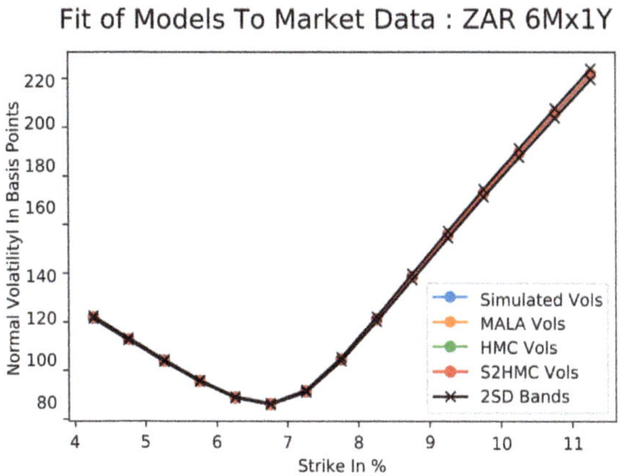

(**a**) Fit over the observed ZAR market volatility skew for the 6M into 1Y swaption using the MALA, HMC, and S2HCM algorithms. We also show the two standard deviation confidence bands using the S2HMC algorithm.

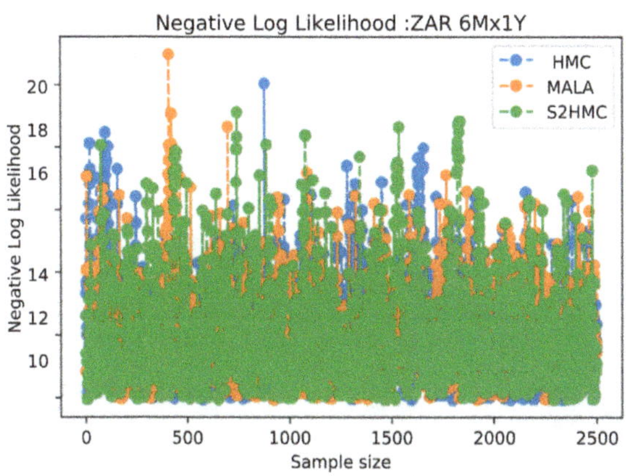

(**b**) Convergence profile based on the negative likelihood for the MALA, HMC, and S2HMC on the ZAR market volatility skew for 6M into 1Y swaption.

Fig. 3.2 Inference results for the Bayesian framework across all the MCMC algorithms on the ZAR market-observed volatility skew as at 28 June 2024

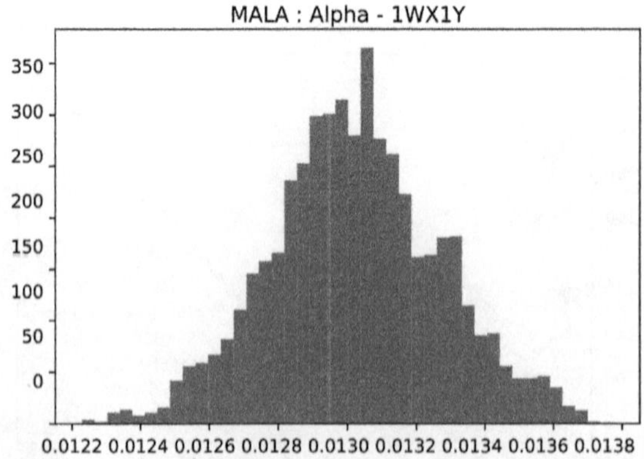

(**a**) Posterior distribution for α on simulated data using MALA algorithm.

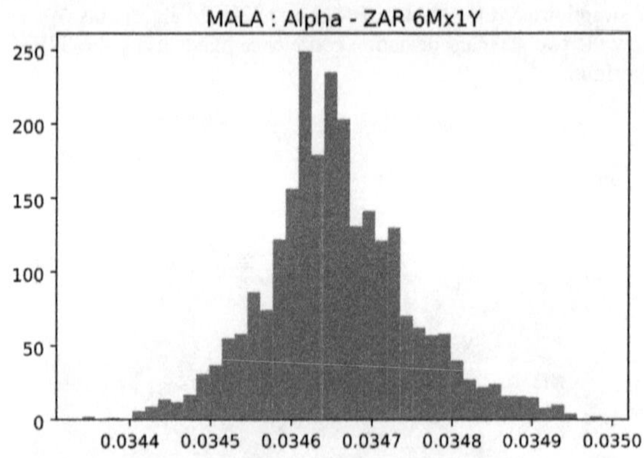

(**b**) Posterior distribution for α on ZAR market observed data using MALA algorithm.

Fig. 3.3 Posterior distribution inference results for the α parameter in the SABR model using the MALA algorithm on both the simulated and the ZAR market swaption data

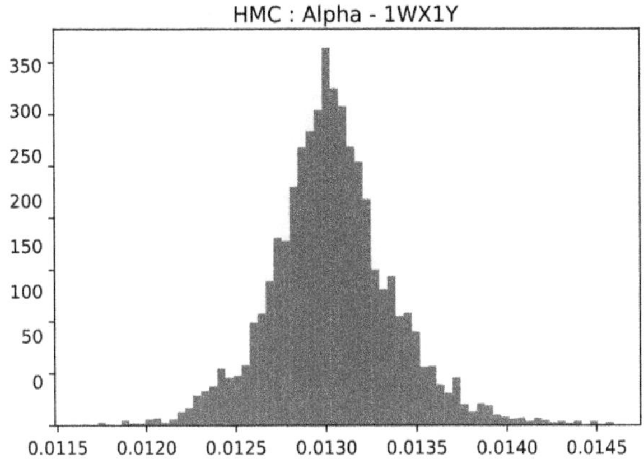

(**a**) Posterior distribution for α on simulated data using HMC algorithm.

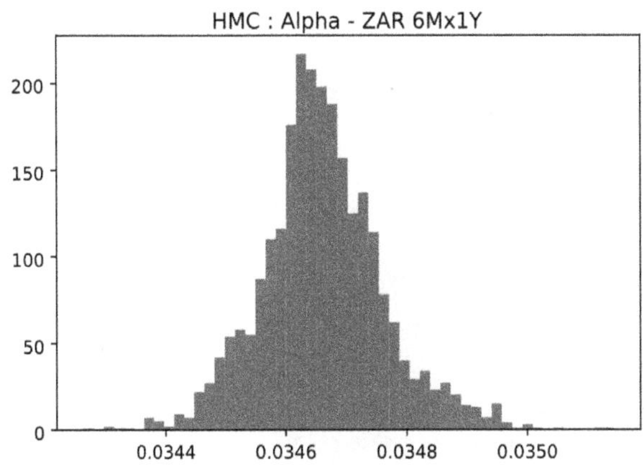

(**b**) Posterior distribution for α on ZAR market data using HMC algorithm.

Fig. 3.4 Posterior distribution inference results for the α parameter in the SABR model using the HMC algorithm on both the simulated and the ZAR market swaption data

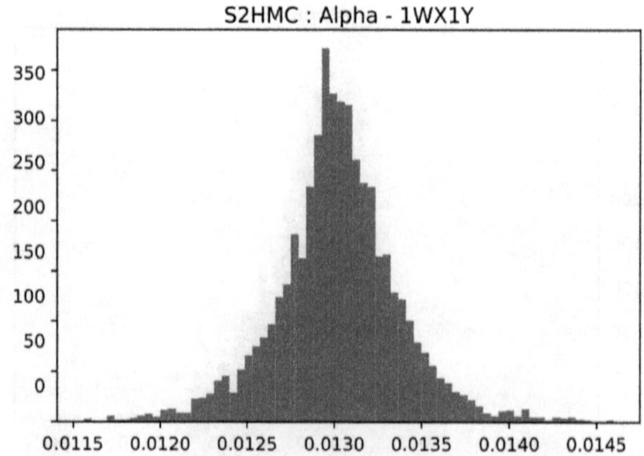

(**a**) Posterior distribution for α on simulated data using S2HMC algorithm.

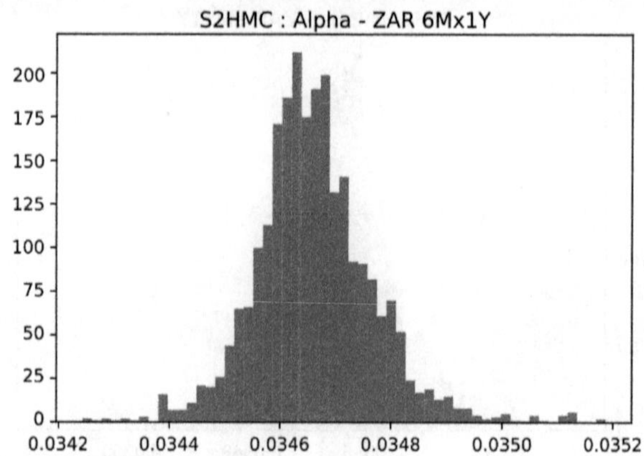

(**b**) Posterior distribution for α on ZAR market data using S2HMC algorithm.

Fig. 3.5 Posterior distribution inference results for the α parameter in the SABR model using the S2HMC algorithm on both the simulated and the ZAR market swaption data

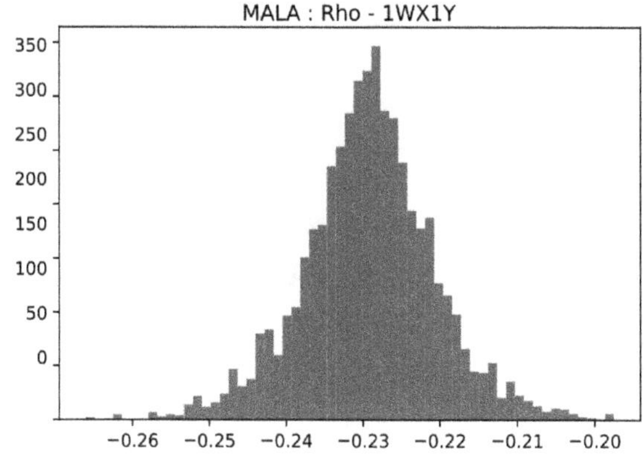

(**a**) Posterior distribution for ρ on simulated data using MALA algorithm.

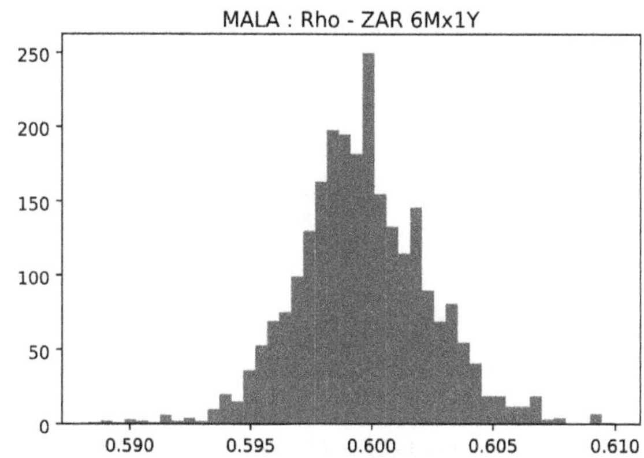

(**b**) Posterior distribution for ρ on ZAR market data using MALA algorithm.

Fig. 3.6 Posterior distribution inference results for the ρ parameter in the SABR model using the MALA algorithm on both the simulated and the ZAR market swaption data

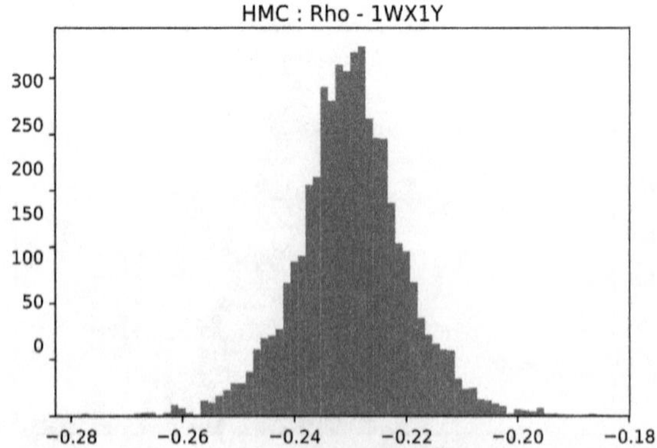

(**a**) Posterior distribution for ρ on simulated data using HMC algorithm.

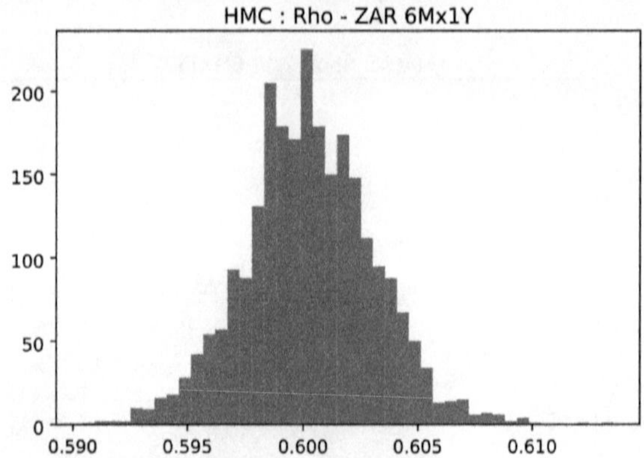

(**b**) Posterior distribution for ρ on ZAR market data using HMC algorithm.

Fig. 3.7 Posterior distribution inference results for the ρ parameter in the SABR model using the HMC algorithm on both the simulated and the ZAR market swaption data

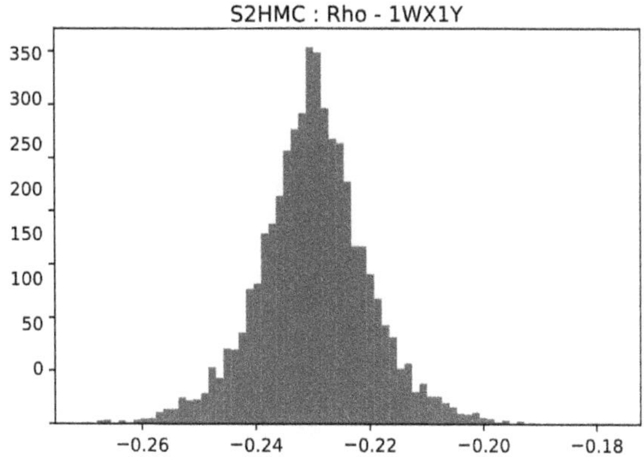

(**a**) Posterior distribution for ρ on simulated data using S2HMC algorithm.

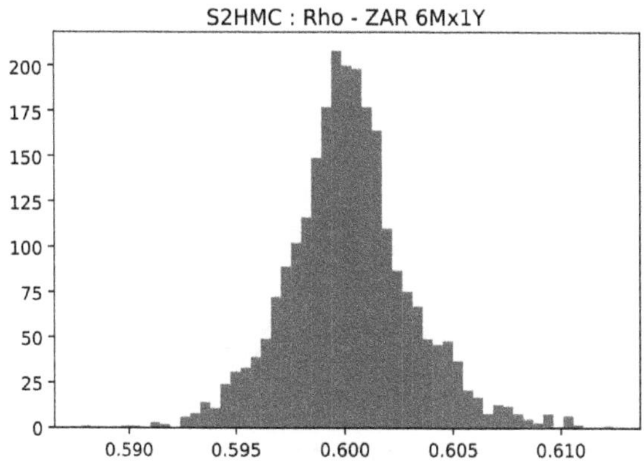

(**b**) Posterior distribution for ρ on ZAR market data using S2HMC algorithm.

Fig. 3.8 Posterior distribution inference results for the ρ parameter in the SABR model using the S2HMC algorithm on both the simulated and the ZAR market swaption data

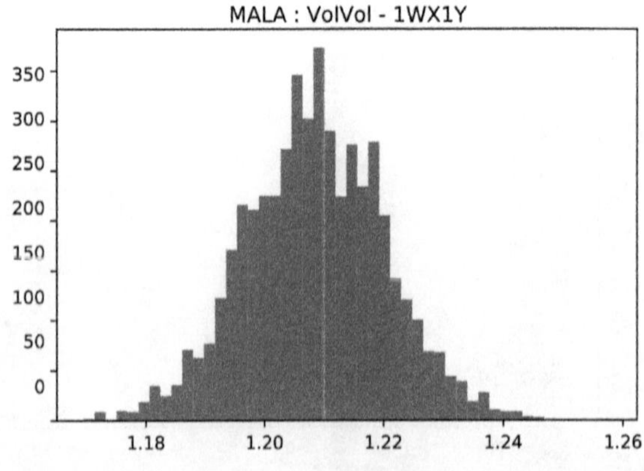

(**a**) Posterior distribution for ν on simulated data using MALA algorithm.

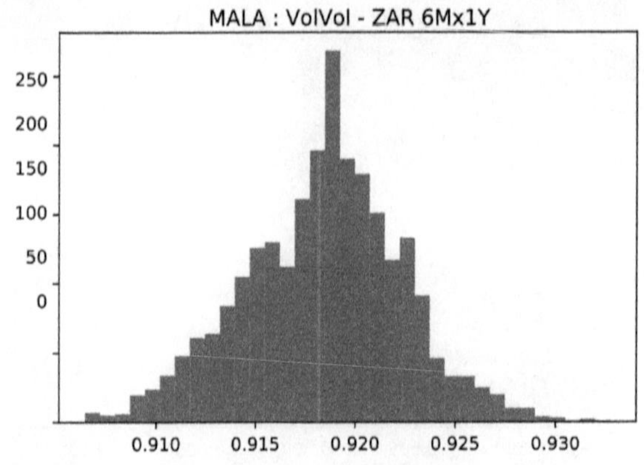

(**b**) Posterior distribution for ν on ZAR market data using MALA algorithm.

Fig. 3.9 Posterior distribution inference results for the ν parameter in the SABR model using the MALA algorithm on both the simulated and the ZAR market swaption data

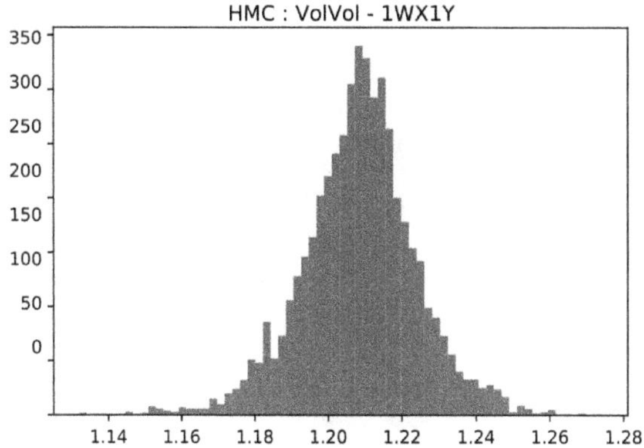

(**a**) Posterior distribution for ν on simulated data using HMC algorithm.

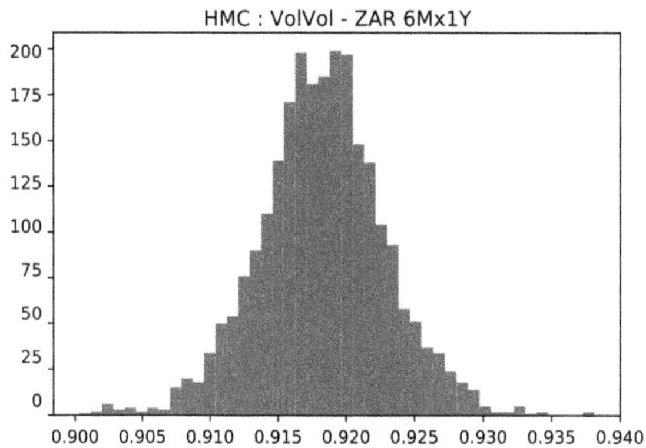

(**b**) Posterior distribution for ν on ZAR market data using HMC algorithm.

Fig. 3.10 Posterior distribution inference results for the ν parameter in the SABR model using the HMC algorithm on both the simulated and the ZAR market swaption data

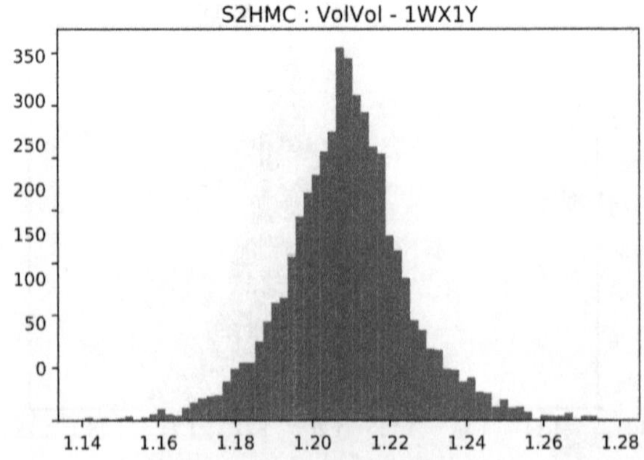

(a) Posterior distribution for ν on simulated data using S2HMC algorithm.

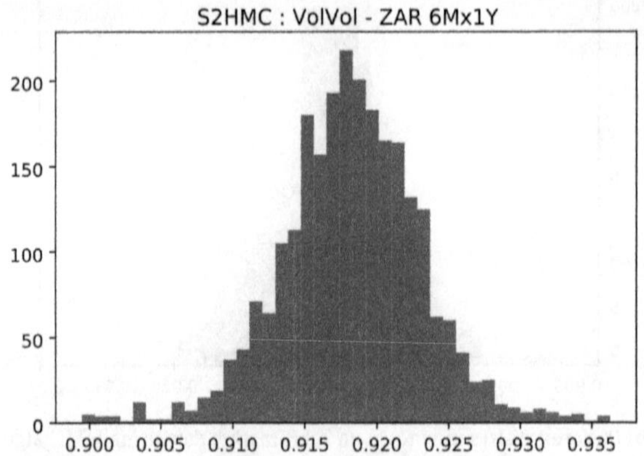

(b) Posterior distribution for ν on ZAR market data using S2HMC algorithm.

Fig. 3.11 Posterior distribution inference results for the ν parameter in the SABR model using the S2HMC algorithm on both the simulated and the ZAR market swaption data chapter presents a first-in-literature probabilistic framework to infer the volatility skew in interest-rate markets using the SABR model on both simulated and ZAR observed market swaption data. The inference of the SABR model is performed using the Metropolis-Adjusted Langevin Algorithm, Hamiltonian Monte Carlo, and the Separable Shadow Hamiltonian Hybrid Monte Carlo methods.

The analysis shows that the methods can reproduce the observed volatility skew on both simulated and market-observed swaption data and produce a similar performance on unseen data across various performance metrics, with S2HMC producing marginal outperformance. We further find that the methods are fairly confident, as measured by the width of the confidence bands of the volatility skew in and around the money point, but get less confident as we move toward the wings of the skew.

The work in this chapter can be enhanced by considering the entire interest-rate volatility surface instead of limiting the data to the 1W into 1Y and 6M into 1Y swaption data. Practitioners could also be interested in comparing other models that can capture the volatility skew. In the next chapter, we explore learning the entire volatility surface using sparse Gaussian processes models in developed and emerging equity option markets.

References

Antonov, A., Konikov, M., & Spector, M. (2015). Mixing SABR models for negative rates. Available at SSRN 2653682.

Black, F., & Scholes, M. (1973). The pricing of options and corporate liabilities. *Journal of Political Economy, 81*(3), 637–654. ISSN: 00223808.

Black, F. (1976). The pricing of commodity contracts. *Journal of Financial Economics, 3*, 167–179.

Choi, J., & Seo, B. K. (2023). Option pricing under the normal SABR model with Gaussian quadratures. Available at SSRN 4265261.

Duane, S., Kennedy, A. D., Pendleton, B. J., & Roweth, D. (1987). Hybrid Monte Carlo. *Physics Letters B, 195*(2), 216–222.

Dupire, B., et al. (1994). Pricing with a smile. *Risk, 7*(1), 18–20.

Girolami, M., & Calderhead, B. (2011). Riemann manifold langevin and Hamiltonian Monte Carlo methods. *Journal of the Royal Statistical Society: Series B (Statistical Methodology), 73*(2), 123–214.

Gu, M., & Sun, S. (2020). Neural langevin dynamical sampling. *IEEE Access, 8*, 31595–31605.

Hagan, P. S., Kumar, D., Lesniewski, A. S., & Woodward, D. E. (2002). Managing smile risk. *The Best of Wilmott, 1*, 249–296.

Hastings, W. K. (1970). Monte Carlo sampling methods using Markov chains and their applications. *Biometrica, 57*(1), 97–109.

Heide, C., Roosta, F., Hodgkinson, L., & Kroese, D. (2021). Shadow manifold Hamiltonian Monte Carlo. In *International conference on artificial intelligence and statistics*. PMLR (pp. 1477–1485).

Hinton, G. E., & Van Camp, D. (1993). Keeping the neural networks simple by minimizing the description length of the weights. In *Proceedings of the sixth annual conference on computational learning theory* (pp. 5–13). ACM.

Hoffman, M. D., & Gelman, A. (2011). *The No-U-Turn Sampler: Adaptively setting path lengths in Hamiltonian Monte Carlo*. arXiv: 1111.4246 [stat.CO]

Hoffman, M. D., Blei, D. M., Wang, C., & Paisley, J. (2013). Stochastic variational inference. *Journal of Machine Learning Research, 14*(5).

Hoffman, M. D., & Gelman, A. (2014). The No-U-turn sampler: Adaptively setting path lengths in Hamiltonian Monte Carlo. *Journal of Machine Learning Research, 15*(1), 1593–1623.

Izaguirre, J. A., & Hampton, S. S. (Nov. 2004). Shadow hybrid Monte Carlo: An efficient propagator in phase space of macromolecules. *Journal of Computational Physics, 200*(2), 581–604. ISSN: 0021-9991. https://doi.org/10.1016/j.jcp.2004.04.016

Kennedy, J. E., Mitra, S., & Pham, D. (2012). On the approximation of the SABR model: A probabilistic approach. *Applied Mathematical Finance, 19*(6), 553–586.

MacKay, D. J. C. (1992). A practical Bayesian framework for backpropagation networks. *Neural Computation, 4*(3), 448–472.

Marwala, T., Mbuvha, R., & Mongwe, W. T. (2023). *Hamiltonian Monte Carlo methods in machine learning*. Elsevier.

Mbuvha, R., & Marwala, T. (2020). Bayesian inference of COVID-19 spreading rates in South Africa. *PloS One, 15*(8), Article e0237126.

Mbuvha, R., Mongwe, W. T., & Marwala, T. (2021). Separable Shadow Hamiltonian hybrid Monte Carlo for Bayesian neural network inference in wind speed forecasting. *Energy and A, 1*, Article 100108.

Mongwe, W. T. (Dec. 2015). *Analysis of equity and interest rate returns in South Africa under the context of jump diffusion processes*. Masters Thesis at University of Cape Town. Last Retrieved: 18 March 2021. https://open.uct.ac.za/bitstream/handle/11427/16600/thesis_com_2015_mongwe_wilson_tsakane.pdf?isAllowed=y&sequence=1

Mongwe, W. T., Mbuvha, R., & Marwala, T. (2021a). Adaptive magnetic Hamiltonian Monte Carlo. *IEEE Access, 9*, 152993–153003. https://doi.org/10.1109/ACCESS.2021.3127931

Mongwe, W. T., Mbuvha, R., & Marwala, T. (2021b). Adaptively setting the path length for separable shadow Hamiltonian hybrid Monte Carlo. *IEEE Access, 9*, 138598–138607.

Mongwe, W. T., Mbuvha, R., & Marwala, T. (2021c). Antithetic magnetic and Shadow Hamiltonian Monte Carlo. *IEEE Access, 9*, 49857–49867.

Mongwe, W. T., Mbuvha, R., & Marwala, T. (2021d). *Bayesian inference of local government audit outcomes*. https://doi.org/10.1371/journal.pone.0261245

Mongwe, W. T., Mbuvha, R., & Marwala, T. (2021e). Locally scaled and stochastic volatility metropolis-hastings algorithms. *Algorithms, 14*(12). ISSN: 1999-4893. https://doi.org/10.3390/a14120351

Mongwe, W. T., Mbuvha, R., & Marwala, T. (2021f). Utilising partial momentum refreshment in separable Shadow Hamiltonian Hybrid Monte Carlo. *IEEE Access, 9*, 151235–151244. https://doi.org/10.1109/ACCESS.2021.3126812

Mongwe, W. T., Mbuvha, R., & Marwala, T. (2022a). Shadow magnetic Hamiltonian Monte Carlo. *IEEE Access, 10*, 34340–34351. https://doi.org/10.1109/ACCESS.2022.3161443

Mongwe, W. T., Sidogi, T., Mbuvha, R., & Marwala, T. (2022b). Probabilistic inference of south african equity option prices under jump-diffusion processes. In *2022 IEEE symposium on computational intelligence for financial engineering and economics (CIFEr)* (pp. 1–8). IEEE.

Neal, R. M. (1993). Bayesian learning via stochastic dynamics. In *Advances in neural information processing systems* (Vol. 5, pp. 475–482). Morgan Kaufmann Publishers Inc. ISBN: 1-55860-274-7. http://dl.acm.org/citation.cfm?id=645753.667903.

Neal, R. M., et al. (2011). MCMC using Hamiltonian dynamics. *Handbook of Markov Chain Monte Carlo, 2*(11), 2.

Ruiz, F., & Titsias, M. (2019). A contrastive divergence for combining variational inference and mcmc. In *International conference on machine learning*. PMLR (pp. 5537–5545).

Salimans, T., Kingma, D., & Welling, M. (2015). Markov chain monte carlo and variational inference: bridging the gap. In *International conference on machine learning*. PMLR (pp. 1218–1226).

Sweet, C. R., Hampton, S. S., Skeel, R. D., & Izaguirre, J. A. (2009). A separable shadow Hamiltonian hybrid Monte Carlo method. *The Journal of Chemical Physics, 131*(17), Article 174106.

Yang, Y., Fabozzi, F. J., & Bianchi, M. L. (2015). Stochastic alpha-beta-rho hedging for foreign exchange options: is it worth the effort? *Journal of Derivatives, 23*(2), 76.

CHAPTER 4

Learning Equity Volatility Surfaces Using Sparse Gaussian Processes

4.1 Introduction

Advances in artificial intelligence, particularly deep learning, have pushed the frontiers of the range of problems and models that can be addressed and deployed in quantitative finance (Sidogi, 2023). These data-driven approaches allow market practitioners to more accurately capture financial markets' stylized facts and frictions compared to traditional methods, allowing for the efficient and optimal portfolio management of derivative books. These learning techniques have been applied to the problems of generating realistic market data (Buehler et al., 2020a; Li et al., 2020; Takahashi et al., 2019; Sidogi et al., 2022), pricing of non-linear derivatives (De Spiegeleer et al., 2018; Frandsen et al., 2022; Ivas et al., 2021), derivative instrument hedging (Buehler et al., 2019; Carbonneau, 2021; Horvath et al., 2021; Lütkebohmert et al., 2022), and model calibration (Cousin et al., 2016; Horvath et al., 2021; Sousa et al., 2012), among others.

Supplementary Information The online version contains supplementary material available at https://doi.org/10.1007/978-3-031-88431-3_4.

W. T. Mongwe et al., *Bayesian Machine Learning in Quantitative Finance*, https://doi.org/10.1007/978-3-031-88431-3_4

Machine learning has fostered new techniques for simulating realistic financial market data time series (Che et al., 2018; Marti, 2020; Wiese et al., 2020). These techniques are based primarily on generative models such as deep generative adversarial networks (GAN) (Buehler et al., 2020a; Che et al., 2018; Sidogi et al., 2022; Takahashi et al., 2019; Wiese et al., 2020), with few studies considering Variational Autoencoders (VAE) (Buehler et al., 2020b). Takahashi et al. (2019) present a GAN model that captures statistical properties of financial time series, such as volatility clustering and leverage (Cont, 2001). On the other hand, Henry-Labordere (2019) presents a primal-dual algorithm for the automatic generation of financial data and anomaly detection. They compare the performance of the primal-dual approach against the Wasserstein-GAN model with good results. A key limitation of deep generative models based on GANs is that they require large amounts of data. Buehler et al. (2020b) present a VAE-based generative model that utilizes rough path signatures. This approach performs well even when the training data is small and oscillatory.

The pricing of options, which are non-linear derivative contracts, using artificial neural networks has been considered extensively in the literature (Ruf & Wang, 2019). Neural networks are preferable for this task as they can capture the non-linear relationship between outputs and inputs and are guaranteed by the universal approximation theorem to provide robust approximations to continuous functions (Ruf & Wang, 2019). Gradojevic et al. (2009) utilize modular neural networks to price European call options on the S&P500 index. Their results show that incorporating modularity improves the performance of feed-forward neural networks, with the limitation that the user has to specify the number of modules to use. Frandsen et al. (2022) utilizes a new differential machine learning technique to price options. Differential machine learning was introduced by Huge et al. (2020) and combines automatic adjoint differentiation with machine learning for managing derivative exposure. In the context of option pricing, differential machine learning involves regularizing the machine learning model using the delta information of the option—which should enhance the learning process. The main drawback of using neural networks for pricing is that most of the methods in the literature do not consider no-arbitrage conditions (Itkin, 2019).

The seminal work of Buehler et al. (2019) utilized deep reinforcement learning to construct hedging strategies using a convex risk measure for a portfolio of derivatives under the Heston (1993b) model. This framework easily incorporates market frictions such as transaction costs and market impact. It is applicable across various hedging instruments with the computational resources related to the hedge instrument universe and not the portfolio size. Horvath et al. (2021) extend this to a non-Markovian scenario, where they present a deep learning framework for hedging under the Rough Bergomi stochastic volatility model. This extension also highlights the importance of selecting the appropriate neural network architecture, with the original architecture used by Buehler et al. (2019) requiring updating for the non-Markovian case to improve performance.

Another quantitative finance problem tackled using deep learning is the model calibration problem (Horvath et al., 2021; Liu et al., 2019; Rosenbaum & Zhang, 2021), which is the focus of this current chapter. For this task, one is interested in setting the model parameters so that they reproduce the observed option market quotes. Horvath et al. (2021) present a deep calibration framework for calibrating stochastic volatility models to option market data. This approach allows one to calibrate complex pricing models (e.g., some of which would require Monte Carlo simulations) in real-time. The authors show that their approach leads to significant orders of magnitude improvement in the execution time of the calibration process. However, it should be noted that this approach does not guarantee that the approximated pricing function is arbitrage-free (Itkin, 2019). Model calibration is an ill-posed problem that frequently necessitates using a regularization method in real-world scenarios (Itkin, 2019). This suggests that Bayesian approaches may be well suited to this problem due to their ability to naturally incorporate regularization through the prior distribution.

Although deep neural network models have been successfully employed to address the calibration problem, thus bringing into the fold more complex methods, one still needs to specify the neural network's architecture—which consists of many possible configurations (Horvath et al., 2021). No canonical techniques exist for determining the optimal architecture for a given calibration problem. Secondly, neural networks are, by their nature, black-box functions and are difficult to interpret, thus limiting their adoption by financial market practitioners. In this chapter, we provide a Bayesian framework for the calibration problem using Gaussian processes to address the issues identified using neural networks.

Gaussian processes provide a non-parametric approach to solving various problems and are priors over functions (Mbuvha et al., 2023; Rasmussen, 2003; Schulz et al., 2018; Williams & Rasmussen, 2006). They have fewer parameters that need to be specified than neural networks, with the benefit that neural networks converge to Gaussian processes in the wide limit (Agrawal et al., 2020; Neal, 1996). In addition, Gaussian processes can provide uncertainties in the calibrated parameters and any predictions thereof. Gaussian processes have the limitation that the training is computationally expensive as it has a cubic complexity to data size (Snelson & Ghahramani, 2005). However, this can be addressed using sparse approaches where instead of using the entire dataset, inducing points are used which are orders of magnitude smaller than the original dataset (Liu et al., 2020; Snelson & Ghahramani, 2005). In addition, there is active research on using distributed approaches for scaling Gaussian processes to larger datasets that do not rely on inducing or variational parameters (Cohen et al., 2020; Deisenroth & Ng, 2015; Liu et al., 2020).

In this chapter, we calibrate the Heston (1993a) stochastic volatility model and the Rough Bergormi stochastic volatility model to option market datasets in developing and developed markets using sparse Gaussian Processes. In particular, we calibrate the models to the FTSE/JSE All Share Index (ALSI) option data and the EuroStoxx 50 index option data. Using simulated data, our approach trains the Gaussian process to learn the pricing function of both stochastic volatility models offline. We then calibrate the models online to real market data. We consider sparse Gaussian processes for each point on the volatility surface and multi-output (i.e., for the whole surface simultaneously) sparse Gaussian processes within our framework and compare our approach with the current start-of-art deep neural networks. This chapter presents a first-in-the-literature Bayesian framework for learning volatility surfaces in developed and developing equity markets. We also present the first use of sparse Gaussian processes to calibrate stochastic volatility models to financial market data.

The remainder of this chapter is structured as follows: We first describe the stochastic volatility models used to model the volatility surface in Sect. 4.2; we then detail the calibration framework that utilizes machine learning techniques methods in Sect. 4.3; we then present the experiment setup, after which we present the results, discuss them, and provide the conclusion in Sects. 4.4–4.6 respectively.

4.2 Stochastic Volatility Models

This section presents the stochastic volatility models we will calibrate to the equity option data. The models considered are the Heston and Rough Bergomi stochastic volatility models. For both dynamics, we consider the usual filtered probability space $(\Omega, \mathcal{F}, (\mathcal{F}_t)_{t\in\mathbb{R}}, \mathbb{Q})$ which supports correlated Brownian motions.

4.2.1 Heston Stochastic Volatility Model

A stochastic volatility model that naturally extends the conventional geometric Brownian motion process is the Heston (1993a) model and is better able to capture the volatility skew. Heston (1993a) presents a model that incorporatesBlack and Scholes (1973) as a special case (Heston, 1993a; Mikhailov & Ulrich Nögel, 2004). Heston's setup is still analytically tractable while considering the non-log-normal distribution of the asset returns, leverage impact, and significant mean-reverting aspect of volatility. The Black-Scholes volatility surfaces produced by Heston's model resemble empirical implied volatility surfaces (Heston, 1993a; Mikhailov & Ulrich Nögel, 2004)

The following system of differential equations gives the Heston (1993a) model dynamics:

$$\begin{aligned} dS_t &= \mu S_t dt + \sqrt{v_t} S_t dW_t^S \\ dv_t &= \kappa(\theta - v_t)dt + \xi(t)\sqrt{v_t} dW_t^v \\ dW_t^v dW_t^S &= \rho dt \end{aligned} \tag{4.1}$$

where μ is the drift term, θ is the long-term average variance, κ is the rate of mean reversion, ξ is the volatility of volatility and ρ is instanteneous correlation between variance and price. Furthermore, we have that $\kappa, \theta, \xi(t) > 0$ and $2\kappa\theta > \xi(t)^2$. The parameters $\{\theta, \kappa, \rho, \xi\}$ affect the level and the shape of the volatility skew . The volatility of the volatility parameter ξ controls the convexity of the skew. A higher ξ generates a more convex function, which leads to more skew. The mean reversion κ and correlation ρ between Brownian motions both control the money skew. The long-term variance θ controls the overall level of skew (Heston, 1993a).

From the dynamics in Eq. 4.1, we note that the underlying asset follows an evolution process similar to theBlack and Scholes (1973) model. Still, it also introduces a stochastic behavior for the volatility process. In particular, Heston assumes that the asset variance v_t follows a mean-reverting Cox-Ingersoll-Ross process, which leads to closed-form formulas for pricing plain vanilla options. However, this increased flexibility makes the Heston model more complex. The model necessitates more complex mathematical calculations to arrive at closed-form prices for vanilla options and more difficult calibration procedures to match observed market prices.

4.2.2 Rough Bergomi Stochastic Volatility Model

Present-day volatility models cannot provide realistic dynamics for the volatility surface while also accurately capturing the implied volatility surface's true shape. In an effort to meet these two requirements, the Rough Bergomi model, a popular rough volatility model, fits a large variety of volatility surfaces with just three parameters, surpassing the majority of traditional stochastic volatility models based on Brownian motion. Within an assets variance process, rough volatility models substitute a fractional Brownian motion for the conventional Brownian motion (Bayer et al., 2016; Bergomi, 2008).

Instead of modeling instantaneous variance, Bergomi (2008) chose to represent the dynamics of forward variance to more correctly reflect forward volatility and forward skew risks. The Bergomi (2008) model was created when he merged his basic framework for predicting forward variances with the proper dynamics of the pricing process. Depending on how many Brownian movements are employed in the forward variance process's dynamics, Bergomi offered a variety of models (Bergomi, 2008).

The Rough Bergomi model was introduced into the literature by Bayer et al. (2016) as an extension of the traditional Bergomi (2008) model, which they formulated when they empirically analyzed log volatility through time. Due to its power-law at-the-money volatility skew, which aligns with empirical data, this model has gained popularity for stochastic volatility modeling (Zhu et al., 2021). The following system of stochastic differential equations gives the dynamics of this model:

$$\begin{aligned} dS_t &= -\frac{1}{2}V_t + \sqrt{V_t}dW_t^S \\ dV_t &= \xi_0(t)\Xi\left(\sqrt{2H\nu}\int_0^t (t-s)^{H-\frac{1}{2}}dW_t^v\right) \\ dW_t^v dW_t^S &= \rho dt \end{aligned} \tag{4.2}$$

where $H \in (0, 1)$ denotes the Hurst parameter, $\nu > 0$, $\Xi(.)$ the stochastic exponential, and $\xi_0(t) > 0$ denotes the initial forward variance curve, and ρ is the instantaneous correlation coefficient between price and variance. It is worth noting that since this volatility model's stochastic process in Eq. 4.2 is rougher than a Brownian motion; in particular, the absence of Markovianity renders traditional pricing techniques impractical (Zhu et al., 2021) for this model.

The parameters of this model are $\{H, \nu, \rho\}$. This model has been praised for its ability to fit a wide range of shapes of volatility surfaces with just these three parameters. The main effect of H is to control the decay of the at-the-money forward skew for short times to maturity. The effects of ρ and ν on the Rough Bergomi model are intertwined. They both impact the shape of the volatility smile.

4.3 Model Calibration Using Bayesian Machine Learning

In this section, we outline the calibration framework used in this chapter and provide details on the Machine learning techniques utilized.

4.3.1 Calibration Framework

In this section, we outline the process we are following in our calibration procedure. These steps are aligned with the two-step procedure outlined in (Horvath et al., 2021). Note that this chapter does not consider the one-step process of using a purely data-driven approach discussed in Horvath et al. (2021) without relying on formal models. We plan to consider this approach in future work. The calibration framework is summarized in Fig. 4.1, with the steps as follows:

1. **Simulate paths from models:** Using the chosen set of parameters, we first simulate synthetic data using the Heston or Rough Bergomi model.
2. **Compute the implied volatilities:** Using the synthetic data, compute the corresponding option price or implied volatility, which is the label for the respective parameter vector. The computation can be done using any numerical method, such as the Monte Carlo simulation.
3. **Train machine learning model:** Learn the approximate pricing map using a machine learning model. We then train the model to learn the pricing model offline.
4. **Calibrate using market data:** After learning the pricing map, we then calibrate the model (using the learned pricing map) to market data using a standard calibration routine.

It is worth noting that since all but the simplest models require numerical approximations of the true option price, this method is conceptually similar to conventional calibration routines (Horvath et al., 2021). The literature has shown that the deep neural network approach typically results in orders of magnitude speed up relative to traditional calibration routines, especially for the models that require Monte Carlo for the pricing (Horvath et al., 2021).

In this chapter, we expand the machine learning models considered to Gaussian processes due to the ability to produce uncertainties in the calibrated parameters and predictions. The main drawback of the GP approach is that they are slower than neural networks for training and evaluation. In future work, we plan to investigate various scaling approaches (such as distributed approaches that have shown good performance in other contexts Cohen et al., 2020) for Gaussian processes within the context of implied volatility surface calibration. In our analysis in this

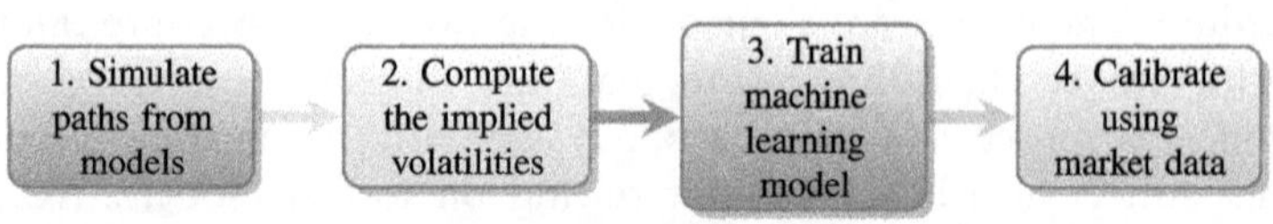

Fig. 4.1 Model calibration framework using machine learning utilized in this chapter

chapter, we compare the performance of our proposed Bayesian framework that utilizes Gaussian processes to deep learning models. We discuss both machine learning models in the next section.

4.3.2 Deep Neural Networks and Gaussian Processes

In this section, we discuss the machine learning techniques that we use to learn the volatility surfaces in both developing and developed equity markets.

4.3.2.1 Deep Neural Networks

Neural networks are universal function approximators inspired by the functioning of the human brain. They have driven various advancements across multiple industries, and quantitative finance is no exception (Horvath et al., 2021; Mbuvha et al., 2021). This deep network consists of a group of neurons arranged in a series of layers, where each layer's input is the previous layer's neuron activations, and each layer's output is a weighted sum of the input followed by a non-linear activation (Montavon et al., 2018).

The network's neurons cooperatively implement a sophisticated non-linear mapping from the input to the output (Montavon et al., 2018). In this chapter, we consider fully connected feed-forward deep neural networks of the form depicted in Fig. 4.2 with the last layer defined as:

$$f_k(x) = b_k + \sum_j v_{jk} h_j(x) \tag{4.3}$$

$$h_j(x) = \Psi\left(a_j + \sum_i w_{ij} x_i\right) \tag{4.4}$$

where w_{ij} is the weight connection for the ith previous layer input to the jth hidden unit and v_{jk} is the weight connection between the jth hidden unit to the kth output. The activation function Ψ provides the non-linearity required to approximate complex non-linear relationships between inputs and outputs.

Selecting the optimal neural network architecture for a given task is still an open research problem. In this chapter, we limit our investigations to a neural network with three hidden layers, each with 30 neurons, and the output nodes corresponding to the size of the volatility surface .

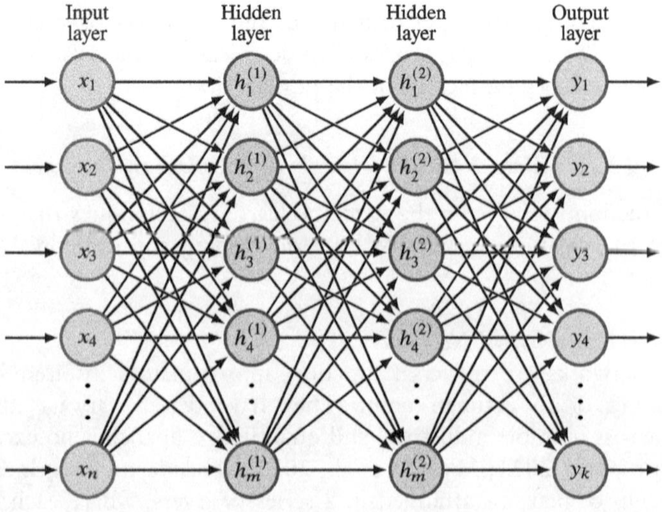

Fig. 4.2 An illustration of the data flow in a deep feed-forward neural network. In this chapter, we limit our investigations to a neural network with three hidden layers (each with 30 neurons) and the output nodes corresponding to the size of the volatility surface

4.3.2.2 Gaussian Processes

Gaussian processes are non-parametric probabilistic models often utilized to solve regression problems. Unlike deep neural networks, Gaussian processes can produce uncertainties in the predictions made from this model. A Gaussian process is a set of random variables, each of a finite subset of which is collectively Gaussian distributed (Mbuvha et al., 2023; Rasmussen & Williams, 2006). Gaussian processes are priors over functions.

Gaussian processes are fully defined by a mean function $\mu(\mathbf{x}')$ and a Kernel function $k(\mathbf{x}'_i, \mathbf{x}'_j)$. Given a training dataset $\{\mathbf{x}'_t, \mathbf{x}_t\}_{t=1}^{t}$ with t noisy observations $\mathbf{x}_t = f(\mathbf{x}'_t) + \epsilon$, where $\epsilon \sim \mathcal{N}(0, \sigma_X^2)$. The Gaussian process prior on f is such that $f(\mathbf{x}') \sim \mathcal{N}(\mu_{x'}, \mathbf{K}_{x'} + \sigma_X^2\mathbf{I})$. The mean and variance of the Gaussian posterior predictive distribution of the function $f(\mathbf{x}'_*)$ at a test point $\mathbf{x}'_*$, are given by:

$$\mathbb{E}(f_*) = \mu_{\mathbf{x}'_*} + k_*(K_{X'} + \sigma_{X'}^2\mathbf{I})^{-1}(\mathbf{X} - \mu_{\mathbf{x}'}), \tag{4.5}$$

$$\mathrm{var}(f_*) = \mathbf{k}_{**} - \mathbf{k}_*^T (K_{X'} + \sigma_{X'}^2 \mathbf{I})^{-1} \mathbf{k}_* \tag{4.6}$$

where $k_{**} = k(\mathbf{x'}_*, \mathbf{x'}_*)$ and $\mathbf{k}_* = k(\mathbf{x'}, \mathbf{x'}_*)$. The kernel hyperparameters θ and the noise parameter $\sigma_{\mathbf{X}}$ are obtained by maximizing the log-marginal likelihood given below:

$$\log p(\mathbf{X}|\mathbf{X'}) = \log \mathcal{N}\left(\mu_{X'}, \mathbf{K}_{\mathbf{X'X'}} + \sigma_{\mathbf{X}}^2 \mathbf{I}\right). \tag{4.7}$$

As can be seen from Eqs. 4.5 and 4.6, traditional Gaussian processes require the inversion of matrices as expressed through the Kernel functions—which is an operation that has cubic complexity (Cohen et al., 2020). Various methods have been investigated to circumvent Gaussian processes' cubic training cost. They primarily rely on two approaches: training dispersed (weak) experts on portions of the whole dataset or using sparse approximations and structure-exploiting assumptions to the covariance matrix (Cohen et al., 2020).

This chapter considers sparse Gaussian processes that use inducing points and not the entire dataset, which assists in reducing the computational burden. Inducing inputs, pseudo-training examples, are used by sparse Gaussian processes to lower the rank of the matrix that has to be inverted (Cohen et al., 2020). The number of inducing points determines the quality of the approximation produced by sparse Gaussian processes; a considerable number of them may be needed to reflect the local structures of some fast-changing functions (Cohen et al., 2020). Crucially, user-defined pseudo-training example count allows for control over memory and computational cost (Leibfried et al., 2020). Sparse Gaussian processes typically lack closed-form solutions, necessitating the use of approximate methods for training. Variational inference , which frames the task of Bayesian inference as an optimization problem (i.e., maximizing a lower bound on the logarithm of the marginal probability), is a useful option for approximate inference in this situation (Cohen et al., 2020; Leibfried et al., 2020). A detailed discussion on variational inference can be found in Chapter 2.

Furthermore, we consider sparse processes where we individually model each point on the volatility surface and multi-output Gaussian processes, allowing for implicit inference of connectivity relationships between various points on the volatility surface. A multi-output Gaussian process extends a Gaussian process to a distribution over vector-valued functions. While an ordinary Gaussian process outputs a scalar Gaussian random variable when evaluated at a specific input location, a multi-output Gaussian process outputs a multidimensional multivariate Gaussian random variable (Leibfried et al., 2020). A multi-output Gaussian process is defined similarly to an ordinary single-output Gaussian process but with a vector-valued mean function and a matrix-valued cross-covariance function (Leibfried et al., 2020). As with a single-output Gaussian process, a multi-output Gaussian process has a sparse analog that utilizes inducing points. The model is then typically trained using variational inference techniques.

In this chapter, we utilized the squared exponential kernel for both versions (i.e., single output and multi-output) of the Gaussian processes. The inducing points and kernels used for the multi-output Gaussian process are shared. We plan to explore various configurations of this setup in future work.

4.4 Numerical Experiments

In this section, we present the numerical experiments conducted. We first describe the datasets used and then outline the experiments, settings, and performance metrics used.

4.4.1 Data Description

The data used consists of data from the FTSE/JSE ALSI options and EuroSToxx 50 option data, which were collected over 100 consecutive trading days in 2019.

FTSE/JSE option data: The data consists of implied volatilities from the ALSI index options. Each sample is a discrete two-dimensional grid point showing the moneyness and time to maturity for each implied volatility observed. Specifically, we look at the collection: $X = f(M * T)$ where $M := \{80\%; 90\%; 100\%; 110\%; 120\%\}$ and $T := \{1M; 2M; 3M; 6M; 9M; 1Y\}$ which results in 30 points on each implied surface.

EuroStoxx 50 option data: The data consists of implied volatilities from the EuroStoxx 50 index options. Each sample is a discrete two-dimensional grid point showing the moneyness and time to maturity for each implied volatility observed. Specifically, we look at the collection: $X = f(M * T)$ where $M :=$

$\{50\%, 60\%, 70\%, 80\%; 90\%; 100\%; 110\%; 120\%, 130\%, 140\%, 150\%\}$ and $T := \{0.1Y, 0.3Y, 0.6Y, 0.9Y, 1.2Y, 1.5Y, 1.8Y, 2.0Y\}$ which results in 88 points on each implied surface.

4.4.2 Experiment Description

For each method's training, we simulated 40,000 training examples: 40,000 Heston smiles, and 40,000 Rough Bergomi smiles. The machine learning models (i.e., deep neural networks, single-output Gaussian process, and multi-output Gaussian process) trained on this data were then calibrated online to the real-world volatility surface data from the FTSE/JSE ALSI and EuroStoxx 50. We calibrate the Heston stochastic volatility model to the FTSE/JSE ALSI data and the Rough Bergomi model to the EuroStoxx 50 data.

We use three hidden layers with 30 neurons with an Elu activation function for the deep neural network model. The output node has linear activation, and the number of points equals the size of the surface. For example, the FTSE/JSE surface has 30 points, while the EuroStoxx 50 would have 88 points. This architecture was chosen to align with that proposed in the deep calibration seminal paper of Horvath et al. (2021). We utilize the squared exponential kernel for the Gaussian processes (GPs). The number of inducing points is set to 1000 for the multi-output and 100 for each point in the single-output GP.

We use the root square mean error across the entire surface to assess the methods' performance and the computational resources required.

4.5 Results and Discussion

All the results in this work were produced in Python using a 64-bit machine. Figure 4.3 shows the Heston calibrated parameters through time on the FTSE/JSE ALSI option data, with similar behavior observed on the EuroStoxx 50 data using the Rough Bergomi model. Figures 4.4 and 4.5 show the calibrated volatility surfaces on the FTSE/JSE ALSI and EuroStoxx 50 data on days where the calibration procedures performed the worst (based of the error metric) on each dataset. Figures 4.6 and 4.7 show the calibrated volatility surfaces on the FTSE/JSE ALSI and EuroStoxx 50 data on days where the calibration performed the best on each dataset. Figures 4.8 and 4.9 show the RMSE across the entire surface on the FTSE/JSE ALSI and EuroStoxx 50 data through time, respectively.

Our analysis found that the fastest method (as expected) to produce results was the deep neural network approach, with the single-output Gaussian process being the slowest by being around 6 times slower than the deep neural network approach. These results indicate some avenues for improving the Gaussian process approach, such as with methods for scaling the performance of the Gaussian processes using distributed approaches (Cohen et al., 2020).

Figure 4.3 shows that the methods produce similar parameter estimates for the Heston model for all the parameters across time, with the deep neural network showing the most instability in the parameter estimate, particularly on the v and θ.

Figures 4.4 and 4.5 show the calibration results on the worst date for each market. In general, we find that all methods produce the same results across both markets, except for the multi-output Gaussian process, whose performance deviates from the other two methods as we increase the maturity. We further see that the GP approaches produce similar confidence bands on the ALSI dataset, while the single-output GP produces a much lower one standard deviation confidence bands than the multi-output GP method. Furthermore, the results show that for the smallest maturity for the Eurostoxx 50 data, all methods fail to capture the skew around the at-the-money point. It should be noted that this skew was very steep compared to the typical skew over the period of study. The ALSI dataset also reveals that the lowest maturity has the lowest narrowest confidence bands, with the confidence bands increasing with maturity. Furthermore, for the lowest maturity—we find that the narrowest confidence bands are around the at-the-money moneyness level, with the bands becoming wider as we move away from at-the-money.

Contrary to Figs. 4.4 and 4.5, 4.6 and 4.7 show that all three methods produce a better fit to the data. This is magnified by the fact that all three methods capture the full volatility skew for the Eurostoxx 50 data for the smallest maturity. However, the multi-output approach deviates from the other approaches as maturity increases. We also observe the phenomenon of narrower confidence bands at the lower maturity and much wider confidence bands at the larger maturities.

Figure 4.8 shows the root means square error across the whole surface through time. These results show that the three methods produce similar performance over time. On the other hand, Fig. 4.9 shows the calibration

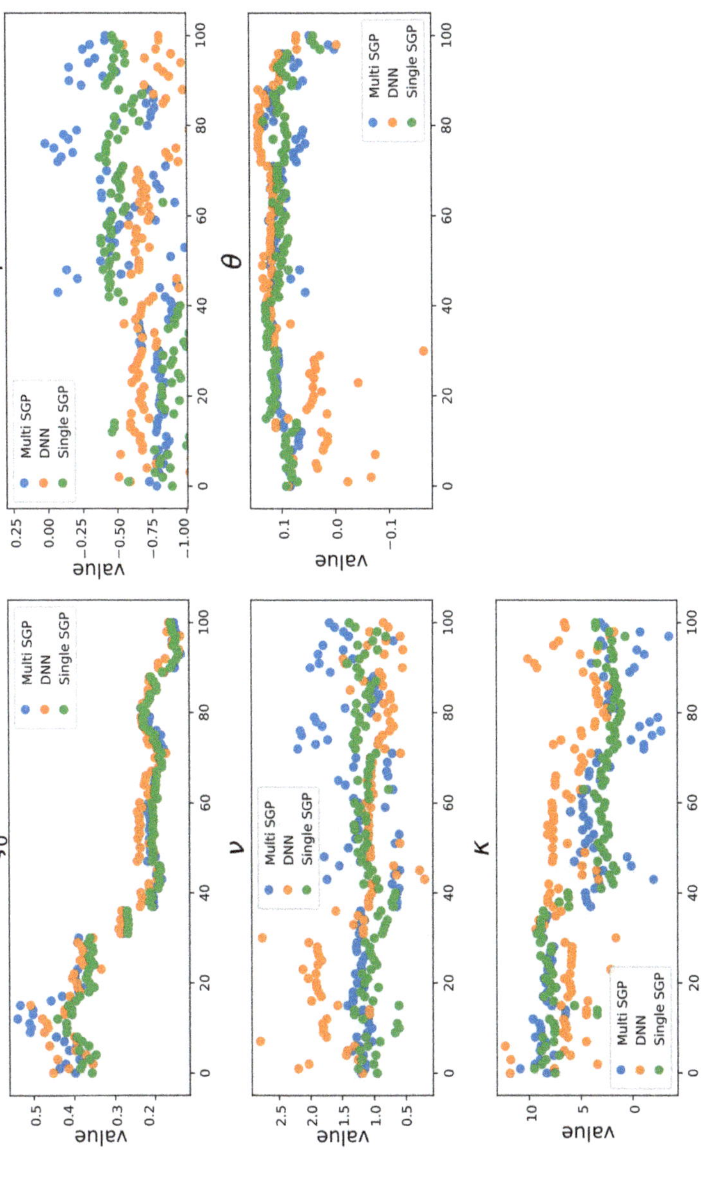

Fig. 4.3 Calibrated Heston parameters over the 100 days. The Heston model was calibrated to the FTSE/JSE equity option volatility data

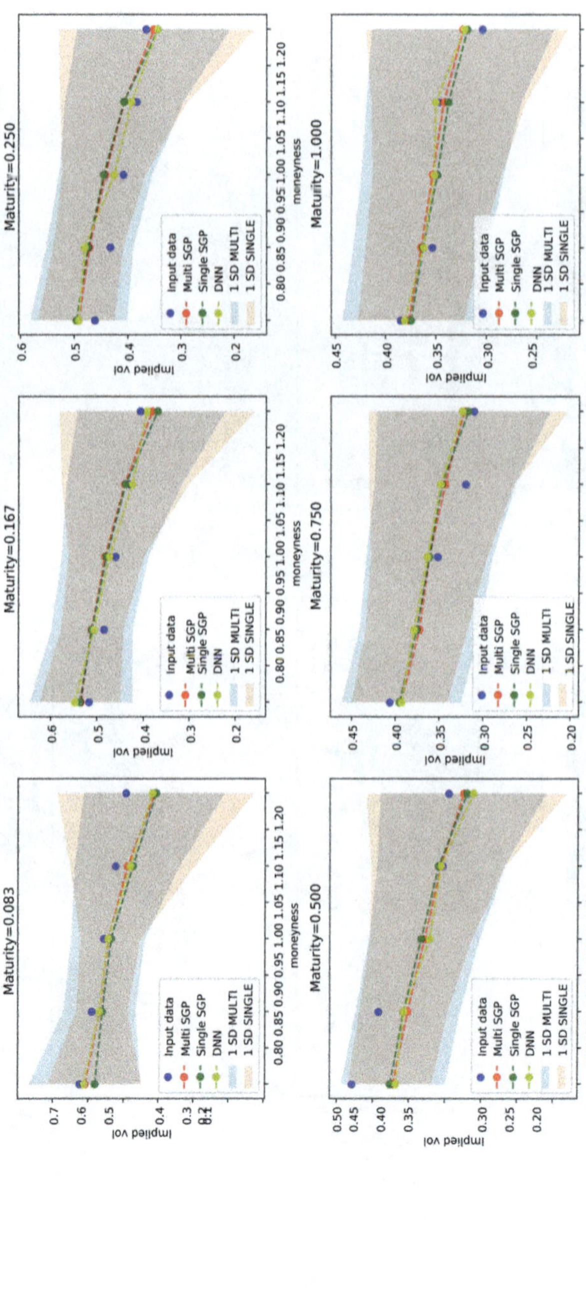

Fig. 4.4 Heston smile on the day with the largest error for FTSE/JSE ALSI

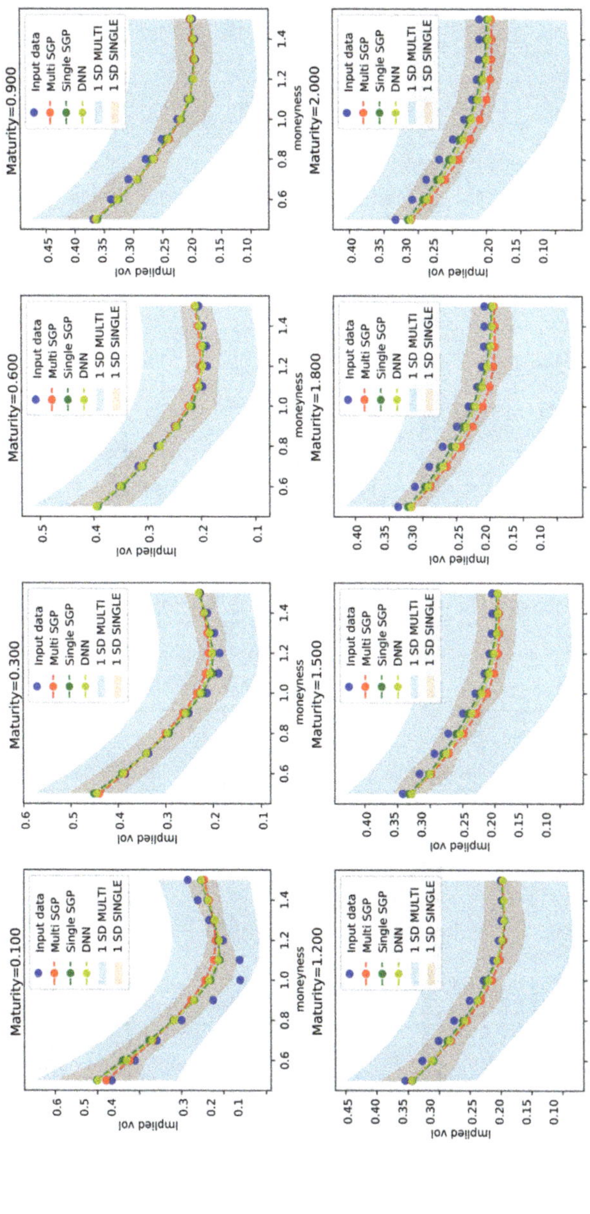

Fig. 4.5 Rough Bergomi smile on the day with the largest error for EuroStoxx 50

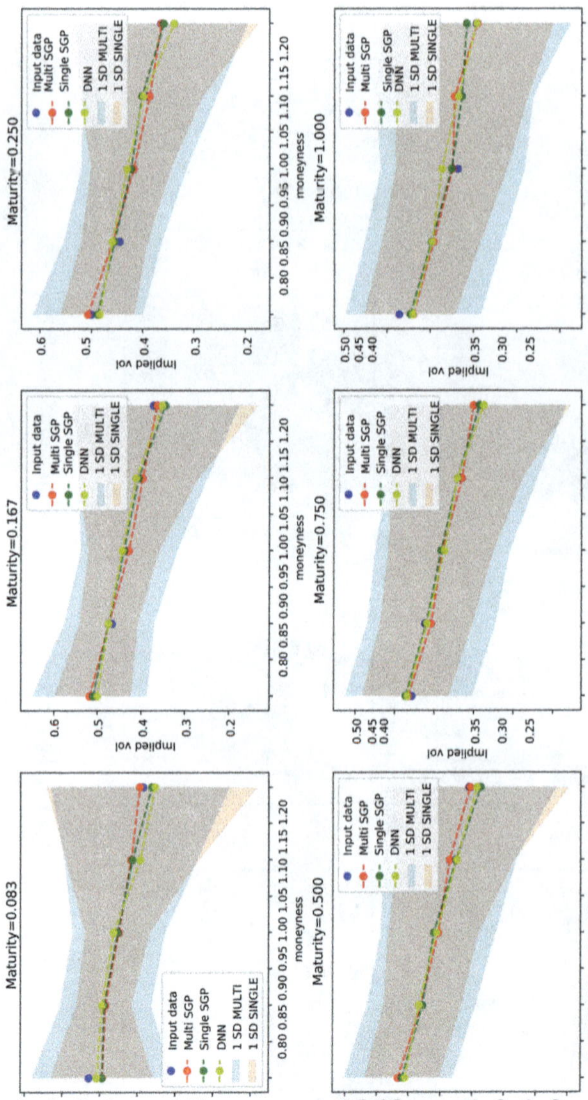

Fig. 4.6 Heston model smile on a day with the lowest error for ALSI

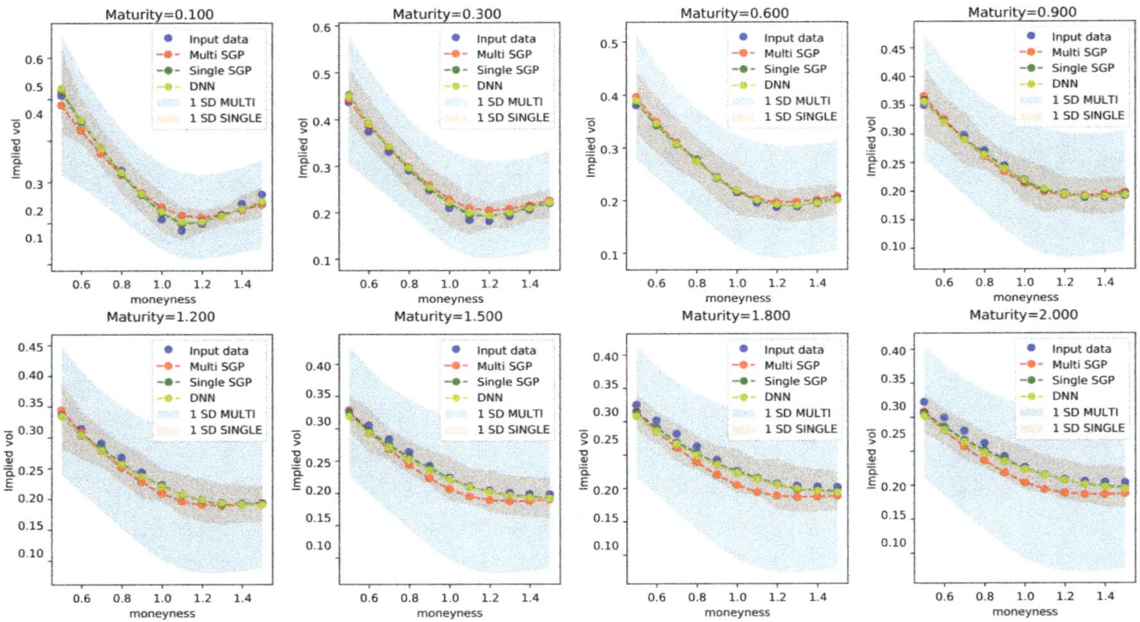

Fig. 4.7 Rough Bergomi model smile on a day with the lowest error for EuroStoxx 50

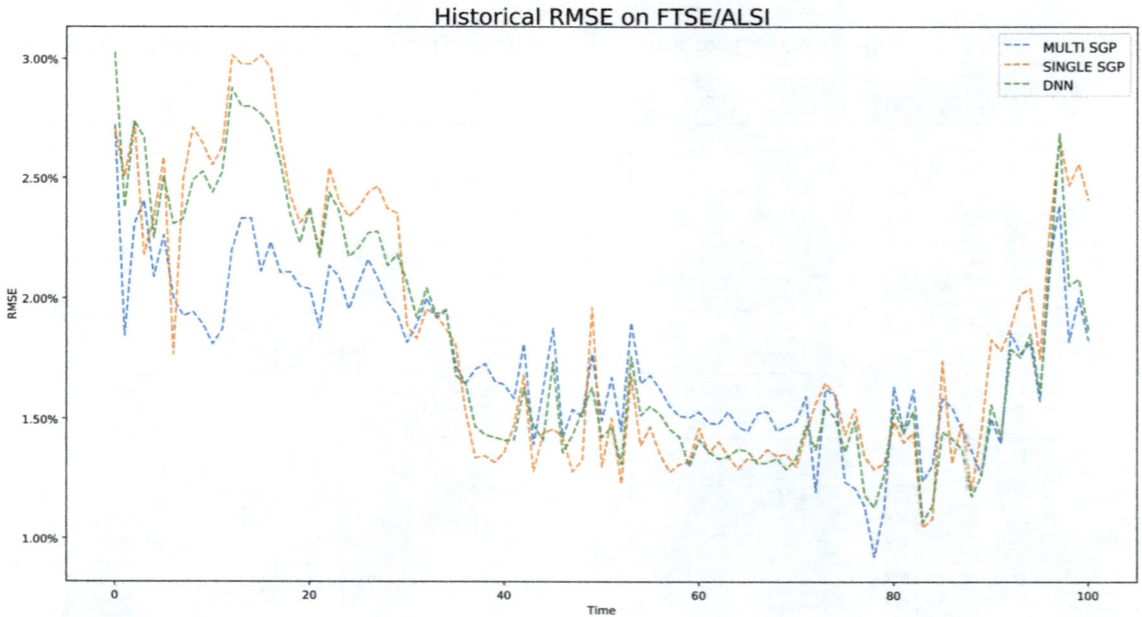

Fig. 4.8 RMSE overtime on ALSI volatility surface across the DNN, single-output GP, and multi-output GP methods

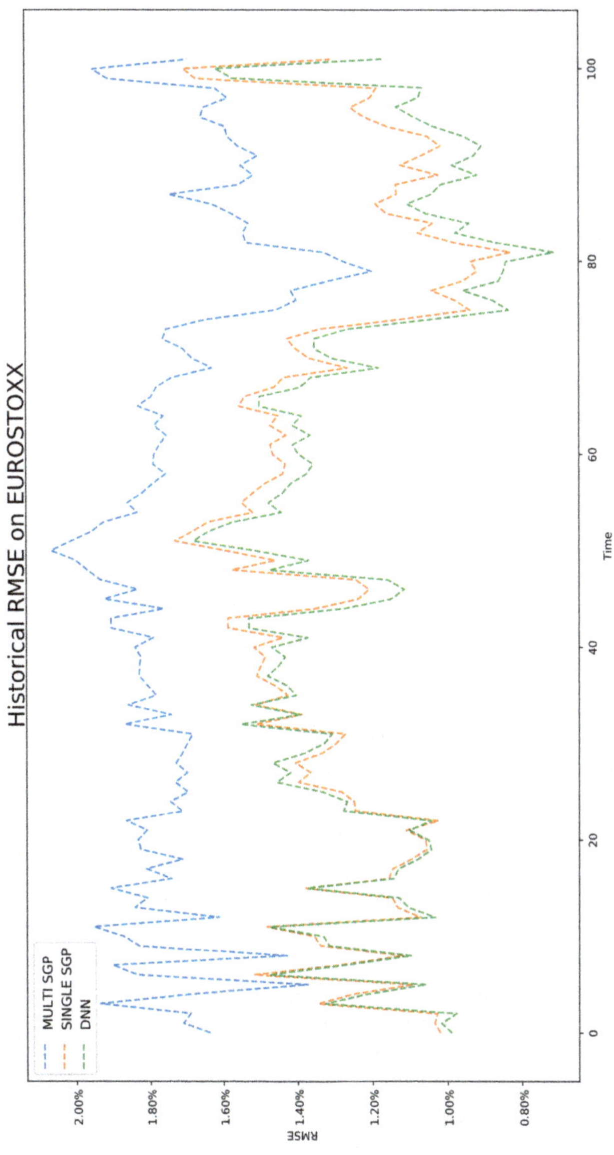

Fig. 4.9 RMSE overtime on EuroStoxx 50 volatility surface across the DNN, single-output GP, and multi-output GP methods

error across the entire surface. This figure shows that the method with the poorest performance is the multi-output GP, with the RMSE being larger than the other two methods through time. This can be explained by the poor performance of the multi-output GP on the large maturities on the vol surface. The calibration error results also show that the calibration error is fairly stable, but there may be periods with large errors. These may indicate that large training data sizes are required or inappropriate models (e.g., not Heston or Rough Bergomi) are being used. We plan to assess these options in future work.

The results in this chapter can prove useful to practitioners in understanding the volatility surface, particularly around the confidence we have in the shape of the smile across all the maturities. The results show the utility one obtains through the uncertainty estimates obtained by using Gaussian processes to calibrate the volatility surface instead of neural networks.

4.6 Conclusion

This chapter utilizes sparse Gaussian processes to calibrate stochastic volatility models to option volatility data across developing and developed markets. We consider both multi-output sparse Gaussian processes and single-output sparse Gaussian processes for each point on the volatility surface . Our results are compared with the current state-of-the-art model, which is deep neural networks.

The results show that the probabilistic approach produces results similar to those of the deep neural network, with the added advantage of capturing uncertainty in the calibration. We find that on the FTSE/JSE ALSI data, the single and multi-output GPs produce similar results, with narrow confidence bands at lower and wider confidence bands as we increase moneyness and maturity. On the Eurostoxx 50 dataset, we find that the poorest performer is the multi-output GP, and the very wide confidence shows this, while the single-output GP produces similar results to the neural network and corresponding narrower confidence bands compared to the multi-output GP.

The results in this work can be improved by ensuring that the inducing points and kernels used for the multi-output GP are not shared, which should improve the results observed on the EuroStoxx 50 data. Furthermore, all the models approximated the pricing function without explicitly incorporating no-arbitrage conditions. In future work, we plan to incorporate no-arbitrage conditions explicitly. A limitation of the GP approach is the computational complexity of the method. We will address this limitation in future work by utilizing start-of-art approaches to scaling GPs, such as distributed GP approaches (e.g., product-of-experts Cohen et al., 2020).

The following chapter presents a normalizing flows-based approach to pricing options in an emerging market. This approach to using machine learning for pricing options is preferable as one learns the risk-neutral density directly and thus does not have to impose no-arbitrage conditions on a loss function as the risk-neutral density already captures these.

References

Agrawal, D., Papamarkou, T., & Hinkle, J. (2020). Wide neural networks with bottlenecks are deep Gaussian processes. *Journal of Machine Learning Research, 21*, 175.

Bayer, C., Friz, P., & Gatheral, J. (2016). Pricing under rough volatility. *Quantitative Finance, 16*(6), 887–904.

Bergomi, L. (2008). Smile dynamics III. Available at SSRN 1493308.

Black, F., & Scholes, M. (1973). The pricing of options and corporate liabilities. *Journal of Political Economy, 81*(3), 637–654. ISSN: 00223808.

Buehler, H., Horvath, B., Lyons, T., Arribas, I. P., & Wood, B. (2020a). A data-driven market simulator for small data environments. arXiv preprint arXiv:2006.14498

Buehler, H., Horvath, B., Lyons, T., Arribas, I. P., & Wood, B (2020b). Generating financial markets with signatures. Available at SSRN 3657366.

Buehler, H., Gonon, L., Teichmann, J., & Wood, B. (2019). Deep hedging. *Quantitative Finance, 19*(8), 1271–1291.

Carbonneau, A. (2021). Deep hedging of long-term financial derivatives. *Insurance: Mathematics and Economics, 99*, 327–340.

Che, Z., Purushotham, S., Li, G., Jiang, B., & Liu, Y. (2018). Hierarchical deep generative models for multi-rate multivariate time series. In *International Conference on Machine Learning*. PMLR (pp. 784–793).

Cohen, S., Mbuvha, R., Marwala, T., & Deisenroth, M. (2020). Healing products of Gaussian process experts. In *International conference on machine learning*. PMLR (pp. 2068–2077).

Cont, R. (2001). Empirical properties of asset returns: Stylized facts and statistical issues. *Quantitative Finance, 1*, 223–236.

Cousin, A., Maatouk, H., & Rullière, D. (2016). Kriging of financial term-structures. *European Journal of Operational Research, 255*(2), 631–648.

De Spiegeleer, J., Madan, D. B., Reyners, S., & Schoutens, W. (2018). Machine learning for quantitative finance: Fast derivative pricing, hedging and fitting. *Quantitative Finance, 18*(10), 1635–1643.

Deisenroth, M., & Ng, J. W. (2015). Distributed gaussian processes. In *International conference on machine learning*. PMLR (pp. 1481–1490).

Frandsen, M. G., Pedersen, T. C., & Poulsen, R. (2022). Delta force: option pricing with differential machine learning. *Digital Finance, 4*(1), 1–15.

Gradojevic, N., Gençay, R., & Kukolj, D. (2009). Option pricing with modular neural networks. *IEEE Transactions on Neural Networks, 20*(4), 626–637.

Henry-Labordere, P. (2019). Generative models for financial data. Available at SSRN 3408007.

Heston, S. L. (1993b). A closed-form solution for options with stochastic volatility with applications to bond and currency options. *The Review of Financial Studies, 6*(2), 327–343. ISSN: 08939454.

Heston, S. L. (1993). A closed-form solution for options with stochastic volatility with applications to bond and currency options. *The Review of Financial Studies, 6*(2), 327–343.

Horvath, B., Muguruza, A., & Tomas, M. (2021). Deep learning volatility: A deep neural network perspective on pricing and calibration in (rough) volatility models. *Quantitative Finance, 21*(1), 11–27.

Huge, B., & Savine, A. (2020). Differential machine learning. arXiv preprint arXiv:2005.02347

Itkin, A. (2019). Deep learning calibration of option pricing models: Some pitfalls and solutions. arXiv preprint arXiv:1906.03507

Ivascu, C. F. (2021). Option pricing using machine learning. *Expert Systems with Applications,163*, Article 113799.

Leibfried, F., Dutordoir, V., John, S. T., & Durrande, N. (2020). A tutorial on sparse Gaussian processes and variational inference. arXiv preprint arXiv:2012.13962

Li, J., Wang, X., Lin, Y., Sinha, A., & Wellman, M. (2020). Generating realistic stock market order streams. In *Proceedings of the AAAI conference on artificial intelligence* (Vol. 34. 01, pp. 727–734).

Liu, S., Borovykh, A., Grzelak, L. A., & Oosterlee, C. W. (2019). A neural network-based framework for financial model calibration. *Journal of Mathematics in Industry, 9*(1), 1–28.

Liu, H., Ong, Y.-S., Shen, X., & Cai, J. (2020). When Gaussian process meets big data: A review of scalable GPs. *IEEE Transactions on Neural Networks and Learning Systems, 31*(11), 4405–4423.

Lütkebohmert, E., Schmidt, T., & Sester, J. (2022). Robust deep hedging. *Quantitative Finance, 22*(8), 1465–1480.

Marti, G. (2020). Corrgan: Sampling realistic financial correlation matrices using generative adversarial networks. In *ICASSP 2020-2020 IEEE international conference on acoustics, speech and signal processing (ICASSP)* (pp. 8459–8463). IEEE.

Mbuvha, R., Mongwe, W. T., & Marwala, T. (2021). Separable Shadow Hamiltonian hybrid Monte Carlo for Bayesian neural network inference in wind speed forecasting. *Energy and A, 1*, Article 100108.

Mbuvha, R., Adounkpe, J. Y. P., Houngnibo, M. C. M., Mongwe, W. T., Nikraftar, Z., Marwala, T., & Newlands, N. K. (2023). A novel workflow for streamflow prediction in the presence of missing gauge observations. *Environmental Data Science, 2*, Article e23.

Mikhailov, S., & Nögel, U. (2004). *Heston's stochastic volatility model: Implementation, calibration and some extensions*. Wiley.

Montavon, G., Samek, W., & Müller, K.-R. (2018). Methods for interpreting and understanding deep neural networks. *Digital Signal Processing, 73*, 1–15.

Neal, R. M. (1996). Priors for infinite networks. In *Bayesian learning for neural networks* (pp. 29–53). Springer.

Rasmussen, C. E. (2003). Gaussian processes in machine learning. In *Summer school on machine learning* (pp. 63–71). Springer.

Rasmussen, C. E., & Williams, C. K. I. (2006). *Gaussian processes for machine learning*. The MIT Press.

Rosenbaum, M., & Zhang, J. (2021). Deep calibration of the quadratic rough Heston model. arXiv preprint arXiv:2107.01611

Ruf, J., & Wang, W. (2019). Neural networks for option pricing and hedging: A literature review. arXiv preprint arXiv:1911.05620

Schulz, E., Speekenbrink, M., & Krause, A. (2018). A tutorial on Gaussian process regression: Modelling, exploring, and exploiting functions. *Journal of Mathematical Psychology, 85*, 1–16.

Sidogi, T. (2023). Machine learning methods for financial data challenges in quatitative finance. PhD thesis. University of Johannesburg.

Sidogi, T., Mongwe, W. T., Mbuvha, R., & Marwala, T. (2022). Creating synthetic volatility surfaces using generative adversarial networks with static arbitrage loss conditions. In *2022 IEEE symposium series on computational intelligence (SSCI)* (pp. 1423–1429). IEEE.

Snelson, E., & Ghahramani, Z. (2005). Sparse Gaussian processes using pseudo-inputs. In *Advances in neural information processing systems* (p. 18).

Sousa, J. B., Esquivel, M. L., & Gaspar, R. M. (2012). Machine learning Vasicek model calibration with Gaussian processes. *Communications in Statistics-Simulation and Computation, 41*(6), 776–786.

Takahashi, S., Chen, Y., & Tanaka-Ishii, K. (2019). Modeling financial time-series with generative adversarial networks. *In Physica A: Statistical Mechanics and its Applications, 527*, Article 121261.

Wiese, M., Knobloch, R., Korn, R., & Kretschmer, P. (2020). Quant GANs: deep generation of financial time series. *Quantitative Finance, 20*(9), 1419–1440.

Williams, C. K. I., & Rasmussen, C. E. (2006). *Gaussian processes for machine learning* (Vol. 2, p. 3). MIT Press.

Zhu, Q., Loeper, G., Chen, W., & Langrené, N. (2021). Markovian approximation of the rough Bergomi model for Monte Carlo option pricing. *Mathematics, 9*(5), 528.

CHAPTER 5

Analyzing South African Equity Option Prices Using Normalizing Flows

5.1 Introduction

It is well known that the geometric Brownian motion model that underlies the Black and Scholes framework does not capture the fat tails of the return distributions as observed in the market (Cont, 2001; Heston, 1993; Merton, 1967; Mongwe, 2015; Mongwe et al., 2022). The mathematical finance community has attempted to address this deficiency in the Black and Scholes model mainly in two ways (Buehler et al., 2019; Heston, 1993; Kou, 2007; Merton, 1967; Mongwe, 2015; Mongwe et al., 2022; Zhu et al., 2021). Firstly, extending the geometric Brownian motion dynamics assumed in the Black-Scholes model by allowing the volatility to be stochastic and have its own dynamics leads to stochastic volatility models such as the Heston (1993) model which we discuss in Chapter 4. Secondly, practitioners also deal with the deficiency of the Black and Scholes model by adding jumps to the stock dynamics, allowing the model to capture the heavy tails and the volatility skew in the options markets. This leads to jump-diffusion models such as the Merton (1967),

---

Supplementary Information The online version contains supplementary material available at https://doi.org/10.1007/978-3-031-88431-3_5.

W. T. Mongwe et al., *Bayesian Machine Learning in Quantitative Finance*, https://doi.org/10.1007/978-3-031-88431-3_5

Marwala et al. (2023), Mongwe et al. (2022), Mongwe (2015) and the double exponential jump-diffusion model of Kou (2007).

Model development within the mathematical finance community is typically based on a set of economic assumptions, from which the dynamics of the driving process are then determined or derived (Bayer et al., 2016; Horvath et al., 2021;Loaiza-Ganem et al., 2022; Yang & Hospedales, 2023). This allows the models to be easily interpretable to the stakeholders who rely on their results. However, this approach to modeling derivative prices makes extending the models by adding more parameters difficult as they lose their economic basis (Yang & Hospedales, 2023). Growing interest has been in exploring the capabilities of data-driven and machine learning-based methods to model option prices. The benefit of machine learning models is that they can be easily extended to better fit the observed market prices, with the limitation that they are less interpretable (for example, when using neural networks) compared to their economics theory-based counterparts (Loaiza-Ganem et al., 2022; Yang & Hospedales, 2023).

In the machine learning formulation of option pricing, models are treated as regression problems with any economic basis typically incorporated after the fact (Loaiza-Ganem et al., 2022; Yang & Hospedales, 2023). Machine learning techniques such as kernel-based methods and neural networks can reproduce the option prices observed in the market almost perfectly (Loaiza-Ganem et al., 2022; Yang & Hospedales, 2023). However, these models are not guaranteed to produce option prices free from arbitrage (Sidogi et al., 2022; Yang & Hospedales, 2023). Furthermore, they tend to behave poorly when there is less data. This makes them less desirable to market practitioners as they might behave unexpectedly (Yang & Hospedales, 2023). Custom loss functions incorporating static arbitrage conditions are required to allow the machine learning models to prevent the possibility of arbitrage in the predicted option prices (Sidogi et al., 2022). However, this approach does not guarantee that the prices will always be arbitrage-free (Yang & Hospedales, 2023). To circumvent this, one can directly model the risk-neutral density implied from market-observed option prices and then use this risk-neutral density to retrieve the option prices. Given their ability to learn target distribution, normalizing flow-based approaches are ideal for this task (Buchen and Kelly, 1996; Loaiza-Ganem et al., 2022; Yang & Hospedales, 2023).

Generative probabilistic models, such as normalizing flows, can model any target distribution. They begin with a simple distribution, such as the standard Gaussian distribution, then work their way up to the target distribution by applying invertible transformations one after the other (Yang & Hospedales, 2023). Yang and Hospedales proposed a normalizing flows-based model for the risk-neutral density (Yang & Hospedales, 2023). This framework yields a deterministic option pricing function at the end. Their approach can generate precise option price estimations and satisfy all financial axiom requirements through a particular architecture and activation function design for the normalizing flow.

This chapter utilizes the mixture of normalizing flows framework discussed in Yang and Hospedales (2023) to model equity option prices on the South African Johannesburg Stock Exchange (JSE) All share Index across various expires and strike prices. We compare the performance of a normalizing flow mixture where the number of components in the mixture is 1, 8, 15, or 30. We find that the normalizing flow mixture framework can capture the observed option prices. Furthermore, we observe a relationship between option expiry and the number of components in the mixture.

The remainder of this chapter is structured as follows: We first explore how the risk-neutral density is implied from option prices in Sect. 5.2 and then explain how normalizing flows can be used to learn this density in Sect. 5.3. We then present the experiment setup used in this chapter in Sect. 5.4, after which we provide the results, discuss them, and conclude in Sects. 5.5 and 5.6.

5.2 Risk-Neutral Density from Option Prices

Option pricing is an active research area in mathematical finance. Since the seminal work of Black and Scholes (1973), there has been interest in better models to price and model options. Data-driven techniques have drawn much interest in recent years (Sidogi et al., 2022; Yang & Hospedales, 2023). A popular data-driven method for pricing options is neural networks—where the option pricing function is learned using option prices observed in the market (Sidogi et al., 2022; Yang & Hospedales, 2023). Neural networks are preferable as they are universal function approximations (Yang & Hospedales, 2023). If $f_w(K)$ is the option pricing function evaluated at strike K with parameters w that approximate option price, the distance between this function and the observed market prices is minimized to obtain w. However, the main limitation of neural network-based methods is that they don't guarantee that the generated option prices are arbitrage-free, a crucial assumption that must be satisfied when pricing options. Typically, a custom loss incorporating no-arbitrage conditions is constructed to enforce no-arbitrage (Sidogi et al., 2022; Yang & Hospedales, 2023).

Carr et al. (2003) outlines the static arbitrage conditions for option pricing curves, which include the following constraints for call options:

$$\frac{\partial f_w(K)}{\partial K} \leq 0 \tag{5.1}$$

$$\frac{\partial^2 f_w(K)}{\partial^2 K} \geq 0 \tag{5.2}$$

$$f_w(\infty) = 0 \tag{5.3}$$

$$\max(0, \exp(-r\tau)(F_\tau - K)) \leq f_w(K) \geq \exp(-r\tau)F_\tau \tag{5.4}$$

where $f_w(K)$ is the function (with parameters w) that approximates the option price for a fixed expiry τ, F_τ is the forward price and $F_\tau = \exp(-r\tau)S_0$, r is the continuously compounded zero-coupon interest rate, K is the strike, S_0 is the initial stock price and q is the continuously paid dividend yield. Thus, any data-driven or machine learning-based method must incorporate these conditions in the loss function to keep the options prices generated by the model arbitrage-free.

The critical finding of Yang and Hospedales (2023) is that, although it is much simpler to describe the risk-neural density, it is difficult for a parametric model (such as neural networks) to satisfy all of the no-arbitrage conditions as described in Carr et al. (2003). They suggest modeling the density of forward log-moneyness, which is also the approach in this chapter. The call option pricing function is then given as follows (Yang & Hospedales, 2023):

$$f_w(K) = \exp(-r\tau)F_\tau \int_{-\infty}^{\infty} \max\left(\exp(x) - \frac{K}{F_\tau}, 0\right) q_w(x)dx \tag{5.5}$$

where $q_w(x)$ is the risk-neutral density estimator. All constraints for the pricing model f_w are reduced to the following three constraints, with the proof provided in Yang and Hospedales (2023), on the density estimator $q_w(x)$:

$$q_w(x) \geq 0 \tag{5.6}$$

$$\int_{-\infty}^{\infty} q_w(x)dx = 1 \tag{5.7}$$

$$\int_{-\infty}^{\infty} \exp(x) q_w(x)dx = 1 \tag{5.8}$$

The first two constraints are constraints for any valid density function, and the last constraint sets the expectation of $\exp(x)$ to be constant 1, which means the expectation of the underlying asset price at the maturity date should be the same as the forward price. Its discounted value should be the spot price adjusted for dividends, corresponding to the upper bound of the call option price given in Eq. 5.4. The density that meets the last constraint above is referred to as risk-neutral density, as it states that the expectation of an asset priced at S_0 will be $S_0 \exp((r-q)\tau)$ after the period of τ. In this chapter, we learn the risk-neutral density using normalizing flows, which will be described in the next section.

5.3 Normalizing Flows

Normalizing flows represent a class of generative probabilistic models that facilitate the determination of a target density from a simple probability distribution. They consist of a series of transformations applied to an initial distribution. A vector w of an unknown distribution $p(w)$ can be expressed through a transformation T of a vector x sampled from a base distribution $q(x)$; $w = T(x)$ where $x \sim q(x)$. The base distribution is often selected to allow for easy sampling and evaluation of its density. For the base distribution, a Gaussian distribution is frequently utilized. The change of variables formula may then be used to obtain the unknown distribution (Polanska et al., 2023):

$$p(w) = q(x)|\det(J_T(x))|^{-1} \tag{5.9}$$

where $J_T(x)$ is the Jacobian corresponding to transformation T. The whole transformation in a flow-based model is invertible and differentiable because T comprises a sequence of transformations, each of which is invertible and differentiable (Polanska et al., 2023; Yang & Hospedales, 2023). This enables us to combine several straightforward transformations with previously learned parameters into a process known as a flow, from which we may sample and assess a normalized approximation of the unknown distribution (Polanska et al., 2023). The design of the transformations is done with great care so that it is easy to compute the determinant of the Jacobian (Polanska et al., 2023). One of the simplest and most commonly used normalizing flows in practice is the real-valued non-volume preserving flow (Polanska et al., 2023).

Loaiza-Ganem et al. (2022) made an early attempt to use normalizing flows for risk-neutral density estimation. The authors used the maximum entropy principle introduced in Buchen and Kelly (1996) to retrieve the implied risk-neutral density from European call options on Apple stocks. Because of the auxiliary loss, which is not guaranteed to be zero, the density is essentially not risk neutral (Yang & Hospedales, 2023). Rather than modeling the option pricing function directly, Yang and Hospedales (2023) re-frame the problem by employing normalizing flows to construct a model for risk-neutral density, which produces a pricing model. They first translate the direct pricing model constraints into models supported by risk-neutral density estimation, as described in the previous section. They then create a normalizing flow architecture that complies with these requirements. They also discovered that a mixture of these normalizing flows greatly enhances performance compared to utilizing a deeper single normalizing flow. They demonstrated the superiority of their approach over mathematical finance solutions by evaluating the framework on five option datasets in a developed market (Yang & Hospedales, 2023). In this chapter, we employ this mixture of normalizing flows framework to analyze the option prices within a developing economy.

We build $q_w(x)$ by a normalizing flows model, which maps a one-dimensional standard Gaussian to the distribution of interest. We have a sample $y \sim N(0, 1)$. After a sequence of invertible transforms, it becomes a sample from the risk neural density, i.e., $y \xrightarrow{q_w} x$ where q_w is the sequence of transforms. To find the best w, we can estimate the pricing function using Monte Carlo methods. The architecture of the normalizing flow utilized in this chapter is further described in detail in Yang and Hospedales (2023).

Yang and Hospedales (2023) also notice that this framework is difficult to scale to larger dimensions as it would require a deeper normalizing flows model. Instead, they propose using a mixture of normalizing flow models rather than a single normalizing flow model. This formulation implies that:

$$q(x) = \sum_{i=1}^{M} \pi_i q_i(x) \tag{5.10}$$

for $\pi_i > 0$ and $\sum_{i=1}^{M} \pi_i = 1$. Behind each q_i is an independent normalizing flow model, realized by $\gamma \xrightarrow{q_{w_i}} x$. Note that all the other conditions are still satisfied so long as π is a probability simplex (Yang & Hospedales, 2023). The mixture of normalizing flows effectively creates M pricing models, and the final price is the re-weighted sum of the outputs of those models. Then, all the parameters in the mixture $\{\pi, w_1, w_2, ..., w_M\}$ can be obtained through gradient-based methods (Yang & Hospedales, 2023). This is the setup that we use in this chapter as well.

5.4 Numerical Experiments

This section presents the data used in all the experiments, describes the experiments performed, and discusses the performance metrics utilized.

5.4.1 Data Description

The data used is for 14-, 20-, 30-, 60—and 90-day European options on the JSE All Share Index expiring on 22 July 2019, using a subset of the data used in Mongwe et a. (2022). It consists of the strikes, 3MJIBAR rate, and time to expiry for both puts and calls. Two hundred call options were divided into train and test using a 90-10 split.

5.4.2 Experiment Setup and Performance Metrics

The performance metrics used in this chapter are predictive performance on unseen data. The predictive performance metrics used are the Mean Square Error (MSE), Mean Absolute Error (MAE), coefficient of determination (R^2), and Mean Percentage Error (MAPE) (Mongwe & Malan, 2020; Sidogi et al., 2023). We utilize a mixture normalizing flows model for the experiments, where each normalizing flow has four layers and the number of components in the set $\{1, 8, 15, 30\}$. We use the same architecture specifications of the normalizing flows as in Yang and Hospedales (2023). Our solution is implemented in Python based on the module provided in Yang and Hospedales (2023). It should be noted that every model is trained to minimize the actual market's mean absolute error compared to the predicted prices.

5.5 Results and Discussions

In this section, we present the results and the discussions from the numerical experiments. Tables 5.1, 5.2, 5.3, 5.4 and 5.5 show the performance results on unseen data for 14, 20, 30, 60, and 90-day options on the JSE All Share Index across the 1,8, 15, and 30 normalizing flows mixture models. Figures 5.1, 5.2, 5.3, 5.4 and 5.5 show the predicted option prices from the models compared to market data and the resultant absolute errors produced by each model.

Tables 5.1 and 5.2—which correspond to options expiring in 14 and 20 days, respectively—show that the model that outperforms all the

Table 5.1 Results on unseen data for 14-day options on the JSE All Share Index. The entries in **bold** indicate outperformance for that performance metric

Metric	*1 mixture*	*8 mixture*	*15 mixture*	*30 mixture*
R2	0.99936833	0.99925830	0.99963457	**0.99989999**
MSE	0.00131217	0.00154073	0.00075910	**0.00020792**
MAPE	0.14248936	0.176270277	0.14951472	**0.07344729**
MAE	0.02642767	0.02970133	0.0228218	**0.01126697**

Table 5.2 Results on unseen data for 20-day options on the JSE All Share Index. The entries in **bold** indicate outperformance for that performance metric

Metric	*1 mixture*	*8 mixture*	*15 mixture*	*30 mixture*
R2	0.99738186	0.99874109	0.99967048	**0.99983906**
MSE	0.00496526	0.00238749	0.00062491	**0.00030521**
MAPE	0.29285721	0.11292648	0.05536494	**0.03841418**
MAE	0.05339091	0.03505068	0.01846331	**0.01131606**

Table 5.3 Results on unseen data for 30-day JSE All Share Index options. The entries in **bold** indicate outperformance for that performance metric

Metric	*1 mixture*	*8 mixture*	*15 mixture*	*30 mixture*
R2	0.99941305	**0.99990101**	0.99938930	0.99984136
MSE	0.00148616	**0.00025062**	0.00154610	0.00040166
MAPE	0.08995644	0.02934196	0.03757242	**0.02122791**
MAE	0.03490084	**0.01289784**	0.02974536	0.01489130

Table 5.4 Results on unseen data for 60-day options on the JSE All Share Index. The entries in **bold** indicate outperformance for that performance metric

Metric	*1 mixture*	*8 mixture*	*15 mixture*	*30 mixture*
R2	0.99065079	**0.99964408**	0.99750925	0.99921971
MSE	0.01183464	**0.00045052**	0.00315288	0.00098771
MAPE	0.11747006	**0.01410177**	0.07385365	0.02503132
MAE	0.08086322	**0.01507402**	0.04882987	0.02420844

Table 5.5 Results on unseen data for 90-day JSE All Share Index options. The entries in **bold** indicate outperformance for that performance metric

Metric	*1 mixture*	*8 mixture*	*15 mixture*	*30 mixture*
R2	0.99713960	**0.99956541**	0.999050502	0.99806153
MSE	0.00518381	**0.00078761**	0.00172074	0.00351303
MAPE	0.10925920	**0.01698751**	0.03629014	0.03546318
MAE	0.06111890	**0.02207337**	0.03577344	0.04499231

models across all the performance metrics on unseen data is the 30 mixture normalizing flow model and is closely followed in second place by the 15 mixture normalizing flow model. On the other hand, we find that for options expiring in 30, 60, and 90 days (as shown in Tables 5.3, 5.4, and 5.5), the model that outperforms is the mixture of 8 normalizing flows. These results show that the best model to use depends on the time to expiry of the option. This suggests a future research direction of jointly modeling the risk-neutral density across all maturities to capture

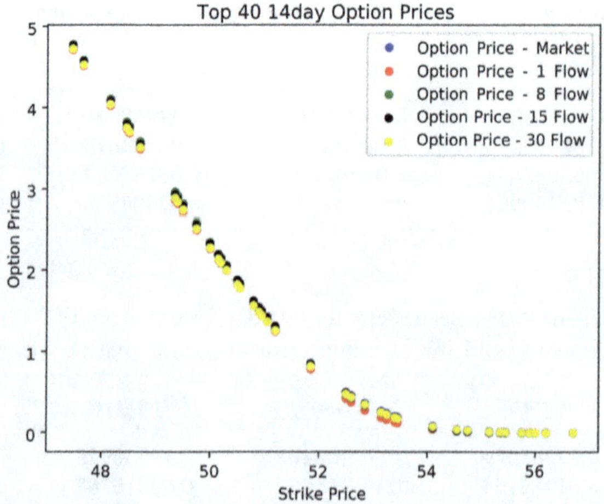

(a) Option prices from models compared to unseen market data for 14-day options on the JSE All Share Index.

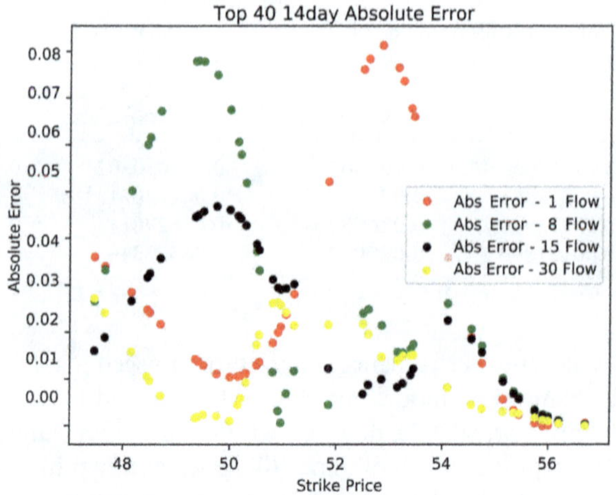

(b) Absolute errors produced by each model for 14-day options on the JSE All Share Index.

Fig. 5.1 Results from normalizing flow mixture models for 14-day options on the JSE All Share Index. **a** Option prices from models compared to market data and **b** Absolute errors produced by each model

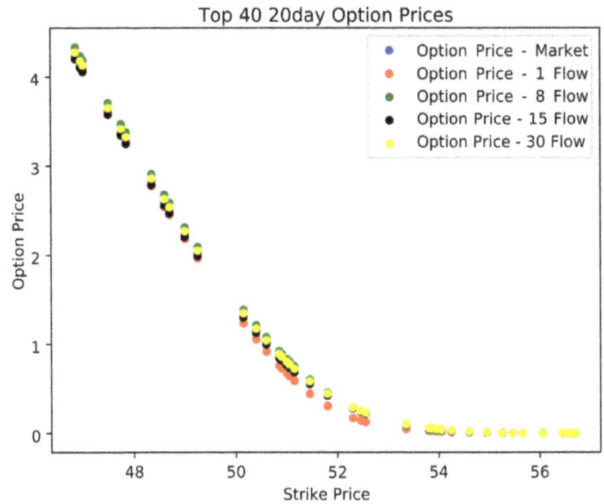

(**a**) Option prices from models compared to unseen market data for 20-day options on the JSE All Share Index.

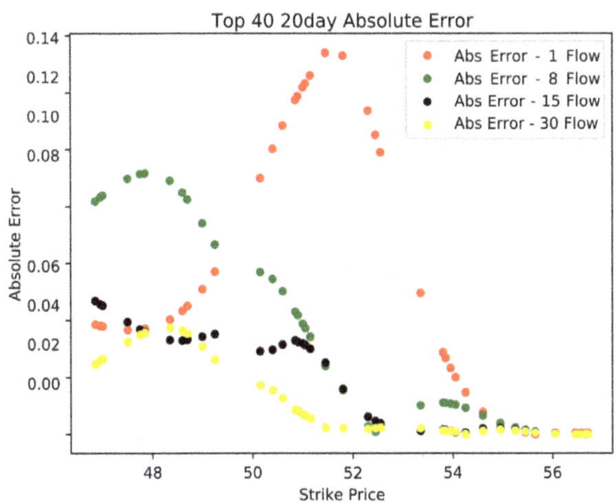

(**b**) Absolute errors produced by each model for 20-day options on the JSE All Share Index.

Fig. 5.2 Results from normalizing flow mixture models for 20-day options on the JSE All Share Index. **a** Option prices from models compared to unseen market data and **b** Absolute errors produced by each model

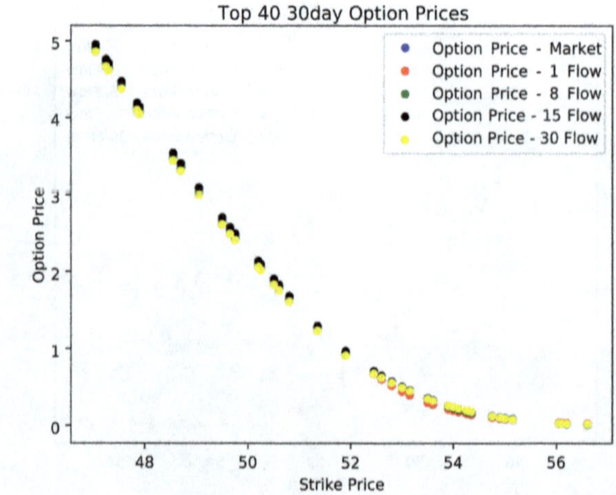

(a) Option prices from models compared to unseen market data for 30-day options on the JSE All Share Index.

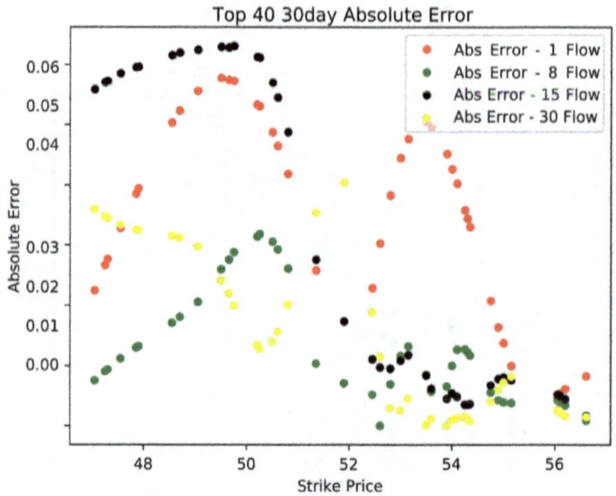

(b) Absolute errors produced by each model for 30-day options on the JSE All Share Index.

Fig. 5.3 Results from normalizing flow mixture models for 30-day options on the JSE All Share Index. **a** Option prices from models compared to unseen market data and **b** Absolute errors produced by each model

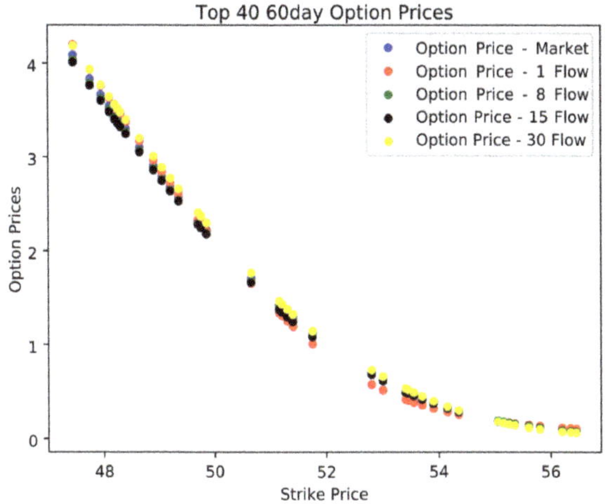

(**a**) Option prices from models compared to unseen market data for 60-day options on the JSE All Share Index.

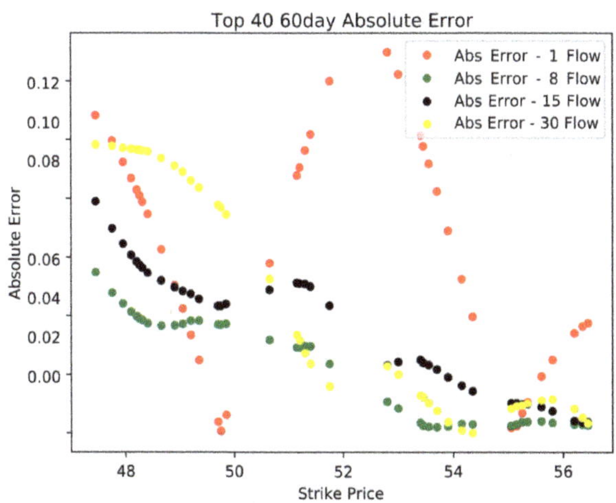

(**b**) Absolute errors produced by each model for 60-day options on the JSE All Share Index.

Fig. 5.4 Results from normalizing flow mixture models for 60-day options on the JSE All Share Index. **a** Option prices from models compared to unseen market data and **b** Absolute errors produced by each model

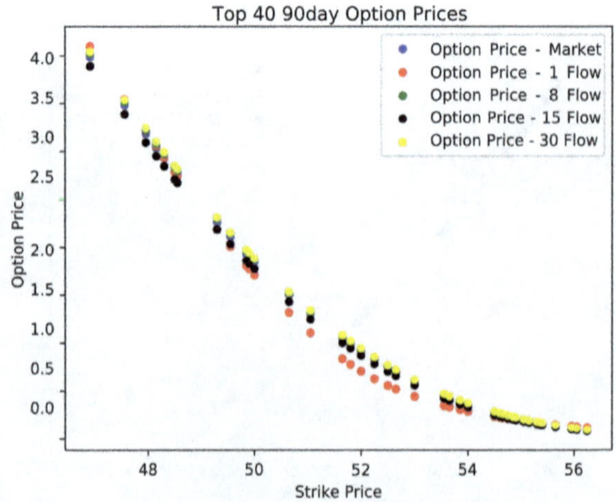

(**a**) Option prices from models compared to test market data for for 90-day options on the JSE All Share Index

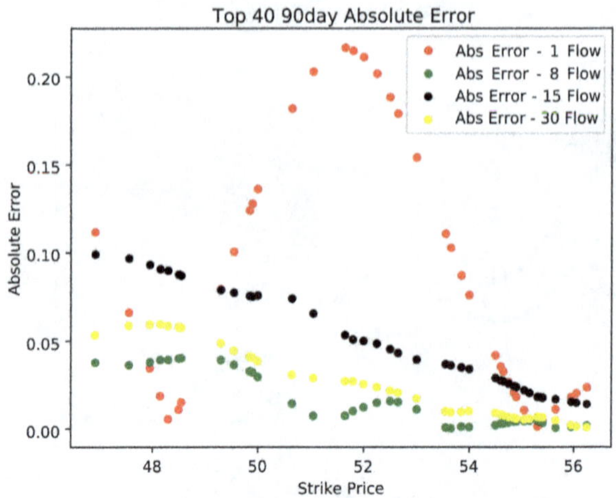

(**b**) Absolute errors produced by each model for 90-day options on the JSE All Share Index.

Fig. 5.5 Results from normalizing flow mixture models for 90-day options on the JSE All Share Index. **a** Option prices from models compared to unseen market data and **b** Absolute errors produced by each model

this effect. Furthermore, it also opens an area of research on optimally selecting the number of components in the normalizing flow mixture.

Figures 5.1, 5.2, 5.3, 5.4, and 5.5 show that the predicted option prices from the models closely fit the market data across the various times to expiry of the options. The results show that the one mixture normalizing flow is typically the worst-performing mixture and thus supports the case for considering some mixture components greater than one. This is also supported by the results displayed in Tables 5.1, 5.2, 5.3 and 5.4. Furthermore, the options closer to expiry approach a payoff with a kink (because for large strikes, the option's value becomes zero). This possibly explains why more components are required in the mixture to capture this highly non-linear payoff (as a function of strike) as we approach the option's expiry. On the other hand, options that are still far from expiry have an almost straight-line payoff as a function of strike, and thus, this can be captured by a few components in the mixture.

We further find that although most models fit the unseen data well, they don't fit option prices perfectly, as shown by the non-zero absolute errors. The results in these figures also show that, on average, the most significant errors are for small strikes (where the option price is large), while the smallest errors are at large strikes (where the option price is approaching zero).

The results in this chapter support the case for considering data-driven approaches for modeling option prices. Furthermore, modeling the risk-neutral density directly and extracting the option prices from it is ideal as it ensures that the no-arbitrage conditions hold and, thus, don't require custom loss functions to incorporate these conditions.

5.6 Conclusions

This chapter analyzed the option prices on the South African JSE All Share Index options across various option maturities and strikes. We model the risk-neutral density directly, which guarantees that the no-arbitrage conditions are satisfied. We undertake the modeling using a mixture of normalizing flows.

The results show that the normalizing flows can fit observed market option prices across different maturities and strikes. We observed that, on average, the largest errors are for small strikes, while the smallest errors are at large strikes. The results further indicate that using a mixture of normalizing flows with only one component leads to underperformance.

Instead, options close to maturity require a higher number of components in the mixture, while options far from expiry require fewer components in the mixture. This indicates a non-negligible relation between the number of components in the mixture and the options' expiry.

The results in this chapter can be extended by comparing various techniques to optimally select the number of components in the normalizing flow mixture. Furthermore, it could be interesting to explore jointly modeling the entire option price surface (i.e., across all expiry and strikes).

The next chapter models corporations' credit ratings using distributed Gaussian processes. Accurately modeling an entity's credit rating is crucial as it can affect, for example, the interest rate at which the entity can borrow funds from the capital markets.

References

Bayer, C., Friz, P., & Gatheral, J. (2016). Pricing under rough volatility. *Quantitative Finance, 16*(6), 887–904.

Black, F., & Scholes, M. (1973). The pricing of options and corporate liabilities. *Journal of Political Economy*, 81(3), 637–654. ISSN: 00223808.

Buchen, P. W., & Kelly, M. (1996). The maximum entropy distribution of an asset inferred from option prices. *Journal of Financial and Quantitative Analysis, 31*(1), 143–159.

Buehler, H., Gonon, L., Teichmann, J., & Wood, B. (2019). Deep hedging. *Quantitative Finance, 19*(8), 1271–1291.

Carr, P., Geman, H., Madan, D. P., & Yor, M. (2003). Stochastic volatility for Lévy processes. *Mathematical Finance, 13*(3), 345–382.

Cont, R. (2001). Empirical properties of asset returns: Stylized facts and statistical issues. *Quantitative Finance, 1*, 223–236.

Heston, S. L. (1993). A closed-form solution for options with stochastic volatility with applications to bond and currency options. *The Review of Financial Studies* 6(2), 327–343. ISSN: 08939454.

Horvath, B., Muguruza, A., & Tomas, M. (2021). Deep learning volatility: A deep neural network perspective on pricing and calibration in (rough) volatility models. *Quantitative Finance, 21*(1), 11–27.

Kou, S. G. (2007). Jump-diffusion models for asset pricing in financial engineering. *Handbooks in operations research and management science, 15*, 73–116.

Loaiza-Ganem, G., Gao, Y., & Cunningham, J. P. (2022). Maximum entropy flow networks. In *International Conference on Learning Representations*.

Marwala, T., Mbuvha, R., & Mongwe, W. T. (2023). *Hamiltonian Monte Carlo methods in machine learning*. Elsevier.

Merton, R. C. (1976). Option pricing when underlying stock returns are discontinuous. *Journal of Financial Economics, 3*(1–2), 125–144. ISSN: 0304-405X.

Mongwe, W. T. (2015). *Analysis of equity and interest rate returns in South Africa under the context of jump diffusion processes*. Masters Thesis at University of Cape Town. Last Retrieved: 18 March 2021. https://open.uct.ac.za/bitstream/handle/11427/16600/thesis_com_2015_mongwe_wilson_tsakane.pdf?isAllowed=y&sequence=1

Mongwe, W. T., & Malan, K. M. (2020). A survey of automated financial statement fraud detection with relevance to the South African context. *South African Computer Journal, 32*(1). https://doi.org/10.18489/sacj.v32i1.777

Mongwe, W. T., Sidogi, T., Mbuvha, R., & Marwala, T. (2022). Probabilistic inference of south african equity option prices under jump-diffusion processes. In *2022 IEEE symposium on computational intelligence for financial engineering and economics (CIFEr)* (pp. 1–8). IEEE.

Polanska, A., Price, M. A., Mancini, A. S., & McEwen, J. D. (2023). Learned harmonic mean estimation of the marginal likelihood with normalizing flows. *Physical Sciences Forum, 9*(1), MDPI, 10.

Sidogi, T., Mongwe, W. T., Mbuvha, R., & Marwala, T. (2022). Creating synthetic volatility surfaces using generative adversarial networks with static arbitrage loss conditions. In *2022 IEEE symposium series on computational intelligence (SSCI)* (pp. 1423–1429). IEEE.

Sidogi, T., Mongwe, W. T., Mbuvha, R., Olukanmi, P., & Marwala, T. (2023). A signature transform of limit order book data for stock price prediction. *IEEE Access*.

Yang, Y., & Hospedales, T. M. (2023). Mixture of normalizing flows for european option pricing. In *Uncertainty in artificial intelligence*. PMLR (pp. 2390–2399).

Zhu, Q., Loeper, G., Chen, W., & Langrené, N. (2021). Markovian approximation of the rough Bergomi model for Monte Carlo option pricing. *Mathematics, 9*(5), 528.

CHAPTER 6

Sparse and Distributed Gaussian Processes for Modeling Corporate Credit Ratings

6.1 Introduction

To draw in investments from the public, H.V. Poor started releasing financial data on railroad firms in 1860, and this is when the concept of credit rating first emerged in the financial markets (Wallis et al., 2019). Following this advancement, J. Moody, the founder of Moody's Investors Service, expanded this concept by grouping this information into alphabetical groups. Currently, at least one credit rating agency in the US rates 100% of all commercial papers and 99% of corporate bonds (Wallis et al., 2019). Across the world, these credit rating companies have grown to meet the demands of corporate borrowers and investors (Wallis et al., 2019).

Assessing a company's risk of default is necessary in several situations (Wallis et al., 2019). A credit rating indicates the level of risk involved in investing with a company's financial instruments and represents the likelihood that the company will pay its financial obligations on time

Supplementary Information The online version contains supplementary material available at https://doi.org/10.1007/978-3-031-88431-3_6.

W. T. Mongwe et al., *Bayesian Machine Learning in Quantitative Finance*, https://doi.org/10.1007/978-3-031-88431-3_6

(Hajek & Michalak, 2013; Huang et al., 2004; Muñoz-Izquierdo et al., 2022; Wallis et al., 2019). Bond investors, debt issuers, government officials, and credit-granting businesses use credit ratings to evaluate the risk of an investment. Since credit rating evaluations are used as inputs into crucial investment decisions, they must be as precise as possible (Wallis et al., 2019). However, this typically means that much information about a company's profile must be considered. Experts can conduct a thorough investigation, but it is frequently expensive and time-consuming (Hajek & Michalak, 2013; Muñoz-Izquierdo et al., 2022; Wallis et al., 2019).

Currently, a lot of emphasis is placed on automated credit rating evaluation techniques since the manual study of a company's profile is slow and expensive (Muñoz-Izquierdo et al., 2022). The credit rating forecasting literature is divided into research using traditional statistical and machine learning techniques (Hajek and Michalak, 2013; Muñoz-Izquierdo et al., 2022; Wallis et al., 2019). Financial ratios have been employed in developing credit rating models in existing credit rating prediction studies (Hajek & Michalak, 2013). The most commonly selected indicators for predicting credit ratings are profitability, liquidity, leverage, and market ratios (Hajek & Henriques, 2017; Muñoz-Izquierdo et al., 2022; Wallis et al., 2019), with some authors incorporating information from the entities audit report as well. The traditional statistical techniques used for forecasting credit ratings include logistic regression, linear discriminant analysis, and Bayesian networks (Hajek and Michalak, 2013; Wallis et al., 2019). The most accurate types are the ordered logistic regression and ordered probit models, as indicated by previous studies that utilized traditional models (Muñoz-Izquierdo et al., 2022; Wallis et al., 2019). These statistical techniques make assumptions around the distribution generating the data, and often struggle to pick up non-linear relationships between inputs and outputs (Hajek and Michalak, 2013; Mongwe & Malan, 2020; Muñoz-Izquierdo et al., 2022). When the input and output mapping are too complicated to explain analytically, machine learning technologies are frequently used (Hajek & Michalak, 2013).

The literature has demonstrated that machine learning techniques accurately predict corporate credit ratings using financial and accounting ratios (Hajek & Michalak, 2013; Huang et al., 2004; Muñoz-Izquierdo et al., 2022; Wallis et al., 2019). The main advantage of these techniques is that they make minimal assumptions about the distribution underlying the data, and they typically improve performance with increased data available (Mongwe & Malan, 2020). The most commonly used machine learning techniques for predicting credit ratings are decision trees, artificial neural networks, Naïve Bayes, support vector machines, ensembles, as well as combining these methods with feature selection strategies (Muñoz-Izquierdo et al., 2022; Wallis et al., 2019). These studies concur that data mining techniques are more effective and precise than conventional statistical models in evaluating credit ratings (Muñoz-Izquierdo et al., 2022; Wallis et al., 2019). However, few studies have considered utilizing Bayesian approaches to analyze credit ratings (Antunes et al., 2017; Huang, 2011; Yu et al., 2022). The Bayesian approaches are preferable as they not only provide point estimate, but also allow one to incorporate uncertainties in any predictions produced by the model.

In this chapter, we provide a first-in-literature analysis of credit ratings of US companies using sparse and distributed Gaussian processes. The sparse Gaussian processes we consider are trained using variational inference by minimizing the log marginal likelihood. For the distributed Gaussian processes, we consider variations of the product of expert models that combine local experts through a tractable product. The kernel used for the distributed Gaussian processes is shared among the experts. The distributed Gaussian processes are also trained using variational inference by minimizing the log marginal likelihood where the kernel parameters are shared. The adopted Bayesian approach also allows us to extract the most relevant inputs through an automatic relevant determination kernel. The ranking of the features, which is based on the reciprocal of the kernel length scales, may provide insight for stakeholders to understand what is driving the credit ratings of US entities. This framework can also be extended to other jurisdictions in the world.

The rest of this chapter is organized as follows: We first present the machine learning models that we train in Sect. 6.2; we then present the numerical experiments we conduct in this chapter in Sect. 6.3, after which we provide the results and the discussion and conclude in Sects. 6.4 and 6.5 respectively.

6.2 Machine Learning Models

This section discusses the sparse and distributed Gaussian processes we use to model corporate credit ratings in this chapter. We also discuss the multinomial logistic regression model used as the benchmark to assess the performance of the Gaussian processes models.

6.2.1 Multinomial Logistic Regression

Multinomial logistic regression (MLR) is a commonly utilized machine learning model in the credit rating literature (Muñoz-Izquierdo et al., 2022; Wallis et al., 2019). The three primary assumptions of MLR are as follows: (1) there is a linear connection between the covariates and the link-function-transformed result; (2) observations are independent of each other; and (3) outcomes follow a categorical distribution produced from the covariates via a link function (Wallis et al., 2019). As MLR generates a chance that an outcome falls into a particular category, it is an extension of logistic regression from binary to multiple categories (Wallis et al., 2019). The logarithm of the chances, or logit, is still the link function that is employed. This appropriately limits the probability to be between 0 and 1.

6.2.2 Sparse Gaussian Processes

Gaussian processes are non-parametric probabilistic models that can solve regression and classification problems (Cohen et al., 2020; Mbuvha et al., 2023; Rasmussen & Williams, 2006;). Unlike deep neural networks, Gaussian processes can produce uncertainties in the predictions made from this model. A Gaussian process is a set of random variables, each of a finite subset of which is collectively Gaussian distributed (Mbuvha et al., 2023; Rasmussen & Williams, 2006). Gaussian processes are priors over functions.

Gaussian processes are fully defined by a mean function $\mu(\mathbf{x}')$ and a Kernel function $k(\mathbf{x}'_i, \mathbf{x}'_j)$. Given a training dataset $\{\mathbf{x}'_t, \mathbf{x}_t\}_{t=1}^{t}$ with t noisy observations $\mathbf{x}_t = f(\mathbf{x}'_t) + \epsilon$, where $\epsilon \sim \mathcal{N}(0, \sigma_X^2)$. The Gaussian process prior on f is such that $f(\mathbf{x}') \sim \mathcal{N}(\mu_{x'}, \mathbf{K}_{\mathbf{x}'} + \sigma_X^2\mathbf{I})$. The mean and variance of the Gaussian posterior predictive distribution of the function $f(\mathbf{x}'_*)$ at a test point $\mathbf{x}'_*$, are given by:

$$\mathbb{E}(f_*) = \mu_{\mathbf{x}'_*} + k_*(K_{x'} + \sigma_{X'}^2\mathbf{I})^{-1}(\mathbf{X} - \mu_{\mathbf{x}'}), \tag{6.1}$$

$$\text{var}(f_*) = k_{**} - \mathbf{k}_*^T(K_{x'} + \sigma_{X'}^2\mathbf{I})^{-1}\mathbf{k}_* \tag{6.2}$$

where $\mathbf{k}_{**} = k(\mathbf{x}'_*, \mathbf{x}'_*)$ and $\mathbf{k}_* = k(\mathbf{x}', \mathbf{x}'_*)$. The kernel hyperparameters θ and the noise parameter $\sigma_{\mathbf{X}}$ are obtained by maximizing the log-marginal likelihood given below:

$$\log p(\mathbf{X}|\mathbf{X}') = \log \mathcal{N}\left(\mu_{x'}, \mathbf{K}_{\mathbf{x}'\mathbf{x}'} + \sigma_{\mathbf{X}}^2 \mathbf{I}\right). \tag{6.3}$$

As can be seen from Eqs. 6.1 and 6.2, traditional Gaussian processes require the inversion of matrices as expressed through the Kernel functions—which is an operation that has cubic complexity (Cohen et al., 2020). Various methods have been investigated to circumvent Gaussian processes' cubic training cost. They primarily rely on two approaches: training dispersed (weak) experts on portions of the whole dataset or using sparse approximations and structure-exploiting assumptions to the covariance matrix (Cohen et al., 2020). In this chapter, we consider both the sparse approximations and utilizing local experts.

Sparse Gaussian processes use inducing points and not the entire dataset, which assists in reducing the computational burden. Inducing inputs, pseudo-training examples, are used by sparse Gaussian processes to lower the rank of the matrix that has to be inverted (Cohen et al., 2020). The number of inducing points determines the approximation quality produced by sparse Gaussian processes; many may be needed to reflect the local structures of some fast-changing functions (Cohen et al., 2020). Crucially, user-defined pseudo-training example count allows for control over memory and computational cost (Leibfried et al., 2020).

Sparse Gaussian processes typically lack closed-form solutions, necessitating approximate methods for training. Variational inference, which frames the task of Bayesian inference as an optimization problem (i.e., maximizing a lower bound on the logarithm of the marginal probability), is a valuable option for approximate inference in this situation (Leibfried et al., 2020). This opens the door to a strong and adaptable framework in which pseudo-training instances are handled as optimization arguments of the approximating posterior that are concurrently identified during training with the hyperparameters of the generative model (i.e., likelihood and prior) (Leibfried et al., 2020). Variational inference is discussed in more detail in Chapter 2 of this book.

6.2.3 Distributed Gaussian Processes

Expert models are a method for scaling Gaussian processes to large datasets. In this case, many Gaussian processes are trained on subsets of the data, either a product-of-expert technique or another approach to recombine the predictions (Cohen et al., 2020). In contrast to the product of experts, a mixture of experts is effective in heteroskedastic and nonstationary environments but usually does not enable tractable posterior inference (Cohen et al., 2020). This chapter concentrates on product-of-expert models, where M experts share the same hyperparameters. We start by outlining how these models are trained. The population of experts is automatically regularized by sharing kernel hyperparameters, assuming that the model we aim to mimic is a complete Gaussian process. Due to this standard set of hyperparameters, individual experts cannot overfit the local subset of their given data (Cohen et al., 2020).

Assuming independence across experts (given the training data), the log marginal likelihood is:

$$\log p(y|X, \theta) = \sum_{j=1}^{J} \log p_j(y|x^j, \theta^j) \tag{6.4}$$

where $\{x^j, y^j\}$ is the data assigned to the jth expert. To train the model, we maximize the log-marginal likelihood with respect to the (shared) kernel hyperparameters. Training can be distributed across diverse compute clusters, which improves the cubic complexity for the full Gaussian processes (Cohen et al., 2020).

The prediction technique using product-of-Gaussian process experts models is now explained. Specifically, we provide various methods for recombining expert predictions that have been trained. One significant unique feature of these models is that all prediction distributions of function values are Gaussians in contrast to the mixture of experts.

6.2.3.1 *Generalized Product of Experts*

The Generalized Product of Experts (gPoE) approach aggregates predictions of M experts at test point x_* via (Cohen et al., 2020):

$$p(f_*|x_*) \propto \prod_{j=1}^{J} p_j^{\beta_j(x_*)}(f_*|x_*, D^j) \tag{6.5}$$

where the predictive mean and precision are given as:

$$m_{(g)poe}(x_*) = \sigma^2_{(g)poe}(x_*) \sum_{j=1}^{J} \beta_j(x_*)\sigma_j^{-2}(x_*)m_j(x_*) \tag{6.6}$$

$$\sigma^{-2}_{(g)poe}(x_*) = (x_*) \sum_{j=1}^{J} \beta_j(x_*)\sigma_j^{-2}(x_*) \tag{6.7}$$

where $D(j) = \{x^j, y^j\}$ is the data assigned to expert j, $\beta_j(x_*)$ controls the contribution of expert j at x_* (typically a measure of its confidence at x_*), and then the Product of Experts (PoE) model is recovered when setting $\beta_j(x_*) = 1$ for all j. As the number of experts increases, the product of experts' aggregated variance vanishes, leading to overconfident predictions.

6.2.3.2 *Robust Bayesian Committee Machine*

The robust Bayesian committee machine (rBCM) assumes conditional independence $D_i \perp\!\!\!\perp D_j|f_*$. By repeated application of Bayes' theorem, we obtain the predictive distribution (Cohen et al., 2020):

$$p(f_*|x_*) = \frac{\prod_{j=1}^{J} p_j^{\beta_j(x_*)}(f_*|x_*, D^j)}{p_j^{-1+\sum_{j=1}^{J}\beta_j(x_*)}(f_*|x_*)} \tag{6.8}$$

at test point x_*. Then, the predictive mean and precision are given as:

$$m_{(r)bcm}(x_*) = \sigma^2_{(r)bcm}(x_*) \sum_{j=1}^{J} \beta_j(x_*)\sigma_j^{-2}(x_*)m_j(x_*) \tag{6.9}$$

$$\sigma^{-2}_{(r)bcm}(x_*) = (x_*) \sum_{j=1}^{J} \beta_j(x_*)(\sigma_j^{-2}(x_*) + \sigma_*^{-2}) + \sigma_*^{-2} \tag{6.10}$$

Bayesian committee machine (BCM) is recovered when $\beta_j(x_*) = 1$ for all j. This predictive distribution guarantees that the model returns to the prior training data.

This chapter considers the following distributed Gaussian process models: PoE, gPoE, BCM, and rBCM. The following section describes the numerical experiments we conducted in this chapter.

6.3 Numerical Experiments

In this section, we present the numerical experiments conducted. We first describe the datasets used and then outline the experiments, settings, and performance metrics used.

6.3.1 Data Description

The dataset comprises 2021 credit rating observations from the three major international rating agencies on US corporations. There are 26 features for each company, of which 25 are financial indicators with the descriptive statistics shown in Table 6.1, and the other indicates the company's sector. The financial indicators can be further divided into:

- **Liquidity Measurement Ratios:** currentRatio, quickRatio, cashRatio, daysOfSalesOutstanding
- **Profitability Indicator Ratios:** grossProfitMargin, operatingProfitMargin, pretaxProfitMargin, netProfitMargin, effectiveTaxRate, returnOnAssets, returnOnEquity, returnOnCapitalEmployed
- **Debt Ratios:** debtRatio, debtEquityRatio
- **Operating Performance Ratios:** assetTurnover
- **Cash Flow Indicator Ratios:** operatingCashFlowPerShare, freeCashFlowPerShare, cashPerShare, operatingCashFlowSalesRatio, freeCashFlowOperatingCashFlowRatio

The target variable is the credit rating, which is encoded as an alphabet from the rating agencies. Using a consistent mapping approach, we map all the ratings to four categories—low risk, medium risk, high risk, and highest risk. The mapping is shown below in Table 6.2.

Note that for our analysis in this chapter, we exclude entities that are in default and those that are AAA (i.e., very low risk) as they were few. The

Table 6.1 Descriptive statistics for the corporate credit rating dataset

Variable	*Mean*	*Std*	*Minimum*	*Median*	*Maximum*
currentRatio	3.5200	44.050	−0.9320	1.4930	1725.500
quickRatio	2.6530	32.944	−1.8930	0.9856	1139.541
cashRatio	0.6673	3.5830	−0.1920	0.2974	125.9170
daysOfSalesOutstanding	333.795	4447.839	−811.845	42.374	115961.63
netProfitMargin	0.27844	6.0641	−101.845	0.0647	198.51700
pretaxProfitMargin	0.431483	8.984982	−124.343612	0.084965	309.69485
grossProfitMargin	0.497968	0.525307	−14.800817	0.414774	2.702533
operatingProfitMargin	0.587322	11.224622	−124.343612	0.107895	410.18221
returnOnAssets	−37.517928	1166.1722	−40213.178	0.045608	0.487826
returnOnCapitalEmployed	−73.97419	2350.2757	−87162.162	0.07442	2.439504
returnOnEquity	143.494296	4406.515045	−63.814815	0.122383	141350.211
assetTurnover	3.678340e+03	9.565410e+04	−9.157477e+00	6.983455e-01	2.553149e+06
fixedAssetTurnover	7.269487e+03	1.889967e+05	−2.679777e+01	3.811684e+00	5.156884e+06
debtEquityRatio	2.328306	87.528880	−2556.419643	1.652456	2561.871795
debtRatio	0.661495	0.208921	0.000000	0.640915	1.927839
effectiveTaxRate	0.397572	10.5950	−100.6110	0.3005	429.9262
freeCashFlowOperatingCashFlowRatio	0.40955	3.79648	−120.9160	0.64452	34.594086
freeCashFlowPerShare	5.094719e+03	1.469156e+05	−4.912742e+03	2.131742e+00	5.753380e+06
cashPerShare	4.227549e+03	1.224000e+05	−1.915035e+01	3.686513e+00	4.786803e+06
companyEquityMultiplier	3.323579	87.52986	−2555.4196	2.6524	2562.87179
ebitPerRevenue	0.437454	8.984299	−124.3436	0.08732	309.69485
enterpriseValueMultiple	48.28798	529.11896	−3749.9213	9.27439	11153.607
operatingCashFlowPerShare	6.515123e+03	1.775290e+05	−1.195049e+04	4.352584e+00	6.439270e+06
operatingCashFlowSalesRatio	1.447653	19.483294	−4.461837	0.133050	688.52659
payablesTurnover	38.002718	758.923588	−76.662850	5.759722	20314.880400

Table 6.2 Credit rating mapping to risk category

Credit rating	*Risk category*
'AAA'	'Lowest Risk'
'AA'	'Low Risk'
'A'	'Low Risk'
'BBB'	'Medium Risk'
'BB'	'High Risk'
'B'	'High Risk'
'CCC'	'Highest Risk'
'CC'	'Highest Risk'
'C'	'Highest Risk'
'D'	'In Default'

distribution of the target variable is shown in Fig. 6.1. A 70-30 train-test split was employed for this dataset, and the dataset was normalized using a min-max scaler.

6.3.2 *Performance Metrics*

The performance metrics used in this chapter are predictive performance on unseen data, including accuracy, recall, precision, and F1 measures (Marwala et al., 2023; Mongwe & Malan, 2020). The higher these measures, the better the model performance on unseen data.

We consider the sparse variation Gaussian process (SVGP) model with 100 and 500 inducing points and the distributed Gaussian process (i.e., PoE, gPoE, BCM, and rBMC) with 100 and 200 experts, respectively. The distributed Gaussian processes all employ 100 inducing points. We use a square exponential kernel for both the distributed GPs and the SVGP. Note that the kernel used for the distributed GP model is shared among the experts. Note that we use an automatic relevance determination kernel for all the models, which allows us to extract the most relevant inputs for the credit rating prediction task.

6.4 Results and Discussions

In this section, we present the results and the discussions from the numerical experiments. Tables 6.3 and 6.4 show the classification report on unseen data for all the models for the case when the SVGP model uses 100 inducing points, and the distributed GPs use 100 experts, as well as

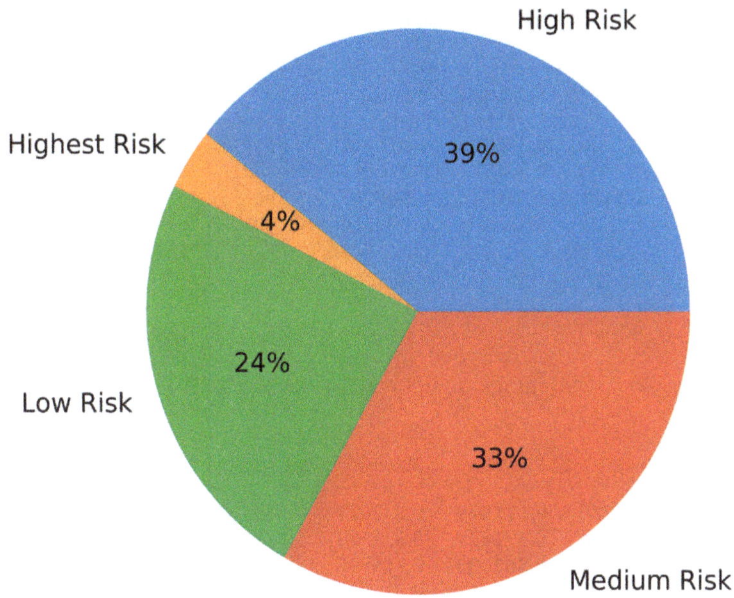

Fig. 6.1 Distribution of the credit ratings from lowest risk to highest risk categories as mapped out in Table 6.2

for the case when the SVGP model uses 500 inducing points, and the distributed GPs use 200 experts. Figures 6.2 and 6.3 show the mean posterior variances from each of the Bayesian models, while Table 6.5 shows the ranking of the top five features (covariates) by each method for the corporate credit rating dataset.

Table 6.3 shows that the PoE model outperforms across all the performance metrics when the SVGP model uses 100 inducing points, and the distributed GPs use 100 experts, with the worst-performing model being MLR. In general, all the distributed GP models outperform the SVGP model. We further find that, as shown in Table 6.4, increasing the number of inducing points for the SVGP model improved its performance (as

Table 6.3 Classification report on unseen data for all the models for the case where the SVGP model uses 100 inducing points, and the distributed GPs use 100 experts. The entries in **bold** indicate outperformance for the given performance metric

Metric	MLR	$SVGP_{100}$	PoE_{100}	$gPoE_{100}$	BCM_{100}	$rBCM_{100}$
Accuracy	0.384236	0.541872	**0.610837**	0.605911	0.600985	0.605911
Recall	0.384236	0.541872	**0.610837**	0.605911	0.600985	0.605911
Precision	0.378414	0.534043	**0.600907**	0.596394	0.590524	0.596394
F1	0.308521	0.537916	**0.604563**	0.600153	0.594459	0.600153

Table 6.4 Classification report on unseen data for all the models for the case where the SVGP model uses 500 inducing points, and the distributed GPs use 200 experts. The entries in **bold** indicate outperformance for the given performance metric

Metric	MLR	$SVGP_{500}$	PoE_{200}	$gPoE_{200}$	BCM_{200}	$rBCM_{200}$
Accuracy	0.384236	**0.571429**	0.532020	0.532020	0.532020	0.532020
Recall	0.384236	**0.571429**	0.532020	0.532020	0.532020	0.532020
Precision	0.378414	**0.562605**	0.516395	0.515777	0.516395	0.515777
F1	0.308521	**0.565572**	0.516891	0.517190	0.516891	0.517190

expected) while increasing the number of experts used in the distributed GPs led to performance degradation. However, it is essential to note that increasing the number of inducing points for the SVGP model led to a substantial increase in the execution time. Furthermore, the results show that the number of experts influences the performance for the distributed GP model, and approaches for selecting the optimal number of experts are still an open research problem.

Figures 6.2 and 6.3 show the relative importance of the 26 features, as extracted as the reciprocal of the kernel length scales for both the SVGP model and the shared kernel in the distributed GP model. All the models could clearly distinguish the necessary variables from the less relevant features for the credit rating prediction task. This can be seen in Figs. 6.2 and 6.3 by some features with near zero importance and some with more considerable importance. Table 6.5 summarizes the top five ranking features. The results show that the models broadly agree on which features are important. The most commonly featured variables in the top

Fig. 6.2 Mean posterior variances for SVGP model with 100 inducing points and for distributed GP model with 100 experts. The higher the value, the more important the variable is to the task of detecting and modeling corporate credit ratings

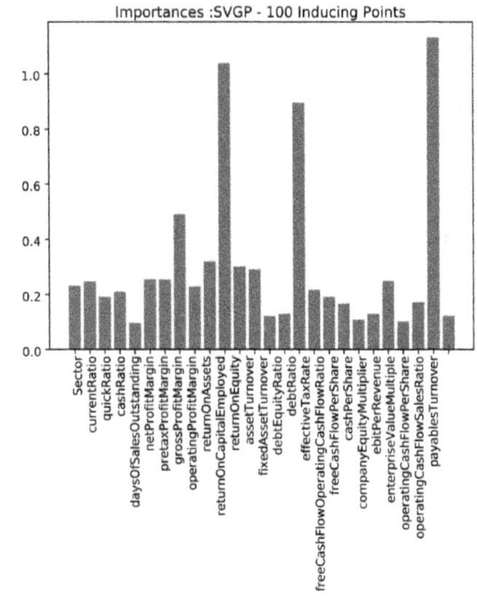

(**a**) Importance's for SVGP with 100 Inducing Points.

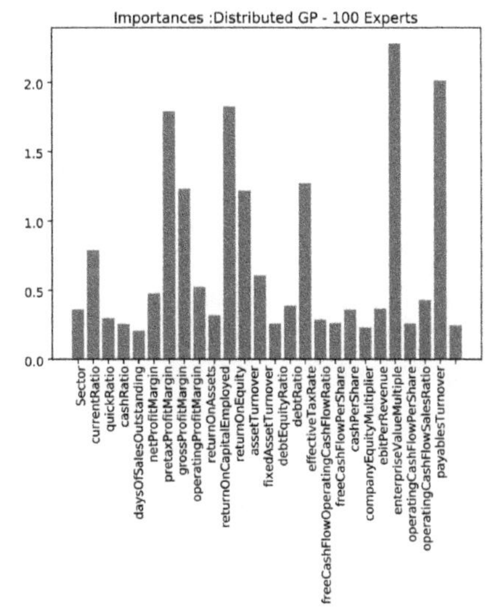

(**b**) Importance's for Distributed GP with 100 experts.

Fig. 6.3 Mean posterior variances for SVGP model with 500 inducing points and for distributed GP model with 200 experts. The higher the value, the more important the variable is to the task of detecting and modeling corporate credit ratings

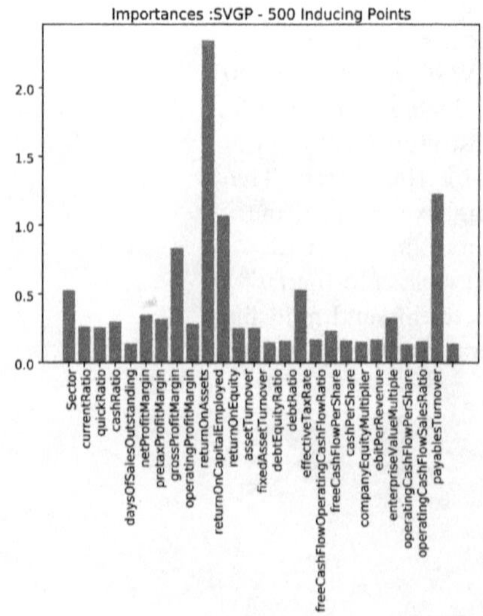

(**a**) Importance's for SVGP with 500 inducing points.

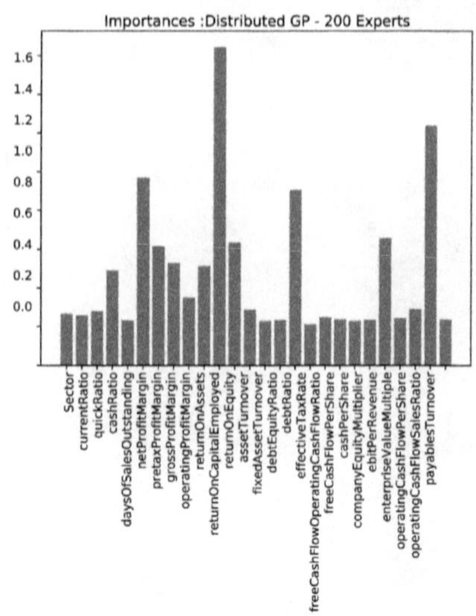

(**b**) Importance's for Distributed GP with 200 experts.

Table 6.5 Ranking of the top five features by each method for the corporate credit rating dataset. For example, $SVGP_{500}$ ranks *returnOnAssets* as the most important, while $DistributedGP_{200}$ ranks *netProfitMargin* as the third most important

Ranking	$SVGP_{100}$	$SVGP_{500}$	$DistributedGP_{100}$	$DistributedGP_{200}$
1	operatingCashFlowSalesRatio	returnOnAssets	ebitPerRevenue	returnOnCapitalEmployed
2	returnOnCapitalEmployed	operatingCashFlowSalesRatio	operatingCashFlowSalesRatio	operatingCashFlowSalesRatio
3	debtRatio	returnOnCapitalEmployed	returnOnCapitalEmployed	netProfitMargin
4	grossProfitMargin	grossProfitMargin	pretaxProfitMargin	debtRatio
5	returnOnAssets	debtRatio	debtRatio	ebitPerRevenue

five rankings are the operatingCashFlowSalesRatio, debtRatio, and profit margin-related metrics.

These results make intuitive sense in that firms with large values for the operatingCashFlowSalesRatio variable and profit margin-related metrics would be less likely to default on obligations and, thus, are likely to have a higher rating. On the other hand, entities with high debt ratios would likely be over-indebted, affecting their ability to repay loans—thus pushing the entity's credit rating down. These results could prove useful for various stakeholders that make use of the credit ratings.

6.5 Conclusion

We provide a first-in-literature application of a Bayesian inference framework to analyze credit rating data from corporations in the USA. Our analyses utilize the sparse and distributed Gaussian processes, with multinomial logistic regression being the benchmark model. The distributed Gaussian processes we consider are the products of experts, the generalized products of experts, the Bayesian committee machines, and the robust Bayesian committee machines.

The results show that the distributed Gaussian processes outperform the sparse Gaussian processes and the benchmark model across all performance metrics. However, we find that the performance of the distributed Gaussian processes degenerates when more experts are utilized. The results from the sparse and distributed Gaussian processes also produce the most essential variables as a by-product. The debt ratio, profit margin-related metrics, and return on capital metrics are the most important for determining the corporate rating of an entity. These results could prove helpful for various stakeholders using the credit ratings.

The work in this chapter can be expanded by considering other distributed Gaussian processes, such as a mixture of experts instead of a product of experts. Furthermore, data from a developing nation such as South Africa could also be utilized to assess the performance of the models. The problem of selecting the number of experts to use for the distributed Gaussian process model would also be of interest.

In the next chapter, we use advanced Hamiltonian Monte Carlo techniques to analyze the recovery rates on charged-off loans on a portfolio of loans. Similarly to analyzing credit ratings, analyzing recovery rates can inform which clients to offer loans to and how to manage better the institution's loan book.

References

Antunes, F., Ribeiro, B., & Pereira, F. (2017). Probabilistic modeling and visualization for bankruptcy prediction. *Applied Soft Computing, 60*, 831–843.

Cohen, S., Mbuvha, R., Marwala, T., & Deisenroth, M. (2020). Healing products of Gaussian process experts. In *International conference on machine learning*. PMLR (pp. 2068–2077).

Hajek, P., & Henriques, R. (2017). Mining corporate annual reports for intelligent detection of financial statement fraud - A comparative study of machine learning methods. *Knowledge-Based Systems, 128*, 139–152. https://doi.org/10.1016/j.knosys.2017.05.001

Hajèk, P., & Michalak, K. (2013). Feature selection in corporate credit rating prediction. *Knowledge-Based Systems, 51*, 72–84.

Huang, S.-C. (2011). Using Gaussian process based kernel classifiers for credit rating forecasting. *Expert Systems with Applications, 38*(7), 8607–8611.

Huang, Z., Chen, H., Hsu, C.-J., Chen, W.-H., & Wu, S. (2004). Credit rating analysis with support vector machines and neural networks: a market comparative study. *Decision Support Systems, 37*(4), 543–558.

Leibfried, F., Dutordoir, V., John, S. T., & Durrande, N. (2020). A tutorial on sparse Gaussian processes and variational inference. arXiv preprint arXiv:2012.13962.

Marwala, T., Mbuvha, R., & Mongwe, W. T. (2023). *Hamiltonian Monte Carlo methods in machine learning*. Elsevier.

Mbuvha, R., Adounkpe, J. Y. P., Houngnibo, M. C. M., Mongwe, W. T., Nikraftar, Z., Marwala, T., & Newlands, N. K. (2023). A novel workflow for streamflow prediction in the presence of missing gauge observations. *Environmental Data Science, 2*, Article e23.

Mongwe, W. T., Malan, K. M. (2020). A survey of automated financial statement fraud detection with relevance to the South African context. *South African Computer Journal, 32*(1). https://doi.org/10.18489/sacj.v32i1.777

Muñoz-Izquierdo, N., Segovia-Vargas, M. J., Camacho-Miñano, M., & Pérez-Pérez, Y. (2022). Machine learning in corporate credit rating assessment using the expanded audit report. *Machine Learning, 111*(11), 4183–4215.

Rasmussen, C. E., & Williams, C. K. I. (2006). *Gaussian processes for machine learning*. The MIT Press.

Wallis, M., Kumar, K., & Gepp, A. (2019). Credit rating forecasting using machine learning techniques. In *Managerial perspectives on intelligent big data analytics* (pp. 180–198). IGI Global.

Yu, B., Li, C., Mirza, N., & Umar, M. (2022). Forecasting credit ratings of decarbonized firms: Comparative assessment of machine learning models. *Technological Forecasting and Social Change, 174*, Article 121255.

CHAPTER 7

Bayesian Detection of Recovery on Charged-Off Loan Accounts

7.1 Introduction

The main activity of retail banks is, by far, lending. A bank's core function is to convert short-term deposits into long-term assets through loans. While most loans are repaid in full and on schedule, some loans experience defaults owing to the borrower's financial position changing (Loang et al., 2023). Non-performing loans (NPLs) grew substantially for most banks during the COVID-19 pandemic (Ari et al., 2021; Loang et al., 2023). This was primarily driven by customers' being retrenched and losing their sources of income. Large NPLs are not good for a bank as they lead to the impairment of their loan assets and negatively impact the bank's profitability (Loang et al., 2023).

Various tactics, including written reminders, more targeted letters, phone calls, and legal action like court orders and marshal dispatch, are typically used to collect debt and recover it after default (Hoechstoetter et al., 2012). The various steps often cause the debtor to take different actions; sometimes, this leads to an agreement on a payment schedule with the customer. During the loan relationship, a lender may consider

Supplementary Information The online version contains supplementary material available at https://doi.org/10.1007/978-3-031-88431-3_7.

W. T. Mongwe et al., *Bayesian Machine Learning in Quantitative Finance*, https://doi.org/10.1007/978-3-031-88431-3_7

any of three fundamental collection methods unless prohibited by the nation's legislative structure (Hoechstoetter et al., 2012). The first option is the internal or in-house collection and recovery procedure. This is typically the first course of action taken by lenders. Second, a lender may keep ownership of the debt while designating an agent to handle collection (Hoechstoetter et al., 2012). The third option is selling the loan to a third party and cutting ties with the borrower. As argued by Hoechstoetter et al. (2012), a potential benefit of internal collection might be that all relevant debt features are known. At the same time, critical information that a third-party buyer lacks (such as loan specifics, borrower repayment patterns, or credit score changes) is exclusive to the original lender (Hoechstoetter et al., 2012).

Banks typically pool their NPLs and sell them to specialized investors, such as debt collection agencies, to limit impairment losses and financial stability concerns (Hoechstoetter et al., 2012). The crucial details on the exact date of the default, the amount owed, and the most recent payment are sent to the third-party buyer. Like the external agency, the third-party buyer might experience a poor selection, though, as he will probably only be able to obtain non-performing debt (Hoechstoetter et al., 2012; Loang et al., 2023). Large bid-ask spreads result from different data availability between banks and investors, and subpar valuation techniques impede the timely disposal of NPLs (Hoechstoetter et al., 2012). The recovery rate, or the portion of exposure that can be retrieved from each borrower via the debt collection procedure, is one of the key variables influencing the pricing of NPL portfolios (Hoechstoetter et al., 2012; Ye & Bellotti, 2019).

At the time of portfolio purchase, the debt collector's potential recovery rates are unknown and must be estimated. To do this, both parties need to determine which factors most accurately represent the possibility for recovery of borrowers as well as a set of efficient forecasting techniques (Hoechstoetter et al., 2012). These are by no means simple problems, and models that concentrate on retail credit products continue to be the focus of a great deal of research. Recoveries are defined as the loan amounts received less administrative expenses, divided by the remaining loan balance (i.e., the exposure at default) (Hoechstoetter et al., 2012; Ye & Bellotti, 2019). The recovery rate less one is the loss given default. The Probability of default (PD), loss given default (LGD), and exposure at default (EAD) are crucial credit parameters that the bank monitors (Ye & Bellotti, 2019).

It is even more critical for the bank to know their recoveries on each book under Basel III's internal ratings-based methodology, as the regulator allows the bank to estimate the LGD internally (Ye & Bellotti, 2019). Financial institutions have placed a greater emphasis on modeling LGD in recent years as Basel III's capital requirement calculation primarily relies on it (Ye & Bellotti, 2019). In contrast to the well-accepted assessment of PD, LGD is still being studied and is not as well known (Bellotti & Crook, 2012; Hlongwane et al., 2024; Ye & Bellotti, 2019). Enhancing LGD modeling can assist financial institutions in more accurately evaluating their risk and regulatory capital needs and in debt management. The bimodal feature with high concentrations at 0 and 1 commonly seen in LGD empirical distributions—where persons either repay in whole or nothing at all—presents the biggest obstacle in estimating LGD (Ye & Bellotti, 2019). In general, the shape of the distribution of the LGD depends on the loan book that one is looking at, and thus, a one-size-fits-all approach does not typically work. In practice, one would generally need to customize the model for the given dataset. In the literature, recoveries from defaulted loans have been studied using conventional statistical approaches and machine learning techniques (Bellotti & Crook, 2012; Calabrese, 2014; Loterman et al., 2012; Ye & Bellotti, 2019; Zhang & Zhao, 2024).

Based on a dataset of UK credit card defaults, Bellotti and Crook (2012) constructed Tobit and decision tree models in addition to Beta and fractional logit transformation of the recovery rate response variable to predict the loss given default. They concluded that the best forecasting performance was achieved using ordinary least squares regression with macroeconomic variables. Calabrese (2014) developed a mixed continuous-discrete model in which a Beta random variable represents the continuous portion of the recovery rate. They used this model to predict the Bank of Italy's loan recovery rate. In a benchmark study of LGD, Loterman et al. (2012) used six datasets taken from international banks to compare twenty-four distinct models. They concluded that non-linear models (such as neural networks) outperform linear models. Using a dataset from a European country, Ye and Bellotti (2019) propose a two-stage model incorporating a Beta mixture model combined with a logistic regression model. The proposed model allowed the authors to accurately capture the multi-modal distribution of recovery rates. There has been little investigation in the literature on the utility of using Bayesian approaches for the recovery modeling task, with Zhang and Zhao (2024) using Markov chain Monte Carlo (MCMC) sampling to draw model coefficients to generate LGD distributions and they found that they were able to capture the multi-modal nature of LGD distributions.

In this chapter, we present the first use of Bayesian logistic regression with automatic relevance determination (BLR-ARD) to detect the presence of recoveries on charged-off loan accounts using a dataset from a peer-to-peer lending platform. By employing the Bayesian approach, we can quantify our predictions' uncertainty, indicating the degree of confidence we have in specific predictions. Using automatic relevance determination allows us to determine which of the most relevant input features, with uncertainty measures around these as well (Mbuvha et al., 2019a; Mongwe et al., 2021c). This results in the model outcomes being more interpretable, allowing stakeholders to understand the model's results better.

Markov Chain Monte Carlo (MCMC) methods are employed to train the BLR-ARD model parameters. MCMC methods possess an advantage over approximate inference methods, such as variational inference and Laplace approximations, in that they are asymptotically guaranteed to converge to the true target posterior distribution. The Metropolis-Adjusted Langevin Algorithm (MALA), Hamiltonian Monte Carlo (HMC), and No-U-Turn Sampler (NUTS) MCMC algorithms are introduced in this chapter for the first time in the training of BLR-ARD models for the inference of recoveries on charged-off accounts. Our results show the added benefit of using a Bayesian framework for analyzing loan recoveries, with the proposed framework being easily extendable to other contexts.

The rest of this chapter is structured as follows: We first discuss the model we use to detect the recovery on defaulted loans in Sect. 7.2 and then the MCMC methods we use to train this model in Sect. 7.3. After this, we discuss the setup of our numerical experiments in Sect. 7.4. We then present and discuss the results, after which we conclude in Sects. 7.5 and 7.6 respectively.

7.2 Model for Bayesian Detection of Recoveries

We model the recovery rates using Bayesian logistic regression. The negative log-likelihood $l(\mathrm{D}|\mathbf{w})$ function for this model is given by (Marwala et al., 2023; Mongwe et al., 2021d; Mongwe, 2022):

$$l(\mathrm{D}|\mathbf{w}) = \sum_{i}^{N} y_i \log(\mathbf{w}^T x_i) + (1 - y_i)\log(1 - \mathbf{w}^T x_i) \tag{7.1}$$

where D ={x, y} is the data, N is the number of observations and $\mathbf{w}$ are the parameters that need to be estimated. Thus, the target un-normalized posterior log distribution is given as (Mongwe et al., 2021d):

$$\ln p(\mathbf{w}|\mathrm{D}) = l(\mathrm{D}|\mathbf{w}) + \ln p(\mathbf{w}|\alpha) + \ln q(\alpha) \tag{7.2}$$

where $\ln p(\mathbf{w}|\alpha)$ is the log of the prior distribution placed on the parameters given the hyperparameters, and $\ln q(\alpha)$ is the distribution of the hyperparameters. As in Marwala et al. (2023), Mongwe et al. (2021d), Mongwe (2022), we model the parameters $\mathbf{w}$ as having a Gaussian prior with each parameter having zero mean and its own standard deviation or regularization parameter α_i, meaning that we are using an automatic relevance determination (ARD) prior within our framework.

The α_i indicates how important the parameter associated with the input feature is. The larger the value of α_i, the more critical the input feature is in predicting the recovery rates (Mongwe et al., 2021d). Thus, this framework automatically ranks the importance of the input features. The α_i will have low values for irrelevant inputs, which will cause their weights to be driven to decay to values around zero (Mbuvha et al., 2021; Mongwe et al., 2021d). Conversely, essential inputs will have weights with high variances while less important inputs will have low variances (Mbuvha et al., 2021). Since the mean for the weight priors is fixed at zero, it follows that weights with high variances can take values far from zero (resulting in a more significant effect), while those with low variances must take values close to zero (thus reduced effect) (Mbuvha et al., 2021).

Due to the multi-modal and non-convex structure of the ARD loss function, inference of ARD prior hyperparameters is a fundamentally hard inverse problem (Mbuvha et al., 2021; Neal, 1993, 1995). Through maximizing the Bayesian evidence metric, Neal (1995) obtains estimates of the ARD hyperparameters, and this is due to the Laplace approximation's simplifying assumptions producing a tractable closed-form calculation of the evidence. On the other hand, Neal (2012) deploys an alternating framework of using Hamiltonian Monte Carlo for network weights and Gibbs sampling for ARD hyperparameters from various posteriors such as the Gamma (Mbuvha et al., 2021). This strategy converges to an asymptotically true posterior based on Markov Chain Monte Carlo. However, a lot of design decisions, such as the choice of the appropriate prior distribution, are still necessary (Mbuvha et al., 2021). The hyperparameter sampling strategy used in this chapter is to jointly infer the α hyperparameters and the $\mathbf{w}$ parameters as in Mongwe et al. (2021d). Although the effective parameter space is doubled in this approach, compared to the Gibbs sampling strategy, this method has the advantage of producing a more stable exploration across the MCMC methods (Mongwe et al., 2021d). As the $\mathbf{w}$ parameters are assumed to be normally distributed, we select the α hyperparameters to be log-normally distributed to make the joint sampling of parameters and hyperparameters mathematically convenient. In particular, the α_is are assumed to follow a log-normal distribution with mean zero, and unit variance as in Marwala et al. (2023), Mongwe et al. (2021d), Mongwe (2022).

7.3 Markov Chain Monte Carlo Algorithms

We now present the details of the MCMC methods that are used to train the Bayesian logistic regression model with an ARD prior in Eq. 7.2. We implemented all the MCMC methods in Python.

7.3.1 Metropolis-Adjusted Langevin Algorithm

The Metropolis-Adjusted Langevin Algorithm (MALA) enhances the Metropolis-Hastings (MH) method through the use of first-order gradient information of the target posterior. MALA reduces the random walk behavior of MH via the use of Langevin dynamics where the drift component is the derivative of the log of the target posterior, and the diffusive component is Brownian motion which is represented as follows (Gu & Sun, 2020; Marwala et al., 2023; Mongwe et al., 2021e, 2022b):

$$d\mathbf{w}_t = \frac{1}{2} f'(\mathbf{w})dt + dZ_t \tag{7.3}$$

where $\mathbf{w}$ are the parameters, $f'(\mathbf{w})$ is the first derivative of the target $f(\mathbf{w})$ with respect to the parameters, and Z_t is a Brownian motion process at a fictitious time t. The Langevin dynamics in Eq. 7.3 typically cannot be solved analytically, and numerical methods such as the Euler-Maruyama integration scheme are typically used (Marwala et al., 2023). This, however, introduces errors that can break the detailed balance condition, which would not guarantee that the method would converge to the correct target distribution (Marwala et al., 2023). To rectify this, a Metropolis acceptance step is incorporated into the algorithm to ensure detailed balance (Marwala et al., 2023). The MALA algorithm converges to the stationary distribution at a faster pace than the MH algorithm because it takes into account the density's first-order gradient data, which is represented by $f'(\mathbf{w})$ (Girolami & Calderhead, 2011; Gu & Sun, 2020; Marwala et al., 2023). The samples produced using the MALA method are still highly correlated. Girolami and Calderhead (2011) incorporate second-order gradient information of the target by extending MALA from being on a Euclidean manifold to a Riemannian manifold (Marwala et al., 2023). Despite a corresponding increase in compute time, this approach demonstrated significant gains in the sampling performance of the MALA method (Marwala et al., 2023).

The sampler converges to the target distribution more quickly with the MALA algorithm than with the MH algorithm because it utilizes the gradient information of the target distribution (Girolami and Calderhead, 2011; Gu & Sun, 2020). The produced samples are still very correlated. The next section discusses the Hamiltonian Monte Carlo and Magnetic Hamiltonian Monte Carlo approaches, which employ Hamiltonian dynamics to traverse the target distribution better.

7.3.2 *Hamiltonian Monte Carlo and the No-U-Turn Sampler*

Hamiltonian Monte Carlo (HMC) is a popular MCMC method for performing Bayesian inference and has been utilized in various disciplines such as finance, health, and energy (Duane et al., 1987; Mbuvha & Marwala, 2020; Mbuvha et al., 2021; Mongwe et al., 2021b, 2021d, 2021f, 2022a, 2022b). The method is premised on using Hamiltonian dynamics, which naturally considers the first-order gradient information of the target posterior. The dynamics that underpin HMC are as follows (Marwala et al., 2023; Neal, 1993):

$$\frac{d\mathbf{w}}{\partial t} = \frac{\partial \mathrm{H}(\mathbf{w}, \mathbf{p})}{\partial \mathbf{p}}; \quad \frac{d\mathbf{p}}{\partial t} = -\frac{\partial \mathrm{H}(\mathbf{w}, \mathbf{p})}{\partial \mathbf{w}} \tag{7.4}$$

where $\mathbf{w}$ are the parameters, $\mathbf{p}$ is the auxiliary momentum variable with the same dimensionality as $\mathbf{w}$, and $\mathrm{H}(\mathbf{w}, \mathbf{p})$ is the Hamiltonian—which represents the total energy (i.e., potential energy defined by the target posterior and kinetic energy which is typically captured through a multivariate Gaussian distribution) from this system (Mongwe et al., 2021b, 2022a). This HMC method allows distant proposals, which results in a significant reduction in the autocorrelations of the generated samples (Marwala et al., 2023).

The HMC technique is composed of two steps. The first step integrates Hamiltonian dynamics in Eq. 7.4 typically using the leapfrog integrator (Duane et al., 1987; Neal, 1993; Marwala et al., 2023), and the second step utilizes a Metropolis-Hastings correction to account for the numerical integration errors arising from the first step (Duane et al., 1987; Hastings et al., 1970; Neal et al., 2011). The parameter and momentum update equations for the leapfrog integration scheme (corresponding to the first step of HMC) are given as follows:

$$\begin{aligned} \mathbf{p}_{t+\frac{\epsilon}{2}} &= \mathbf{p}_t + \frac{\epsilon}{2}\frac{\partial H\left(\mathbf{w}_t, \mathbf{p}_t\right)}{\partial \mathbf{w}} \\ \mathbf{w}_{t+\epsilon} &= \mathbf{w}_t + \epsilon \mathbf{M}^{-1}\mathbf{p}_{t+\frac{\epsilon}{2}} \\ \mathbf{p}_{t+\epsilon} &= \mathbf{p}_{t+\frac{\epsilon}{2}} + \frac{\epsilon}{2}\frac{\partial H\left(\mathbf{w}_{t+\epsilon}, \mathbf{p}_{t+\frac{\epsilon}{2}}\right)}{\partial \mathbf{w}} \end{aligned} \tag{7.5}$$

where ϵ is the discretization step size and $\mathbf{M}$ is a covariance matrix emanating from the kinetic energy component in $\mathrm{H}(\mathbf{w}, \mathbf{p})$. If the integration of the Hamiltonian dynamics in the first step were solved precisely, the second step would not be required. However, due to the discretization errors, a Metropolis-Hastings acceptance step is typically required where the $\mathbf{w}^*$ proposed by the first step are accepted with probability:

$$\mathrm{P}(\text{accept } \mathbf{w}^*) = \min\left(1, \frac{\exp(-\mathrm{H}(\mathbf{w}^*, \mathbf{p}^*))}{\exp(-\mathrm{H}(\mathbf{w}, \mathbf{p}))}\right). \tag{7.6}$$

The parameters of HMC are the discretization step size ϵ, which is required for the first step in HMC, and the trajectory length, which determines the number of times the integration is performed. The step size parameter is typically set to obtain a user-specified target acceptance rate using the dual averaging method (Hoffman & Gelman, 2014; Marwala et al., 2023) while tuning the trajectory length parameter is a more complex problem (Hoffman & Gelman, 2014). It can further be shown that when the trajectory length parameter is set to 1, the HMC method becomes the MALA method. The overall HMC sampling process follows a Gibbs sampling scheme, where we sample **p** auxiliary momentum variable and then sample a new set of parameters **w** given the drawn momentum **p**. This procedure is repeated until the required number of samples are generated (Marwala et al., 2023; Mongwe et al., 2021a, 2021b). The pseudo-code for HMC can be found in Algorithm 3.1 in Chapter 3 of this book.

The step size and trajectory length are numerous parameters that necessitate tuning to achieve efficient sampling in the HMC algorithm. A trajectory length that is too short leads to a random walk behavior similar to the Metropolis-Hasting method (Hoffman & Gelman, 2014; Marwala et al., 2023; Mbuvha & Marwala, 2020; Mongwe et al., 2021a, 2021b). A trajectory length that is too long results in a trajectory that inefficiently traces back (Hoffman & Gelman, 2014; Mbuvha & Marwala, 2020; Mongwe, 2022; Marwala et al., 2023). The step size is also a critical parameter for sampling. Small step sizes are computationally inefficient, leading to correlated samples and poor mixing, while large step sizes compound discretization errors, leading to low acceptance rates (Hoffman & Gelman, 2014; Mbuvha & Marwala, 2020). Tuning these parameters requires multiple time-consuming pilot runs (Hoffman & Gelman, 2014; Marwala et al., 2023; Mbuvha & Marwala, 2020, Mongwe et al., 2021a, 2021b). The leapfrog step size and trajectory length are automatically adjusted by the No-U-Turn Sampler (NUTS) (Hoffman & Gelman, 2014; Marwala et al., 2023). In NUTS, the step size is tuned through primal-dual averaging during an initial burn-in phase by targeting a particular sample acceptance rate (Hoffman & Gelman, 2014; Marwala et al., 2023; Mbuvha & Marwala, 2020). The trajectory length is adjusted by iteratively adding steps until the chain begins to trace back (U-turn) or the Hamiltonian reaches infinity (Hoffman & Gelman, 2014; Mbuvha & Marwala, 2020).

Primal-dual averaging is used in NUTS to adjust the step size parameter during the burn-in phase (Marwala et al., 2023). Primal-dual averaging is used to achieve a user-specified Metropolis-Hastings acceptance rate δ which is expressed as (Andrieu & Thoms, 2008; Marwala et al., 2023; Mbuvha et al., 2019b; Mongwe, 2022):

$$\begin{aligned} \epsilon_{t+1} &\leftarrow \mu - \frac{\sqrt{t}}{\gamma} \frac{1}{t+t_0} \sum_{i=1}^{t} H_i \\ \bar{\epsilon}_{t+1} &\leftarrow \eta_t \epsilon_{t+1} + (1-\eta_t)\bar{\epsilon}_t \end{aligned} \tag{7.7}$$

where η_t is a decaying rate of adaptation in accordance with (Andrieu and Thoms, 2008), γ regulates the convergence toward μ, H_t is the difference between the target acceptance rate and the actual acceptance rate (Hoffman & Gelman, 2014; Mbuvha et al., 2021), and μ is a free parameter that ϵ_t gravitates to Marwala et al. (2023). The updates from primal-dual averaging are such that (Mbuvha et al., 2021; Marwala et al., 2023):

$$\mathbb{E}[H_t] = \mathbb{E}[\delta - \alpha_t] = 0. \tag{7.8}$$

As a result, the step size is updated toward the desired acceptance rate δ. Setting $\mu = \log(10\epsilon_0)$, $\bar{\epsilon}_0 = 1$, $\bar{H}_0 = 0$, $\gamma = 0.05$, $t_0 = 10$, $\kappa = 0.75$, and $\epsilon_0 = 0.0001$ as the initial step size yields acceptable performance across a variety of target posterior distributions (Hoffman & Gelman, 2014; Marwala et al., 2023; Mongwe, 2022). As outlined above, the settings used in this chapter are the same as those in Marwala et al. (2023).

Iteratively increasing the trajectory length until the Hamiltonian becomes infinite or the chain begins to trace back is how NUTS automatically adjusts the trajectory length parameter (Afshar et al., 2021; Mbuvha & Marwala, 2020). At that point, the final suggested position state $\mathbf{w}^*$ begins to resemble the starting position $\mathbf{w}$, and this is also when $(\mathbf{w}^* - \mathbf{w}) \times \mathbf{p} \leq 0$. This approach breaks down the detailed balancing criterion and is rectified through the use of a slice sampling technique (Hoffman & Gelman, 2011; Marwala et al., 2023).

NUTS operates at least as efficiently as and occasionally more efficiently than a well-tuned standard HMC method without necessitating user intervention or a costly tuning run (Hoffman & Gelman, 2014). This makes the NUTS method more accessible to non-expert audiences.

A detailed exposition of the NUTS, HMC, MALA, and MH algorithms can be found in Marwala et al. (2023).

7.4 Numerical Experiments

In this section, we present the numerical experiments conducted. We first describe the dataset and then outline the experiments, settings, and performance metrics used.

7.4.1 Data Description

We perform the recovery rate on charged-off loans analysis using data from the *Lending Club* peer-to-peer lending platform in 2018. The description of the variables is presented below.

1. **tot-coll-amt**—Total collection amounts ever owed.
2. **tot-cur-bal**—Total current balance of all accounts.
3. **open-acc-6m**—Number of open trades in last 6 months.
4. **total-bal-il**—Total current balance of all installment accounts.
5. **max-bal-bc**—Maximum current balance owed on all revolving accounts.
6. **all-util**—Balance to credit limit on all trades.
7. **total-rev-hi-lim**—Total revolving high credit/credit limit.
8. **inq-fi**—Number of personal finance inquiries.
9. **total-cu-tl**—Number of finance trades.
10. **inq-last-12m**—Number of credit inquiries in past 12 months.
11. **acc-open-past-24mths**—Number of trades opened in the past 24 months.
12. **avg-cur-bal**—Average current balance of all accounts.
13. **delinq-amnt**—The past-due amount owed for the accounts on which the borrower is now delinquent.
14. **mort-acc** —Number of mortgage accounts.
15. **num-accts-ever-120-pd**—Number of accounts ever 120 or more days past due.
16. **application-type**—Indicates whether the loan is an individual application or a joint application with two co-borrowers.
17. **num-actv-bc-tl**—Number of currently active bankcard accounts.
18. **num-actv-rev-tl**—Number of currently active revolving trades.

19. **num-bc-sats**—Number of satisfactory bankcard accounts.
20. **num-bc-tl**—Number of bankcard accounts.
21. **num-il-tl**—Number of installment accounts.
22. **num-op-rev-tl**—Number of open revolving accounts.
23. **num-rev-accts**—Number of revolving accounts.
24. **loan-amnt**—The listed amount of the loan applied for by the borrower. If, at some point in time, the credit department reduces the loan amount, then it will be reflected in this value.
25. **term**—The number of payments on the loan. Values are in months and can be either 36 or 60.
26. **int-rate**—Interest Rate on the loan.
27. **installment**—The monthly payment owed by the borrower if the loan originates.
28. **purpose**—A category provided by the borrower for the loan request.
29. **title**—The loan title provided by the borrower.
30. **addr-state**—The state provided by the borrower in the loan application.
31. **dti**—A ratio calculated using the borrower's total monthly debt payments on the total debt obligations, excluding mortgage and the requested LC loan, divided by the borrower's self-reported monthly income.
32. **delinq-2yrs**—The number of 30+ days past-due incidences of delinquency in the borrower's credit file for the past 2 years.
33. **fico-range-low**—The lower boundary of the range the borrower's FICO belongs to.
34. **fico-range-high**—The higher boundary of range the borrower's FICO belongs to.
35. **inq-last-6mths**—The number of inquiries in the past 6 months (excluding auto and mortgage inquiries)
36. **open-acc**—The number of open credit lines in the borrower's credit file.
37. **pub-rec**—Number of derogatory public records
38. **revol-bal**—Total credit revolving balance.
39. **grade**—Lending Club assigned loan grade.
40. **subgrade**—Lending Club assigned loan subgrade.
41. **emp-length**—Employment length in years. Possible values are between 0 and 10, where 0 means less than one year and 10 means ten or more years.

42. **home-ownership**—The home-ownership status provided by the borrower during registration or obtained from the credit report. The values are: RENT, OWN, MORTGAGE, OTHER.
43. **annual-inc**—The self-reported annual income provided by the borrower during registration.

The full dataset had 658 records and was split using a train-test split of 70-30. The distribution of the recovery rates is shown in Fig. 7.1, which shows that most recoveries are zero, with a long tail to the right.

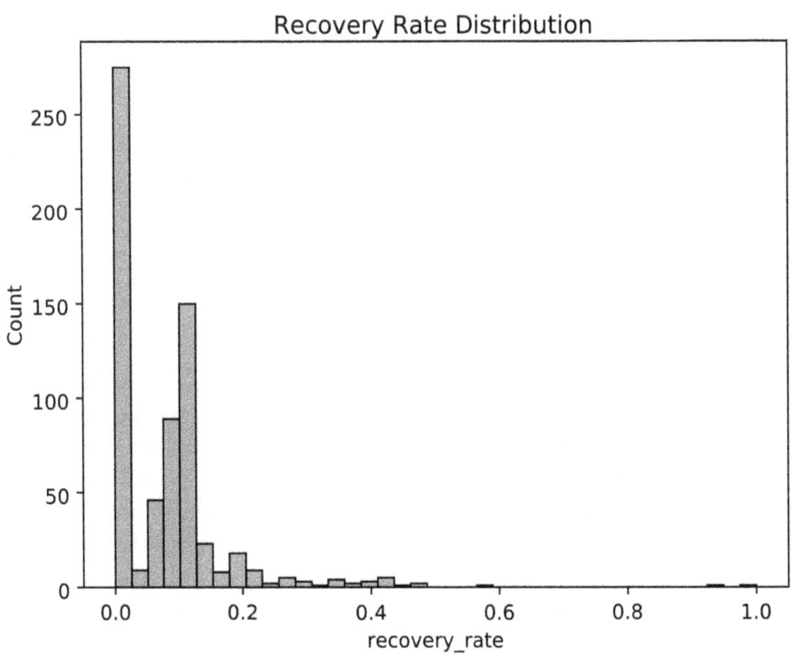

Fig. 7.1 Distribution of the recovery rates (in decimal) on charged-off loan accounts

7.4.2 *Experiment Description*

For the recovery analysis, we fit the Bayesian logistic regression model. We consider the binary classification problem of whether a given defaulted loan account will recover more than 10% or not. Thus, we encode the target as zero when there is less than 10% recovery and one otherwise. We split the data into a train and test set using a 70-30 split.

When fitting the Bayesian model, we generate a total of ten thousand samples, of which five thousand formed the burn-in period where tuning was performed for all the MCMC methods considered in this chapter. The step size parameters of all the methods were tuned using the primal-dual averaging methodology outlined in Hoffman and Gelman (2011), targeting an acceptance rate of 60% for MALA and 80% for both HMC and NUTS. Note that the path length of HMC was fixed at 25.

The next section discusses the performance metrics used to assess the MCMC methods.

7.4.3 *Performance Metrics for MCMC Methods*

We assess the performance of the algorithms by generating the trace plots of the un-normalized target posterior distribution, the effective sample sizes of the generated samples, the effective sample sizes of the generated samples normalized by execution time, and predictive performance on unseen data. It is important to note that the execution time is required to create the samples after the burn-in period. We utilize the multivariate effective sample size metric developed by Vats et al. (2019) as our effective sample size measure (Marwala et al., 2023; Mongwe, 2022; Mongwe et al., 2021b, 2021e).

The Receiver Operating Curve (ROC) and Area Under the ROC are the predictive performance metrics we employ to evaluate the outcomes of the Bayesian analysis. The model's true positives are shown on the y-axis against false positives on the x-axis on the ROC. The Area Under the ROC, or AUC, measures the average rate of misclassifications. When it comes to measuring performance when the costs of misclassification are unclear, AUC is useful (Bradley, 1997; Gaganis, 2009; Mongwe & Malan, 2020), which is the case for the recovery detection task at hand.

7.5 Results and Discussions

In this section, we present the results and the discussions from the numerical experiments conducted in this chapter. Table 7.1 shows the relative ranking of the importance of the input variables across the MALA, HMC, and NUTS methods. Figures 7.2 to 7.3 show the inference results indicating the effective sample size, the effective sample size normalized by execution time, the diagnostic trace plots of the negative log-likelihood and the predictive performance on unseen data using the Area Under the Receiver Operating Curve (AUC) metric.

Figures 7.2 to 7.3 show the inference results indicating the effective sample size, the effective sample size normalized by execution time, the diagnostic negative log-likelihood trace plots, and the predictive performance on unseen data. Figures 7.4, 7.5 and 7.6 show the features' ranking across the MALA, HMC, and NUTS MCMC algorithms.

Figure 7.2a shows that the NUTS algorithm outperforms all the other MCMC methods on an effective sample size basis, indicating the ability of NUTS not to produce correlated samples. HMC has the second-highest effective sample size, with MALA's low effective sample size suggesting that MALA produces correlated samples. However, Fig. 7.2b shows that, on a normalized (by execution time) effective sample size basis, the MALA outperforms all the methods. This is a testament that MALA has a low execution time compared to the methods driven by Hamiltonian dynamics. We found that MALA had the lowest execution time of all the methods, followed by HMC. NUTS had the largest execution time due to the extra computations required to tune the path length. Furthermore, Fig. 7.3a shows that all the MCMC methods have converged. Figure 7.3b indicates that the HMC and NUTS have similar predictive performance, with MALA producing the highest predictive performance as measured by the AUC.

The relevance or importance of each feature, as indicated by α_i from Eq. 7.2, for each MCMC method, is shown in Figs. 7.4, 7.5, and 7.6. The analysis of the results reveals that all three MCMC algorithms could clearly distinguish the important variables from the less relevant features

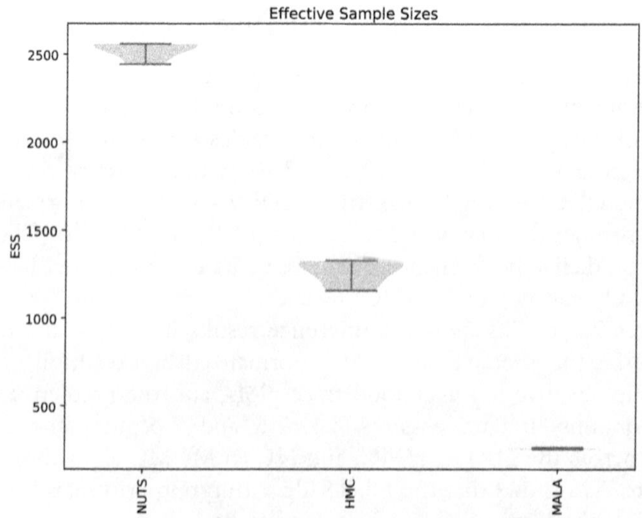

(**a**) Effective sample sizes across all the MCMC methods.

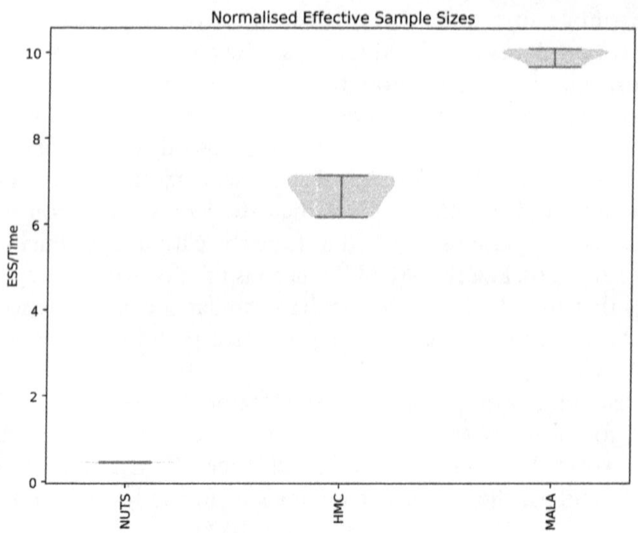

(**b**) Effective sample sizes normalized by execution time.

Fig. 7.2 Inference results for the Bayesian Framework across all the MCMC algorithms. **a** Effective sample sizes, and **b** Effective sample sizes normalized by execution time

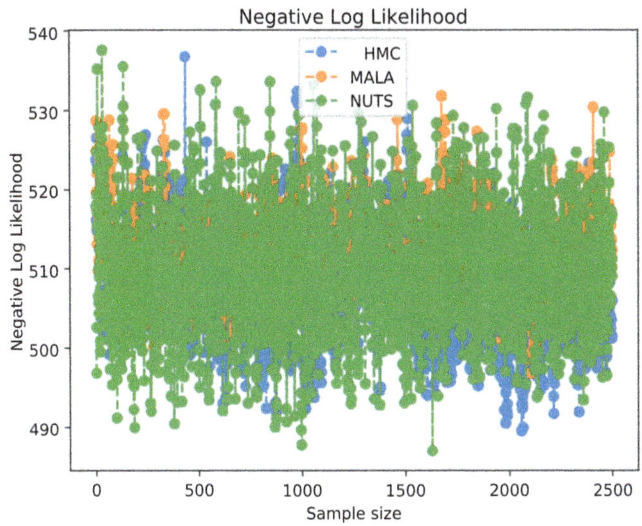

(**a**) Diagnostic negative log-likelihood trace plots.

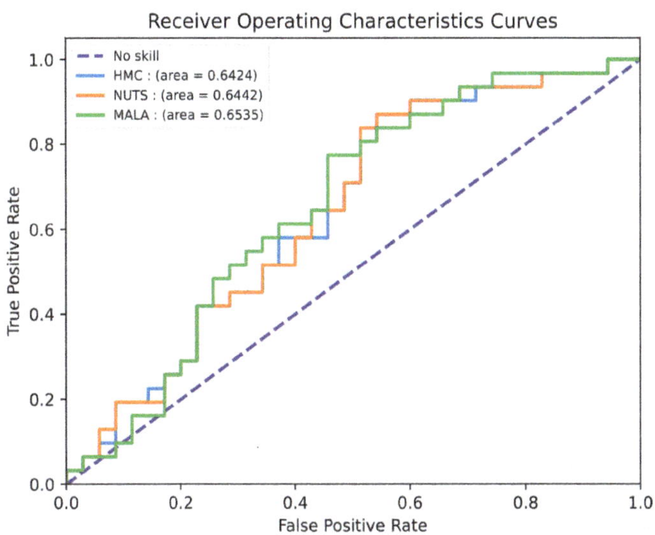

(**b**) Predictive performance based on the Area under the Receiver Operating Curve

Fig. 7.3 Inference results for the Bayesian Framework across all the MCMC algorithms. **a** Diagnostic negative log-likelihood trace plots, and **b** Predictive performance based on the Area Under the Receiver Operating Curve

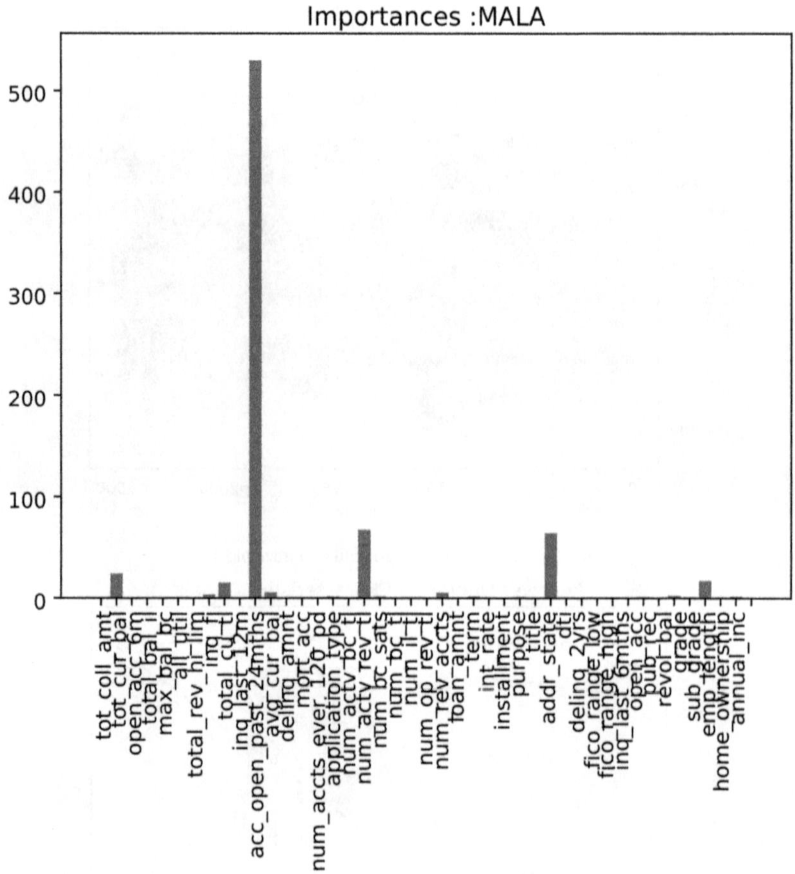

Fig. 7.4 Mean posterior variances from the MALA method. The higher the value, the more important the variable

for the recovery detection problem. This can be seen in Figs. 7.4, 7.5, and 7.6 by some features having near zero importance and some having more considerable significance for the three MCMC.

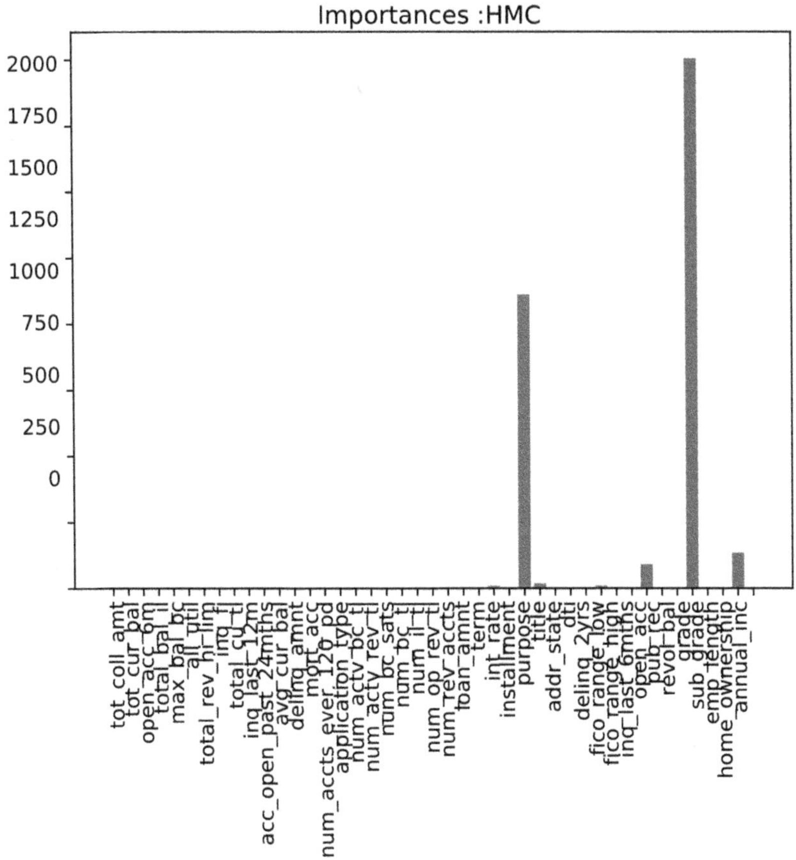

Fig. 7.5 Mean posterior variances from the HMC method. The higher the value, the more important the variable

Table 7.1 shows the top ten rankings of the importance of the features produced by each of the methods. The most commonly featured variable in the top ten rankings are *purpose*, *title*, *home-ownership*, *interest rate*, *number of bank accounts*, and *grade* related features. These results make intuitive sense since, for example, if the purpose of the loan is for debt consolidation, there might be a higher chance of default (and increasing the chances of no or low recoveries) compared to if the purpose of the loan is to improve the house. Similarly, loans with higher interest rates are

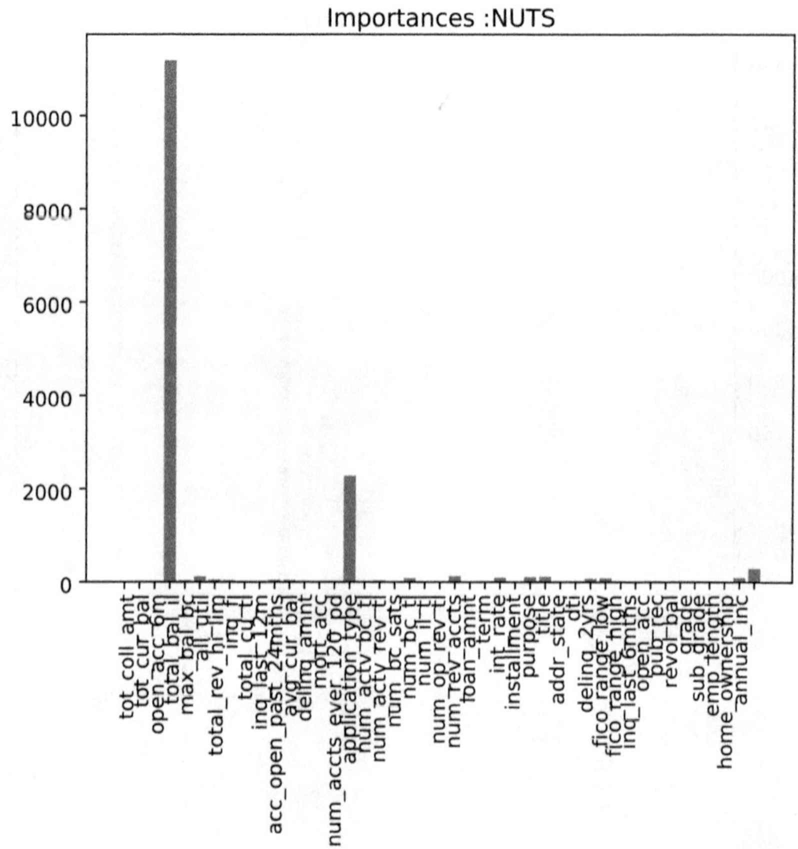

Fig. 7.6 Mean posterior variances from each the NUTS method. The higher the value, the more important the variable

riskier and more likely to default and, hence, have lower recoveries than loans with lower interest rates. Similar arguments can be made about the other variables.

Table 7.1 Ranking of the top five features by each method for the loan recovery detection dataset. For example, HMC ranks *purpose* as the second most important, while NUTS ranks *title* as the sixth most important

Ranking	*MALA*	*HMC*	*NUTS*
1	acc-open-past-24mths	grade	total-bal-il
2	num-actv-rev-tl	purpose	application-type
3	addr-state	home-ownership	annual-inc
4	tot-cur-bal	open-acc	num-rev-accts
5	sub-grade	title	all-util
6	total-cu-tl	fico-range-low	title
7	avg-cur-bal	int-rate	purpose
8	num-rev-accts	num-op-rev-tl	home-ownership
9	inq-fi	sub-grade	int-rate
10	revol-bal	num-bc-tl	num-bc-tl

7.6 Conclusion

We provide a first-in-literature application of a Bayesian inference framework to analyze recovery data from a peer-to-peer lending platform. We utilize Bayesian logistic regression with an automatic relevance determination (ARD) prior in the Bayesian framework. We train this Bayesian model using the Metropolis-Hastings Adjusted Langevin Algorithm (MALA), Hamiltonian Monte Carlo (HMC), and the No-U-Turn Sampler (NUTS) Markov Chain Monte Carlo (MCMC) methods.

The MALA algorithm has the lowest execution time, followed by the HMC, with NUTS having the longest execution time. On an effective sample size (ESS) basis, we find that NUTS produces the highest ESS, followed by HMC, with MALA producing the lowest ESS. On a time-normalized ESS basis, we find that MALA outperforms all the methods, with NUTS being the laggard. We further find that MALA produced the best predictive performance on unseen data, with NUTS and HMC producing similar performance. When analyzing the results of the sampled ARD prior variance, we find that the MCMC methods broadly agree on which variables are essential. In particular, we find that *purpose*, *how ownership*, and *interest rate* are some of the critical features in determining which charged-off account will have recoveries.

The work in this chapter can be extended by considering more complex models, such as deep neural networks. Furthermore, instead of only detecting whether recoveries are present, modeling the actual recovery on the charged-off loan using Bayesian techniques would be of interest, and this aspect is yet to be explored in detail in the literature.

In the next chapter, we employ Bayesian evidence metrics based on using normalizing flows to select and compare models that predict audit outcomes for South African municipalities.

References

Afshar, H. M., Oliveira, R., & Cripps, S. (2021). Non-volume preserving Hamiltonian Monte Carlo and No-U-Turn Samplers. In *International conference on artificial intelligence and statistics*. PMLR (pp. 1675–1683).

Andrieu, C., & Thoms, J. (2008). A tutorial on adaptive MCMC. *Statistics and Computing, 18*(4), 343–373.

Ari, A., Chen, S., & Ratnovski, L. (2021). The dynamics of non-performing loans during banking crises: A new database with post-COVID-19 implications. *Journal of Banking and Finance,133*, Article 106140.

Bellotti, T., & Crook, J. (2012). Loss given default models incorporating macroeconomic variables for credit cards. *International Journal of Forecasting, 28*(1), 171–182.

Bradley, A. P. (1997). The use of the area under the ROC curve in the evaluation of machine learning algorithms. *Pattern Recognition, 30*(7), 1145–1159. https://doi.org/10.1016/s0031-3203(96)00142-2

Calabrese, R. (2014). Predicting bank loan recovery rates with a mixed continuous-discrete model. *Applied Stochastic Models in Business and Industry, 30*(2), 99–114.

Duane, S., Kennedy, A. D., Pendleton, B. J., & Roweth, D. (1987). Hybrid monte carlo. *Physics Letters B, 195*(2), 216–222.

Gaganis, C. (July2009). Classification techniques for the identification of falsified financial statements: A comparative analysis. *Intelligent Systems in Accounting, Finance & Management, 16*(3), 207–229. https://doi.org/10.1002/isaf.303

Girolami, M., & Calderhead, B. (2011). Riemann manifold langevin and hamiltonian monte carlo methods. *Journal of the Royal Statistical Society: Series B (Statistical Methodology), 73*(2), 123–214.

Gu, M., & Sun, S. (2020). Neural Langevin dynamical sampling. *IEEE Access, 8*, 31595–31605.

Hastings, W. K. (1970). Monte Carlo sampling methods using Markov chains and their applications. *Biometrica, 57*(1), 97–109.

Hlongwane, R., Ramabao, K., & Mongwe, W. (2024). A novel framework for enhancing transparency in credit scoring: Leveraging Shapley values for interpretable credit scorecards. *Plos One,19*(8), Article e0308718.

Hoechstoetter, M., Nazemi, A., Rachev, S. T., & Bozic, C. (2012). Recovery rate modelling of non-performing consumer credit using data mining algorithms. *Review of*.

Hoffman, M. D., & Gelman, A. (2011). *The No-U-Turn sampler: Adaptively setting path lengths in Hamiltonian Monte Carlo.* arXiv:1111.4246 [stat.CO].

Hoffman, M. D., & Gelman, A. (2014). The No-U-turn sampler: Adaptively setting path lengths in Hamiltonian Monte Carlo. *Journal of Machine Learning Research, 15*(1), 1593–1623.

Loang, O. K., Ahmad, Z., & Naveenan, R. V. (2023). Non-performing loans, macroeconomic and bank-specific variables in Southeast Asia during COVID-19 pandemic. *The Singapore Economic Review, 68*(03), 941–961.

Loterman, G., Brown, I., Martens, D., Mues, C., & Baesens, B. (2012). Benchmarking regression algorithms for loss given default modeling. *International Journal of Forecasting, 28*(1), 161–170.

Marwala, T., Mbuvha, R., & Mongwe, W. T. (2023). *Hamiltonian Monte Carlo methods in machine learning*. Elsevier.

Mbuvha, R., & Marwala, T. (2020). Bayesian inference of COVID-19 spreading rates in South Africa. *PloS One,15*(8), Article e0237126.

Mbuvha, R., Boulkaibet, I., & Marwala, T. (2019a). *Automatic relevance determination Bayesian neural networks for credit card default modelling*. arXiv: 1906.06382. [stat.ML].

Mbuvha, R., Boulkaibet, I., & Marwala, T. (2019b). Bayesian automatic relevance determination for feature selection in credit default modelling. In *International conference on artificial neural networks* (pp. 420–425). Springer.

Mbuvha, R., Mongwe, W. T., & Marwala, T. (2021). Separable shadow Hamiltonian hybrid Monte Carlo for Bayesian neural network inference in wind speed forecasting. *Energy and A,I*, Article 100108.

Mongwe, W. T. (2022). *Hybrid Monte Carlo methods in machine learning: stochastic volatility methods, shadow Hamiltonians, adaptive approaches and variance reduction techniques*. University of Johannesburg (South Africa).

Mongwe, W. T., & Malan, K. M. (2020). A survey of automated financial statement fraud detection with relevance to the South African Context. *South African Computer Journal, 32*(1). https://doi.org/10.18489/sacj.v32i1.777

Mongwe, W. T., Mbuvha, R., & Marwala, T. (2021a). Adaptive magnetic Hamiltonian Monte Carlo. *IEEE Access, 9*, 152993–153003. https://doi.org/10.1109/ACCESS.2021.3127931

Mongwe, W. T., Mbuvha, R., & Marwala, T. (2021b). Adaptively setting the path length for separable shadow Hamiltonian hybrid Monte Carlo. *IEEE Access, 9*, 138598–138607.

Mongwe, W. T., Mbuvha, R., & Marwala, T. (2021c). Antithetic Riemannian manifold and quantum-inspired Hamiltonian Monte Carlo. arXiv preprint arXiv:2107.02070

Mongwe, W. T., Mbuvha, R., & Marwala, T. (2021d). Bayesian inference of local government audit outcomes. *Plos One*. https://doi.org/10.1371/journal.pone.0261245

Mongwe, W. T., Mbuvha, R., & Marwala, T. (2021e). Locally scaled and stochastic volatility metropolis-hastings algorithms. *Algorithms, 14*(12). ISSN: 1999-4893. https://doi.org/10.3390/a14120351. https://www.mdpi.com/1999-4893/14/12/351

Mongwe, W. T., Mbuvha, R., & Marwala, T. (2021f). Utilising partial momentum refreshment in separable shadow Hamiltonian hybrid Monte Carlo. *IEEE Access, 9*, 151235–151244. https://doi.org/10.1109/ACCESS.2021.3126812

Mongwe, W. T., Mbuvha, R., & Marwala, T. (2022a). Shadow magnetic Hamiltonian Monte Carlo. *IEEE Access, 10*, 34340–34351. https://doi.org/10.1109/ACCESS.2022.3161443

Mongwe, W. T., Sidogi, T., Mbuvha, R., & Marwala, T. (2022b). Probabilistic inference of South African equity option prices under jump-diffusion processes. In *2022 IEEE symposium on computational intelligence for financial engineering and economics (CIFEr)* (pp. 1–8). IEEE.

Neal, R. M. (1993). Bayesian learning via stochastic dynamics. In *Advances in neural information processing systems* (Vol. 5, pp. 475–482). Morgan Kaufmann Publishers Inc. ISBN: 1-55860-274-7. http://dl.acm.org/citation.cfm?id=645753.667903

Neal, R. M. (1995). Probable networks and plausible predictions—a review of practical Bayesian methods for supervised neural networks. *Network: Computation in Neural Systems, 6*(3), 469–505.

Neal, R. M. (2012). *Bayesian learning for neural networks* (Vol. 118). Springer Science & Business Media.

Neal, R. M., et al. (2011). MCMC using Hamiltonian dynamics. *Handbook of Markov Chain Monte Carlo, 2*(11), 2.

Vats, D., Flegal, J. M., & Jones, G. L. (Apr. 2019). Multivariate output analysis for Markov chain Monte Carlo. *Biometrika, 106*(2), 321–337. ISSN: 0006-3444. eprint: https://academic.oup.com/biomet/article-pdf/106/2/321/28575440/asz002.pdf

Ye, H., & Bellotti, A. (2019). Modelling recovery rates for non-performing loans. *Risks, 7*(1), 19.

Zhang, X., & Zhao, X. (2024). Using the Bayesian sampling method to estimate corporate loss given default distribution. *Journal of Empirical Finance*, 101540.

CHAPTER 8

Bayesian Audit Outcome Model Selection Using Normalizing Flows

8.1 Introduction

The annual audit opinions formulated by the Auditor General South Africa (AGSA) on South African municipalities often reveal the poor state of South African municipality financial management (Auditor-General South Africa, 2023; Mongwe et al., 2020b, 2021e). In a recent report, the AGSA found that most of the municipalities were still struggling to obtain clean audits, indicating that some questions need to be answered around the financial management of the municipalities and whether the current controls in place are adequate (Auditor-General South Africa, 2023). Understanding the drivers of the poor performance of a given municipality is essential, particularly if one can assess this using unaudited financials or before the audit has to be done (Mabelane et al., 2023; Mongwe et al., 2020a, 2021e). This will allow the AGSA or any auditor to allocate resources to entities optimally, especially for entities where there are likely to be red flags and more time would be required to scrutinize

Supplementary Information The online version contains supplementary material available at https://doi.org/10.1007/978-3-031-88431-3_8.

W. T. Mongwe et al., *Bayesian Machine Learning in Quantitative Finance*, https://doi.org/10.1007/978-3-031-88431-3_8

the financials (Mabelane et al., 2023; Mongwe et al., 2020a, 2021e). Artificial intelligence tools can assist auditors and other stakeholders in this regard.

The developments in artificial intelligence, particularly machine learning, have resulted in the possibility of performing a reliable risk-rating exercise before the audit can begin (Mabelane et al., 2023; Mongwe et al., 2020a). Machine learning has been utilized to successfully predict the audit opinions of municipalities and highlight which variables are essential. Marwala et al. (2023), Mongwe (2022), Mongwe et al. (2021e) utilize a Bayesian framework to model outcomes in South African municipalities. This framework utilized Markov Chain Monte Carlo techniques to train a Bayesian logistic regression model. The results showed that the framework could predict the audit outcomes while providing uncertainties in the predictions. The framework was further able to detect which variables are most relevant for predicting audit outcomes. In Mabelane et al. (2023), various traditional machine learning models, such as logistic regression, random forests, and support vector machines (SVM), were used to model audit opinions successfully. The authors found that the debt to operating ratio, current ratio, and net operating surplus margin financial ratios are the three most commonly important financial ratios across the various feature selection techniques employed (Mabelane et al., 2023).

Various studies, including those in Greece, China, the USA, and South Africa, have been conducted worldwide on utilizing machine learning to model audit outcomes in the listed entity space. Spathis et al. (2022) utilize discriminant analysis and logit analysis, with correlation and t-tests as feature selection methods, to model fraud (where fraud is defined as obtaining a qualified or worse audit opinion) for listed companies in Greece. Kotsiantis et al. (2006) also used financial ratios as features for listed companies in Greece to detect qualified audit opinions. The authors utilize Bayesian networks, decision trees, SVM, artificial neural networks (ANN), logistic regression , and k-nearest neighbors (kNN) and found that a stacking ensemble outperforms all the other methods. On the other hand, Gaganis et al. (2007) used kNN, discriminant analysis, and logit models to model audit outcomes for UK-listed companies. The authors found that kNN outperforms, and the credit rating variable is significant.

Deng and Mei (2009) utilize an unsupervised learning approach where they combine a self-organizing map with k-means clustering to analyze audit opinions for listed entities in China. The authors found this approach helpful in distinguishing financial statements with clean audit opinions from the rest. Deng (2010) later compared Naïve Bayes, SVM, and ANN methods for modeling audit outcomes in China-listed entities and found that the Naïve Bayes classifier outperforms. Moepya et al. (2014) analyzed the audit opinions of South African listed entities and found that the linear SVM classifier outperforms kNN and logistic regression. These papers show that machine learning has provided good results for the audit opinion modeling task but raises the question of how one can reliably select between various models. This chapter aims to address this model selection task using a probabilistic framework.

The Bayesian inference framework provides a mechanism for calibrating the model's parameters and estimating the marginal likelihood (or evidence)—which can be used to compare between models (Marwala et al., 2023). Parameter estimation is typically conducted through Markov Chain Monte Carlo (MCMC) algorithms, which are theoretically guaranteed to converge to the true posterior, or variational techniques (which approximate the true posterior). The MCMC approaches and variational inference do not require explicitly computing the normalizing constant (or the marginal likelihood) (Marwala et al., 2023). However, this normalizing constant is necessary for the model comparison task as this is the subject of interest.

Numerous techniques have been explored in the literature for calculating the normalizing constant, also known as the evidence. These techniques include variations of nested sampling such as static, diffusive, and dynamic nested sampling and importance sampling-based algorithms such as the harmonic mean evidence estimation method (McEwen et al., 2021; Polanska et al., 2023; Skilling, 2006). The nested sampling algorithm of Skilling (2004) and its variations are by far the most commonly used technique, with the harmonic mean approach less utilized due to the exploding variance issue typically encountered with this method. The nested sampling methods are typically computationally inefficient and can thus only be used in low-dimensional problems. This chapter focuses on the Bayesian evidence technique based on the advancements made to improve the harmonic mean estimator.

Newton and Raftery (1994) proposed the harmonic mean estimator of the Bayesian evidence, which offers considerably more flexibility as it simply takes samples from the posterior, which can be obtained using any MCMC approach, for example. Newton and Raftery (1994), however, quickly discovered that this approach might fail catastrophically since the estimator's variance can become significant. McEwen et al. (2021) recently proposed the learnt harmonic mean estimator as a solution to this problem, wherein machine learning techniques were developed to learn an appropriate internal importance sampling target distribution. Unlike nested sampling, the estimator takes samples from the posterior and is therefore independent of the method used to produce samples, making it simple to apply with any MCMC sampling strategy, including stored MCMC chains or any variational inference approach (Polanska et al., 2023). The learned harmonic mean estimator based on normalizing flows is the focus of the contributions in this chapter.

The remainder of this chapter is structured as follows: we first present the Bayesian logistic regression models in Sect. 8.2, which we will compare using the Bayesian evidence metric discussed in Sect. 8.3. We then discuss the learnt harmonic mean Bayesian evidence estimator based on normalizing flows and briefly discuss the MCMC methods we use to generate the samples in Sect. 8.4. We proceed to present the numerical experiments we conduct in this chapter in Sect. 8.5, followed by the results and the discussions of the results and the conclusion in Sects. 8.6 and 8.7 respectively.

8.2 Models

This section presents the Bayesian models we analyze in this chapter. The audit opinion models we consider in this chapter are variations of the Bayesian logistic regression model with different covariates or financial ratios used.

8.2.1 Bayesian Logistic Regression Models

The negative log-likelihood $l(\mathrm{D}|\mathbf{w})$ function for the Bayesian logistic regression model is given by (Marwala et al., 2023; Mongwe, 2022; Mongwe et al., 2021e, 2021f, 2021g)

$$l(\mathrm{D}|\mathbf{w}) = \sum_{i}^{N} y_i \log(\mathbf{w}^T x_i) + (1 - y_i)\log(1 - \mathbf{w}^T x_i) \tag{8.1}$$

where D ={x, y} is the data with x being the covariates and y being the target, N is the number of observations and $\mathbf{w}$ are the parameters that need to be estimated. Thus, the target un-normalized posterior log distribution is given as (Mongwe et al., 2021e):

$$\ln p(\mathbf{w}|\mathrm{D}) = l(\mathrm{D}|\mathbf{w}) + \ln p(\mathbf{w}|\alpha) \tag{8.2}$$

where $\ln p(\mathbf{w}|\alpha)$ is the log of the prior distribution placed on the parameters $\mathbf{w}$ given the hyperparameters α. Following the methodology used in Mongwe et al. (2021e), we model the parameters $\mathbf{w}$ as having a Gaussian prior, with each parameter having a zero mean and a standard deviation of $\alpha = 10$.

Using the same dataset described in Mongwe et al. (2021e), we consider various combinations of the covariates (financial ratios) to arrive at the following models:

1. **Model 1:** covariates = {'Debt to Community Wealth/Equity', 'Capital Expenditure % Total Expenditure', 'Debt to Total Operating Revenue', 'Current Ratio', 'Net Operating Surplus Margin %'}
2. **Model 2:** covariates = {Capital Expenditure % Total Expenditure', 'Debt to Total Operating Revenue', 'Current Ratio', 'Net Operating Surplus Margin %'}
3. **Model 3:** covariates = {'Debt to Total Operating Revenue', 'Current Ratio', 'Net Operating Surplus Margin %'}
4. **Model 4:** covariates = {'Debt to Total Operating Revenue', 'Current Ratio'}
5. **Model 5:** covariates = {'Debt to Total Operating Revenue'}

As seen above, Model 1 has the highest number of parameters with five parameters (excluding the intercept term), and each subsequent model has one fewer parameter. In contrast, Model 5 only has one parameter. This means that the models are subsets of each other. The move from Model 5 to Model 4 assesses the impact of adding the "Current Ratio" covariate. In contrast, Model 3 assesses the effect of adding the "Net Operating Surplus Margin %" variable, and Model 2 tests the impact of the "Capital Expenditure % Total Expenditure" covariate. In contrast, Model 1 assesses the effect of adding the "Debt to Community Wealth/ Equity" variable.

In the next section, we present the Bayesian evidence metric that we will utilize to compare the five models we highlighted above.

8.3 Bayesian Evidence Metric

Estimating the posterior distribution $P(\theta|D, M)$ of a collection of parameters θ for a given model M and data D is one of the core interests in Bayesian inference . Bayes theorem can be used to express this inference problem:

$$P(\theta|D, M) = \frac{P(D|\theta, M)P(\theta|M)}{P(D|M)} \tag{8.3}$$

where $P(D|\theta, M)$ is the likelihood of the data, $P(\theta|M)$ is the prior for the parameters, and

$$P(D|M) = \int_{\Omega_\theta} P(D|\theta, M)P(\theta|M)d\theta \tag{8.4}$$

is the evidence or marginal likelihood for the data supplied M, where θ may have a large dimension. The integral is taken across the whole domain Ω_θ of θ. It is important to note that the prior distribution in this evidence metric inherently penalizes overly complicated models. Even though the likelihood of the two models is the same, their levels of complexity might differ greatly. The evidence metric naturally embodies Occam's Razor, which penalizes overly complicated models in favor of simpler ones (Bishop, 1997; MacKay, 1992; Rasmussen & Ghahramani, 2001).

For ease of reference, the shorthand notation below will be used in the rest of this chapter (Speagle, 2020):

$$P(\theta_M) = \frac{L(\theta_M)\pi(\theta_M)}{Z_M} \tag{8.5}$$

where $P(\theta_M) := P(\theta|D, M)$ is the posterior, $L(\theta_M) := P(D|\theta, M)$ is the likelihood, $\pi(\theta_M) := P(\theta|M)$ is the prior, $Z_M := P(D|M)$ is the evidence. From the posterior $P(\theta_M)$ one gets the parameter estimates for a given model M, while Z_M allows one to compare models using the Bayes factor (Kass & Raftery, 1995):

$$B_{ij} := \frac{Z_{M_i}}{Z_{M_j}} \frac{\pi(M_i)}{\pi(M_j)} \tag{8.6}$$

where $\pi(M_i)$ is the prior belief for model i. Values of the Bayes factor greater than one are considered as evidence in favor of model M_1

Table 8.1 The values of both the linear and the logarithmic Jeffreys' scale with a description of the strength of the evidence

B_{ij}	$\ln B_{ij}$	*Evidence*
$1 \leq B_{ij} < 3$	$0 \leq B_{ij} < 1.1$	Weak
$3 \leq B_{ij} < 20$	$1.1 \leq B_{ij} < 3$	Definite
$20 \leq B_{ij} < 150$	$3 \leq B_{ij} < 5$	Strong
$150 \leq B_{ij}$	$5 \leq B_{ij}$	Very strong

and vice versa (Kass & Raftery, 1995). Suppose one has no prior belief that one model is better than another, which is usually the case in practice. In that case, the prior probabilities of all the models are equal, so comparing models amounts to comparing the model evidences (Kass & Raftery, 1995; Nesseris & Garcia-Bellido, 2013). As outlined in Nesseris and Garcia-Bellido (2013), the interpretation of Bayes factors for the linear and logarithmic Jeffreys' scale are shown in Table 8.1.

The posterior $P(\theta_M)$ is usually analytically intractable for complicated models. The posterior distribution must then be estimated using numerical methods (Higson et al., 2019; MacKay, 1992; Speagle, 2020). The main focus of this chapter is not on assessing the posterior of the parameters but rather on calculating the evidence of a given model. The evidence will be the metric used to compare between different models. We then utilize the estimated posterior $P(\theta_M)$ to estimate the model's predictive performance on unseen data. The following section outlines the method used to calculate the evidence metric.

8.4 Harmonic Mean Bayesian Evidence Estimator

Due to the parameters for most models of interest being frequently high dimensional, computing the Bayesian evidence can be difficult (Polanska et al., 2023; Skilling, 2006; Speagle, 2020). Therefore, computing the evidence requires assessing a multidimensional integral over a function that may be quite variable. The typical Markov Chain Monte Carlo integration of the posterior might theoretically be used to accomplish this; however, even in very low dimensions, this method is unreliable (Polanska et al., 2023).

Numerous alternative approaches for computing the Bayesian evidence have been suggested, including nested sampling variations such as static, diffusive, and dynamic nested sampling (Polanska et al., 2023).

The nested sampling method of Skilling (2006) is the most widely used technique for calculating the evidence. However, the method used to generate samples is severely limited in its flexibility by nested sampling. Custom nested sampling methods must be created for each task at hand and are usually limited to settings with low dimensions (Higson et al., 2019; Polanska et al., 2023; Speagle, 2020).

Recently, a useful method for calculating the marginal likelihood was proposed: the learnt harmonic mean estimator (Polanska et al., 2023). Unlike nested sampling, the estimator needs samples from the posterior, hence independent of the sample generation technique. As a result, combining the acquired harmonic mean with other variational inference or Markov Chain Monte Carlo sampling strategies is simple (Polanska et al., 2023). Because of this feature, the estimator may also be modified to handle the selection of Bayesian models for simulation-based inference when an explicit likelihood is unavailable or cannot be implemented (Polanska et al., 2023). This section briefly reviews the learned harmonic mean estimator we utilize to estimate the Bayesian evidence metric in this chapter.

Newton and Raftery (1994) were the first to propose the harmonic mean estimator. He demonstrated that, given posterior samples, the marginal likelihood Z_M (for a given model M) could be estimated from the harmonic mean of the likelihood. The estimator of the reciprocal of the marginal likelihood is obtained by considering the expectation of the reciprocal of the likelihood with respect to the posterior distribution $\rho_M = \frac{1}{Z_M}$ that is as follows:

$$\hat{\rho_M} = \frac{1}{N} \sum_{i=0}^{N} \frac{1}{L(\theta_M^i)} \tag{8.7}$$

where N specifies the number of samples θ_M^i drawn from the posterior $P(\theta_M)$. Then, estimating the marginal likelihood from its reciprocal is simple (Polanska et al., 2023). It was quickly discovered that the original harmonic mean estimator was susceptible to an explosive variance, which may lead to a catastrophic failure (Newton & Raftery, 1994).

Another way to think about the estimator is as importance sampling, where the sampling density is the posterior and the importance sampling target distribution is the prior. The sample density must have more probability mass in the distribution's tails than the target distribution for importance sampling to be effective (Polanska et al., 2023). Since the posterior modifies our original knowledge of the underlying parameters contained in the prior in the presence of new data, the prior often has broader tails than the posterior (Polanska et al., 2023). Importance sampling is ineffective for the harmonic mean estimator because the importance sampling density (the posterior) usually does not have broader tails than the target (the prior) (Polanska et al., 2023).

McEwen et al. (2021) present the learned harmonic mean estimator, which employs machine learning techniques to determine the target density. McEwen et al. (2021) show that the posterior distribution is the optimal target. The normalized posterior is not directly accessible due to the normalizing constant; the term of interest in McEwen et al. (2021), Polanska et al. (2023) is the exact reason for its inaccessibility. Using a normalized trained model, the learned harmonic mean estimator estimates the posterior's ideal objective. While the approximation need not be exact, the learned distribution's probability mass must fall within the posterior to avoid enormous variance. The study by McEwen et al. (2021) proposes a specialized optimization problem to train models, ensuring this property is met (McEwen et al., 2021; Polanska et al., 2023).

8.4.1 Normalizing Flows

This section explores how one may learn the target distribution of the learnt harmonic mean estimator using normalizing flows. Since normalizing flows offer a sophisticated means of guaranteeing that the probability mass of the learned distribution is contained within the posterior, they eliminate the need for the bespoke approach to training and produce a more flexible and robust learnt harmonic mean estimator that was introduced in McEwen et al. (2021), Polanska et al. (2023). Moreover, the possibility of scaling to higher dimensional settings is provided by normalizing flows (Polanska et al., 2023).

Normalizing flows represent a class of generative probabilistic models that facilitate the assessment of a sample's density from an acquired probability distribution. They consist of a series of transformations applied to an initial distribution. A vector θ of an unknown distribution $p(\theta)$ can be expressed through a transformation T of a vector z sampled from a base distribution $q(z)$; $\theta = T(z)$ where $z \sim q(z)$. The base distribution is often selected to allow for easy sampling and evaluation of its density. For the base distribution, a Gaussian is frequently utilized. The change of variables formula may then be used to obtain the unknown distribution (Polanska et al., 2023):

$$p(\theta) = q(z)|\det(J_T(z))|^{-1} \tag{8.8}$$

where $J_T(z)$ is the Jacobian corresponding to transformation T. The whole transformation in a flow-based model is invertible and differentiable because T comprises a sequence of transformations, each of which is invertible and differentiable (Polanska et al., 2023). This enables us to combine several straightforward transformations with previously learned parameters into a process known as a flow, from which we may sample and assess a normalized approximation of the unknown distribution (Polanska et al., 2023). The design of the transformations is done with great care so that it is easy to compute the determinant of the Jacobian (Polanska et al., 2023).

Introduced in Dinh et al. (2016), the real-valued non-volume preserving (real NVP) flow is an elementary example of a normalizing flow. It is composed of affine coupling layers-given bijective transformations. Consider the D dimensional input z, split into elements up to and following d, respectively, $z_{1:d}$ and $z_{d+1:D}$, for $d < D$. Given input z, the output y of an affine couple layer is calculated by:

$$y_{1:d} = z_{1:d} \tag{8.9}$$

$$y_{d+1:D} = z_{d+1:D} \odot \exp(s(z_{1:d})) + t(z_{1:d}) \tag{8.10}$$

where $\odot$ denotes elementwise Hadamard multiplication. The scale s and translation t are usually expressed by artificial neural networks with learnable parameters that take as input $z_{1:d}$. This chapter utilizes this real NVP flow formulation, which utilizes neural networks.

8.4.2 *Markov Chain Monte Carlo Algorithms*

We now present the MCMC methods used to train the Bayesian logistic regression model and whose samples will be passed to the learnt harmonic mean estimator for the Bayesian evidence calculation.

8.4.2.1 Metropolis-Hastings and the Metropolis-Adjusted Langevin Algorithm

One of the classical MCMC methods is the random walk Metropolis-Hastings (MH) technique, which uses a Gaussian distribution centered at the current state as the proposal distribution (Hastings, 1970; Mbuvha et al., 2021; Mongwe et al., 2021f). This results in samples that are strongly autocorrelated, which causes slow convergence. Large sample sizes must be created to do this. Methods that apply additional information about the target posterior distributions and lessen the random walk behavior enhance the traditional MH method (Girolami & Calderhead, 2011; Marwala et al., 2023). The standard extension considers the posterior's local curvature using the second-order gradient information and the first-order gradient information to direct the target's sampling (Girolami & Calderhead, 2011; Marwala et al., 2023). The Langevin and the Hamiltonian dynamics on the Euclidean manifold are two approaches that use the first-order gradient information (Marwala et al., 2023). On the other hand, techniques on the Riemannian and other manifolds employ the second-order gradient information (Girolami and Calderhead, 2011). In practice, methods utilizing Hamiltonian dynamics in Euclidean spaces have shown great promise and are also relatively more straightforward to implement than those on other manifolds (Marwala et al., 2023; Mongwe et al., 2021c).

The Metropolis-Adjusted Langevin Algorithm (MALA) enhances the Metropolis-Hastings (MH) method through the use of first-order gradient information of the target posterior. MALA reduces the random walk behavior of MH via the use of Langevin dynamics where the drift component is the derivative of the log of the target posterior, and the diffusive component is Brownian motion which is represented as follows (Gu & Sun, 2020; Marwala et al., 2023; Mongwe et al., 2022b, 2021f):

$$d\mathbf{w}_t = \frac{1}{2} f'(\mathbf{w})dt + dZ_t \tag{8.11}$$

where $\mathbf{w}$ are the parameters, $f'(\mathbf{w})$ is the first derivative of the target $f(\mathbf{w})$ with respect to the parameters, and Z_t is a Brownian motion process at a fictitious time t. The Langevin dynamics in Eq. 8.11 typically cannot be solved analytically, and numerical methods such as the Euler-Maruyama integration scheme are typically used (Marwala et al., 2023). This, however, introduces errors that can break the detailed balance condition, which would not guarantee that the method would converge to the correct target distribution (Marwala et al., 2023). To rectify this, a Metropolis acceptance step is incorporated into the algorithm to ensure detailed balance (Marwala et al., 2023). The MALA algorithm converges to the stationary distribution at a faster pace than the MH algorithm because it takes into account the density's first-order gradient data, which is represented by $f'(\mathbf{w})$ (Girolami & Calderhead, 2011; Gu & Sun, 2020; Marwala et al., 2023). The samples produced using the MALA method are still highly correlated. Girolami and Calderhead (2011) incorporate second-order gradient information of the target by extending MALA from being on a Euclidean manifold to a Riemannian manifold (Marwala et al., 2023). Despite a corresponding increase in compute time, this approach demonstrated significant gains in the sampling performance of the MALA method (Marwala et al., 2023).

The sampler converges to the target distribution more quickly with the MALA algorithm than with the MH algorithm because it utilizes the gradient information of the target distribution (Girolami & Calderhead, 2011; Gu & Sun, 2020). The produced samples are still very correlated. The next section discusses the Hamiltonian Monte Carlo and Magnetic Hamiltonian Monte Carlo approaches, which employ Hamiltonian dynamics to traverse the target distribution better.

8.4.2.2 Hamiltonian Monte Carlo and the No-U-Turn Sampler

Hamiltonian Monte Carlo (HMC) is a popular MCMC method for performing Bayesian inference and has been utilized in various disciplines such as finance, health, and energy (Duane et al., 1987; Mbuvha & Marwala, 2020; Mbuvha et al., 2021; Mongwe et al., 2021a, 2021b, 2021e, 2022b). The method is premised on using Hamiltonian dynamics, which naturally considers the first-order gradient information of the target posterior. The dynamics that underpin HMC are as follows (Marwala et al., 2023, Neal, 1993):

$$\frac{d\mathbf{w}}{\partial t} = \frac{\partial \mathrm{H}(\mathbf{w}, \mathbf{p})}{\partial \mathbf{p}}; \quad \frac{d\mathbf{p}}{\partial t} = -\frac{\partial \mathrm{H}(\mathbf{w}, \mathbf{p})}{\partial \mathbf{w}} \tag{8.12}$$

where $\mathbf{w}$ are the parameters, $\mathbf{p}$ is the auxiliary momentum variable with the same dimensionality as $\mathbf{w}$, and $\mathrm{H}(\mathbf{w}, \mathbf{p})$ is the Hamiltonian—which represents the total energy (i.e. potential energy defined by the target posterior and kinetic energy which is typically captured through a multivariate Gaussian distribution) from this system (Mongwe et al., 2022a; Mongwe et al., 2021b). This HMC method allows distant proposals, which results in a significant reduction in the autocorrelations of the generated samples (Marwala et al., 2023).

The HMC technique is composed of two steps. The first step integrates Hamiltonian dynamics in Eq. 8.12 typically using the leapfrog integrator (Duane et al., 1987; Marwala et al., 2023; Neal, 1993), and the second step utilizes a Metropolis-Hastings correction to account for the numerical integration errors arising from the first step (Duane et al., 1987; Hastings, 1970; Neal et al., 2011). The parameter and momentum update equations for the leapfrog integration scheme (corresponding to the first step of HMC) are given as follows:

$$\begin{aligned}
\mathbf{p}_{t+\frac{\epsilon}{2}} &= \mathbf{p}_t + \frac{\epsilon}{2}\frac{\partial H(\mathbf{w}_t, \mathbf{p}_t)}{\partial \mathbf{w}} \\
\mathbf{w}_{t+\epsilon} &= \mathbf{w}_t + \epsilon \mathbf{M}^{-1}\mathbf{p}_{t+\frac{\epsilon}{2}} \\
\mathbf{p}_{t+\epsilon} &= \mathbf{p}_{t+\frac{\epsilon}{2}} + \frac{\epsilon}{2}\frac{\partial H\left(\mathbf{w}_{t+\epsilon}, \mathbf{p}_{t+\frac{\epsilon}{2}}\right)}{\partial \mathbf{w}}
\end{aligned} \tag{8.13}$$

where ϵ is the discretization step size and $\mathbf{M}$ is a covariance matrix emanating from the kinetic energy component in $\mathrm{H}(\mathbf{w}, \mathbf{p})$. If the integration of the Hamiltonian dynamics in the first step were solved precisely, the second step would not be required. However, due to the discretization errors, a Metropolis-Hastings acceptance step is typically required where the $\mathbf{w}^*$ proposed by the first step are accepted with probability:

$$\mathrm{P}(\text{accept } \mathbf{w}^*) = \min\left(1, \frac{\exp(-\mathrm{H}(\mathbf{w}^*, \mathbf{p}^*))}{\exp(-\mathrm{H}(\mathbf{w}, \mathbf{p}))}\right). \tag{8.14}$$

The parameters of HMC are the discretization step size ϵ, which is required for the first step in HMC, and the trajectory length, which determines the number of times the integration is performed. The step size parameter is typically set to obtain a user-specified target acceptance rate using the dual averaging method (Hoffman & Gelman, 2014; Marwala et al., 2023) while tuning the trajectory length parameter is a more complex problem (Hoffman & Gelman, 2014). It can further be shown that when the trajectory length parameter is set to 1, the HMC method becomes the MALA method. The overall HMC sampling process follows a Gibbs sampling scheme, where we sample **p** auxiliary momentum variable and then sample a new set of parameters **w** given the drawn momentum **p**. This procedure is repeated until the required number of samples are generated (Marwala et al., 2023; Mongwe et al., 2021a, 2021b). The pseudo-code for HMC can be found in Algorithm 3.1 in Chapter 3 of this book.

The step size and trajectory length are numerous parameters that necessitate tuning to achieve efficient sampling in the HMC algorithm. A trajectory length that is too short leads to a random walk behavior similar to the Metropolis-Hasting method (Hoffman & Gelman, 2014; Marwala et al., 2023; Mbuvha & Marwala, 2020; Mongwe et al., 2021a, 2021b). A trajectory length that is too long results in a trajectory that inefficiently traces back (Hoffman & Gelman, 2014; Marwala et al., 2023; Mbuvha & Marwala, 2020; Mongwe, 2022). The step size is also a critical parameter for sampling. Small step sizes are computationally inefficient, leading to correlated samples and poor mixing, while large step sizes compound discretization errors, leading to low acceptance rates (Hoffman & Gelman, 2014; Mbuvha & Marwala, 2020). Tuning these parameters requires multiple time-consuming pilot runs (Hoffman & Gelman, 2014; Marwala et al., 2023; Mbuvha & Marwala, 2020; Mongwe et al., 2021a, 2021b). The leapfrog step size and trajectory length are automatically adjusted by the No-U-Turn Sampler (NUTS) (Hoffman & Gelman, 2014; Marwala et al., 2023). In NUTS, the step size is tuned through primal-dual averaging during an initial burn-in phase by targeting a particular sample acceptance rate (Hoffman & Gelman, 2014; Marwala et al., 2023; Mbuvha & Marwala, 2020). The trajectory length is adjusted by iteratively adding steps until the chain begins to trace back (U-turn) or the Hamiltonian reaches infinity (Hoffman & Gelman, 2014; Mbuvha & Marwala, 2020).

Primal-dual averaging is used in NUTS to adjust the step size parameter during the burn-in phase (Marwala et al., 2023). Primal-dual averaging is used to achieve a user-specified Metropolis-Hastings acceptance rate δ which is expressed as (Andrieu & Thoms, 2008; Marwala et al., 2023; Mbuvha et al., 2019; Mongwe, 2022):

$$\begin{aligned} \epsilon_{t+1} &\leftarrow \mu - \frac{\sqrt{t}}{\gamma} \frac{1}{t + t_0} \sum_{i=1}^{t} H_i \\ \bar{\epsilon}_{t+1} &\leftarrow \eta_t \epsilon_{t+1} + (1 - \eta_t) \bar{\epsilon}_t \end{aligned} \tag{8.15}$$

where η_t is a decaying rate of adaptation in accordance with Andrieu and Thoms (2008), γ regulates the convergence toward μ, H_t is the difference between the target acceptance rate and the actual acceptance rate (Hoffman & Gelman, 2014; Mbuvha et al., 2021), and μ is a free parameter that ϵ_t gravitates to Marwala et al. (2023). The updates from primal-dual averaging are such that (Mbuvha et al., 2021; Marwala et al., 2023):

$$\mathbb{E}[H_t] = \mathbb{E}[\delta - \alpha_t] = 0. \tag{8.16}$$

As a result, the step size is updated toward the desired acceptance rate δ. Setting $\mu = \log(10\epsilon_0)$, $\bar{\epsilon}_0 = 1$, $\bar{H}_0 = 0$, $\gamma = 0.05$, $t_0 = 10$, $\kappa = 0.75$, and $\epsilon_0 = 0.0001$ as the initial step size yields acceptable performance across a variety of target posterior distributions (Hoffman & Gelman, 2014; Marwala et al., 2023; Mongwe, 2022). As outlined above, the settings used in this chapter are the same as those in Marwala et al. (2023).

Iteratively increasing the trajectory length until the Hamiltonian becomes infinite or the chain begins to trace back is how NUTS automatically adjusts the trajectory length parameter (Afshar et al., 2021; Mbuvha & Marwala, 2020). At that point, the final suggested position state $\mathbf{w}^*$ begins to resemble the starting position $\mathbf{w}$, and this is also when $(\mathbf{w}^* - \mathbf{w}) \times \mathbf{p} \leq 0$. This approach breaks down the detailed balancing criterion and is rectified through the use of a slice sampling technique (Hoffman & Gelman, 2011; Marwala et al., 2023).

NUTS operates at least as efficiently as and occasionally more efficiently than a well-tuned standard HMC method without necessitating user intervention or a costly tuning run (Hoffman & Gelman, 2014). This makes the NUTS method more accessible to non-expert audiences. A detailed exposition of the NUTS, HMC, MALA, and MH algorithms can be found in Marwala et al. (2023).

8.5 Numerical Experiments

In this section, we present the numerical experiments conducted. We first describe the dataset and then outline the experiments, settings, and performance metrics used.

8.5.1 Data Description

We perform model selection on a South African municipal finance dataset. We employ the same data that Mongwe et al. (2020b) used to examine how well financial ratios identify financial statement fraud. The dataset (Mongwe et al., 2020b, 2021e) was obtained from the South African National Treasury website, https://municipaldata.treasury.gov.za/. From 2012 to 2018, a sample of 1560 observations was collected from South African municipalities' audited financial statements and audit findings. The descriptive statistics for the dataset is shown in Table 8.2, with the description of the variables presented in Mongwe et al. (2020b). Our analysis uses a train-test split of 70-30 based on time. Figure 8.1 shows the distribution of the audit opinions categories for this dataset. In our modeling, we convert the target variable into a binary target that only consists of the *unqualified* and the *not unqualified* classes. This leads to a 55% allocation to the unqualified audit opinion category, indicating that the dataset is fairly balanced.

8.5.2 Performance Metrics

The performance metrics used in this chapter are predictive performance on unseen data. The Area Under the Receiver Operating Curve (AUC) is the predictive performance metric used in this chapter. For all the MCMC algorithms, we set the pre-conditioning matrix $\mathbf{M} = \mathbf{I}$, which is the typical approach in practice (Marwala et al., 2023; Mongwe et al., 2021b; Mongwe, 2022).

We generated ten chains with 6000 samples for all the datasets with a burn-in period of 1000 samples. This was adequate for all the methods converging across all the models. The number of steps required to create each sample was 25 for HMC. The step sizes were chosen by targeting an acceptance rate of 60% for MALA and 80% for HMC and NUTS

Table 8.2 Descriptive statistics across all the variables for the audit opinion dataset

Variable	*Mean*	*Std*	*Minimum*	*Median*	*Maximum*
Debt to community wealth/equity	36.850597	254.099229	–2046.452017	19.426493	6640.183971
Capital expenditure % total expenditure	19.112776	11.113937	–3.814135	17.856319	77.659687
Impairment of PPE, IP, and IA %	6.381171	9.502630	–15.346032	4.940701	159.269195
Repairs and maintenance % PPE +IP	1.763209	6.472785	–1.862655	0.834512	170.67029
Debt to total operating revenue	0.507699	0.331572	–0.092095	0.433360	2.642195
Current ratio	1.762651	2.008214	–0.880299	1.163037	23.061255
Capital cost % total operating expenditure	1.600531	1.905377	–0.311002	0.980238	13.968485
Net operating surplus margin %	3.183214	20.758087	–147.327938	4.705661	81.071917
Remuneration % total operating expenditure	35.943978	17.365554	–67.607058	32.508621	159.977247
Contracted services % total operating expen	3.514189	5.969999	–11.319593	0.977132	51.831705
Own source revenue to total operating rev	97.215221	7.536901	7.870721	99.851701	103.543054
Net surplus/deficit water %	–2.257200e+08	3.290739e+09	–1.141189e+11	0.000000e+00	1.435856e+09
Net surplus/deficit elec %	–6.266644e+08	1.426661e+10	–5.554223e+11	0.000000e+00	1.496614e+10

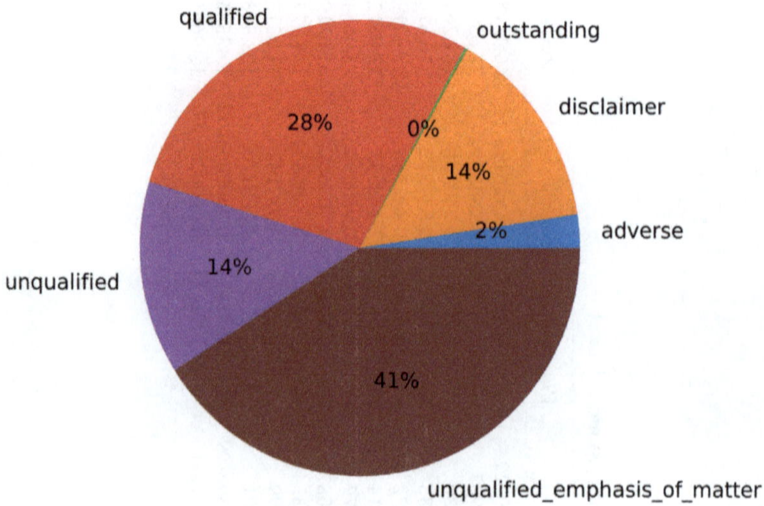

Fig. 8.1 Distribution of the audit opinions across the different categories on the South African audit opinion dataset

methods through the dual averaging (Hoffman & Gelman, 2011). These samples were then used in the learnt harmonic mean evidence calculation to produce the evidence. We train an actual NVP flow consisting of six scaled layers followed by two unscaled ones, with a temperature of 0.8.

8.6 Results and Discussion

In this section, we present the results and the discussions from the numerical experiments. Table 8.3 shows the log evidence metric as calculated on the training data using all the MCMC methods and across all the models. Table 8.4 shows the pair-wise model comparisons through computation of the Bayes factor across all the models using the log evidence from the MALA method.

Figures 8.2, 8.3 and 8.4 show the inference results in the form of effective sample sizes and effective sample sizes normalized by execution time across all inference algorithms. Figures 8.5, 8.6 and 8.7 show the predictive performance on unseen data for each model using all the MCMC methods and the convergence profile on training data across all models and MCMC methods. Figures 8.8, 8.9 and 8.10 show the corner plots of the samples posterior overlayed with the normalized flow across all the MCMC methods and models. Note that the $x_i s$ that appear in these corner plots in Figs. 8.8, 8.9 and 8.10 correspond to the covariates in the order presented in Sect. 8.2.

Table 8.3 Log evidence on training data and AUC on unseen data across the various MCMC algorithms. The entries in **bold** indicate outperformance on that metric. The lower the log evidence, the better the model. The higher the AUC, the better the model

Metric	*Model 1*	*Model 2*	*Model 3*	*Model 4*	*Model 5*
Log evidence (MALA)	-909.8554	**-908.9116**	-921.2695	-923.2310	-950.6296
Log evidence (HMC)	-910.1528	**-908.9963**	-921.3057	-923.2002	-950.6219
Log evidence (NUTS)	-910.1562	**-908.9949**	-921.3277	-923.2058	-950.6200
Test AUC (MALA)	0.7391	**0.7419**	0.7386	0.7358	0.6734
Test AUC (HMC)	**0.7402**	0.7401	0.7385	0.7358	0.6734
Test AUC (NUTS)	**0.7401**	**0.7401**	0.7383	0.7355	0.6734

Table 8.4 Pair-wise model comparisons through the natural log Bayes factor for all models using the log evidence from the MALA method. The comparison is between the columns and the rows. For example, the Bayes factor for Model 2 vs Model 4 is 14.3194. Note that we only show the pair-wise comparisons for the MALA method because all the MCMC methods produce similar log evidence results across all the models as shown in Table 8.3

	Model 1	*Model 2*	*Model 3*	*Model 4*	*Model 5*
Model 1	x				
Model 2	–0.9438	x			
Model 3	11.4141	12.3579	x		
Model 4	13.3756	14.3194	1.9615	x	
Model 5	40.7742	41.718	29.3601	27.3986	x

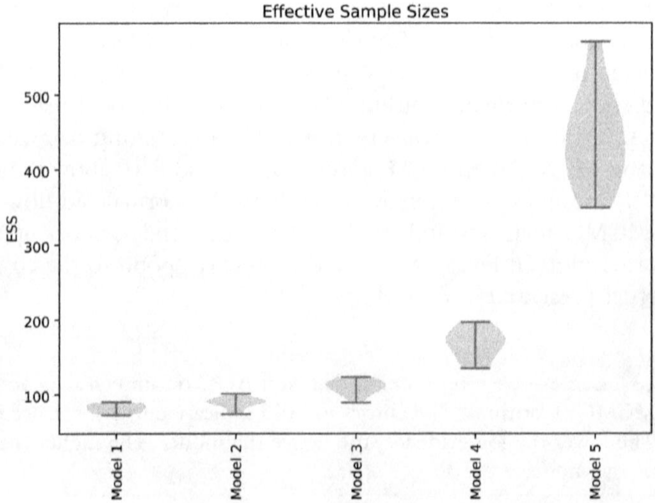

(**a**) Effective sample size from MALA algorithm across all the models.

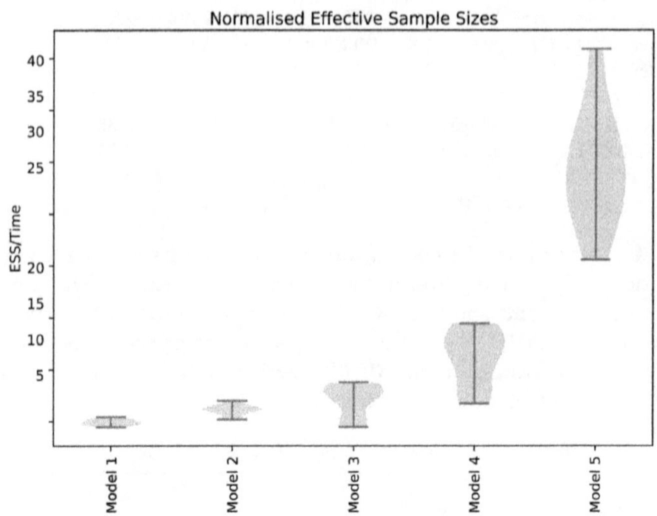

(**b**) Effective sample size normalized by execution time from MALA algorithm across all the models.

Fig. 8.2 Inference results for the Bayesian framework for the MALA algorithm. The left panels show the effective sample sizes, while the right panel shows the effective sample sizes normalized by execution time for each model

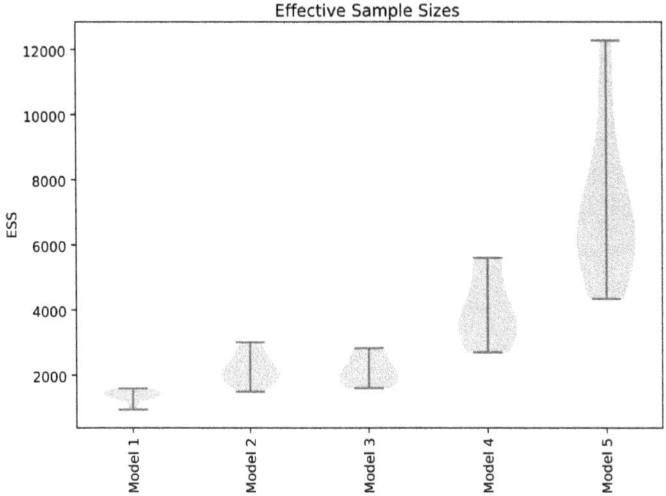

(**a**) Effective sample size from HMC algorithm across all the models.

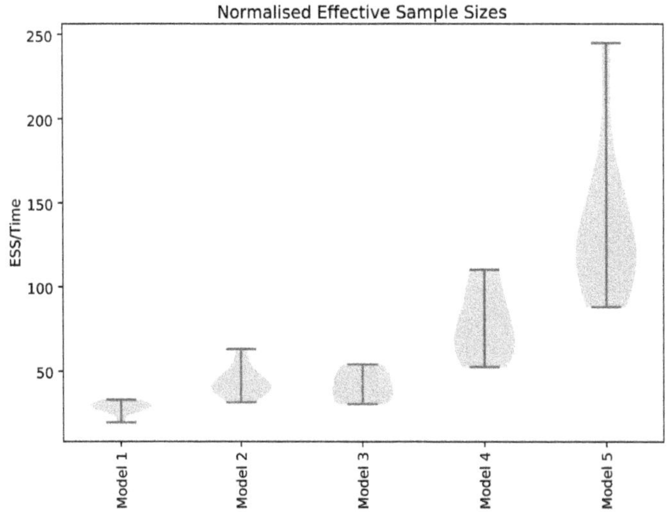

(**b**) Effective sample size normalized by execution time from HMC algorithm across all the models.

Fig. 8.3 Inference results for the Bayesian framework for the HMC algorithm. The left panels show the effective sample sizes, while the right panel shows the effective sample sizes normalized by execution time for each model

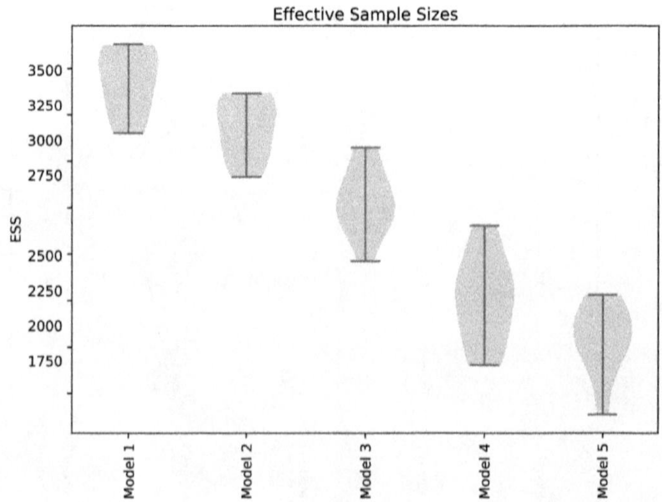

(**a**) Effective sample size from NUTS algorithm across all the models.

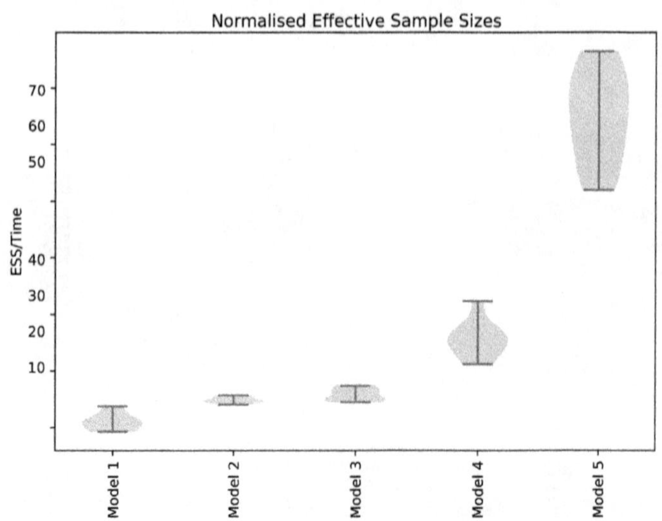

(**b**) Effective sample size normalized by execution time from NUTS algorithm across all the models.

Fig. 8.4 Inference results for the Bayesian framework for the NUTS algorithm. The left panels show the effective sample sizes, while the right panel shows the effective sample sizes normalized by execution time for each model

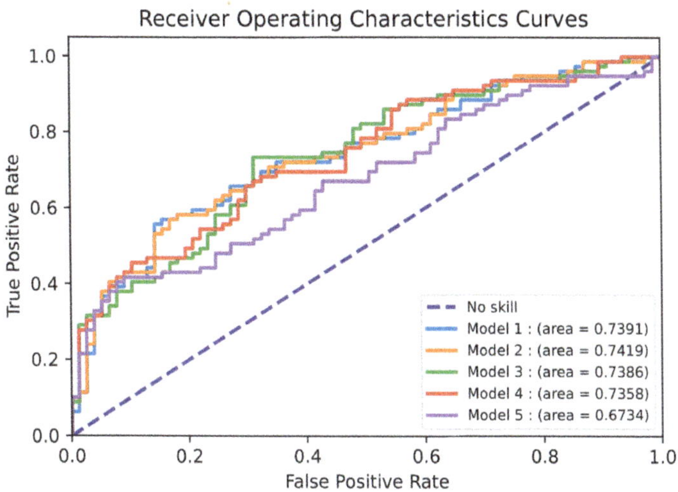

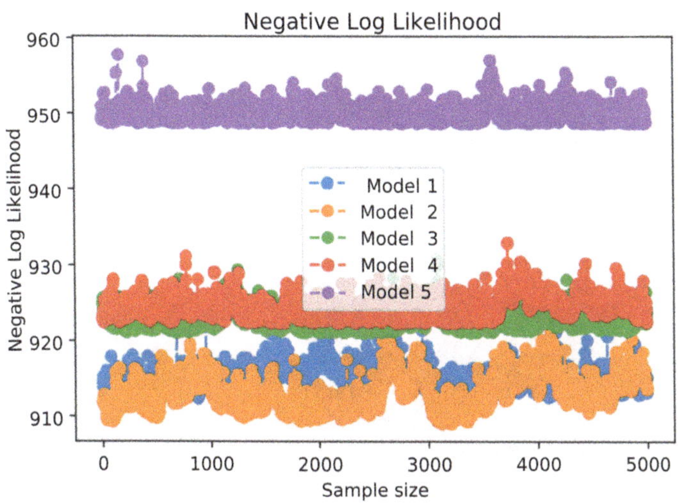

Fig. 8.5 Inference results for the Bayesian framework for the MALA method. The left panels show the predictive performance based on the Area Under the Receiver Operating Curves. In contrast, the right panel shows all models' Diagnostic negative log-likelihood trace plots

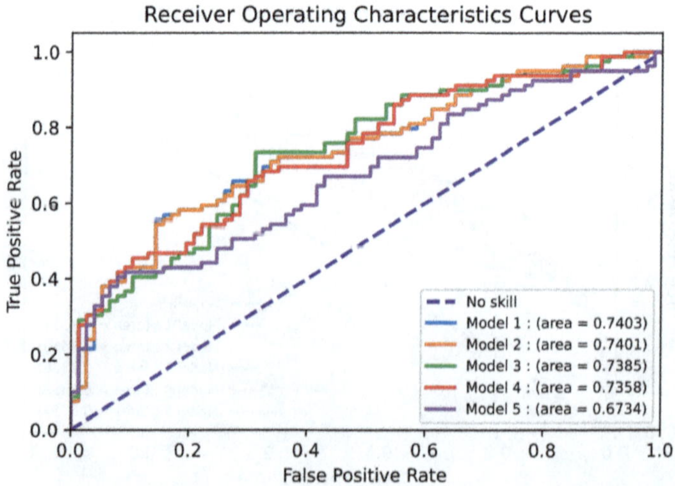

(**a**) Predictive performance based on the Area under the Receiver Operating Curves for MALA method.

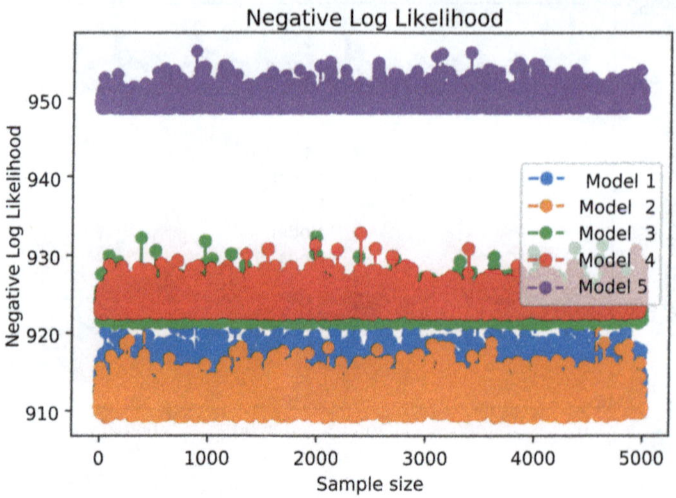

(**b**) Diagnostic negative log-likelihood trace plots for MALA method.

Fig. 8.6 Inference results for the Bayesian framework for the HMC method. The left panels show the predictive performance based on the Area Under the Receiver Operating Curves. In contrast, the right panel shows all models' Diagnostic negative log-likelihood trace plots

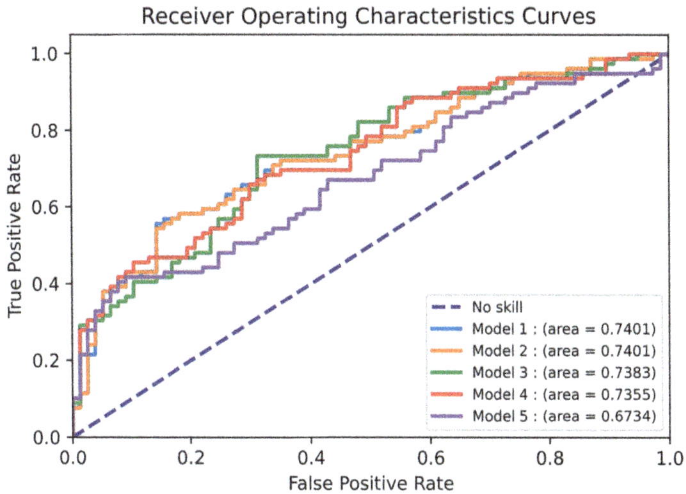

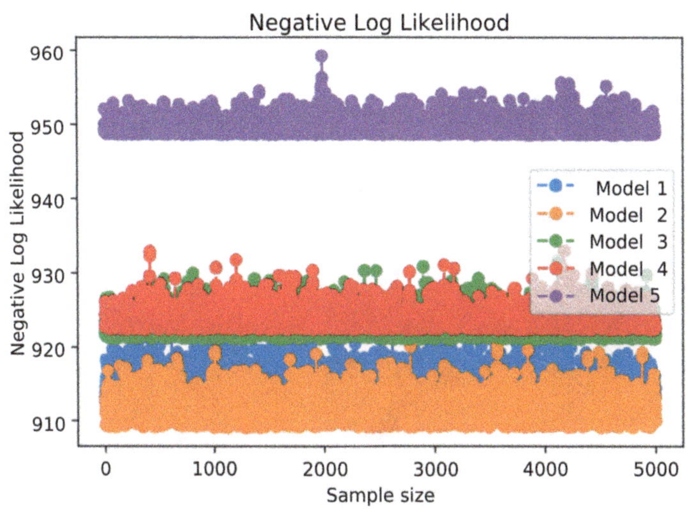

(b) Diagnostic negative log-likelihood trace plots for HMC method.

Fig. 8.7 Inference results for the Bayesian framework for the NUTS method. The left panels show the predictive performance based on the Area Under the Receiver Operating Curves. In contrast, the right panel shows all models' Diagnostic negative log-likelihood trace plots

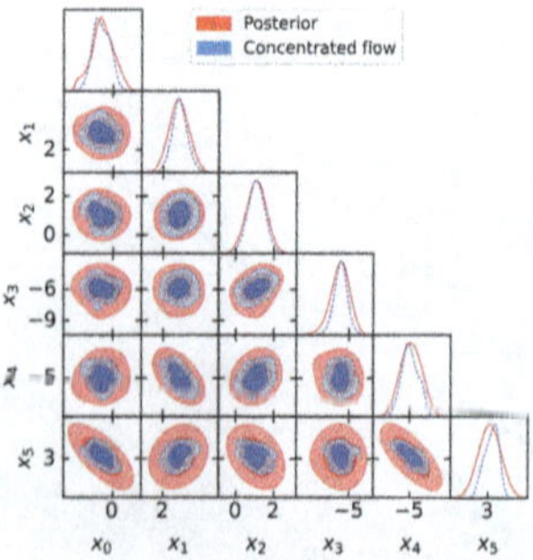

(a) Plots of the sampled posterior using the MALA method (solid red) and a real NVP flow (dashed blue) for Model 1.

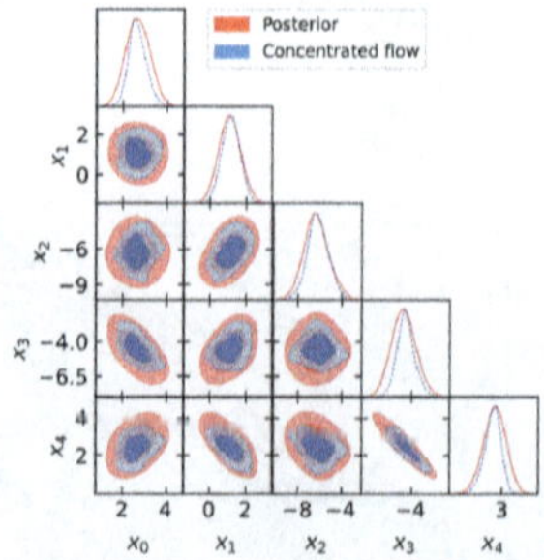

(b) Plots of the sampled posterior using the MALA method (solid red) and a real NVP flow (dashed blue) for Model 2.

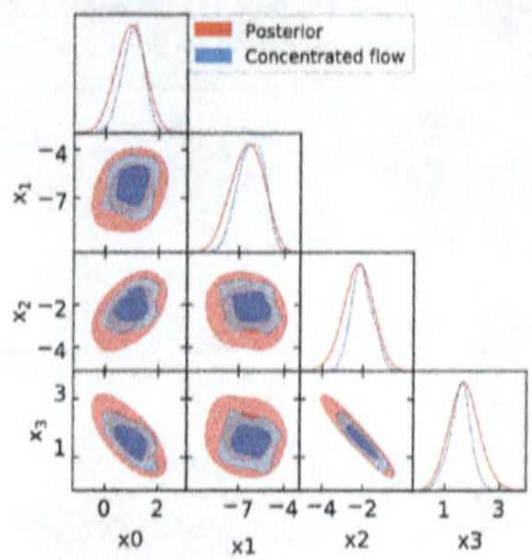

(c) Plots of the sampled posterior using the MALA method (solid red) and a real NVP flow (dashed blue) for Model 3.

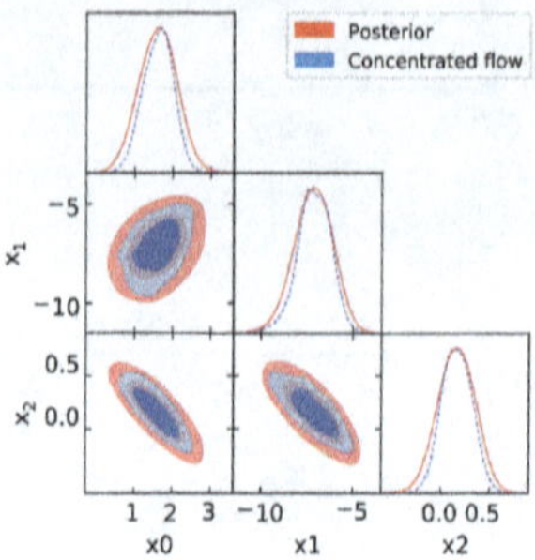

(d) Plots of the sampled posterior using the MALA method (solid red) and a real NVP flow (dashed blue) for Model 4.

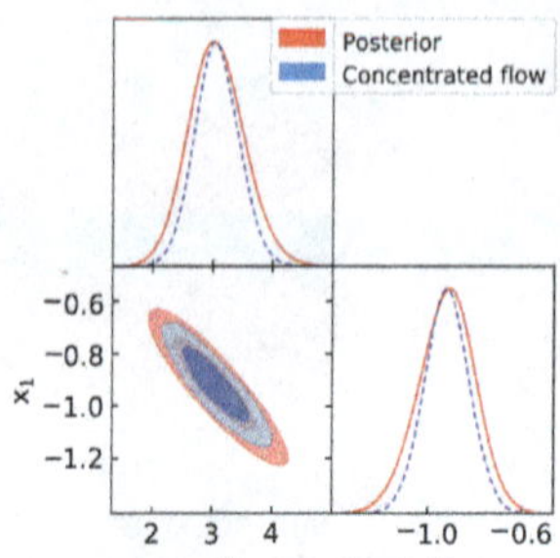

(e) Plots of the sampled posterior using the MALA method (solid red) and a real NVP flow (dashed blue) for Model 5.

Fig. 8.8 Plots of the sampled posterior using the MALA method (solid red) and a real NVP flow (dashed blue) for the five models

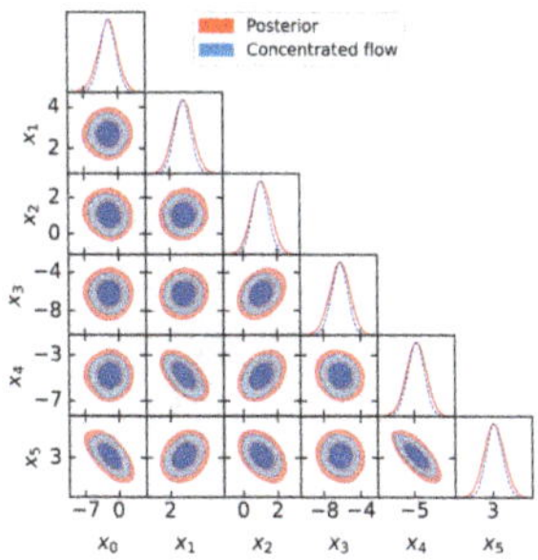

(**a**) Plots of the sampled posterior using the HMC method (solid red) and a real NVP flow (dashed blue) for Model 1.

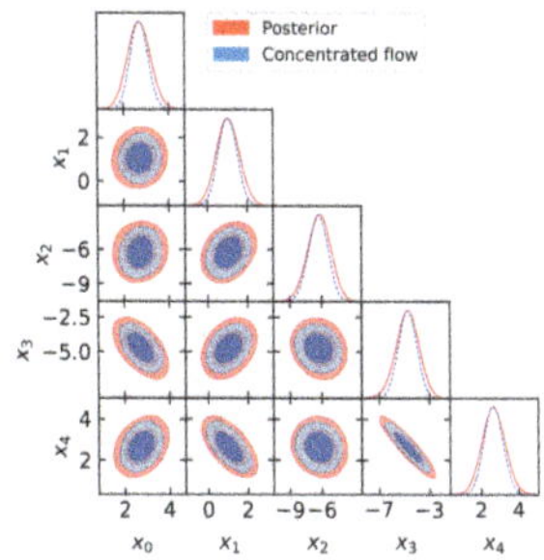

(**b**) Plots of the sampled posterior using the HMC method (solid red) and a real NVP flow (dashed blue) for Model 1.

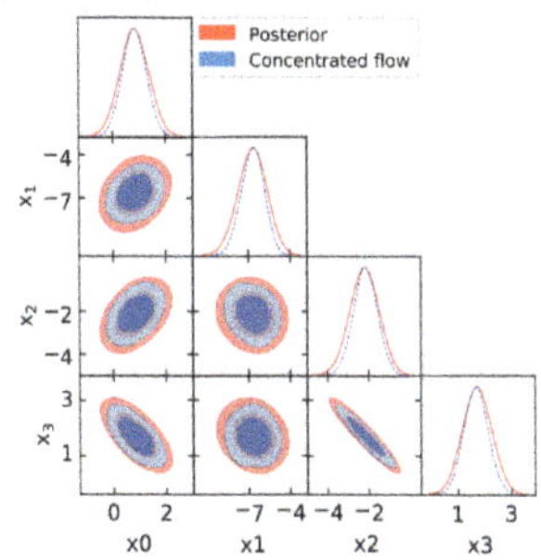

(**c**) Plots of the sampled posterior using the HMC method (solid red) and a real NVP flow (dashed blue) for Model 3.

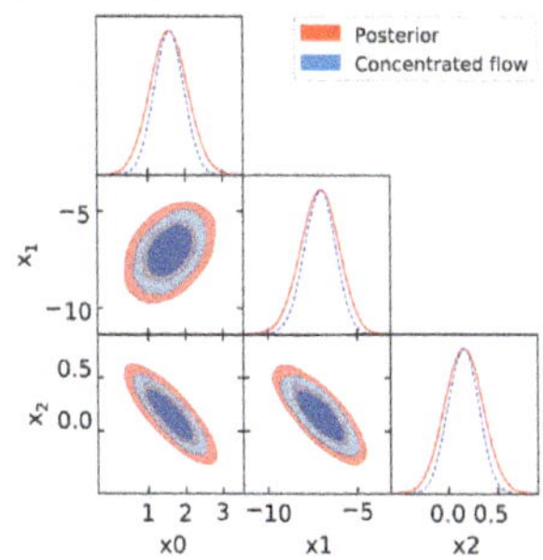

(**d**) Plots of the sampled posterior using the HMC method (solid red) and a real NVP flow (dashed blue) for Model 4.

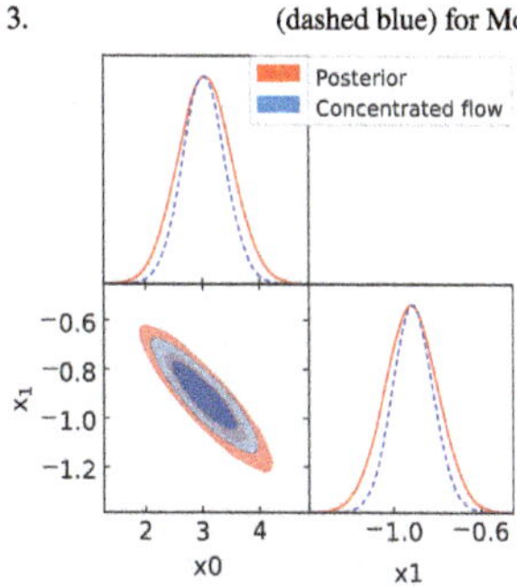

(**e**) Plots of the sampled posterior using the HMC method (solid red) and a real NVP flow (dashed blue) for Model 5.

Fig. 8.9 Plots of the sampled posterior using the HMC method (solid red) and a real NVP flow (dashed blue) for each of the five models

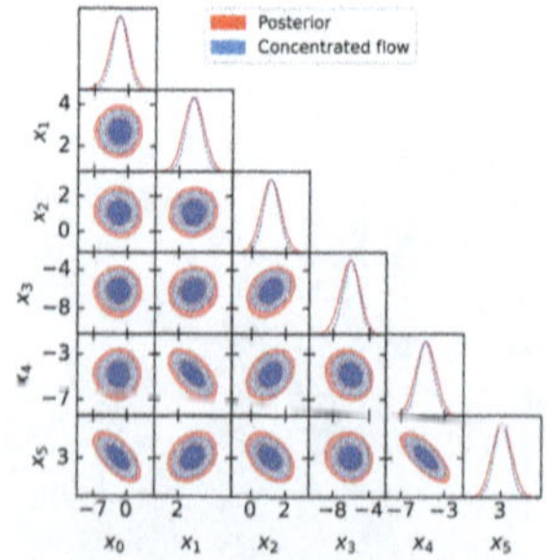

(**a**) Plots of the sampled posterior using the NUTS method (solid red) and a real NVP flow (dashed blue) for model 1.

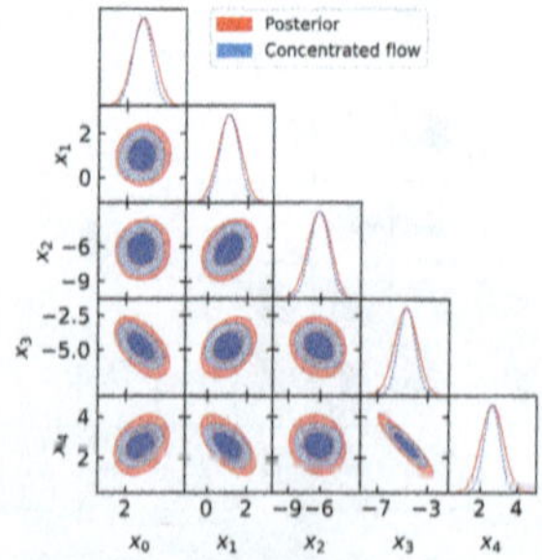

(**b**) Plots of the sampled posterior using the NUTS method (solid red) and a real NVP flow (dashed blue) for model 2.

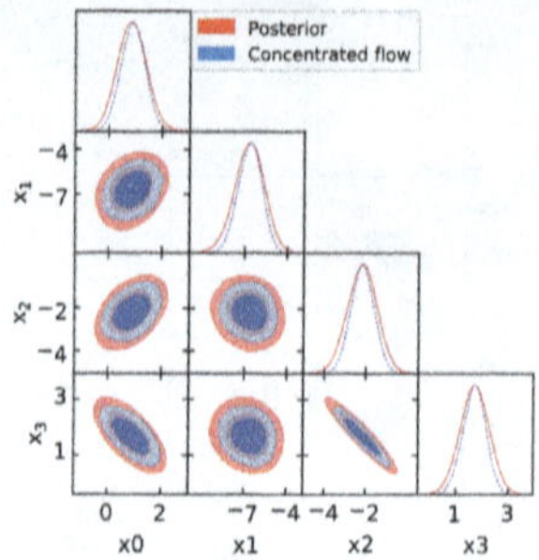

(**c**) Plots of the sampled posterior using the NUTS method (solid red) and a real NVP flow (dashed blue) for Model 3.

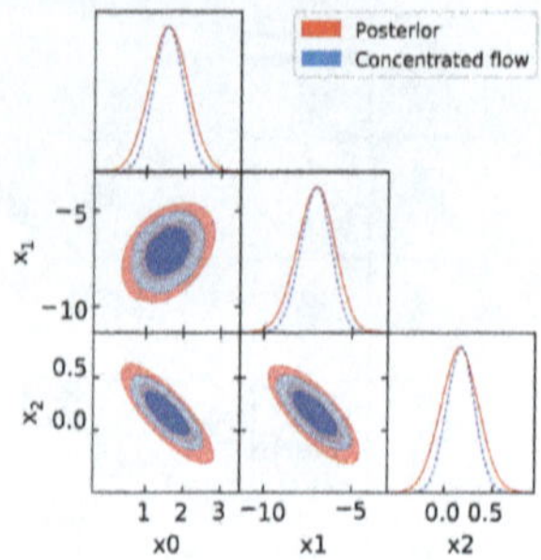

(**d**) Plots of the sampled posterior using the NUTS method (solid red) and a real NVP flow (dashed blue) for Model 4.

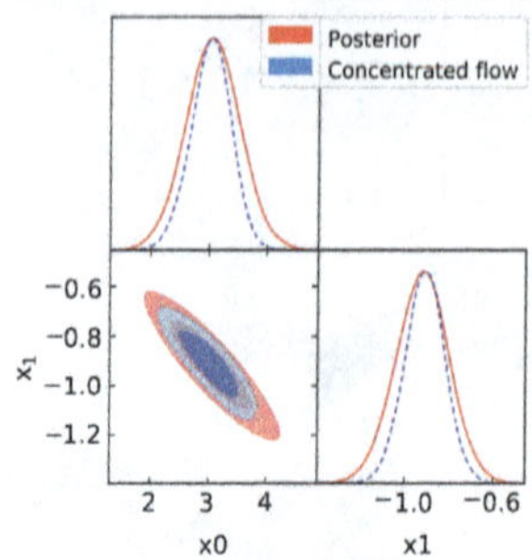

(**e**) Plots of the sampled posterior using the NUTS method (solid red) and a real NVP flow (dashed blue) for Model 5.

Fig. 8.10 Plots of the sampled posterior using the NUTS method (solid red) and a real NVP flow (dashed blue) for each of the five models

Table 8.3 shows that the MALA, HMC, and NUTS methods produce similar values of the log evidence across all the models. This table further indicates that Model 2 is the model that has the highest log evidence across all the MCMC methods, followed in close second place by Model 1, and Model 5 has the lowest evidence as computed on the training dataset. We further note that Model 2 produces the highest or second-highest AUC on unseen data, with Model 1 being a close second (or first). This shows that the log evidence metric computed on training data can select the best-performing method on unseen data. It is worth noting that Model 1 has more parameters than Model 2, and the log evidence metric captures this by penalizing Model 1 with lower evidence than Model 2, even though they have similar performance on unseen data. We further find that Model 5, which has the lowest evidence on training data, has the lowest AUC on the unseen data, showing that the evidence metric can also detect poor-performing models.

Table 8.4 shows the pair-wise comparison across all the models using the log evidence from the MALA method. The results show that Model 2 better represents the data than all the other models, with solid evidence of differences and a weak difference detected against Model 1 based on Jeffreys' scale in Table 8.1. We further note that Model 5 is the laggard. As Models 1 to 4 are extensions of Model 5, these results also indicate the impact of variables as they are added to the models. For example, adding the "Current Ratio" covariate to Model 5 (to create Model 4) results in a significant improvement of the model, as seen by the AUC metric on unseen data, while adding the "Debt to Community Wealth/Equity" financial ratio to Model 2 (to create Model 1) has minimal impact, with Models 1 and 2 being very similar both in terms of log evidence on training data and predictive performance using the AUC metric on unseen data.

Figures 8.2, 8.3, and 8.4 show the sampling results across all the MCMC methods and all the models. The results show that Model 5 has the highest effective sample size when using MALA and HMC and produces the lowest using the NUTS algorithm. The MALA, HMC, and NUTs methods agree that Model 5 has the highest execution time-normalized effective sample size—which makes sense as Model 5 has the lowest number of parameters and thus has the lowest execution time.

Figures 8.5, 8.6, and 8.7 show the predictive performance across all the models and the MCMC methods. All MCMC methods have converged across all the models, as indicated by the diagnostic negative log-likelihood trace plots across all the methods. Furthermore, the MCMC techniques produce a similar predictive performance on unseen data, as demonstrated by the Area Under the Receiver Operating Curves (AUC) plots for all the methods. We find that Model 2 and Model 1 produce the highest AUC, with Model 5 producing the lowest AUC and Model 3 and Model 4 producing results in between the two extremes. These results align with Table 8.3.

Figures 8.8, 8.9, and 8.10 show the corner plots of the samples posterior overlayed with the normalized flow across all the MCMC algorithms and models. The findings demonstrate that, as needed by the learnt harmonic mean estimator, the internal significance target distribution provided by the real NVP flow is confined inside the posterior and has narrower tails. This guarantees the reliability of the calculated evidence metrics for all models and across all the MCMC techniques.

8.7 Conclusion

In this chapter, we considered the problem of model comparison and selection for modeling audit opinions in South African municipalities. This is an important question to be able to answer, given the increase in the number of machine learning models used for this task. We compare five Bayesian logistic regression models using the Bayesian evidence metric. The evidence metric is calculated using the learnt Harmonic mean based on normalizing flows, with the posterior samples generated from the Metropolis-Adjusted Langevin Algorithm, Hamiltonian Monte Carlo, and No-U-Turn Sampler Markov Chain Monte Carlo algorithms.

Our results show that Bayesian evidence can select the model performing well on unseen data as measured by the Area Under the Receiver Operating Curve (AUC) metric. Furthermore, the evidence metric naturally penalizes complex models that don't add significant outperformance—this is seen by the metric not necessarily selecting the model with the most considerable number of parameters. The framework presented in this chapter can be extended to more complicated models, such as deep neural networks, and by employing more advanced sampling techniques, such as those based on Riemannian manifolds (Mongwe et al., 2020d).

In the next chapter, we model unauthorized expenditures in South African municipalities using a Bayesian framework based on Markov Chain

Monte Carlo methods. This framework also allows us to identify the most relevant variables to detect unauthorized expenditures from ***unaudited*** financial statements.

References

Afshar, H. M., Oliveira, R., & Cripps, S. (2021). Non-volume preserving Hamiltonian Monte Carlo and No-U-TurnSamplers. In *International conference on artificial intelligence and statistics*. PMLR (pp. 1675–1683).

Andrieu, C., & Thoms, J. (2008). A tutorial on adaptive MCMC. *Statistics and Computing, 18*(4), 343–373.

Auditor-General South Africa (2023). *Consololidated general report on local government audit outcomes - mfma 2021-22.* https://mfma-2022.agsareports.co.za/report/mfma_report_2021_22_final_31_may_2023.pdf. Last Retrieved: 16 November 2023.

Bishop, C. M. (July 1997). Bayesian neural networks. *Journal of the Brazilian Computer Society, 4*. ISSN: 0104-6500.

Deng, Q. (Aug. 2010). Detection of fraudulent financial statements based on Naıve Bayes classifier. In *2010 5th international conference on computer science & education* (pp. 1032–1035). IEEE. https://doi.org/10.1109/iccse.2010.5593407

Deng, Q., & Mei G. (Aug. 2009). Combining self-organizing map and K-means clustering for detecting fraudulent financial statements. In *2009 IEEE international conference on granular computing* (pp. 126–131). IEEE. https://doi.org/10.1109/grc.2009.5255148

Dinh, L., Sohl-Dickstein, J., & Bengio, S. (2016). Density estimation using real nvp. arXiv preprint arXiv:1605.08803

Duane, S., Kennedy, A. D., Pendleton, B. J., & Roweth, D. (1987). Hybrid Monte Carlo. *Physics Letters B, 195*(2), 216–222.

Gaganis, C., Pasiouras, F., Spathis, C., & Zopounidis, C. (Jan. 2007). A comparison of nearest neighbours, discriminant and logit models for auditing decisions. *Intelligent Systems in Accounting, Finance and Management, 15*(1–2), 23–40. https://doi.org/10.1002/isaf.283

Girolami, M., & Calderhead, B. (2011). Riemann manifold langevin and hamiltonian monte carlo methods. *Journal of the Royal Statistical Society: Series B (Statistical Methodology), 73*(2), 123–214.

Gu, M., & Sun, S. (2020). Neural Langevin dynamical sampling. *IEEE Access, 8*, 31595–31605.

Hastings, W. K. (1970). Monte Carlo sampling methods using Markov chains and their applications. *Biometrica, 57*(1), 97–109.

Higson, E., Handley, W., Hobson, M., & Lasenby, A. (2019). Dynamic nested sampling: An improved algorithm for parameter estimation and evidence calculation. *Statistics and Computing, 29*, 891–913.

Hoffman, M. D., & Gelman, A. (2011). *The No-U-Turn Sampler: Adaptively setting path lengths in Hamiltonian Monte Carlo.* arXiv:1111.4246 [stat.CO]

Hoffman, M. D., & Gelman, A. (2014). The No-U-turn sampler: adaptively setting path lengths in Hamiltonian Monte Carlo. *Journal of Machine Learning Research, 15*(1), 1593–1623.

Kass, R. E., & Raftery, A. E. (1995). Bayes factors. *Journal of the American Statistical Association, 90*(430), 773–795.

Kotsiantis, S., Koumanakos, E., Tzelepis, D., & Tampakas, V. (2006). Financial application of neural networks: Two case studies in Greece. In *Artificial neural networks – ICANN 2006* (pp. 672–681). Springer. https://doi.org/10.1007/11840930_70

Mabelane, K., Mongwe, W. T., Mbuvha, R., & Marwala, T. (2023). An analysis of local government financial statement audit outcomes in a developing economy using machine learning. *Sustainability, 15*(1), 12.

MacKay, D. J. C. (1992). Bayesian interpolation. *Neural Computation, 4*(3), 415–447.

Marwala, T., Mbuvha, R., & Mongwe, W. T. (2023). *Hamiltonian Monte Carlo methods in machine learning*. Elsevier.

Mbuvha, R., Illyes Boulkaibet, and Marwala, T. (2019). Bayesian automatic relevance determination for feature selection in credit default modelling. In *International conference on artificial neural networks* (pp. 420–425). Springer.

Mbuvha, R., & Marwala, T. (2020). Bayesian inference of COVID-19 spreading rates in South Africa. *PloS One, 15*(8), Article e0237126.

Mbuvha, R., Mongwe, W. T., & Marwala, T. (2021). Separable Shadow Hamiltonian hybrid Monte Carlo for Bayesian neural network inference in wind speed forecasting. *Energy and A, 1*, Article 100108.

McEwen, J. D., Wallis, C. G. R., Price, M. A., & Mancini, A. S. (2021). Machine learning assisted Bayesian model comparison: Learnt harmonic mean estimator. arXiv preprint arXiv:2111.12720

Moepya, S. O., Akhoury, S. S., & Nelwamondo, F. V. (Dec. 2014). Applying cost-sensitive classification for financial fraud detection under high class-imbalance. In *2014 IEEE international conference on data mining workshop* (pp. 183–192). IEEE.https://doi.org/10.1109/icdmw.2014.141

Mongwe, W. T. (2022). *Hybrid Monte Carlo methods in machine learning: Stochastic volatility methods, shadow Hamiltonians, adaptive approaches and variance reduction techniques*. University of Johannesburg (South Africa).

Mongwe, W. T., & Malan, K. M. (2020a). A survey of automated financial statement fraud detection with relevance to the South African context. *South African Computer Journal, 32*(1). https://doi.org/10.18489/sacj.v32i1.777

Mongwe, W. T., & Malan, K. M. (2020b). The efficacy of financial ratios for fraud detection using self organising maps. In *2020 IEEE symposium series on computational intelligence (SSCI)* (pp. 1100–1106). IEEE.

Mongwe, W. T., Mbuvha, R., & Marwala, T. (2021a). Adaptive magnetic Hamiltonian Monte Carlo. *IEEE Access, 9*, 152993–153003. https://doi.org/10.1109/ACCESS.2021.3127931

Mongwe, W. T., Mbuvha, R., & Marwala, T. (2021b). Adaptively setting the path length for separable shadow Hamiltonian hybrid Monte Carlo. *IEEE Access, 9*, 138598–138607.

Mongwe, W. T., Mbuvha, R., & Marwala, T. (2021c). Antithetic magnetic and Shadow Hamiltonian Monte Carlo. *IEEE Access, 9*, 49857–49867.

Mongwe, W. T., Mbuvha, R., & Marwala, T. (2021d). Antithetic Riemannian manifold and quantum-inspired Hamiltonian Monte Carlo. arXiv preprint arXiv:2107.02070

Mongwe, W. T., Mbuvha, R., & Marwala, T. (2021e). Bayesian inference of local government audit outcomes. *Plos One*. https://doi.org/10.1371/journal.pone.0261245

Mongwe, W. T., Mbuvha, R., & Marwala, T. (2021f). Locally scaled and stochastic volatility metropolis-hastings algorithms. *Algorithms, 14*(12). ISSN: 1999-4893. https://doi.org/10.3390/a14120351

Mongwe, W. T., Mbuvha, R., & Marwala, T. (2021g). Quantum-inspired magnetic Hamiltonian Monte Carlo. *Plos One, 16*(10), Article e0258277.

Mongwe, W. T., Mbuvha, R., & Marwala, T. (2022a). Shadow magnetic Hamiltonian Monte Carlo. *IEEE Access, 10*, 34340–34351. https://doi.org/10.1109/ACCESS.2022.3161443

Mongwe, W. T., Sidogi, T., Mbuvha, R., & Marwala, T. (2022b). Probabilistic inference of south african equity option prices under jump-diffusion processes. In *2022 IEEE symposium on computational intelligence for financial engineering and economics (CIFEr)* (pp. 1–8). IEEE.

Neal, R. M. (1993). Bayesian learning via stochastic dynamics. In *Advances in neural information processing systems* (Vol. 5, pp. 475–482). Morgan Kaufmann Publishers Inc. ISBN: 1-55860-274-7. http://dl.acm.org/citation.cfm?id=645753.667903

Neal, R. M., et al. (2011). MCMC using Hamiltonian dynamics. *Handbook of Markov Chain Monte Carlo, 2*(11), 2.

Nesseris, S., & Garcia-Bellido, J. (2013). Is the Jeffreys' scale a reliable tool for Bayesian model comparison in cosmology? *Journal of Cosmology and Astroparticle Physics, 2013*(08), 036.

Newton, M. A., & Raftery, A. E. (1994). Approximate Bayesian inference with the weighted likelihood bootstrap. *Journal of the Royal Statistical Society Series B: Statistical Methodology, 56*(1), 3–26.

Polanska, A., Price, M. A., Mancini, A. S., & McEwen, J. D. (2023). Learned harmonic mean estimation of the marginal likelihood with normalizing flows. In *Physical sciences forum* (Vol. 9. 1. p. 10). MDPI.

Rasmussen, C. E., & Ghahramani, Z. (2001). Occam's razor. In *Advances in neural information processing systems* (pp. 294–300).

Skilling, J. (2004). Nested sampling. In *AIP conference proceedings* (Vol. 735. 1, pp. 395–405). American Institute of Physics.

Skilling, J. (2006). Nested sampling for general Bayesian computation. *Bayesian Analysis, 1*(4), 833–859.

Spathis, C., Doumpos, M., & Zopounidis, C. (Sept. 2002). Detecting falsified financial statements: A comparative study using multicriteria analysis and multivariate statistical techniques. *European Accounting Review, 11*(3), 509–535. https://doi.org/10.1080/0963818022000000966

Speagle, J. S. (2020). Dynesty: A dynamic nested sampling package for estimating bayesian posteriors and evidences. *Monthly Notices of the Royal Astronomical Society, 493*(3), 3132–3158.

CHAPTER 9

Bayesian Detection of Unauthorized Expenditure Using Langevin and Hamiltonian Monte Carlo

9.1 Introduction

Staying within budget is crucial to successfully running a local government entity. According to a recent South African Auditor General study, 68% of municipalities expended R25,47 billion in unauthorized spending in the fiscal year 2021–2022 (Auditor-General South Africa, 2023). This illustrates the dismal status of South African municipalities and provides a plausible explanation for the poor service delivery witnessed in municipalities (Sikhosana, 2021). Financially sound municipalities would have clean audits and no irregular, unproductive, or wasteful expenditure (Auditor-General South Africa, 2011, 2023) and are better positioned to deliver quality service to the public. The unauthorized, irregular, fruitful, and wasteful expenditures are collectively considered unlawful expenditures (Sikhosana, 2021).

Unauthorized expenditure is defined as municipalities spending money that the council had not budgeted for, or that did not match the terms of a certain grant (Auditor-General South Africa, 2011, 2023; Sikhosana, 2021). A wasteful and fruitless expenditure is one that was made in

Supplementary Information The online version contains supplementary material available at https://doi.org/10.1007/978-3-031-88431-3_9.

W. T. Mongwe et al., *Bayesian Machine Learning in Quantitative Finance*, https://doi.org/10.1007/978-3-031-88431-3_9

vain and might have been avoided if reasonable care had been exercised (Auditor-General South Africa, 2011, 2023; Sikhosana, 2021). Irregular expenditure is defined as spending that was not incurred in the manner required by law, and it does not always imply that money was squandered or that fraud was perpetrated (Auditor-General South Africa, 2011, 2023; Sikhosana, 2021). Understanding the behavior and drivers of these expenditures is critical. Artificial intelligence is a technology that may be used for the detection and analysis of these expenditures.

Artificial intelligence (AI) has opened opportunities for stakeholders to better understand the operation of municipalities—with a critical branch of AI that has shown significant success in practice being machine learning (Mongwe & Malan, 2020a, 2020b; Mongwe et al., 2021d). In Mabelane et al. (2023), machine learning techniques are used to understand and analyze the audit outcomes of South African municipalities and found that neural networks outperform in the task of predicting audit outcomes. More generally, various authors have used machine learning to model audit outcomes of both public and private entities across the globe with good success (Chandrashekar & Sahin, 2014; Kirkos et al., 2007; Moepya et al., 2014; Mongwe & Malan, 2020a). Moepya et al. (2014) used support vector machines to analyze the presence of fraud in publicly listed entities in South Africa, while Kirkos et al. (2007) used various machine learning techniques for entities listed in Greece.

More recently, there have been advances in using Bayesian techniques to analyze these audit outcomes. Mongwe et al. (2021d) use a Bayesian logistic regression model trained with variants of Hamiltonian Monte Carlo to predict whether a particular financial report from a municipality had a clean audit or not in a probabilistically sound fashion while also using an automatic relevance determination prior distribution. Their results also identified the current ratio and debt to operating income as critical financial ratios for the audit opinion prediction task. However, a key issue yet to be analyzed in the literature is the potential of using machine learning in predicting unlawful expenditure. This is the focus of this chapter.

In the current chapter, we aim only to detect the presence of expenditures, while in future work, we strive to predict the absolute amount of the expenditure. For this analysis, we collect data on all South African municipalities over the last 10 years. We collect each entity's audited and unaudited financial statements for each financial year. The aim is to use the unaudited financial statements to predict the expenditures that the Auditor-General will flag on the audited financial statements. In this chapter, we present a Bayesian framework for detecting the presence of unauthorized expenditures in audited financial statements using unaudited financials of South African municipalities as inputs. We use a Bayesian logistic regression model trained with Hamiltonian and Langevin Monte Carlo techniques, and we also identify the most relevant financial ratios for detecting the presence of expenditures.

The remainder of this chapter is structured as follows: We first provide a background into unlawful expenditure analysis in municipalities in Sect. 9.2; we then detail the Bayesian logistic regression model that we use in Sect. 9.3 and the Markov Chain Monte Carlo methods that we utilize to train the model in Sect. 9.4; we then present the experiment setup, after which we present the results, discuss them, and provide the conclusion in Sects. 9.5–9.7 respectively.

9.2 Background to Unlawful Expenditure Analysis

The South African Parliament passed the Public Finance Management Act No. 1 of 1999 (PFMA) in 1999. This act aimed to improve the effectiveness and efficiency of government financial administration. The Act requires government entities to implement methods to reduce wasteful expenditure (Dlomo, 2017). On the other hand, the Auditor General reports year after year that most South African municipalities have billions of Rands in unauthorized expenditure (Auditor-General South Africa, 2023).

South Africa has 257 municipalities, including eight metropolitan municipalities, 44 district municipalities, and 205 local municipalities (Motubatse & Ngwakwe, 2020). The South African Constitution requires these municipalities to provide essential services such as water and sanitation, power, roads and transportation, and garbage collection. However, providing the mandated services necessitates providing resources such as infrastructure and human capital, as well as adequate funding (Motubatse & Ngwakwe, 2020).

Municipalities get subsidies from the provincial and national governments, which may be conditional or unconditional. Conditional payments are allocated to specific national purposes (Motubatse & Ngwakwe, 2020). An unconditional grant, also known as the equitable share, is the amount of revenue received by institutions in all branches of government as an entitlement to enable them to provide basic services and carry out their tasks. However, their equal share is inadequate to assure the communities' long-term existence (Motubatse & Ngwakwe, 2020). As a result, each municipality must generate its revenue by levying taxes and selling the services it offers to its citizens (Auditor-General South Africa, 2023; Motubatse & Ngwakwe, 2020).

The study by Sikhosana (2021) explored theories about the link between unlawful spending and municipal financial performance factors. To understand the correlations (rather than forecast them), all factors were described, regardless of their relevance. There were statistically significant negative connections between unauthorized expenditure and cost coverage, current ratio, compensation as a proportion of total expenditure, and net operating surplus margin. Furthermore, a statistically significant positive relationship was discovered between irregular expenditure and net operating surplus, and a statistically significant negative relationship was found between fruitless and wasteful expenditure and outstanding service debtors to revenue and cost coverage. These results indicate that it is sensible to attempt to predict expenditures based on the financial ratios. However, a fundamental limitation of the work by Sikhosana (2021) is that the expenditures are not predicted, and both the inputs (i.e., the financial ratios) and the target (i.e., the expenditures) are extracted from the audited financials. This limits the usefulness of the results from a risk-screening perspective before the audit is performed. In this chapter, we aim to address these weaknesses.

This chapter provides the first-in-literature approach to using artificial intelligence techniques for analyzing the financial performance metrics that may indicate the presence or absence of unauthorized expenditure. Our approach is a Bayesian approach, which was selected for two main reasons. The Bayesian framework provides a probabilistically sound basis for performing predictions as we can also produce uncertainty bounds. Furthermore our approach also provides us with the relative ranking of the importance of the input variables, which will make our results interpretable for the various stakeholders. The results of this work can provide valuable insights to auditors as it provides a mechanism for them to flag municipalities that are likely to have unlawful expenditures—and hence, more resources can be deployed for this purpose.

9.3 Model for Bayesian Detection of Expenditure

We model the unauthorized expenditure using Bayesian logistic regression. The negative log-likelihood $l(\mathrm{D}|\mathbf{w})$ function for this model is given by (Marwala et al., 2023; Mongwe, 2022; Mongwe et al., 2021d, 2022a):

$$l(\mathrm{D}|\mathbf{w}) = \sum_{i}^{N} y_i \log(\mathbf{w}^T x_i) + (1 - y_i)\log(1 - \mathbf{w}^T x_i) \tag{9.1}$$

where $\mathrm{D} = \{\mathrm{x}, \mathrm{y}\}$ is the data, N is the number of observations and $\mathbf{w}$ are the parameters that need to be estimated. Thus, the target un-normalized posterior log distribution is given as (Mongwe et al., 2021d):

$$\ln p(\mathbf{w}|\mathrm{D}) = l(\mathrm{D}|\mathbf{w}) + \ln p(\mathbf{w}|\alpha) + \ln q(\alpha) \tag{9.2}$$

where $\ln p(\mathbf{w}|\alpha)$ is the log of the prior distribution placed on the parameters given the hyperparameters, and $\ln q(\alpha)$ is the distribution of the hyperparameters. As in Marwala et al. (2023), Mongwe et al. (2021d); Mongwe (2022), we model the parameters $\mathbf{w}$ as having a Gaussian prior with each parameter having zero mean and its own standard deviation or regularization parameter α_i, meaning that we are using an automatic relevance determination (ARD) prior within our framework.

The α_i indicates how important the parameter associated with the input feature is. The larger the value of α_i, the more critical the input feature is in predicting the expenditures (Mongwe et al., 2021d). Thus, this framework automatically ranks the importance of the input features. The α_i will have low values for irrelevant inputs, which will cause their weights to be driven to decay to values around zero (Mbuvha et al., 2021; Mongwe et al., 2021d). Conversely, essential inputs will have weights with high variances while less important inputs will have low variances (Mbuvha et al., 2021). Since the mean for the weight priors is fixed at zero, it follows that weights with high variances can take values far from zero (resulting in a more significant effect), while those with low variances must take values close to zero (thus reduced effect) (Mbuvha et al., 2021).

Due to the multi-modal and non-convex structure of the ARD loss function, inference of ARD prior hyperparameters is a fundamentally hard inverse problem (MacKay, 1995; Mbuvha et al., 2021; Neal, 1993).

Through maximizing the Bayesian evidence metric, MacKay (1995) obtains estimates of the ARD hyperparameters, and this is due to the Laplace approximation's simplifying assumptions producing a tractable closed-form calculation of the evidence. On the other hand, Neal (2012) deploys an alternating framework of using Hamiltonian Monte Carlo for network weights and Gibbs sampling for ARD hyperparameters from various posteriors such as the Gamma (Mbuvha et al., 2021). This strategy converges to an asymptotically true posterior based on Markov Chain Monte Carlo. However, a lot of design decisions, such as the choice of the appropriate prior distribution, are still necessary (Mbuvha et al., 2021). The hyperparameter sampling strategy used in this chapter is to jointly infer the α hyperparameters and the $\mathbf{w}$ parameters as in Mongwe et al. (2021d). Although the effective parameter space is doubled in this approach, compared to the Gibbs sampling strategy, this method has the advantage of producing a more stable exploration across the MCMC methods (Mongwe et al., 2021d). As the $\mathbf{w}$ parameters are assumed to be normally distributed, we select the α hyperparameters to be log-normally distributed to make the joint sampling of parameters and hyperparameters mathematically convenient. In particular, the α_is are assumed to follow a log-normal distribution with mean zero, and unit variance as in Marwala et al. (2023), Mongwe et al. (2021d), Mongwe (2022).

9.4 Markov Chain Monte Carlo Algorithms

We now present the details of the MCMC methods that are used to train the Bayesian logistic regression model with an ARD prior in Eq. 9.2. We implemented all the MCMC methods in Python.

9.4.1 *Metropolis-Hastings and the Metropolis-Adjusted Langevin Algorithm*

One of the classical MCMC methods is the random walk Metropolis-Hastings (MH) technique, which uses a Gaussian distribution centered at the current state as the proposal distribution (Hastings, 1970; Mbuvha et al., 2021; Mongwe et al., 2021e). This results in samples that are strongly autocorrelated, which causes slow convergence. Large sample sizes must be created to do this. Methods that apply additional information about the target posterior distributions and lessen the random walk behavior enhance the traditional MH method (Girolami & Calderhead, 2011; Marwala et al., 2023). The standard extension considers the posterior's local curvature using the second-order gradient information and the first-order gradient information to direct the target's sampling (Girolami & Calderhead, 2011; Marwala et al., 2023). The Langevin and the Hamiltonian dynamics on the Euclidean manifold are two approaches that use the first-order gradient information (Marwala et al., 2023). On the other hand, techniques on the Riemannian and other manifolds employ the second-order gradient information (Girolami & Calderhead, 2011). In practice, methods utilizing Hamiltonian dynamics in Euclidean spaces have shown great promise and are also relatively more straightforward to implement than those on other manifolds (Marwala et al., 2023; Mongwe et al., 2021c).

The Metropolis-Adjusted Langevin Algorithm (MALA) enhances the Metropolis-Hastings (MH) method through the use of first-order gradient information of the target posterior. MALA reduces the random walk behavior of MH via the use of Langevin dynamics where the drift component is the derivative of the log of the target posterior, and the diffusive component is Brownian motion which is represented as follows (Gu & Sun, 2020; Marwala et al., 2023; Mongwe et al., 2021e, 2022b):

$$d\mathbf{w}_t = \frac{1}{2} f'(\mathbf{w})dt + dZ_t \tag{9.3}$$

where $\mathbf{w}$ are the parameters, $f'(\mathbf{w})$ is the first derivative of the target $f(\mathbf{w})$ with respect to the parameters, and Z_t is a Brownian motion process at a fictitious time t. The Langevin dynamics in Eq. 9.3 typically cannot be solved analytically, and numerical methods such as the Euler-Maruyama integration scheme are typically used (Marwala et al., 2023). This, however, introduces errors that can break the detailed balance condition, which would not guarantee that the method would converge to the correct target distribution (Marwala et al., 2023). To rectify this, a Metropolis acceptance step is incorporated into the algorithm to ensure detailed balance (Marwala et al., 2023). The MALA algorithm converges to the stationary distribution at a faster pace than the MH algorithm because it takes into account the density's first-order gradient data, which is represented by $f'(\mathbf{w})$ (Girolami & Calderhead, 2011; Gu & Sun, 2020; Marwala et al., 2023). The samples produced using the MALA method are still highly correlated. Girolami and Calderhead (2011) incorporate second-order gradient information of the target by extending MALA from being on a Euclidean manifold to a Riemannian manifold (Marwala et al., 2023). Despite a corresponding increase in compute time, this approach demonstrated significant gains in the sampling performance of the MALA method (Marwala et al., 2023).

The sampler converges to the target distribution more quickly with the MALA algorithm than with the MH algorithm because it utilizes the gradient information of the target distribution (Girolami & Calderhead, 2011; Gu & Sun, 2020). The produced samples are still very correlated. The next section discusses the Hamiltonian Monte Carlo and Magnetic Hamiltonian Monte Carlo approaches, which employ Hamiltonian dynamics to traverse the target distribution better.

9.4.2 Hamiltonian Monte Carlo and Magnetic Hamiltonian Monte Carlo

Hamiltonian Monte Carlo (HMC) is a popular MCMC method for performing Bayesian inference and has been utilized in various disciplines such as finance, health, and energy (Duane et al., 1987; Mbuvha & Marwala, 2020; Mbuvha et al., 2021; Mongwe et al., 2021d, 2021h; 2022b). The method is premised on using Hamiltonian dynamics, which naturally considers the first-order gradient information of the target posterior. The dynamics that underpin HMC are as follows (Marwala et al., 2023; Neal, 1993):

$$\frac{d\mathbf{w}}{\partial t} = \frac{\partial \mathrm{H}(\mathbf{w}, \mathbf{p})}{\partial \mathbf{p}}; \quad \frac{d\mathbf{p}}{\partial t} = -\frac{\partial \mathrm{H}(\mathbf{w}, \mathbf{p})}{\partial \mathbf{w}} \tag{9.4}$$

where $\mathbf{w}$ are the parameters, $\mathbf{p}$ is the auxiliary momentum variable with the same dimensionality as $\mathbf{w}$, and $\mathrm{H}(\mathbf{w}, \mathbf{p})$ is the Hamiltonian—which represents the total energy (i.e., potential energy defined by the target posterior and kinetic energy which is typically captured through a multivariate Gaussian distribution) from this system (Mongwe et al., 2021b, 2022a). This HMC method allows distant proposals, which results in a significant reduction in the autocorrelations of the generated samples (Marwala et al., 2023).

The HMC technique is composed of two steps. The first step integrates Hamiltonian dynamics in Eq. 9.4 typically using the leapfrog integrator (Duane et al., 1987; Marwala et al., 2023; Neal, 1993), and the second step utilizes a Metropolis-Hastings correction to account for the numerical integration errors arising from the first step (Duane et al., 1987; Hastings, 1970; Neal et al., 2011). The parameter and momentum update equations for the leapfrog integration scheme (corresponding to the first step of HMC) are given as follows:

$$\begin{aligned}
\mathbf{p}_{t+\frac{\epsilon}{2}} &= \mathbf{p}_t + \frac{\epsilon}{2}\frac{\partial H(\mathbf{w}_t, \mathbf{p}_t)}{\partial \mathbf{w}} \\
\mathbf{w}_{t+\epsilon} &= \mathbf{w}_t + \epsilon \mathbf{M}^{-1}\mathbf{p}_{t+\frac{\epsilon}{2}} \\
\mathbf{p}_{t+\epsilon} &= \mathbf{p}_{t+\frac{\epsilon}{2}} + \frac{\epsilon}{2}\frac{\partial H\left(\mathbf{w}_{t+\epsilon}, \mathbf{p}_{t+\frac{\epsilon}{2}}\right)}{\partial \mathbf{w}}
\end{aligned} \tag{9.5}$$

where ϵ is the discretization step size and $\mathbf{M}$ is a covariance matrix emanating from the kinetic energy component in $\mathrm{H}(\mathbf{w}, \mathbf{p})$. If the integration of the Hamiltonian dynamics in the first step were solved precisely, the second step would not be required. However, due to the discretization errors, a Metropolis-Hastings acceptance step is typically required where the $\mathbf{w}^*$ proposed by the first step are accepted with probability:

$$\mathrm{P}(\text{accept } \mathbf{w}^*) = \min\left(1, \frac{\exp(-\mathrm{H}(\mathbf{w}^*, \mathbf{p}^*))}{\exp(-\mathrm{H}(\mathbf{w}, \mathbf{p}))}\right). \tag{9.6}$$

The parameters of HMC are the discretization step size ϵ, which is required for the first step in HMC, and the trajectory length, which determines the number of times the integration is performed. The step size parameter is typically set to obtain a user-specified target acceptance rate using the dual averaging method (Marwala et al., 2023; Hoffman & Gelman, 2014) while tuning the trajectory length parameter is a more complex problem (Hoffman & Gelman, 2014). It can further be shown that when the trajectory length parameter is set to 1, the HMC method becomes the MALA method. The overall HMC sampling process follows a Gibbs sampling scheme, where we sample $\mathbf{p}$ auxiliary momentum variable and then sample a new set of parameters $\mathbf{w}$ given the drawn momentum $\mathbf{p}$. This procedure is repeated until the required number of samples are generated (Marwala et al., 2023; Mongwe et al., 2021a, 2021b). The pseudo-code for HMC can be found in Algorithm 3.1 in Chapter 3 of this book.

Magnetic Hamiltonian Monte Carlo (MHMC) adds a magnetic field $\mathbf{G}$ to the force field already present in HMC. This magnetic field makes

MHMC more flexible than HMC and promotes a more efficient investigation of the posterior (Gu & Sun, 2020; Marwala et al., 2023; Mongwe et al., 2021a, 2021f, 2021g, 2022, 2022a; Tripuraneni et al., 2017). Compared to HMC, this reduces autocorrelations in the produced samples. MHMC employs the same Hamiltonian as HMC but makes use of non-canonical Hamiltonian dynamics in which the canonical matrix now contains a non-zero element on the diagonal. These dynamics, like HMC, cannot be integrated precisely. Thus, we use a numerical integration technique with a Metropolis-Hastings acceptance step to achieve detailed balance (Tripuraneni et al., 2017). The MHMC dynamics are given as:

$$\frac{d}{\partial t}\begin{bmatrix}\mathbf{w}\\ \mathbf{p}\end{bmatrix}=\begin{bmatrix}\mathbf{0} & \mathbf{I}\\ -\mathbf{I} & \mathbf{G}\end{bmatrix}\begin{bmatrix}\nabla_w \mathrm{H}(\mathrm{w},\mathrm{p})\\ \nabla_p \mathrm{H}(\mathrm{w},\mathrm{p})\end{bmatrix} \tag{9.7}$$

where **G** is a skew-symmetric[1] (or antisymmetric) matrix and is the term that represents the magnetic field. This representation further demonstrates that the sole way MHMC dynamics vary from HMC dynamics is that **G** is non-zero. The dynamics of MHMC and HMC are identical for $\mathbf{G} = \mathbf{0}$. According to Tripuraneni et al. (2017), these dynamics represent Newtonian mechanics of a charged particle in a magnetic field in three dimensions. The degree of sampling efficiency of MHMC over HMC will depend on how this magnetic field interacts with the force field (for example, are they orthogonal?) (Gu and Sun, 2020; Marwala et al., 2023).

The matrix **G** provides an extra degree of freedom for the MHMC algorithm. It is not clear as to how one should set this matrix. In this chapter, we follow the authors' directions (Tripuraneni et al., 2017) and select only a few dimensions to be influenced by the magnetic field. In particular, **G** was set such that $\mathbf{G_{1i}} = \mathbf{G_{5i}} = g$, $\mathbf{G_{i1}} = \mathbf{G_{i5}} = -g$ and zero elsewhere for $g = 0.2$. We also ensure that **G** is anti-symmetric (Brofos & Lederman, 2020; Marwala et al., 2023). A detailed exposition of the MHMC, HMC, MALA, and MH algorithms can be found in Marwala et al. (2023).

[1] That is: $\mathbf{G}^T = -\mathbf{G}$.

9.5 Numerical Experiments

In this section, we present the numerical experiments conducted. We first describe the dataset and then outline the experiments, settings, and performance metrics used.

9.5.1 Data Description

We perform the unauthorized expenditure analysis on a South African municipal finance dataset. The dataset was obtained from the South African National Treasury website, https://municipaldata.treasury.gov.za/. From 2012 to 2019, a sample of 1430 observations was collected from South African municipalities' unaudited financial statements with the expenditures collected from the corresponding audited financials. The specific ratios considered in this chapter are a subset of the variables described in Mongwe and Malan (2020b), with the only difference being that these variables are calculated based on unaudited financial statements, unlike in Mongwe and Malan (2020b) where audited financial statements are used. The variables are: (1) *Debt to Community Wealth/Equity*, (2) *Debt to Total Operating Revenue*, (3) *Current Ratio*, (4) *Net Operating Surplus Margin*, (5) *Remuneration to Total Operating Expenditure*, (6) *Contracted Services to Total Operating Expenditure*, (7) *Net Surplus/Deficit Water*, and (8) *Net Surplus/Deficit Electricity*. The descriptive statistics for the dataset are shown in Table 9.1.

The distribution of the absolute expenditure amounts is shown in Fig. 9.1, which indicates that, as expected, most of the expenditures are zero, with a long tail to the right. When the absolute expenditures are converted into binary output, we find that there are 66% instances where there was expenditure, with the remaining 34% being the case where there was no expenditure.

9.5.2 Experiment Description

We fit the Bayesian logistic regression model for the expenditure analysis. We consider the binary classification problem of whether a given financial has unauthorized expenditures. Thus, we encode the target as zero when there is no expenditure and one otherwise. We split the data into a train and test set using a 70-30 split.

Table 9.1 Descriptive statistics for the municipal expenditure dataset

Variable	*Mean*	*Std*	*Minimum*	*Median*	*Maximum*
Debt to community wealth/equity	1.918638e+04	7.245860e+05	–5.432387e+04	1.981498e+01	2.733321e+07
Debt to total operating revenue	0.543626	1.542988	0.000420	0.420812	57.019927
Current ratio	1.941543	2.272127	–4.651994	1.317792	39.337924
Net operating surplus margin %	3.642827	63.614750	–1988.345733	6.067438	93.920706
Remuneration % total operating expenditure	33.629575	26.419790	–529.064443	32.736612	511.085609
Contracted services % total operating expen	4.257592	7.523553	–38.771366	1.555004	81.189164
Net surplus/deficit water %	–8.865480e+07	1.041600e+09	–1.988261e+10	0.000000e+00	4.533188e+08
Net surplus/deficit elec %	–1.479726e+08	1.616702e+09	–4.777450e+10	0.000000e+00	1.632101e+09
Unauthorized expenditure	5.426093e+07	1.727075e+08	0.000000	6.105852e+06	3.244888e+09

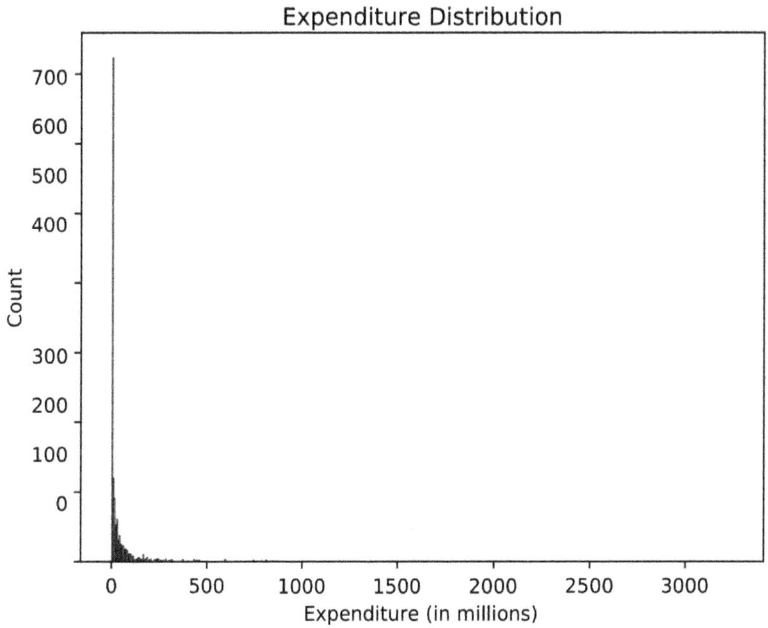

Fig. 9.1 Distribution of the expenditures on the South African municipality expenditure dataset

When fitting the Bayesian model, we generate a total of ten thousand samples, of which five thousand formed the burn-in period where tuning was performed for all the MCMC methods considered in this chapter. The step size parameters of all the methods were tuned using the primal-dual averaging methodology outlined in Hoffman and Gelman (2011) targeting an acceptance rate of 25% for MH, 60% for MALA and 80% for both HMC and MHMC. Note that the path length of HMC and MHMC was fixed at 100.

The following section discusses the performance metrics used to assess the MCMC methods.

9.5.3 Performance Metrics for MCMC Methods

We assess the performance of the algorithms by generating the trace plots of the un-normalized target posterior distribution, the effective sample sizes of the generated samples, the effective sample sizes of the generated samples normalized by execution time, and predictive performance on unseen data. Note that the execution time is the time taken to generate the samples after the burn-in period. We utilize the multivariate effective sample size metric developed by Vats et al. (2019) as our effective sample size measure (Marwala et al., 2023; Mongwe, 2022; Mongwe et al., 2021e).

The Receiver Operating Curve (ROC) and Area Under the ROC are the predictive performance metrics we employ to evaluate the outcomes of the Bayesian analysis. The model's true positives are shown on the y-axis against false positives on the x-axis on the ROC. The area under the ROC, or AUC, measures the average rate of misclassifications. When it comes to measuring performance when the costs of misclassification are unclear, AUC is useful (Bradley, 1997; Gaganis, 2009; Marwala et al., 2023; Mongwe & Malan, 2020a), which is the case for the expenditure detection task at hand.

9.6 Results and Discussion

In this section, we present the results and the discussions from the numerical experiments conducted in this chapter. Table 9.2 shows the relative ranking of the importance of the input variables across the MH, MALA, HMC, and MHMC methods. Figures 9.2, 9.3 show the inference results indicating the effective sample size, the effective sample size normalized by execution time, the diagnostic trace plots of the negative log-likelihood, and the predictive performance on unseen data using the Area Under the Receiver Operating Curve (AUC) metric.

Figures 9.2 and 9.3 show that the HMC algorithm outperforms all the other MCMC methods on an effective sample size basis, indicating the ability of HMC not to produce correlated samples. MALA has the second-highest effective sample sizes, with MH and MHMC having low effective sample sizes, indicating that these two methods produce very correlated samples. The poor performance of MHMC is likely due to a poor choice of the magnetic field for this particular task. This indicates the likely need to tune this parameter. However, Fig. 9.2b shows that, on a normalized (by execution time) effective sample size basis, the MALA outperforms all the methods. This is a testament to the fact that MALA has a very low execution time compared to the methods driven by Hamiltonian dynamics. We found that MH had the lowest execution time of all the methods, followed by MALA and HMC. MHMC had the largest execution time due to the extra computations required to take into account the magnetic field.

Figure 9.3a shows that all the MCMC methods have converged, albeit to different negative log-likelihoods. The MH algorithm converges to a higher and different negative log-likelihood than the other methods. This highlights the very poor exploration capabilities of the MH algorithm, as shown by its very low effective sample size. Figure 9.3b shows that the MH algorithm has the lowest predictive performance. HMC has the highest predictive performance, which aligns with the high effective sample sizes produced by this algorithm.

The relevance or importance of each feature, as indicated by α_i from Eq. (9.2), for each MCMC method, is shown in Figs. 9.4, 9.5. The analysis of the results reveals that the Metropolis-Hastings method cannot clearly rank the input features based on their importance due to its poor exploration of the target posterior (as it does not incorporate gradient information from the posterior, unlike the other three MCMC methods). This is shown by the importance of having similar magnitudes for the MH method. The other three MCMC algorithms could clearly distinguish the important variables from the less relevant features for the expenditure prediction problem. This can be seen in Figs. 9.4 and 9.5 by some features having near zero importance and some having larger importance for the three MCMC methods than the MH algorithm.

Table 9.2 shows the top three rankings of the importance of the features produced by each of the methods. The most commonly featured variable in the top three rankings are:

- Variable 3—*Current Ratio*: This is selected by MALA, MHMC, and HMC
- Variable 2—*Debt to Total Operating Revenue*: This is selected by MALA, HMC
- Variable 4—*Net Operating Surplus Margin %*: This is selected by MALA, HMC
- Variable 1—*Debt to Community Wealth/Equity*: This is selected by MH, MHMC

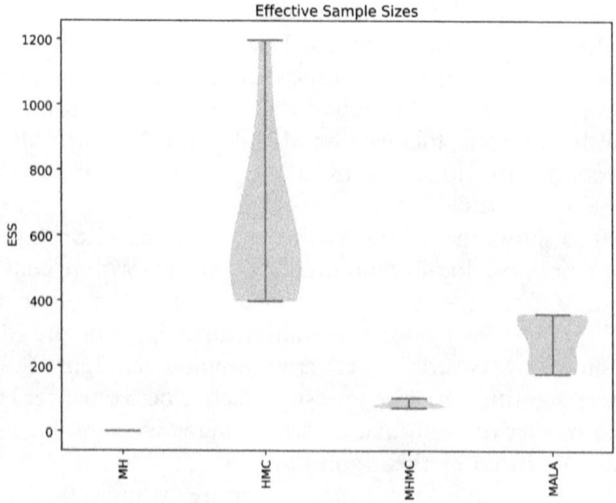

(a) Effective sample sizes across the MCMC methods.

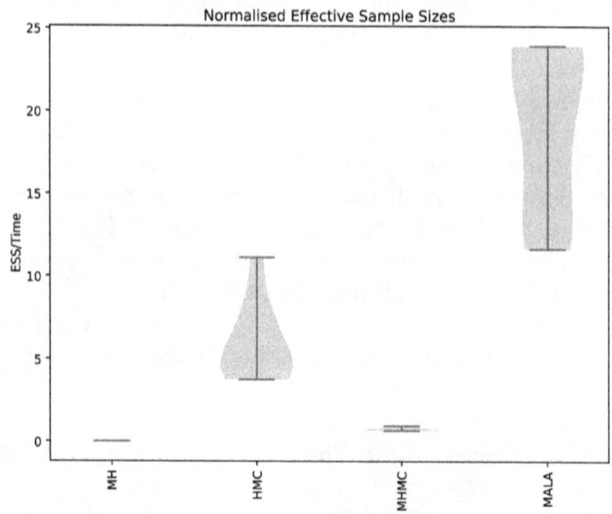

(b) Effective sample sizes normalized by execution time across the MCMC methods.

Fig. 9.2 Inference results for the Bayesian Framework across all the MCMC algorithms. **a** Effective sample sizes, and **b** Effective sample sizes normalized by execution time

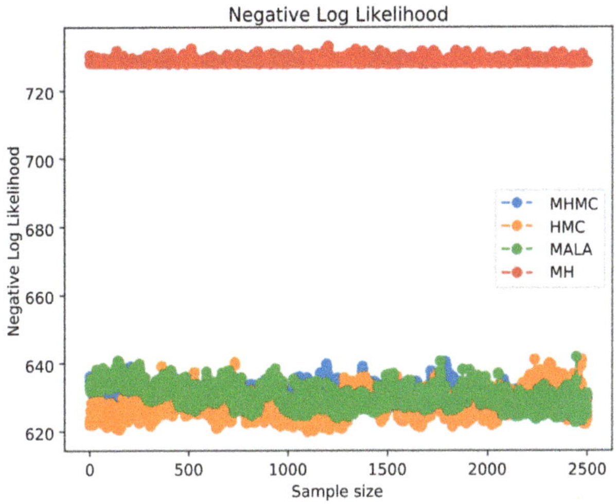

(**a**) Diagnostic negative log-likelihood trace plots across the MCMC methods.

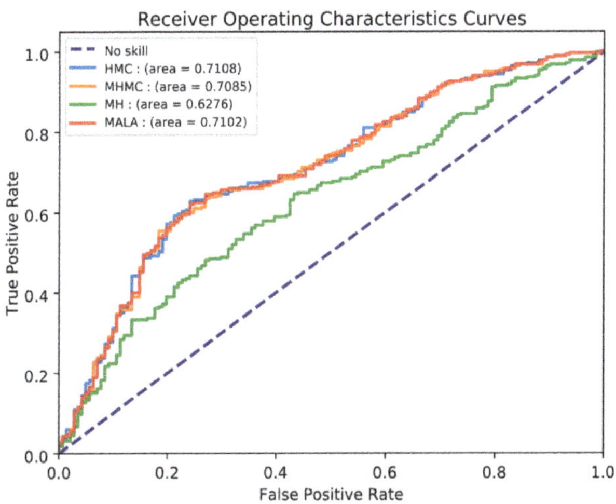

(**b**) Predictive performance across all the MCMC methods based on the Area under the Receiver Operating Curve metric.

Fig. 9.3 Inference results for the Bayesian Framework across all the MCMC algorithms. **a** Diagnostic negative log-likelihood trace plots, and **b** Predictive performance based on the Area Under the Receiver Operating Curve

Fig. 9.4 Mean posterior variances from each of the methods. The higher the value, the more important the variable is to the task of detecting modeling expenditures. **a** Importance for MH and **b** Importance for MALA

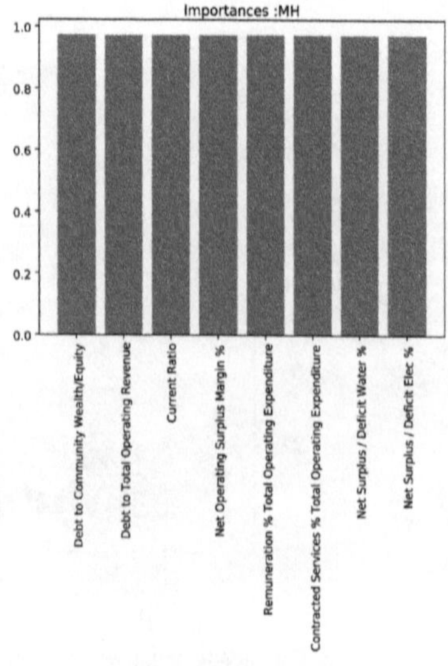

(**a**) Importance's for MH.

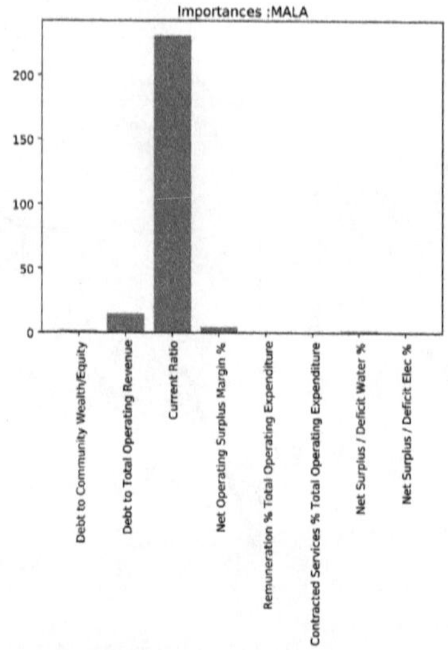

(**b**) Importance's for MALA.

Fig. 9.5 Mean posterior variances from each of the methods. The higher the value, the more important the variable is to the task of detecting modeling expenditures.
a Importance for MHMC and
b Importance for HMC

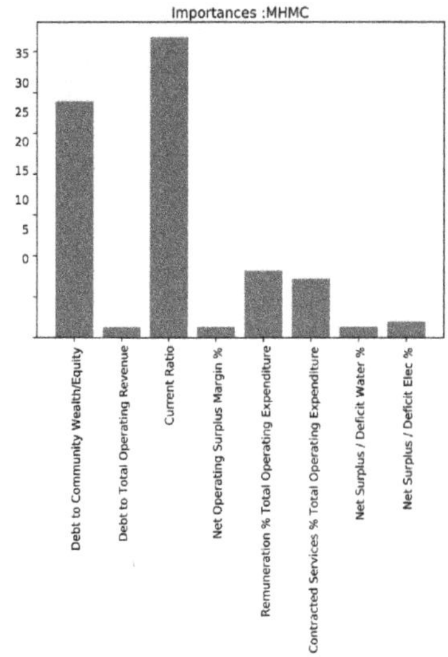

(a) Importance's for MHMC.

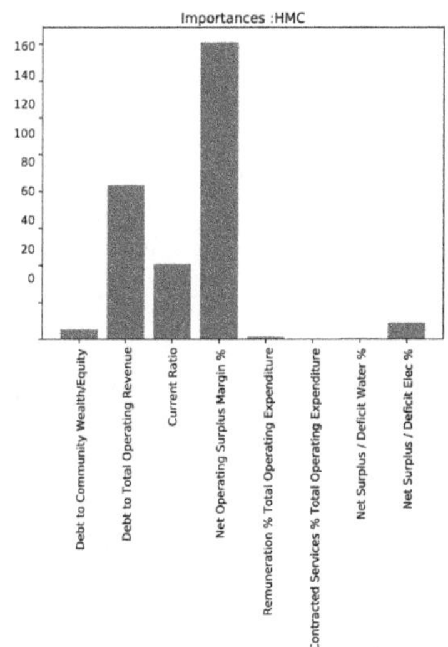

(b) Importance's for HMC.

Table 9.2 Ranking of the top three features by each method for the expenditure dataset. For example, HMC ranks variable four as the most important, while MH ranks variable six as the third most important

Ranking	*MH*	*MALA*	*MHMC*	*HMC*
1	6	3	3	4
2	1	2	1	2
3	5	4	5	3

- Variable 5—*Remuneration % Total Operating Expenditure*: This is selected by MH, MHMC

These results show that the three MCMC methods that incorporate gradient information from the target posterior broadly agree on which features are important. In particular, the analysis shows that some of the variables important for modeling the expenditure are based on *current ratio* and *debt to operating revenue*—which is consistent with results from the analysis of audit opinions conducted in Marwala et al. (2023), Mabelane et al. (2023), Mongwe (2022), Mongwe et al. (2021d).

The overall results suggest that the MCMC methods that can intelligently explore the posterior can result in better predictive performance on unseen data and more insightful information about which features are the most relevant for the unauthorized expenditure prediction task at hand. This can be seen by HMC and MALA producing better results than MH across various metrics, even on a time-normalized basis.

9.7 Conclusions

We provide a first-in-literature application of a Bayesian inference framework to analyze local government expenditure data from a developing democracy. In the Bayesian framework, we utilize Bayesian logistic regression with an automatic relevance determination (ARD) prior. We train this Bayesian model using the Metropolis-Hastings (MH), Metropolis-Hastings Adjusted Langevin Algorithm (MALA), Hamiltonian Monte Carlo (HMC), Magnetic Hamiltonian Monte Carlo (MHMC), and Markov Chain Monte Carlo (MCMC) methods.

We find that the MH algorithm has the lowest execution time, followed by the MALA, with MHMC having the longest execution time.

On an effective sample size (ESS) basis, we find that HMC produces the highest ESS, followed by MALA, with MH producing the lowest ESS. On a time-normalized ESS basis, we find that HMC outperforms all the methods followed by MALA—with MH still being the laggard. We further find that HMC produced the best predictive performance on unseen data, while MH produced the poorest performance. MHMC and MALA produce predictive performance similar to HMC, with MALA coming in at second and MHMC third.

When analyzing the results of the sampled ARD prior variance, we find that the MCMC methods agree on which variables are important. In particular, we find that *current ratio* and *debt to operating revenue* delivery are key in determining which entity has unauthorized expenditure. The work in this chapter can be expanded by considering the case of detecting the absolute value of the unauthorized expenditure and jointly modeling the other unlawful spending, such as irregular, fruitless, and wasteful expenditures.

The following chapter will model motor insurance claims within a Bayesian framework. Our framework also allows us to select between different Bayesian neural network architectures using the Bayesian evidence metric and highlight which inputs are the most relevant for the claim prediction task.

References

Auditor-General South Africa. (2011). *Background to the three aspects we audit.* https://www.agsa.co.za/portals/0/AGSA_Terminology.pdf. Last Retrieved: 16 August 2020.

Auditor-General South Africa. (2023). *Consololidated general report on local government audit outcomes - mfma 2021-22.* https://mfma-2022.agsareports.co.za/report/mfma_report_2021_22_final_31_may_2023.pdf. Last Retrieved: 16 November 2023.

Bradley, A. P. (1997). The use of the area under the ROC curve in the evaluation of machine learning algorithms. *Pattern Recognition, 30*(7), 1145–1159. https://doi.org/10.1016/s0031-3203(96)00142-2

Brofos, J. A., & Lederman, R. R. (2020). Non-canonical Hamiltonian Monte Carlo. arXiv preprint arXiv:2008.08191

Chandrashekar, G., & Sahin, F. (Jan. 2014). A survey on feature selection methods. *Computers & Electrical Engineering, 40*(1), 16–28. https://doi.org/10.1016/j.compeleceng.2013.11.024

Dlomo, P. A. (2017). The impact of irregular expenditure in the South African public finance with specific reference to the National Department of Public Works. PhD thesis. Cape Peninsula University of Technology.

Duane, S., Kennedy, A. D., Pendleton, B. J., & Roweth, D. (1987). Hybrid Monte Carlo. *Physics Letters B, 195*(2), 216–222.

Gaganis, C. (July2009). Classification techniques for the identification of falsified financial statements: A comparative analysis. *Intelligent Systems in Accounting, Finance & Management, 16*(3), 207–229. https://doi.org/10.1002/isaf.303

Girolami, M., & Calderhead, B. (2011). Riemann manifold langevin and hamiltonian monte carlo methods. *Journal of the Royal Statistical Society: Series B (Statistical Methodology), 73*(2), 123–214.

Gu, M., & Sun, S. (2020). Neural Langevin dynamical sampling. *IEEE Access, 8*, 31595–31605.

Hastings, W. K. (1970). Monte Carlo sampling methods using Markov chains and their applications. *Biometrica, 57*(1), 97–109.

Hoffman, M. D., & Gelman, A. (2011). *The No-U-Turn Sampler: Adaptively setting path lengths in Hamiltonian Monte Carlo.* arXiv:1111.4246 [stat.CO]

Hoffman, M. D., & Gelman, A. (2014). The No-U-turn sampler: Adaptively setting path lengths in Hamiltonian Monte Carlo. *Journal of Machine Learning Research, 15*(1), 1593–1623.

Kirkos, E., Spathis, C., & Manolopoulos, Y. (May 2007). Data mining techniques for the detection of fraudulent financial statements. *Expert Systems with Applications, 32*(4), 995–1003. https://doi.org/10.1016/j.eswa.2006.02.016

Mabelane, K., Mongwe, W. T., Mbuvha, R., & Marwala, T. (2023). An analysis of local government financial statement audit outcomes in a developing economy using machine learning. *Sustainability, 15*(1), 12.

MacKay, D. J. C. (1995). Probable networks and plausible predictions—a review of practical Bayesian methods for supervised neural networks. *Network: Computation in Neural Systems, 6*(3), 469–505.

Marwala, T., Mbuvha, R., & Mongwe, W. T. (2023). *Hamiltonian Monte Carlo methods in machine learning*. Elsevier.

Mbuvha, R., & Marwala, T. (2020). Bayesian inference of COVID-19 spreading rates in South Africa. *PloS One, 15*(8), Article e0237126.

Mbuvha, R., Mongwe, W. T., & Marwala, T. (2021). Separable Shadow Hamiltonian Hybrid Monte Carlo for Bayesian neural network inference in wind speed forecasting. *Energy and A, 1*, Article 100108.

Moepya, S. O., Akhoury, S. S., & Nelwamondo, F. V. (Dec. 2014). Applying cost-sensitive classification for financial fraud detection under high class-imbalance. In *2014 IEEE international conference on data mining workshop* (pp. 183–192). IEEE. https://doi.org/10.1109/icdmw.2014.141

Mongwe, W. T. (2022). *Hybrid Monte Carlo methods in machine learning: Stochastic volatility methods, shadow Hamiltonians, adaptive approaches and variance reduction techniques*. University of Johannesburg (South Africa).

Mongwe, W. T., & Malan, K. M. (2020a). A survey of automated financial statement fraud detection with relevance to the South African Context. *South African Computer Journal, 32*(1). https://doi.org/10.18489/sacj.v32i1.777

Mongwe, W. T., & Malan, K. M. (2020b). The efficacy of financial ratios for fraud detection using self organising maps. In *2020 IEEE symposium series on computational intelligence (SSCI)* (pp. 1100–1106). IEEE.

Mongwe, W. T., Mbuvha, R., & Marwala, T. (2021a). Adaptive magnetic Hamiltonian Monte Carlo. *IEEE Access, 9*, 152993–153003. https://doi.org/10.1109/ACCESS.2021.3127931

Mongwe, W. T., Mbuvha, R., & Marwala, T. (2021b). Adaptively setting the path length for separable shadow Hamiltonian hybrid Monte Carlo. *IEEE Access, 9*, 138598–138607.

Mongwe, W. T., Mbuvha, R., & Marwala, T. (2021c). Antithetic magnetic and Shadow Hamiltonian Monte Carlo. *IEEE Access, 9*, 49857–49867.

Mongwe, W. T., Mbuvha, R., & Marwala, T. (2021d). Bayesian inference of local government audit outcomes. *Plos One*. https://doi.org/10.1371/journal.pone.0261245

Mongwe, W. T., Mbuvha, R., & Marwala, T. (2021e). Locally scaled and stochastic volatility metropolis-hastings algorithms. *Algorithms, 14*(12). ISSN: 1999-4893. https://doi.org/10.3390/a14120351. https://www.mdpi.com/1999-4893/14/12/351

Mongwe, W. T., Mbuvha, R., & Marwala, T. (2021f). Magnetic Hamiltonian Monte Carlo with partial momentum refreshment. *IEEE Access, 9*, 108009–108016. https://doi.org/10.1109/ACCESS.2021.3101810

Mongwe, W. T., Mbuvha, R., & Marwala, T. (2021g). Quantum-Inspired Magnetic Hamiltonian Monte Carlo. *Plos One, 16*(10), Article e0258277.

Mongwe, W. T., Mbuvha, R., & Marwala, T. (2021h). Utilising partial momentum refreshment in separable Shadow Hamiltonian Hybrid Monte Carlo. *IEEE Access, 9*, 151235–151244. https://doi.org/10.1109/ACCESS.2021.3126812

Mongwe, W. T., Mbuvha, R., & Marwala, T. (2022a). Shadow magnetic Hamiltonian Monte Carlo. *IEEE Access, 10*, 34340–34351. https://doi.org/10.1109/ACCESS.2022.3161443

Mongwe, W. T., Sidogi, T., Mbuvha, R., & Marwala, T. (2022b). Probabilistic inference of south african equity option prices under jump-diffusion processes. In *2022 IEEE symposium on computational intelligence for financial engineering and economics (CIFEr)* (pp. 1–8). IEEE.

Motubatse, K. N., & Ngwakwe, C. (2020). Factors associated with the risk of irregular expenditure in the public sector. *Southern African Journal of Accountability and Auditing Research, 22*(1), 51–58.

Neal, R. M. (1993). Bayesian learning via stochastic dynamics. In *Advances in neural information processing systems* (Vol. 5, pp. 475–482). Morgan Kaufmann Publishers Inc. ISBN: 1-55860-274-7. http://dl.acm.org/citation.cfm?id=645753.667903.

Neal, R. M. (2012). *Bayesian learning for neural networks* (Vol. 118). Springer Science & Business Media.

Neal, R. M., et al. (2011). MCMC using Hamiltonian dynamics. *Handbook of Markov Chain Monte Carlo, 2*(11), 2.

Sikhosana, M. J. (2021). The relationship between unlawful expenditure and municipal financial performance in a South African context. PhD thesis.

Tripuraneni, N., Rowland, M., Ghahramani, Z., & Turner, R. (2017). Magnetic hamiltonian monte carlo. In *International conference on machine learning*. PMLR (pp. 3453–3461).

Vats, D., Flegal, J. M., & Jones, G. L (Apr. 2019). Multivariate output analysis for Markov chain Monte Carlo. *Biometrika, 106*(2), 321–337. ISSN: 0006-3444. eprint: https://academic.oup.com/biomet/article-pdf/106/2/321/28575440/asz002.pdf

CHAPTER 10

Bayesian Neural Network Inference of Motor Insurance Claims

10.1 Introduction

Insurance is a type of risk management that provides cover against unforeseen losses brought on by unfavorable circumstances (Huyssteen & Rudansky-Kloppers, 2024). Insurance covers numerous causes of loss, such as death and property damage. While general insurance covers all non-life insurance, life insurance is specific to an individual or group of individuals' lives. General insurance is usually short-term, while life insurance is typically long-term. The motor insurance subset of general insurance is the subject of this chapter (Huyssteen & Rudansky-Kloppers, 2024).

Motor insurance is a request for financial coverage caused by an automobile-related potential loss (Fauzan & Murfi, 2018; Huyssteen & Rudansky-Kloppers, 2024). A motor insurance policy typically provides comprehensive cover, including theft, accidents, and third-party cover (Fauzan & Murfi, 2018). This business has grown due to more demand for insurance as more people have access to vehicles. South Africa has the highest insurance penetration rate in Africa, notwithstanding the

---

Supplementary Information The online version contains supplementary material available at https://doi.org/10.1007/978-3-031-88431-3_10.

W. T. Mongwe et al., *Bayesian Machine Learning in Quantitative Finance*, https://doi.org/10.1007/978-3-031-88431-3_10

continent's low level of penetration in general (Huyssteen & Rudansky-Kloppers, 2024). Motor vehicle insurance is the most significant contributor to the African non-life insurance industry. However, this is mostly due to the mandatory third-party insurance requirements in nations like Morocco, Kenya, Nigeria, and Egypt (Olayungbo & Akinlo, 2016). South Africa is one of the few countries that do not obligate motorists to have motor vehicle insurance, not even third-party insurance—with the road accident fund covering aspects of this within the South African context (Huyssteen & Rudansky-Kloppers, 2024).

Motor insurance is one of the insurance products that generates massive amounts of data. Understanding the frequency, size, and cause of claims is essential for insurance companies as it determines the profitability of the basis and is also a step in detecting possibly fraudulent claims (Clemente et al., 2023; Mohd Yunos et al., 2013; Huyssteen & Rudansky-Kloppers, 2024). Claim modeling in motor insurance is typically undertaken using generalized linear models (GLM) modeling claim frequency and severity. Traditional GLM frequency-severity models assume a linear input-output mapping and independence between the claim frequency and severity (Clemente et al., 2023). Due to increased computing power and data, machine learning techniques are gaining traction for modeling motor insurance claims.

The machine learning models typically used to model claim severity and frequency are gradient-boosted trees and artificial neural networks (Clemente et al., 2023; Mohd Yunos et al., 2013). Clemente et al. (2023) employed gradient boosting with decision trees as base learners to model the claim frequency and severity distributions of a significant auto insurance dataset, comparing the results with those derived from a standard GLM model and concluded that the superior trees outperformed the latter. Their results indicate that gradient-boosted models are an invaluable asset for insurers in feature engineering and the development of a data-driven strategy for risk management and insurance, as they effectively capture complex interactions and non-linear relationships between the response variable and feature variables (Clemente et al., 2023). On the other hand, Mohd Yunos et al. (2013) utilized artificial neural networks and the ANFIS method to model data from the Malaysian motor insurance sector and found that both models produce a reliable prediction of insurance claims frequency and severity.

It is also possible to re-frame the motor insurance claim prediction problem as a classification problem in which our goal is to forecast the likelihood of a policyholder filing a claim. Machine learning has been applied to the problem of claim prediction in several papers. Weerasinghe and Wijegunasekara (Weerasinghe & Wijegunasekara, 2016) compared which machine learning method performs best in predicting the claim size of a policyholder. They compared neural networks, decision trees, and multinomial logistic regression. Their results indicated that neural networks were the best predictor. Smith et al. (2000) used decision trees and neural networks to predict whether a policyholder will file a claim. Fauzan and Murfi (2018) compared XGBoost, Adaboost, random forest, and neural networks for the claim prediction task. They found that XSGBoost outperformed their dataset. The literature indicates that neural networks are one of the commonly used techniques for claim prediction tasks. However, very little attention has been paid in the literature to Bayesian approaches, which allow uncertainty to be incorporated into predictions. We aim to fill this gap in this chapter.

In this chapter, we utilize a Bayesian framework for predicting claims on motor insurance policy. We use Bayesian neural networks with automatic relevance determination prior distributions to predict the motor claims. The automatic relevance determination prior also allows us to rank the importance of the input variables. Typically, the posterior of BNNs does not exist in closed form and has to be approximated using numerical methods. Normally, this inference can be undertaken using variational inference or Markov chain Monte Carlo (MCMC) methods. MCMC methods are preferable as they are guaranteed to converge to the true posterior but have the disadvantage of being computationally expensive compared to variational approaches (Mongwe et al., 2022). In this chapter we focus on a variant of variation inference to train the neural network models.

Bayesian inference can be implemented for parameter estimation and model selection. With parameter estimation, one is concerned about attaining the most plausible parameters for a given model. This is usually carried out using sampling approaches such as MCMC (Neal, 1993). Model selection involves calculating each model's marginal over the parameters likelihood (or the evidence). This Bayesian evidence indicates how well a given model fits the observed dataset compared to another model (MacKay, 1992). The evidence metric is not trivial to evaluate analytically and requires numerical methods (Marwala et al., 2016; Russel et al., 2019). This is the case for complex models where the parameter space has a high dimension, such as neural networks. Many techniques have been proposed for calculating the marginal likelihood, including Bayesian quadrature (Osborne et al., 2012), nested sampling (Mthembu et al., 2011; Skilling, 2004), and the Laplace approximation of MacKay (1992).

The Bayesian quadrature approach uses a small number of likelihood observations to infer a distribution of the marginal likelihood (Gunter et al., 2014; Marwala et al., 2023; Mongwe, 2022; Osborne et al., 2012). This approach offers improved sample efficiency, which is essential for samples drawn from complex and computationally expensive models. Bayesian quadrature has, however, displayed high variance around the evidence estimate and convergence diagnostics due to variations in the sample observations selected (Gunter et al., 2014). The nested sampling approach of Skilling (2006) provides advantages over other evidence approximation techniques in that it transforms the evidence integral into a 1-dimensional integral, thus reducing the computational burden. It further calculates the evidence and provides the posterior parameter estimates all in one run at no extra cost. MacKay (1992) uses the evidence framework in the context of multi-layer perceptrons where the posterior distribution of the parameters was approximated using a Gaussian Laplace approximation. This approximation simplifies the calculation of the Bayesian evidence metric. The Laplace approximation has been found to provide inferior evidence estimates due to approximation errors of the Laplace approximation to the true multi-modal posterior (Mbuvha et al., 2017). This leads to trivial or extremely regularized model selection. However, compared to the alternative evidence methods, the place approximations allow one to scale to larger models—which would not be practical with other approaches. The Laplace approximation is the approach that we employ in this chapter.

The remainder of this chapter is structured as follows: We first discuss the Bayesian neural network models in Sect. 10.2 and the corresponding Laplace approximation we use to train the neural networks in Sect. 10.3. We then present the numerical experiments we conducted in Sect. 10.4, after which we present and discuss the results and provide the conclusion in Sects. 10.5–10.6 respectively.

10.2 Bayesian Neural Network Models

Neural networks are universal function approximators inspired by the functioning of the human brain. They have driven various advancements across multiple industries (Horvath et al., 2021; Marwala et al., 2023; Mongwe, 2022). Neural networks consist of a group of neurons arranged in a series of layers, where each layer's input is the previous layer's neuron activations, and each layer's output is a weighted sum of the input followed by a non-linear activation (Montavon et al., 2018).

The network's neurons cooperatively implement a sophisticated non-linear mapping from the input to the output (Montavon et al., 2018). In this chapter, we consider fully connected feed-forward neural networks of

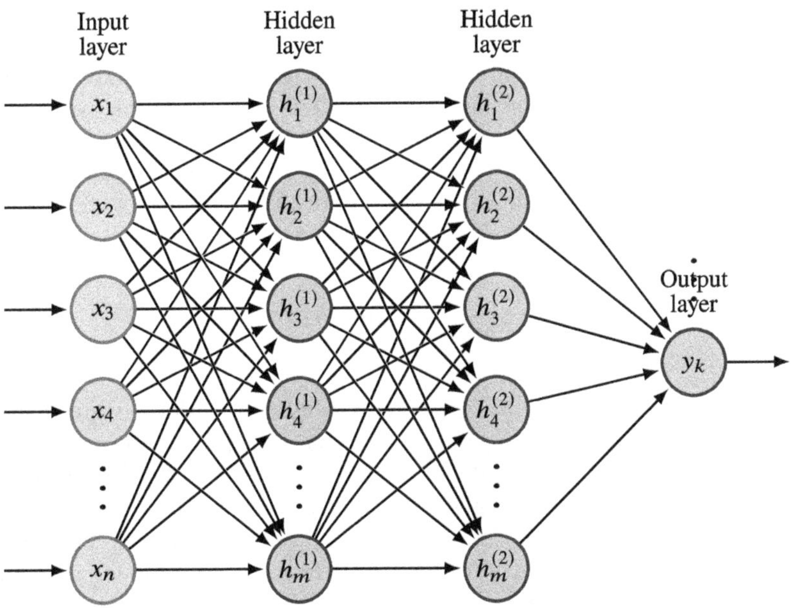

Fig. 10.1 An illustration of the data flow in a feed-forward neural network. In this chapter, we consider various architectures of Bayesian neural networks and compare their performance

the form depicted in Fig. 10.1 with the layers defined as:

$$f_k(x) = b_k + \sum_j v_{jk} h_j(x) \tag{10.1}$$

$$h_j(x) = \Psi\left(a_j + \sum_i w_{ij} x_i\right) \tag{10.2}$$

where w_{ij} is the weight connection for the ith previous layer input to the jth hidden unit and v_{jk} is the weight connection between the jth hidden unit to the kth output, with $k = 1$ in this chapter. The activation function Ψ provides the non-linearity required to approximate complex non-linear relationships between inputs and outputs. This chapter uses the *tanh* activation function across all the hidden layers.

The Bayesian framework facilitates the incorporation of prior conditions regarding the distribution of network weights. These conditions may be specified individually or universally for all weights within the network. The Bayesian framework's foundation emanates from Bayes theorem, which defines the posterior distribution of parameters given the data and prior distributional assumptions. In the context of a neural network model with architecture H, weights $\mathbf{w}$, and training dataset D, Bayes theorem translates to (MacKay, 1995b; Mbuvha et al., 2017, 2021):

$$P(\mathbf{w}|D, H) = \frac{P(D|\mathbf{w}, H)P(\mathbf{w}|H)}{P(D|H)} \tag{10.3}$$

where $P(\mathbf{w}|D, H)$ is the posterior probability of the weights given the data and model architecture, and $P(D|\mathbf{w}, H)$ is the likelihood of the data given the model. $P(\mathbf{w}|H)$ is the prior probability of the weights. $P(D|H)$ is the probability of the data given the model—referred to as the Bayesian evidence (Mbuvha et al., 2017; Mongwe, 2022). From the posterior $P(\mathbf{w}|D, H)$ one gets the parameter estimates for a given model M_i with architecture H_i, while the evidence for model M_i given by $P(D|H_i)$ allows one to compare models using the Bayes factor (Kass & Raftery, 1995):

$$BF := \frac{P(D|H_1)}{P(D|H_2)} \frac{\pi(M_1)}{\pi(M_2)} \tag{10.4}$$

where $\pi(M_i)$ is the prior belief for model i. Values of the Bayes factor greater than one are considered as evidence in favor of model M_1 and vice versa (Kass & Raftery, 1995). If one has no prior belief that one model is better than another (which is usually the case in practice), the prior probabilities of all the models are made equal so that comparing models amounts to comparing the model evidence. The posterior $P(\mathbf{w}|D, H)$ is usually analytically intractable for complicated models. The posterior distribution must then be estimated using numerical methods (MacKay, 1992; Speagle, 2020). In this chapter, we use the Laplace approximation of the posterior. The neural network architectures that we compare in this chapter are as follows:

- **Model 1:** Bayesian neural network with a single hidden layer and five hidden neurons. This model has a total of 137 parameters for the dataset under consideration.
- **Model 2:** Bayesian neural network with a single hidden layer and ten hidden neurons. For the dataset under consideration, this model has 272 parameters.
- **Model 3:** Bayesian neural network with a single hidden layer and 50 hidden neurons. For the dataset under consideration, this model has 1352 parameters.
- **Model 4:** Bayesian neural network with two hidden layers and five hidden neurons in each hidden layer. For the dataset under consideration, this model has 162 parameters.
- **Model 5:** Bayesian neural network with two hidden layers and ten hidden neurons in each hidden layer. For the dataset under consideration, this model has 372 parameters.
- **Model 6:** Bayesian neural network with three hidden layers and ten hidden neurons in each hidden layer. This model has a total of 472 parameters for the dataset under consideration.

As seen above, we compare neural network architectures with one hidden layer, two hidden layers, and three hidden layers. The next section discusses the Laplace approximation used in this chapter.

10.3 Laplace Approximation to Bayesian Neural Networks

For inference in Bayesian deep learning, the Laplace approximation (LA) provides a straightforward, economical, and competitive approximation technique (Daxberger et al., 2021). It approximates the posterior locally using a Gaussian distribution centered at a local maximum and a covariance matrix matching the local curvature. The local maximum can be easily obtained from standard maximum a posteriori (MAP) training of NNs, one of the LA's main advantages (Daxberger et al., 2021; MacKay, 1995a). Curvature estimates can also be obtained quickly and effectively with the help of recent developments in second-order optimization, which include more effective Hessian approximations and user-friendly software libraries (Daxberger et al., 2021). These factors make LA an easy-to-use and practical approach to consider. It is also readily applicable to already trained neural network models, enabling practitioners to turn their already high-performing deep learning models from producing point estimates to producing distributions of predictions (Daxberger et al., 2021). The LA also produces the marginal likelihood that can be used for model selection , neural network training, or both (Daxberger et al., 2021).

The Laplace approximation to the posterior distribution was first proposed by MacKay (1995a) in the context of Bayesian neural networks. In this framework, the prior distribution is assumed to be Gaussian with mean zero and precision α, which results in the exact posterior distribution of the parameters having the form (MacKay, 1995a):

$$P(\mathbf{w}|\alpha, \beta, D, H) = \frac{1}{Z_M(\alpha, \beta)} \exp\left(-(\alpha E_{\mathbf{w}} + \beta E_D)\right) \tag{10.5}$$

$$P(\mathbf{w}|\alpha, \beta, D, H) = \frac{1}{Z_M(\alpha, \beta)} \exp\left(-M(\mathbf{w})\right) \tag{10.6}$$

where D is the data, H is the model specification, $M(\mathbf{w}) = \alpha E_{\mathbf{w}} + \beta E_D$, $\alpha E_{\mathbf{w}}$ is the kernel of the prior distribution on the parameters, βE_D is the kernel of the likelihood and $Z_M(\alpha, \beta)$ is the normalizing constant. The posterior distribution is not computationally tractable in closed form. The Gaussian approximation to the posterior of MacKay (1995a) is based on performing a second-order Taylor approximation of the posterior around the mode of the posterior. The approximation is given as:

$$P(\mathbf{w}|\alpha, \beta, D, H) \approx \frac{1}{Z'_M(\alpha, \beta)} \exp\left(-M(\mathbf{w}) - \frac{1}{2}W(\alpha, \beta)\right) \tag{10.7}$$

where

$$W(\alpha, \beta) = (\mathbf{w} - \mathbf{w}_{MP})^T \mathbf{A}(\mathbf{w} - \mathbf{w}_{MP}) \tag{10.8}$$

$\mathbf{w}_{MP}$ is the mode of the posterior, and $\mathbf{A}$ is the matrix of second derivatives of the negative log posterior. The normalizing constant $Z'_M(\alpha, \beta)$ can then be evaluated as follows (Bishop, 1997; MacKay, 1992):

$$Z'_M(\alpha, \beta) = \int \exp\left(-M(\mathbf{w}) - \frac{1}{2}(\mathbf{w} - w_{MP})^T \mathbf{A}(\mathbf{w} - \mathbf{w}_{MP})\right) d\mathbf{w} \tag{10.9}$$

$$= \exp\left(-M(\mathbf{w})\right)(2\pi)^{-g/2} det(\mathbf{A})^{-\frac{1}{2}} \tag{10.10}$$

where g represents the number of parameters for the neural network. Using this formulation, one can learn the precision α of the prior distribution. The precision of the prior is the one that maximizes the evidence. Using the Gaussian approximation above, the evidence becomes computationally feasible, and α and β can be approximated by alternating between the gradient descent for the parameters and maximizing the evidence. The optimal α and β can be found by taking derivatives of the log evidence. In this chapter, we use the **Laplace** package in Python (Daxberger et al., 2021).

10.4 Numerical Experiments

In this section, we present the numerical experiments conducted in this chapter. We describe the dataset and then outline the experiments, settings, and performance metrics.

10.4.1 Data Description

The data consists of 3000 records of insurance data from a Spanish insurance company concerning a non-life motor insurance portfolio described in Segura-Gisbert et al. (2024). The features of the dataset are shown below (Segura-Gisbert et al., 2024):

1. **ID**—Unique identification number allocated to each annual contract established by an insured party. Each policyholder may possess multiple entries in the dataset, indicating various product annuities.
2. **Date start contract**—Commencement date of the policyholder's contract (DD/MM/YYYY).
3. **Date last renewal**—Last contract renewal date (DD/MM/YYYY).
4. **Date next renewal**—Next contract renewal date (DD/MM/YYYY).
5. **Distribution channel**—Classifies the medium through which the policy was established. 0 denotes Agents, and 1 signifies Insurance Brokers.
6. **Date birth**—The insured's date of birth specified in the policy (DD/MM/YYYY).
7. **Date driving license** Date of issuance of the insured individual's driver's license (DD/MM/YYYY).
8. **Seniority**—The total duration of the insured's affiliation with the insurance entity, reflecting their degree of seniority.
9. **Policies in force** —The aggregate number of policies the insured maintains within the organization during the specified timeframe.
10. **Max policies**—Greatest quantity of policies that the insured has previously maintained with the insurance entity.
11. **Max products**—Maximum quantity of products the insured has concurrently possessed at any moment.
12. **Lapse**—The count of policies the customer has terminated or been annulled due to nonpayment in the current maturity year, excluding those substituted by another policy.
13. **Date lapse**—Date of contract cessation (DD/MM/YYYY).
14. **Payment**—Final payment method of the reference policy. One signifies a semiannual administrative procedure, while 0 denotes an annual payment method.
15. **Premium**—Net premium amount related to the policy for the current year.
16. **R Claims history**—Proportion of claims submitted for the specific policy relative to the total duration (in complete years) of the policy's validity. It denotes the historical frequency of claims associated with the policy. It excludes claims from the current year.

17. **Type risk**—Category of risk linked to the policy. Each value is associated with a particular risk category: 1 for motorcycles, 2 for vans, 3 for automobiles, and 4 for agricultural vehicles.
18. **Area**—A dichotomous variable denotes the area. Assign 0 for rural areas and 1 for urban areas (populations exceeding 30,000) regarding traffic conditions.
19. **Second driver**—1 if multiple regular drivers are declared, or 0 if only one driver is declared.
20. **Year matriculation**—Registration of the vehicle year (YYYY).
21. **Power**—Vehicle power measured in horsepower.
22. **Cylinder capacity**—Vehicle Cylinder capacity.
23. **Value vehicle**—Market value of the vehicle on 31/12/2019.
24. **N doors**—Number of vehicle doors.
25. **Type fuel**—Specific energy source used to power a vehicle. Petrol (P) or Diesel (D).
26. **Length**—Length, in meters, of the vehicle.
27. **Weight**—Weight, in kilograms, of the vehicle.

The target variable was encoded as whether or not the policy had a claim for the given year. All features are normalized using the min-max scaler before being utilized. Only 18% of the instances were claims, which means that the dataset is highly imbalanced.

10.4.2 Experiment Setup and Performance Metrics

We compute the log evidence for each model on the training data. The log evidence allows us to select between the different models–the higher the log evidence, the better the model. The Receiver Operating Curve (ROC) and Area Under the ROC are the predictive performance metrics we employ to evaluate the outcomes of the Bayesian analysis. The model's true positives are shown on the y-axis against false positives on the x-axis on the ROC. The Area Under the ROC, or AUC, measures the average rate of misclassifications. When measuring performance when misclassification costs are unclear, AUC is applicable (Bradley, 1997; Gaganis, 2009; Marwala et al., 2023; Mongwe, 2022; Mongwe & Malan, 2020). We also compute the accuracy of each model on unseen data.

Note that we use a standard Gaussian distribution as the prior for the weights. We ran the steps of the algorithm for 150 iterations. All our computations were performed in Python using the **Laplace** PyTorch package.

10.5 Results and Discussions

In this section, we present the results and the discussions from the numerical experiments conducted in this chapter. Table 10.1 shows the log Bayesian evidence on training data and performance on unseen for all the six BNN models. Table 10.2 shows all the models' pair-wise model comparisons using the natural log Bayes factor. Figure 10.2 shows the predictive performance on unseen data across all the models and the marginal likelihood convergence profile across all the models. Figure 10.3 relative ranking of the input features for each of the models, and Table 10.3 shows the top six variable ranking from each model.

Table 10.1 shows that Model 5 (a two-layer neural network with ten hidden nodes) has the highest log evidence on training data and outperformed on the AUC and accuracy metrics on unseen data. This shows the robustness of using the evidence metric for model selection. Furthermore, we note that Model 5 has 372 parameters, with the model with the largest number of parameters being Model 3. This shows that the log evidence metric can also penalize unnecessarily complex models to end up with a parsimonious model that best explains the variability in the data. Table 10.2 shows in the pair-wise comparisons that Model 6 has the

Table 10.1 Log evidence on training data and AUC and Accuracy on unseen data across the various models. The entries in **bold** indicate outperformance on that metric. The higher the log evidence, the better the model. The higher the AUC and Accuracy, the better the model

Metric	*Model 1*	*Model 2*	*Model 3*	*Model 4*	*Model 5*	*Model 6*
Number of parameters	137	272	1352	162	372	472
Log evidence	−379.2679	−375.7517	−390.8010	−377.9036	**−336.2736**	−363.4986
AUC	0.777896	0.782822	0.803480	0.756140	**0.8406886**	0.7679519
Accuracy	0.890762	0.891538	0.896153	0.891538	**0.9130769**	0.8938461

Table 10.2 Pair-wise model comparisons through the natural log Bayes factor for all models using the log evidence. The comparison is between the columns and the rows. For example, the Bayes factor for Model 5 vs Model 2 is 39.47

	Model 1	*Model 2*	*Model 3*	*Model 4*	*Model 5*	*Model 6*
Model 1	x	3.51	−11.53	1.36	42.99	15.76
Model 2		x	−15.04	−2.15	39.47	12.25
Model 3			x	12.89	54.52	27.30
Model 4				x	41.63	14.40
Model 5					x	−27.22
Model 6						x

highest support based on the evidence across all models except Model 5, with Model 3 being the model with the lowest Bayesian evidence. This table shows that all pair-wise model comparisons show a significant difference in the models as per Jeffreys' scale (Nesseris and Garcia-Bellido, 2013). This analysis suggests that deeper neural network architectures are preferred to wider (but shallow) architectures.

Figure 10.2 shows that all the models have converged, as shown by each model's marginal likelihood convergence profile. Furthermore, Fig. 10.2 also visually shows the predictive performance on unseen data results shown in Table 10.1 for the AUC metric. Figure 10.3 shows the relative ranking of the variables across all the models. The results show that the models broadly agree on which variables are the most important for the motor claim prediction task. The top six rankings of the variables across the models are shown in Table 10.3. The results show that the most critical variable across all the models is claim history, followed by features related to the vehicle, such as the type of fuel and power, as well as the number of policies and products the client has with the insurance company.

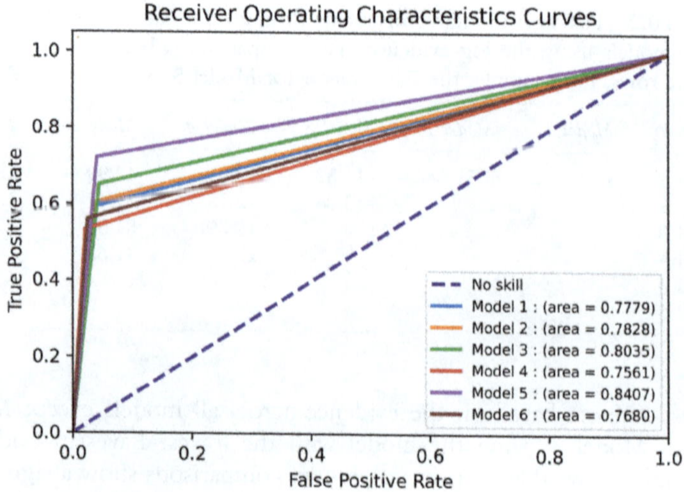

(**a**) Predictive performance based on the Area under the Receiver Operating Curve across all the models.

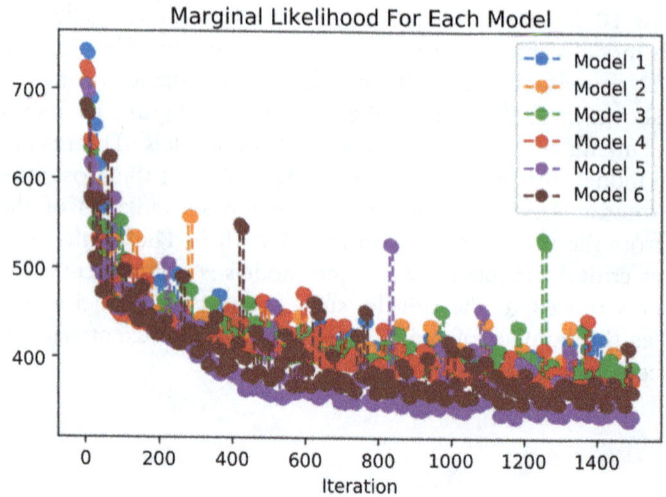

(**b**) Marginal likelihood convergence profile across all the models.

Fig. 10.2 Inference results for the Bayesian neural networks on the motor insurance claims dataset. **a** Predictive performance based on the Area Under the Receiver Operating Curve across all the models and **b** Marginal likelihood convergence profile across all the models

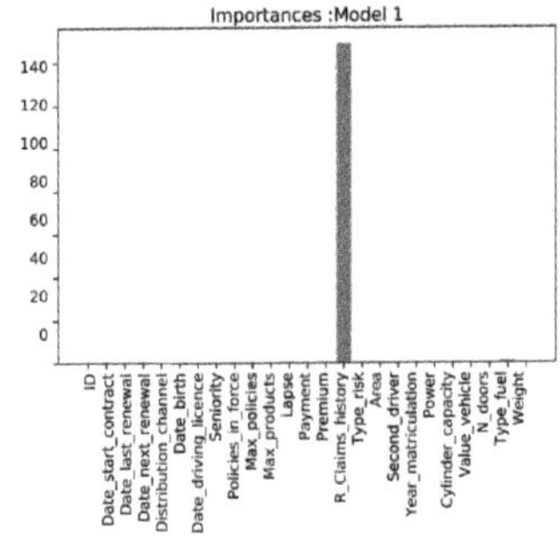

(**a**) Importance's for Model 1 which has 137 parameters.

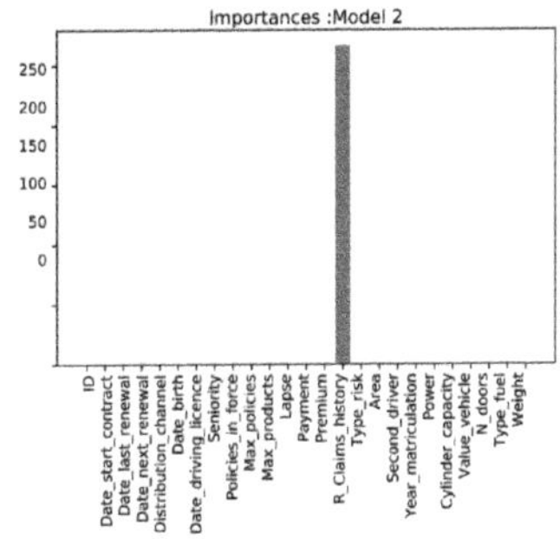

(**b**) Importance's for Model 2 which has 272 parameters.

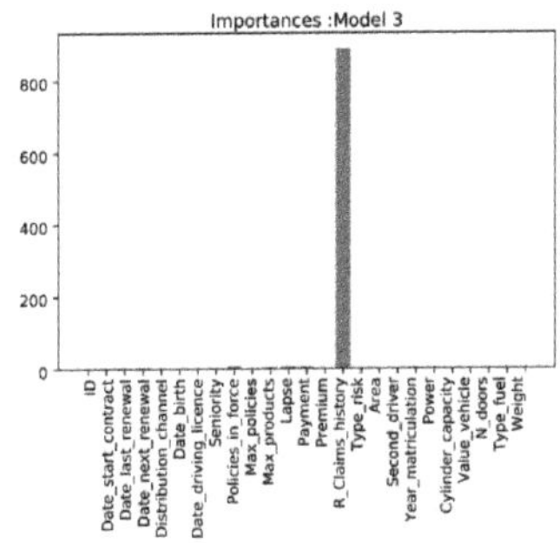

(**c**) Importance's for Model 3 which has 1352 parameters.

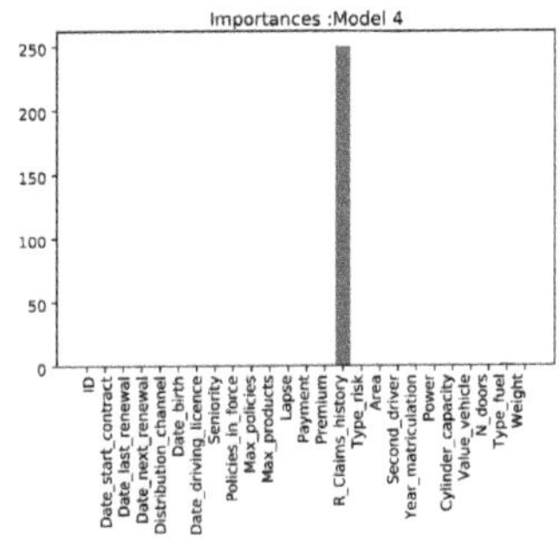

(**d**) Importance's for Model 4 which has 162 parameters.

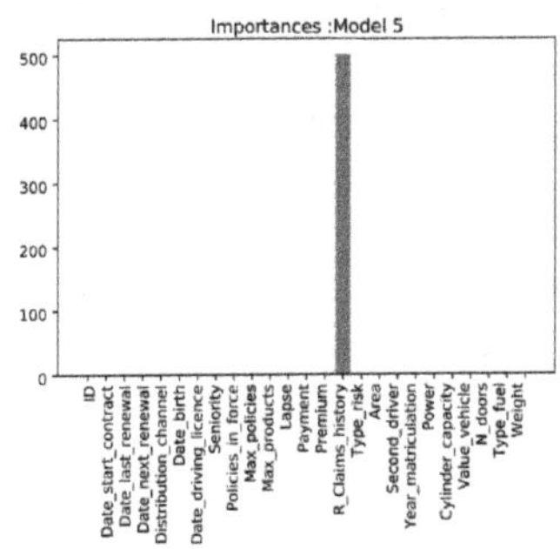

(**e**) Importance's for Model 5 which has 372 parameters.

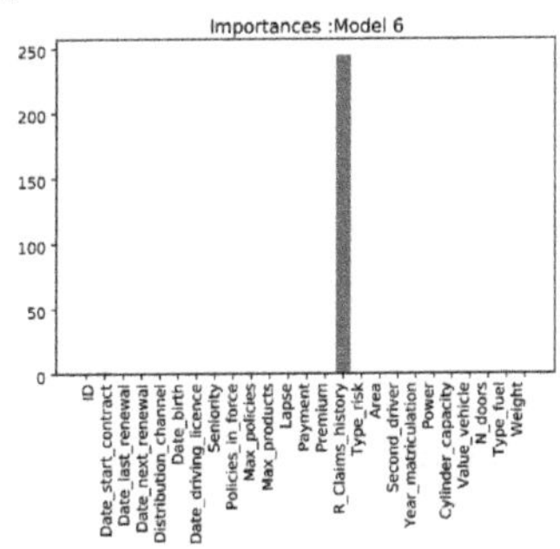

(**f**) Importance's for Model 6 which has 472 parameters.

Fig. 10.3 Mean posterior variances from each of the six neural network models. The higher the value, the more important the variable

Table 10.3 Ranking of the top six features across the five models. For example, *Type fuel* was the second most important feature from Model 1, while *Policies in force* is ranked as the third most important from Model 4

Ranking	*Model 1*	*Model 2*	*Model 3*	*Model 4*	*Model 5*	*Model 6*
1	R Claims history	R Claims history	R Claims history	R Claims history	R Claims history	R Claims history
2	Type fuel	Type fuel	Policies in force	Type fuel	Type fuel	Date start contract
3	Lapse	Date next renewal	Lapse	Policies in force	Type risk	Type fuel
4	Power	Max products	Payment	Max policies	N doors	Cylinder capacity
5	Date last renewal	Power	Max products	N doors	Cylinder capacity	Policies in force
6	Max policies	Date last renewal	Date next renewal	Seniority	Lapse	Power

10.6 Conclusion

We explored a first-in-literature approach for modeling motor insurance claims using a Bayesian framework. We train Bayesian neural networks with automatic relevance determination priors in this framework using the Laplace approximation. This framework allows us to select between neural network architectures using the Bayesian evidence metric and highlight which variables are the most important for the claim forecasting task.

Our results show that the Bayesian evidence metric from the Laplace approximation can be used to reliably select between different models that outperform on test data based on the accuracy and the Area Under the Receiver Operating Curve metrics. Our results suggest that deeper neural network architectures are preferred to wider (but shallow) architectures. We further find that the most critical variables across all the Bayesian neural network models are *claim history*, followed by features related to the vehicle, such as the *type of fuel* and *power*, as well as the *number of policies and products* the client has with the insurance company.

The work in this chapter can be expanded by considering other methods of training the Bayesian neural network, such as Markov Chain Monte Carlo methods, that ensure convergence to the true target posterior. In addition, instead of forecasting whether a claim will occur, we intend to extend the work in this chapter by modeling the absolute value of claims through the analysis of claim frequency and severity.

The next chapter uses shadow and adaptive Hamiltonian Monte Carlo methods to calibrate the Nelson and Siegel yield curve model. This Bayesian approach has advantages because it produces uncertainties in the calibrated parameters and the model's predictions.

References

Bishop, C. M. (July 1997). Bayesian neural networks. *Journal of the Brazilian Computer Society,* 4. ISSN: 0104-6500.

Bradley, A. P. (1997). The use of the area under the ROC curve in the evaluation of machine learning algorithms. *Pattern Recognition, 30*(7), 1145–1159. https://doi.org/10.1016/s0031-3203(96)00142-2

Clemente, C., Guerreiro, G. R., & Bravo, J. M. (2023). Modelling motor insurance claim frequency and severity using gradient boosting. *Risks, 11*(9), 163.

Daxberger, E., Kristiadi, A., Immer, A., Eschenhagen, R., Bauer, M., & Hennig, P. (2021). Laplace redux-effortless bayesian deep learning. *Advances in Neural Information Processing Systems, 34*, 20089–20103.

Fauzan, Muhammad Arief, & Murfi, Hendri. (2018). The accuracy of XGBoost for insurance claim prediction. *International Journal of Advances in Soft Computing and Its Applications, 10*(2), 159–171.

Gaganis, C. (July 2009). Classification techniques for the identification of falsified financial statements: A comparative analysis. *Intelligent Systems in Accounting, Finance & Management, 16*(3), 207–229. https://doi.org/10.1002/isaf.303

Gunter, T., Osborne, M. A., Garnett, R., Hennig, P., & Roberts, S. J. (2014). Sampling for inference in probabilistic models with fast Bayesian quadrature. *Advances in Neural Information Processing Systems*, 2789–2797.

Horvath, B., Muguruza, A., & Tomas, M. (2021). Deep learning volatility: A deep neural network perspective on pricing and calibration in (rough) volatility models. *Quantitative Finance, 21*(1), 11–27.

Kass, R. E., & Raftery, A. E. (1995). Bayes factors. *Journal of the American Statistical Association, 90*(430), 773–795.

MacKay, D. J. C. (1995a). *Probable networks and plausible predictions – a review of practical Bayesian methods for supervised neural networks.*

MacKay, D. J. C. (1995b). Probable networks and plausible predictions—a review of practical Bayesian methods for supervised neural networks. *Network: Computation in Neural Systems, 6*(3), 469–505.

MacKay, D. J. C. (1992). Bayesian interpolation. *Neural Computation, 4*(3), 415–447.

Marwala, T., Boulkaibet, I., & Adhikari, S. (2016). *Probabilistic finite element model updating using Bayesian statistics: Applications to aeronautical and mechanical engineering*. Wiley.

Marwala, T., Mbuvha, R., & Mongwe, W. T. (2023). *Hamiltonian Monte Carlo methods in machine learning*. Elsevier.

Mbuvha, R., Jonsson, M., Ehn, N., & Herman, P. (2017). Bayesian neural networks for one-hour ahead wind power forecasting. In *2017 IEEE 6th international conference on renewable energy research and applications (ICRERA)* (pp. 591–596). IEEE.

Mbuvha, R., Mongwe, W. T., & Marwala, T. (2021). Separable Shadow Hamiltonian Hybrid Monte Carlo for Bayesian neural network inference in wind speed forecasting. *Energy and A, 1*, Article 100108.

Mohd Yunos, Z., Shamsuddin, S. M., Ismail, N., & Sallehuddin, R. (2013). Modeling the Malaysian motor insurance claim using artificial neural network and adaptive neurofuzzy inference system. In *AIP conference proceedings* (Vol. 1522. 1, pp. 1431–1437). American Institute of Physics.

Mongwe, W. T. (2022). *Hybrid Monte Carlo methods in machine learning: Stochastic volatility methods, Shadow Hamiltonians, adaptive approaches and variance reduction techniques*. University of Johannesburg (South Africa).

Mongwe, W. T., & Malan, K. M. (2020). A survey of automated financial statement fraud detection with relevance to the South African context. *South African Computer Journal, 32*(1). https://doi.org/10.18489/sacj.v32i1.777

Mongwe, W. T., Sidogi, T., & Mbuvha, R., & Marwala, T. (2022). Probabilistic inference of South African equity option prices under jump-diffusion processes. In *2022 IEEE symposium on computational intelligence for financial engineering and economics (CIFEr)* (pp. 1–8). IEEE.

Montavon, G., Samek, W., & Müller, K.-R. (2018). Methods for interpreting and understanding deep neural networks. *Digital Signal Processing, 73*, 1–15.

Mthembu, L., Marwala, T., Friswell, M. I., & Adhikari, S. (2011). Model selection in finite element model updating using the Bayesian evidence statistic. *Mechanical Systems and Signal Processing, 25*(7), 2399–2412.

Neal, R. M. (Jan. 1993). *Probabilistic inference using Markov chain Monte Carlo methods*. Technical report. CRG-TR-93-1. University of Toronto, Department of Computer Science.

Nesseris, S., & Garcia-Bellido, J. (2013). Is the Jeffreys' scale a reliable tool for Bayesian model comparison in cosmology? *Journal of Cosmology and Astroparticle Physics, 2013*(08), 036.

Olayungbo, D. O., & Akinlo, A. E. (2016). Insurance penetration and economic growth in Africa: Dynamic effects analysis using Bayesian TVP-VAR approach. *Cogent Economics & Finance, 4*(1), 1150390.

Osborne, M., Garnett, R., Ghahramani, Z., Duvenaud, D. K., Roberts, S. J., & Rasmussen, C. E. (2012). Active learning of model evidence using Bayesian quadrature. *Advances in Neural Information Processing Systems*, 46–54.

Russel, P. M., Brewer, B. J., Klaere, S., & Bouckaert, R. R. (2019). Model selection and parameter inference in phylogenetics using nested sampling. *Systematic Biology, 68*(2), 219–233.

Segura-Gisbert, J., Lledó, J., & Pavía, J. M. (2024). Dataset of an actual motor vehicle insurance portfolio. *European Actuarial Journal*, 1–13.

Skilling, J. (2004). Nested sampling. In *AIP conference proceedings* (Vol. 735. 1, pp. 395–405). American Institute of Physics.

Skilling, J. (2006). Nested sampling for general Bayesian computation. *Bayesian Analysis, 1*(4), 833–859.

Smith, K. A., Willis, R. J., & Brooks, M. (2000). An analysis of customer retention and insurance claim patterns using data mining: A case study. *Journal of the Operational Research Society, 51*(5), 532–541.

Speagle, J. S. (2020). Dynesty: A dynamic nested sampling package for estimating Bayesian posteriors and evidences. *Monthly Notices of the Royal Astronomical Society, 493*(3), 3132–3158.

van Huyssteen, N., & Rudansky-Kloppers, S. (2024). Factors influencing consumers' purchase decisions regarding personal motor vehicle insurance in South Africa. *Cogent Business & Management, 11*(1), 2293488.

Weerasinghe, K. P. M. L., & Wijegunasekara, M. C. (2016). A comparative study of data mining algorithms in the prediction of auto insurance claims.

CHAPTER 11

Shadow and Adaptive Hamiltonian Monte Carlo Methods for Calibrating the Nelson and Siegel Model

11.1 Introduction

The term structure of interest rates, often known as yield curves, is a measure of the market's forecast of future interest rate structure and refers to the connection between yields and the period to maturity of fixed-income contracts (Duffee, 2013; Kazemie, 2014; Hull & White, 2001; Mongwe, 2015; Vasicek, 1977). Two widely used term structure modeling methods are no-arbitrage and equilibrium models. The no-arbitrage models emphasize the need to accurately align the term structure at a particular moment to exclude any potential for arbitrage. This is particularly crucial when pricing interest-rate derivatives like swaps, swaptions, caps, and bonds with embedded options (Duffee, 2013; Kazemie, 2014; Hull & White, 2001). The equilibrium framework primarily concerns modeling the dynamics of the instantaneous rate. This is commonly done using affine models. From these models, yields at other maturities may be obtained by making different assumptions about the risk premium (Cox et al., 1979; Kazemie, 2014; Vasicek, 1977). The use of equilibrium models for pricing is limited as time-homogeneous models

Supplementary Information The online version contains supplementary material available at https://doi.org/10.1007/978-3-031-88431-3_11.

W. T. Mongwe et al., *Bayesian Machine Learning in Quantitative Finance*, https://doi.org/10.1007/978-3-031-88431-3_11

do not perfectly match a market yield curve (Hölzermann, 2021; Hull & White, 2001; Kladívko & Rusý, 2023). Prominent contributions in the no-arbitrage models of the yield curve include Hull and White (2001). In contrast, some seminal work on equilibrium models of term structure consists of the models by Vasicek (1977) and Cox et al. (1979).

Through analyzing the term structure of interest rates, it is possible to deduce the discount function, which represents the price of a zero coupon bond. This function is regarded as a fundamental element in finance (Gürkaynak, 2007). Financial market players, politicians, and academics are concerned with modeling the yield curve (Duffee, 2013). The central bank may use the yield curve to accurately assess the suitability of its monetary policy position (Department, 2005). Several central banks use parsimonious data-driven models for this objective (Department, 2005).

The Nelson and Siegel (NS) model, proposed by Nelson and Siegel in 1987, is widely used in academic research and practical applications for simulating the term structure of interest rates (Nelson & Siegel, 1987). This model is flexible enough to capture various yield curve shapes and ensures continuous forward rates. However, it does not, theoretically, provide the absence of arbitrage opportunities (Nelson and Siegel, 1987). This model and its extensions, the Svensson, Bliss, and Diebold-Li models, are widely accepted by the industry for forecasting the yield curve due to their ability to capture various shapes of the yield curve while also being easy to explain to stakeholders (Diebold & Li, 2006; Wahlstrøm et al., 2022). Wealth managers specializing in fixed-income investments in public organizations, investment banks, and central banks substantially depend on Nelson and Siegel type models to accurately analyze and predict yield curves (Bernadell et al., 2005; Department, 2005). The central banks of Belgium, Finland, France, Germany, Italy, Norway, Spain, and Switzerland use these models, as stated by the Bank of International Settlements, to estimate zero-coupon yield curves (Department, 2005). The European Central Bank (ECB) releases daily Eurosystem-wide yield curves using the Svensson (1995) model, which is an expansion of the Nelson and Siegel (1987) model. The ECB employs a regime-switching variant of the NS model in its foreign reserve management framework (Bernadell et al., 2005). The Nelson and Siegel (1987) model has been used as a parametric model for the term structure of implied volatility on S&P 500 index call options by Guo et al. (2014). These authors demonstrate that the three elements of the NS model, which represent the level, slope, and curvature of the volatility term structure, can be understood as the volatility over the long-, medium-, and short-term, respectively. This shows that the NS model and its extensions are versatile and extensively used in practice and the literature. Thus, it is essential to understand how this model is calibrated to market data.

The NS model is typically calibrated using ordinary least squares methods. Model calibration, i.e., obtaining parameter values such that model yields produced by the NS model correspond with market yields, is complex. Numerous authors have reported numerical difficulties when working with the model (Annaert et al., 2013; Gürkaynak et al., 2006; Lakhany et al., 2021). Calibrating these models presents a dual challenge. Firstly, the objective function used in the calibration procedure is nonlinear and exhibits several local optima (Annaert et al., 2013; Gürkaynak et al., 2006; Lakhany et al., 2021). Furthermore, there exists a significant interdependence among the model parameters. Consequently, their estimated values exhibit unpredictable fluctuations over time. Thus, Gilli et al. (2010) investigate the use of a global optimization technique, such as differential evolution, and demonstrate its reliable capability in solving the model. In addition, Lakhany et al. (2021) use a heuristic optimization technique known as the Genetic Algorithm to demonstrate the ability to generate interest rate curves and maintain stable model parameters throughout time, irrespective of the curve's form. On the other hand, Annaert et al. (2013) suggest using ridge regression instead of ordinary least squares (OLS) regression when they identify significant multicollinearity during the calibration of the NS model using a conventional grid search approach. While ridge regression can enhance the ability to predict future outcomes at both the beginning and end of the term structure, resulting in lower prediction errors and reduced volatility compared to traditional grid search, the estimation of the shape parameter still exhibits unpredictable patterns over time. In this chapter, we explore reformulating the NS model calibration within a Bayesian framework—which amounts to estimating the posterior distribution of the parameters of the NS model. This framework also enforces a regularization term through the prior distribution similar to that utilized by Annaert et al. (2013) in their ridge-regression framework, which has the added advantage of capturing the uncertainties in the different parameters. Various approaches can be used to estimate the posterior distribution, which is often intractable. Examples of such approaches are variational inference and Markov Chain Monte Carlo methods, which we discuss in detail in Chapter 2 of this book.

For our analysis, we consider simulated yield curve data where we know the underlying NS model parameters that generated the data; we look at the Swap curve in South Africa and also a time series of yield curves from the USA corporate bond market. Our results show that our Bayesian approach utilizes Markov Chain Monte Carlo methods: Hamiltonian Monte Carlo, Separable Shadow Hybrid Hamiltonian Monte Carlo, and No-U-Turn Sampler. This Bayesian framework produces results that are in line with or better than OLS techniques, with the added advantage of capturing uncertainties in the model parameters and predictions.

The remainder of this chapter is structured as follows: We first describe the Nelson and Siegel model used to model the yield curve in Sect. 11.2; we then detail the Markov Chain Monte Carlo methods used to train the model in Sect. 11.3; we then present the experiment setup, after which we present the results, discuss them, and provide the conclusion in Sects. 11.4–11.6 respectively.

11.2 The Nelson and Siegel Model

TheNelson and Siegel (1987) model and its extension being the Diebold and Li (2006) are widely accepted by industry for forecasting the yield curve due to their ability to capture various shapes of the yield curve while also being easy to explain. The Nelson and Siegel model assumes that the forward rate curve can be described by:

$$f_t(\tau) = \beta_0 + \beta_1 \exp(-\lambda\tau) + \beta_2 \lambda \exp(-\lambda\tau) \tag{11.1}$$

where $\{\beta_0, \beta_1, \beta_2, \lambda\}$ are the parameters of the model, t is the current time (or valuation date in some contexts) and τ is the time period between now and the point of interest on the yield curve. Note that $\beta_0 > 0$ and $\lambda > 0$, and this must be factored into the calibration. In our Bayesian setting, we set the prior distribution to be Gaussian for β_1 and β_2 and LogNormal for β_0 and λ.

If we combine this with the relationship between the yield to maturity and the forward rate—which is that the spot rate is the integral or average of the forward rates, it gives this yield curve function:

$$y_t(\tau) = \beta_0 + \beta_1\left(\frac{1 - \exp(-\lambda\tau)}{\lambda\tau}\right) + \beta_2\left(\frac{1 - \exp(-\lambda\tau)}{\lambda\tau} - \exp(-\lambda\tau)\right) \tag{11.2}$$

This functional form is a convenient and economical three-component exponential approximation, which works very well to predict the yield curve, as shown in Diebold and Li (2006). The three factors β_0, β_1, and β_2 are of special interest. The loading on β_0 is 1, a constant that does not approach zero in the limit; therefore, β_0 may be considered a long-term factor. The loading on β_1 is $\left(\frac{1-\exp(-\lambda\tau)}{\lambda\tau}\right)$, a function that starts at 1, however, decays monotonically and rapidly to 0, and hence may be considered as a short-term factor. The loading on β_2 is $\left(\frac{1-\exp(-\lambda\tau)}{\lambda\tau} - \exp(-\lambda\tau)\right)$, which begins at 0, increases, and then converges to zero; therefore, it may be considered as a medium-term factor. Additionally, Diebold and Li (2006) show that these three factors may also be interpreted according to the yield curve's level, slope, and curvature. They additionally demonstrate that this simple model is more effective than many other yield curve models in-sample fitting and out-of-sample forecasting.

11.3 Advanced Hamiltonian Monte Carlo Methods

We now describe the HMC, S2HMC, and NUTS Markov Chain Monte Carlo methods that we use to calibrate the Nelson and Siegel model to yield curve data.

11.3.1 Hamiltonian Monte Carlo and The No U-Turn Sampler

Hamiltonian Monte Carlo (HMC) is a popular MCMC method for performing Bayesian inference and has been utilized in various disciplines such as finance, health, and energy (Duane et al., 1987; Mbuvha & Marwala, 2020; Mbuvha et al., 2021; Mongwe et al., 2021b, 2022b). The method is premised on using Hamiltonian dynamics, which naturally considers the first-order gradient information of the target posterior. The dynamics that underpin HMC are as follows (Marwala et al., 2023; Neal et al., 1993):

$$\frac{d\mathbf{w}}{\partial t} = \frac{\partial H(\mathbf{w}, \mathbf{p})}{\partial \mathbf{p}}; \quad \frac{d\mathbf{p}}{\partial t} = -\frac{\partial H(\mathbf{w}, \mathbf{p})}{\partial \mathbf{w}}. \tag{11.3}$$

where **w** are the parameters, p is the auxiliary momentum variable with the same dimensionality as **w**, and H(**w**, **p**) is the Hamiltonian—which represents the total energy (i.e. potential energy defined by the target posterior and kinetic energy which is typically captured through a multivariate Gaussian distribution) from this system (Mongwe et al., 2021b, 2022a). This method allows distant proposals, which results in a significant reduction in the auto-correlations of the generated samples (Marwala et al., 2023).

HMC is composed of two steps. The first step integrates Hamiltonian dynamics in Eq. 11.3 typically using the leapfrog integrator (Duane et al., 1987; Marwala et al., 2023; Neal et al., 1993), and the second step utilizes a Metropolis-Hastings correction to account for the numerical integration errors arising from the first step (Duane et al., 1987; Hastings, 1970; Neal et al., 2011). The parameter and momentum update equations for the leapfrog integration scheme (corresponding to the first step of HMC) are given as follows:

$$\begin{aligned}
\mathbf{p}_{t+\frac{\epsilon}{2}} &= \mathbf{p}_t + \frac{\epsilon}{2}\frac{\partial H\left(\mathbf{w}_t, \mathbf{p}_t\right)}{\partial \mathbf{w}} \\
\mathbf{w}_{t+\epsilon} &= \mathbf{w}_t + \epsilon \mathbf{M}^{-1}\mathbf{p}_{t+\frac{\epsilon}{2}} \\
\mathbf{p}_{t+\epsilon} &= \mathbf{p}_{t+\frac{\epsilon}{2}} + \frac{\epsilon}{2}\frac{\partial H\left(\mathbf{w}_{t+\epsilon}, \mathbf{p}_{t+\frac{\epsilon}{2}}\right)}{\partial \mathbf{w}}
\end{aligned} \tag{11.4}$$

where ϵ is the discretization step size and **M** is a covariance matrix emanating from the kinetic energy component in H(**w**, **p**). If the integration in the first step were solved precisely, the second step would not be required. However, due to the discretization errors, a Metropolis-Hastings acceptance step is typically required where the $\mathbf{w}^*$ proposed by the first step are accepted with probability:

$$\mathrm{P}(\text{accept } \mathbf{w}^*) = \min\left(1, \frac{\exp(-\mathrm{H}(\mathbf{w}^*, \mathbf{p}^*))}{\exp(-\mathrm{H}(\mathbf{w}, \mathbf{p}))}\right). \tag{11.5}$$

The parameters of HMC are the discretization step size ϵ, which is required for the first step in HMC, and the trajectory length L, which determines the number of times the integration is performed. The step size parameter is typically set to obtain a user-specified target acceptance rate using the dual averaging method (Marwala et al., 2023; Neal et al., 2011) while tuning the trajectory length parameter is a more complex problem (Neal et al., 2011). It can further be shown that when the trajectory length parameter is set to 1, the HMC method becomes the MALA method. The overall HMC sampling process follows a Gibbs sampling scheme, where we sample **p** auxiliary momentum variable and then sample a new set of parameters **w** given the drawn momentum **p**. This procedure is repeated until the required number of samples are generated.

The step size and trajectory length are numerous parameters that necessitate tuning to achieve efficient sampling in the HMC algorithm. A trajectory length that is too short leads to a random walk behavior similar to the Metropolis-Hasting method (Hoffman & Gelman, 2014; Marwala et al., 2023; Mbuvha & Marwala, 2020; Mongwe et al., 2021a, 2021b). A trajectory length that is too long results in a trajectory that inefficiently traces back (Hoffman & Gelman, 2014; Mbuvha & Marwala, 2020). The step size is also a critical parameter for sampling. Small step sizes are computationally inefficient, leading to correlated samples and poor mixing, while large step sizes compound discretization errors, leading to low acceptance rates (Hoffman & Gelman, 2014; Mbuvha & Marwala, 2020). Tuning these parameters requires multiple time-consuming pilot runs (Hoffman & Gelman, 2014; Marwala et al., 2023; Mbuvha & Marwala, 2020; Mongwe et al., 2021a, 2021b). The leapfrog step size and trajectory length are automatically adjusted by the No-U-Turn Sampler (NUTS) (Hoffman & Gelman, 2014; Marwala et al., 2023). In NUTS, the step size is tuned through primal-dual averaging during an initial burn-in phase by targeting a particular sample acceptance rate (Hoffman & Gelman, 2014; Marwala et al., 2023; Mbuvha & Marwala, 2020). The trajectory length is adjusted by iteratively adding steps until the chain begins to trace back (U-turn) or the Hamiltonian reaches infinity (Hoffman & Gelman, 2014; Mbuvha & Marwala, 2020).

Primal-dual averaging is used in NUTS to adjust the step size parameter during the burn-in phase (Marwala et al., 2023). Primal-dual averaging is used to achieve a user-specified Metropolis-Hastings acceptance rate δ which is expressed as (Andrieu & Thoms, 2008; Marwala et al., 2023; Mbuvha et al., 2019b):

$$\begin{aligned} \epsilon_{t+1} &\leftarrow \mu - \frac{\sqrt{t}}{\gamma}\frac{1}{t+t_0}\sum_{i=1}^{t} H_i \\ \bar{\epsilon}_{t+1} &\leftarrow \eta_t \epsilon_{t+1} + (1-\eta_t)\bar{\epsilon}_t \end{aligned} \tag{11.6}$$

where η_t is a decaying rate of adaptation in accordance with Andrieu and Thoms (2008), γ regulates the convergence towards μ, H_t is the difference between the target acceptance rate and the actual acceptance rate (Hoffman & Gelman, 2014; Mbuvha et al., 2021), and μ is a free parameter that ϵ_t gravitates to Marwala et al. (2023). The updates from primal-dual averaging are such that (Marwala et al., 2023; Mbuvha et al., 2021):

$$\mathbb{E}[H_t] = \mathbb{E}[\delta - \alpha_t] = 0. \tag{11.7}$$

As a result, the step size is updated toward the desired acceptance rate δ. Setting $\mu = \log(10\epsilon_0)$, $\bar{\epsilon}_0 = 1$, $\bar{H}_0 = 0$, $\gamma = 0.05$, $t_0 = 10$, $\kappa = 0.75$, and ϵ_0 as the initial step size yields acceptable performance across a variety of target posterior distributions (Hoffman & Gelman, 2014; Marwala et al., 2023). The $\epsilon_0 = 0.0001$ settings used in this chapter are the same as those in Marwala et al. (2023).

Iteratively increasing the trajectory length until the Hamiltonian becomes infinite or the chain begins to trace back is how NUTS automatically adjusts the trajectory length parameter (Afshar et al., 2021; Mbuvha & Marwala, 2020). At that point, the final suggested position state $\mathbf{w}^*$ begins to resemble the starting position $\mathbf{w}$, and this is also when $(\mathbf{w}^* - \mathbf{w}) \times \mathbf{p} \leq 0$. This approach breaks down the detailed balancing criterion and is rectified through the use of a slice sampling technique (Marwala et al., 2023; Neal et al., 2011).

NUTS operates at least as efficiently as and occasionally more efficiently than a well-tuned standard HMC method without necessitating user intervention or a costly tuning run (Hoffman & Gelman, 2014). This makes the NUTS method more accessible to non-expert audiences.

11.3.2 Separable Shadow Hamiltonian Hybrid Monte Carlo

Although significantly better than MALA, the HMC method still produces auto-correlated samples (Heide et al., 2021; Marwala et al., 2023). This is mainly driven by the fact that the leapfrog integration scheme in Eq. 11.4 only preserves the Hamiltonian only to up to second order $\mathcal{O}(\epsilon^2)$. This causes the change in the Hamiltonian in step 5 of Algorithm 3.1 to become large, thus leading to more rejections in step 8 of Algorithm 3.1 (Heide et al., 2021; Marwala et al., 2023). There are two possibilities to address this issue; one can either create more accurate (i.e., better than $\mathcal{O}(\epsilon^2)$) integration schemes to integrate the Hamiltonian dynamics, or only run the integration scheme for small step sizes ϵ and short path lengths L—or a combination of these two approaches. However, all these approaches attract longer execution times (Marwala et al., 2023).

It can be shown that when one runs a backward error analysis through the leapfrog integrator in Eq. 11.4, we can derive a modified Hamiltonian (which is called the shadow Hamiltonian) whose energy is better preserved by the leapfrog integrator than the true Hamiltonian (Marwala et al., 2023). By design, the numerical integrator precisely conserves the perturbations of the Hamiltonian of the shadow Hamiltonians. However, as this Hamiltonian is not the true Hamiltonian, we would effectively be sampling from an importance distribution, which we would need to correct so as not to introduce bias in the generated samples (Heide et al., 2021; Mongwe et al., 2021b, 2022a).

At its core, the shadow or modified Hamiltonian is an asymptotic expansion in the powers of the discretization step size ϵ around the Hamiltonian:

$$\tilde{\mathrm{H}} = \mathrm{H} + \epsilon \mathrm{H}_2 + \epsilon^2 \mathrm{H}_3 + \epsilon^3 \mathrm{H}_4 + \ldots \tag{11.8}$$

However, to ensure that this expansion does not diverge, a kth order truncation of the expansion is utilized in practice:

$$\begin{aligned} \tilde{\mathrm{H}}^{[k]} &= \mathrm{H} + \epsilon \mathrm{H}_2 + \epsilon^2 \mathrm{H}_3 + \epsilon^3 \mathrm{H}_4 + \ldots \\ &= \tilde{\mathrm{H}} + \mathcal{O}(\epsilon^k) \end{aligned} \tag{11.9}$$

Through comparing the associated elements of the Taylor series in terms of ϵ and the extended precise flow of the modified differential equation of the Hamiltonian, the H_k terms can be found. For symplectic integrators like the leapfrog integrator, these altered equations can be regarded as being Hamiltonian (Marwala et al., 2023). This chapter considers a fourth-order truncation of the shadow Hamiltonian under the leapfrog integrator. The fourth-order truncation is conserved with more accuracy ($\mathcal{O}^4$) than the true Hamiltonian since the leapfrog is second-order accurate ($\mathcal{O}^2$). The fourth-order shadow Hamiltonian for the leapfrog integrator after matching coefficients from the flow and the asymptotic expansion is expressed as:

$$\tilde{H}^{[4]} = U(\mathbf{w}) + K(\mathbf{p}) + \frac{\epsilon^2}{12} K_{\mathbf{p}}^T U_{\mathbf{ww}} K_{\mathbf{p}} - \frac{\epsilon^2}{24} U_{\mathbf{w}}^T K_{\mathbf{pp}} U_{\mathbf{w}} + \mathcal{O}(\epsilon^4) \quad (11.10)$$

where $U_{\mathbf{w}}$, $U_{\mathbf{ww}}$, $K_{\mathbf{p}}$ and $K_{\mathbf{pp}}$ are Jacobians and Hessians of the potential and kinetic energies respectively. It can be noted that the modified Hamiltonian in Eq. 11.10 is non-separable in terms of the parameter and momentum vectors. This is problematic as it requires potential tuning of additional parameters and momentum acceptance criterion that is computationally expensive (Izaguirre & Hampton, 2004; Marwala et al., 2023; Sweet et al., 2009).

Separable Shadow Hamiltonian Hybrid Monte Carlo (S2HMC) utilizes a processed leapfrog integrator to create a separable Hamiltonian (Sweet et al., 2009). Before passing through the leapfrog integrator, the parameter vector and momenta are pre-processed to minimize computational overhead. The resultant separable Hamiltonian in S2HMC is

$$\tilde{H}(\mathbf{w}, \mathbf{p}) = U(\mathbf{w}) + K(\mathbf{p}) + \frac{\epsilon^2}{24} U_{\mathbf{w}}^T M^{-1} U_{\mathbf{w}} + \mathcal{O}(\epsilon^4) \quad (11.11)$$

The positions and momenta are propagated on the shadow Hamiltonian after performing the reversible mapping $(\hat{\mathbf{w}}, \hat{\mathbf{p}}) = \mathcal{X}(\mathbf{w}, \mathbf{p})$, where $(\hat{\mathbf{w}}, \hat{\mathbf{p}})$ is found through fixed point iterations as:

$$\hat{\mathbf{p}} = \mathbf{p} - \frac{\epsilon}{24}\left[U_{\mathbf{w}}(\mathbf{w} + \epsilon\, \mathbf{M}^{-1}\hat{\mathbf{p}}) - U_{\mathbf{w}}(\mathbf{w} - \epsilon\, \mathbf{M}^{-1}\hat{\mathbf{p}})\right] \quad (11.12)$$

$$\hat{\mathbf{w}} = \mathbf{w} + \frac{\epsilon^2\, \mathbf{M}^{-1}}{24}\left[U_{\mathbf{w}}(\mathbf{w} + \epsilon\, \mathbf{M}^{-1}\hat{\mathbf{p}}) + U_{\mathbf{w}}(\mathbf{w} - \epsilon\, \mathbf{M}^{-1}\hat{\mathbf{p}})\right] \quad (11.13)$$

After the leapfrog is performed, this mapping is reversed using post-processing of the following fixed point iterations:

$$\mathbf{w} = \hat{\mathbf{w}} - \frac{\epsilon^2\mathbf{M}^{-1}}{24}\left[\mathrm{U}_{\mathbf{w}}(\mathbf{w} + \epsilon\mathbf{M}^{-1}\hat{\mathbf{p}}) + \mathrm{U}_{\mathbf{w}}(\mathbf{w} - \epsilon\mathbf{M}^{-1}\hat{\mathbf{p}})\right] \tag{11.14}$$

$$\mathbf{p} = \hat{\mathbf{p}} + \frac{\epsilon}{24}\left[\mathrm{U}_{\mathbf{w}}(\mathbf{w} + \epsilon\mathbf{M}^{-1}\hat{\mathbf{p}}) - \mathrm{U}_{\mathbf{w}}(\mathbf{w} - \epsilon\mathbf{M}^{-1}\hat{\mathbf{p}})\right] \tag{11.15}$$

Importance weights are computed after the samples are obtained using the S2HMC (Marwala et al., 2023; Mongwe et al., 2021c) to guarantee that the shadow canonical density is used rather than the true density. The differences between the true and shadow Hamiltonians are the basis for determining the importance weights. It is worth noting that S2HMC degenerates to HMC when the shadow Hamiltonian is set to equal the true Hamiltonian. A detailed exposition on S2HMC, HMC, and NUTS can be found in Marwala et al. (2023).

11.4 Numerical Experiments

In this section, we present the numerical experiments conducted. We first describe the dataset and then outline the experiments, settings, and performance metrics used.

11.4.1 Data Description and Experiment Setup

The performance of the OLS, HMC, S2HMC, and NUTS algorithms in calibrating the NS model is compared to real-world and simulated datasets. The simulated data is from the NS model with known parameters being $\{\beta_0 = 0.04, \beta_1 = -0.05, \beta_2 = 0.2, \lambda = 1.3\}$, while the real-world data is from the South African Swap Curve as at 29 March 2024, and the time series of USA corporate bond yield curves from 2018 to 2024.

11.4.2 Performance Metrics

The performance metrics used in this chapter are predictive performance on unseen data. The predictive performance metrics used are the Mean Square Error (MSE) , Mean Absolute Error (MAE), coefficient of determination (R^2), and Mean Percentage Error (MAPE) (Mongwe and Malan, 2020). For all the MCMC algorithms, we set the pre-conditioning matrix $\mathbf{M} = \mathbf{I}$, which is the common approach in practice.

We generated five chains with 2000 samples for all the datasets with a burn-in period of 1000. This was sufficient for all the algorithms to converge on all the datasets. The number of steps used to generate each sample was fixed at 25 for HMC and S2HMC. The step-sizes were chosen by targeting an acceptance rate of 80% through the dual averaging methodology (Marwala et al., 2023; Neal et al., 2011).

11.5 Results and Discussions

In this section, we present the results and the discussions from the numerical experiments. Table 11.1 shows the calibrated parameters from the three MCMC methods on the simulated yield curve data. Table 11.2 shows the predictive performance of the MCMC methods across various performance metrics, Table 11.3 shows the calibrated parameters on the ZAR swap curve data using the OLS and NUTS algorithms and Table 11.4 shows the predictive performance of the OLS and NUTS methods on the ZAR swap Curve data across various metrics.

Figures 11.1 and 11.2 show the calibration results across simulated market data as well as on the ZAR swap curve. Figures 11.3, 11.4 and 11.5 show the posterior distribution of the calibrated NS model parameters on the simulated data using HMC, S2HMC, and NUTS algorithms respectively, while Figure 11.6 shows the calibrated parameter distributions using the NUTS algorithm on the ZAR swap curve data. Figure 11.7 shows the mean square error on the USA Corporate Bond Yield Data between 2018 and 2024 using the NUTS and OLS methods.

Table 11.1 Results on simulated yield curve data. The simulated data was generated from the NS model with $\{\beta_0 = 0.04, \beta_1 = -0.05, \beta_2 = 0.2, \lambda = 1.3\}$. The parameter values for the MCMC methods are the average values from the posterior parameter distribution. The results indicate that the MCMC methods can reproduce the true parameters

Parameter	*True Parameters*	*NUTS*	*HMC*$_{25}$	*S2HMC*$_{25}$
β_0	0.040	0.040	0.040	0.040
β_1	-0.050	-0.050	-0.050	-0.051
β_2	0.200	0.200	0.200	0.200
λ	1.300	1.295	1.295	1.292

Table 11.2 Predictive performance on simulated yield curve data. The entries in **bold** indicate the MCMC method that outperforms on that particular performance metric

Metric	*NUTS*	*S2HMC*$_{25}$	*HMC*$_{25}$
R2	0.999988	0.99998	**0.999992**
MSE	2.925e-05	4.420e-05	**1.871e-05**
MAPE	0.000854	0.001092	**0.000718**
MAE	0.004398	0.005338	**0.003197**

Table 11.1 shows that the HMC, S2HMC, and NUTS are all able to reproduce the true parameters that generated the simulated yield curve. Furthermore, Table 11.2 shows that the MCMC methods produce similar predictive performance on unseen data from the simulated yield curve, with HMC producing the overall best performance across all the performance metrics. On the ZR swap curve data, we find that the OLS and NUTS algorithms produce similar parameters as shown in Table 11.3, while Table 11.4 shows that the NUTS algorithm outperforms the OLS

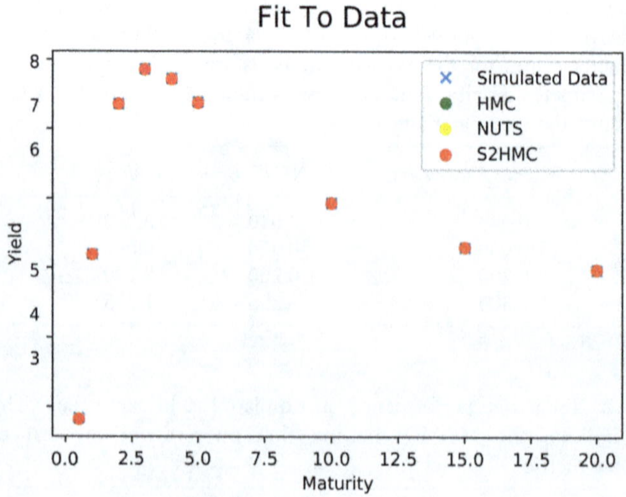

(a) Simulated yield curve from NS model where $\{\beta_0 = 0.04, \beta_1 = -0.05, \beta_2 = 0.2, \lambda = 1.3\}$ with the estimated yield curve using the MCMC methods.

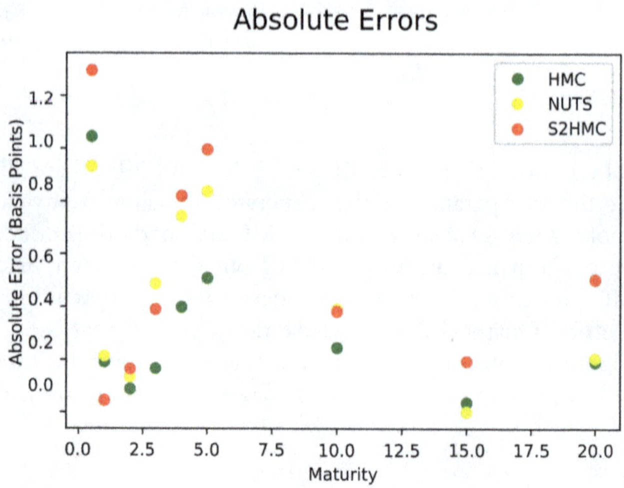

(b) Absolute errors (in basis points) on the simulated market data across the three MCMC methods.

Fig. 11.1 Inference results for the Bayesian framework on unseen simulated data. **a** Comparison to simulated market rates, **b** Absolute errors on simulated market rates

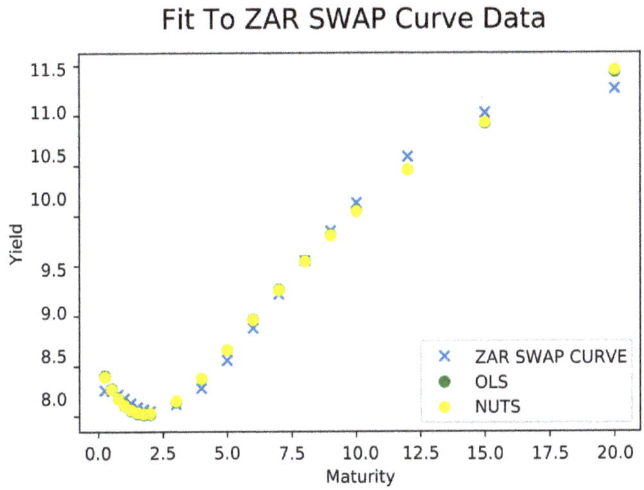

(**a**) ZAR swap curve data as at 29 March 2024 with the estimated yield curves using the OLS and NUTS algorithms.

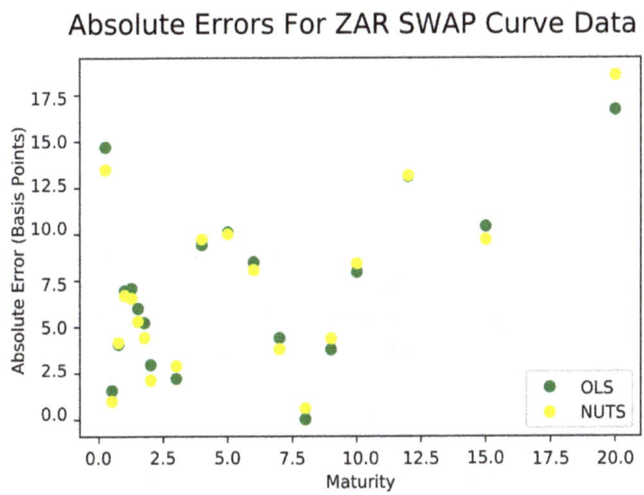

(**b**) Absolute errors (in basis points) on the ZAR swap curve yield data using the OLS and NUTS methods.

Fig. 11.2 Inference results for the Bayesian framework on unseen real market data. **a** Comparison to simulated market rates, and **b** Absolute errors on ZAR Swap market rates

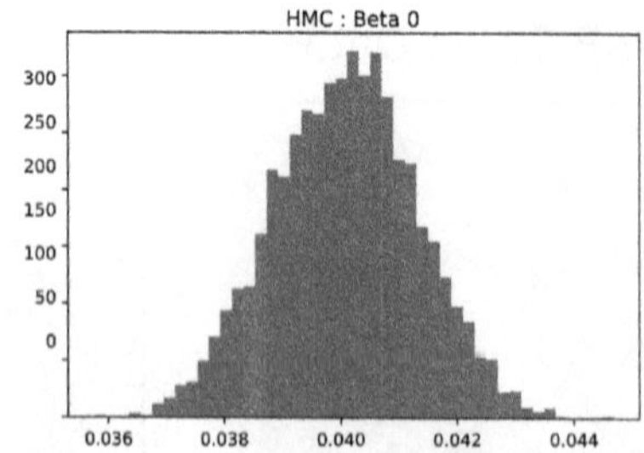

(a) Calibrated β_0 parameter on the simulated data using the HMC algorithm.

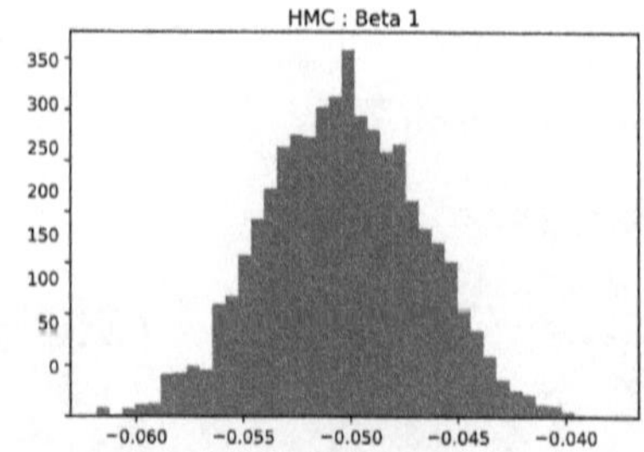

(b) Calibrated β_1 parameter on the simulated data using the HMC algorithm.

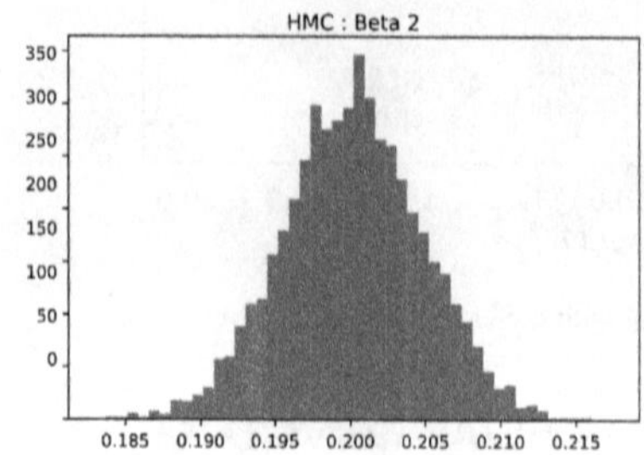

(c) Calibrated β_2 parameter on the simulated data using the HMC algorithm.

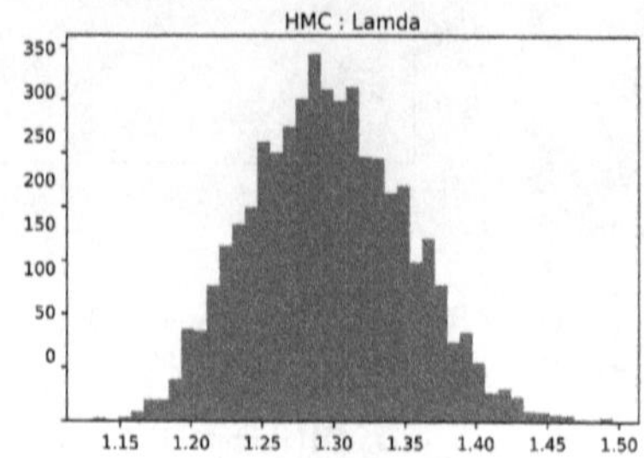

(d) Calibrated λ parameter on the simulated data using the HMC algorithm.

Fig. 11.3 Calibrated parameters using the HMC algorithm on simulated market data

algorithm across all the performance metrics on unseen data from the ZAR swap curve data. The simulated and ZAR swap curve data results are also summarized in Figs. 11.1 and 11.2. We find that the performance of the OLS and NUTS algorithms on the ZAR Swap curve data becomes less accurate with increasing maturity, as shown in Fig. 11.2b.

Figures 11.3, 11.4 and 11.5 show the posterior distribution of the calibrated NS model parameters on the simulated data using HMC, S2HMC, and NUTS algorithms respectively. These figures show that the three

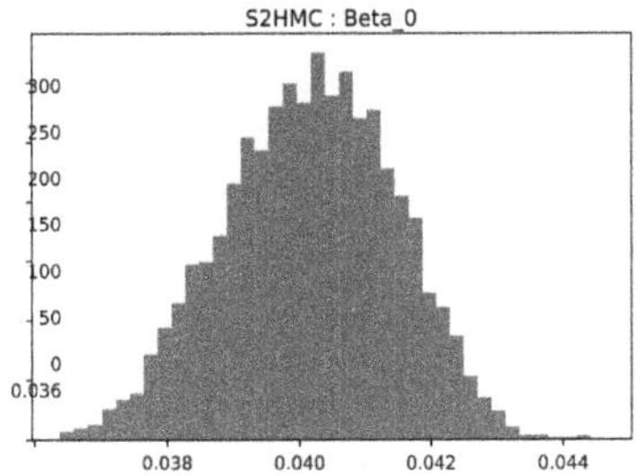

(**a**) Calibrated β_0 parameter on the simulated data using the S2HMC algorithm.

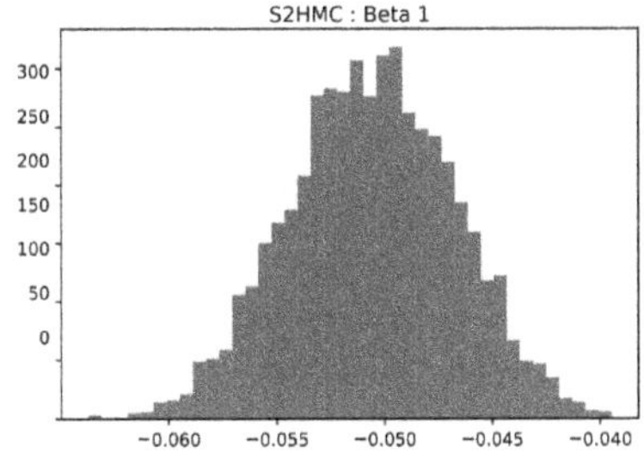

(**b**) Calibrated β_1 parameter on the simulated data using the S2HMC algorithm.

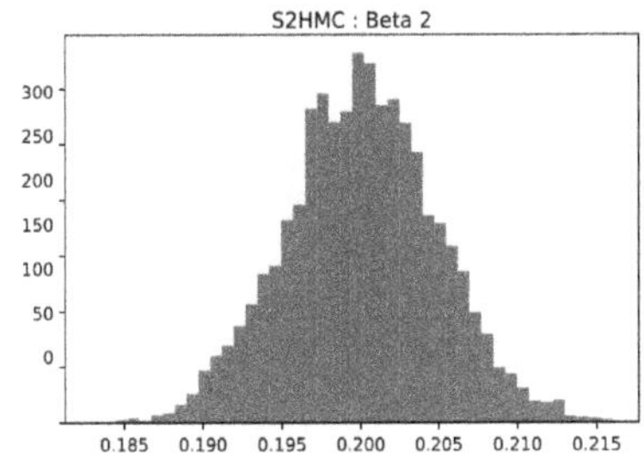

(**c**) Calibrated β_2 parameter on the simulated data using the S2HMC algorithm.

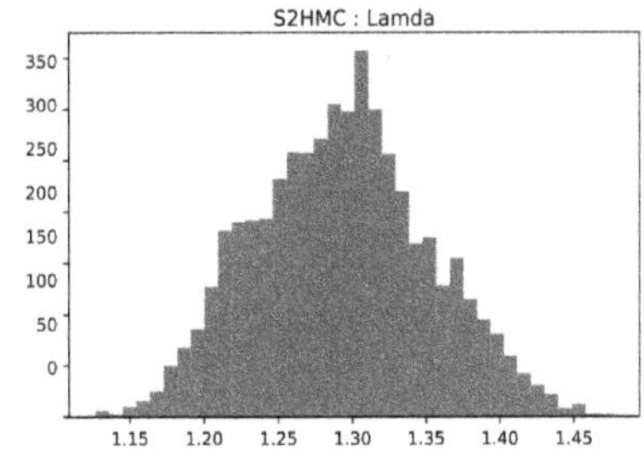

(**d**) Calibrated λ parameter on the simulated data using the S2HMC algorithm.

Fig. 11.4 Calibrated parameters using the S2HMC algorithm on simulated market data

algorithms produce similar posterior distributions across all four parameters on the simulated market data. Furthermore, Fig. 11.6 shows the calibrated parameters from the NUTS algorithm on the ZAR swap curve data. These distributions can then be utilized to create confidence intervals on any predictions made, which is what we explore on the time series data from the USA Corporate bond yield curve data.

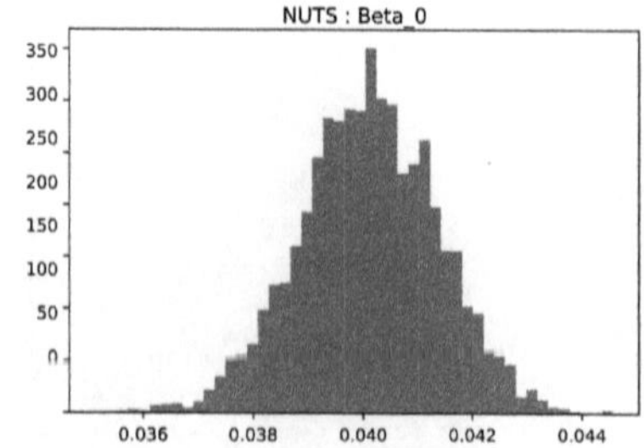

(**a**) Calibrated β_0 parameter on the simulated data using the NUTS algorithm.

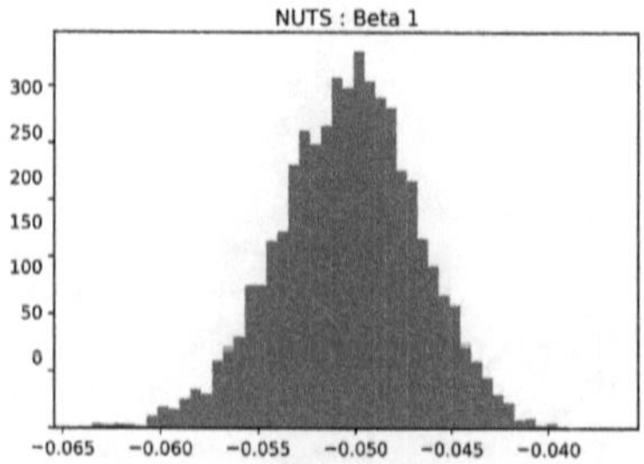

(**b**) Calibrated β_1 parameter on the simulated data using the NUTS algorithm.

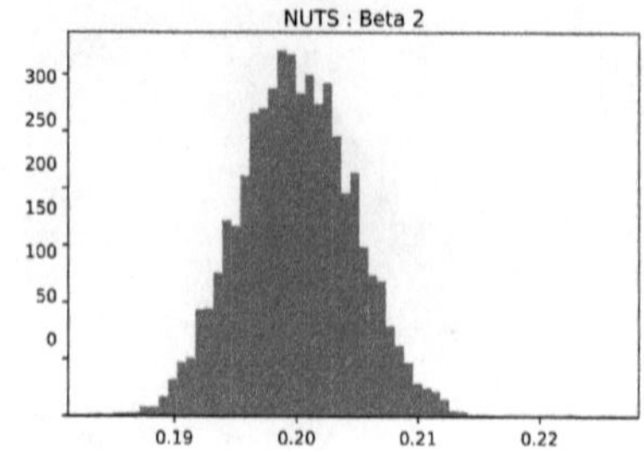

(**c**) Calibrated β_2 parameter on the simulated data using the NUTS algorithm.

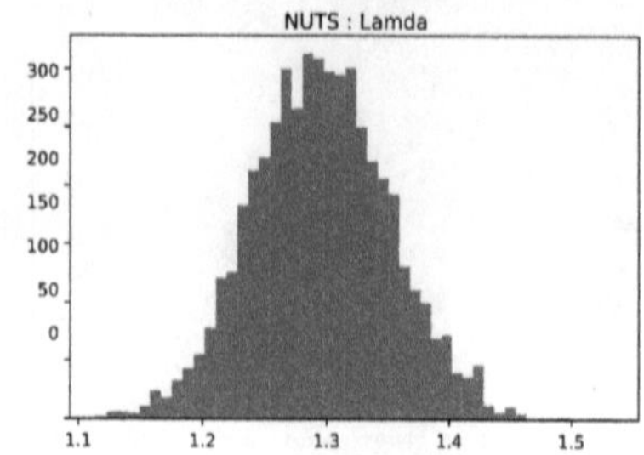

(**d**) Calibrated λ parameter on the simulated data using the NUTS algorithm.

Fig. 11.5 Calibrated parameters using the NUTS algorithm on simulated market data

Figure 11.7 shows the calibrated parameters through time for the β_0, β_1, β_2 and λ parameters on the USA Corporate bond yield curve data between 2018 and 2024 using both the NUTS and the OLS algorithms. In addition, Fig. 11.7 also shows the mean square error through time on unseen data. For each parameter, we show the 1.96 standard deviation confidence bands for the NUTS algorithm. We note the following patterns from Fig. 11.7:

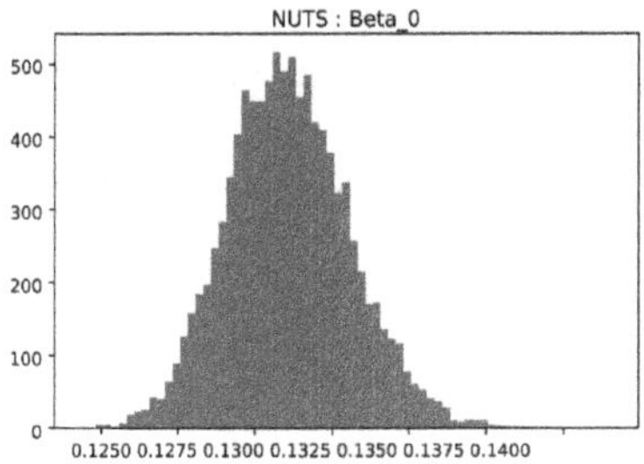

(**a**) Calibrated β_0 parameter on the ZAR swap curve market data as at 28 March 2024 using the NUTS algorithm.

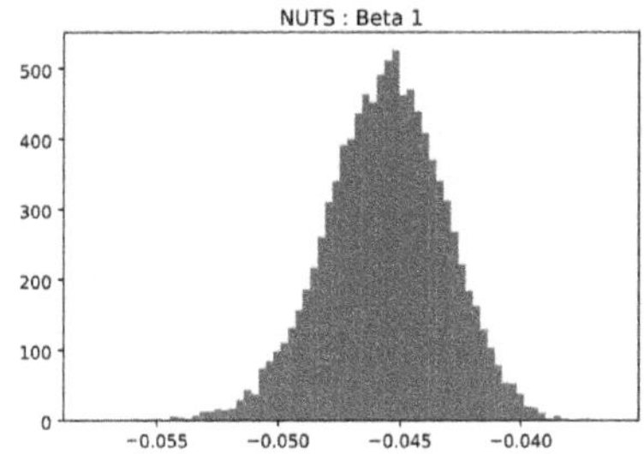

(**b**) Calibrated β_1 parameter on the ZAR swap curve market data as at 28 March 2024 using the NUTS algorithm.

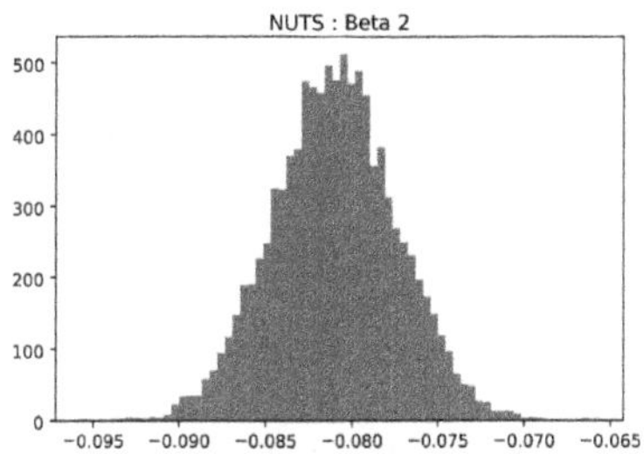

(**c**) Calibrated β_2 parameter on the ZAR swap curve market data as at 28 March 2024 using the NUTS algorithm.

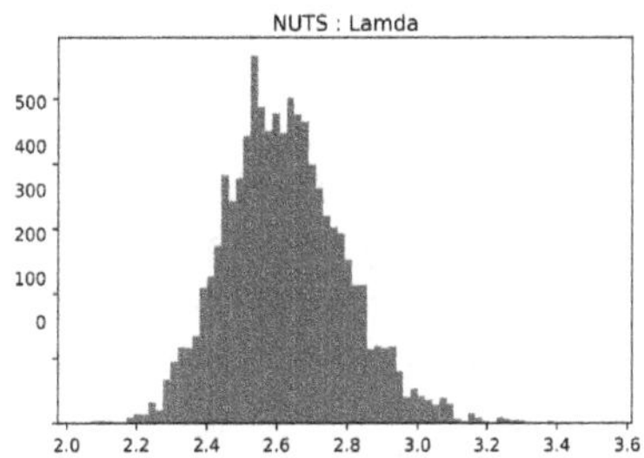

(**d**) Calibrated λ parameter on the ZAR swap curve market data as at 28 March 2024 using the NUTS algorithm.

Fig. 11.6 Calibrated parameters from the NS model using the NUTS algorithm on the ZAR swap curve market data as at 28 March 2024

Table 11.3 Calibrated NS model parameters using OLS and NUTS algorithms on the ZAR Swap Yield Curve Data as at 29 March 2024

Parameter	*OLS*	*NUTS*
β_0	0.1304	0.1311
β_1	−0.7444	−0.0456
β_2	−0.0812	−0.0810
λ	2.5599	2.6179

Table 11.4 Predictive performance on the ZAR Swap Yield Curve data as at 29 March 2024 using the OLS and NUTS algorithms. The entries in **bold** indicate the method that is outperforming the particular performance metric. The results show that the methods produce similar results, with marginal outperformance from the NUTS algorithm

Metric	*OLS*	*NUTS*
R2	0.993763	**0.993787**
MSE	0.007017	**0.006990**
MAPE	0.007804	**0.007636**
MAE	0.071268	**0.070161**

- The OLS and NUTS produce similar parameters for β_0 and β_2. In addition, the NUTS confidence bands are narrow for these parameters, indicating that we are fairly confident that the true parameter values lie in this range.
- The OLS and NUTS algorithms estimate diverge for the β_2 parameter at the start of the period but later align. Furthermore, the confidence bands are also wider for this parameter, indicating that the uncertainty is large for this parameter. In addition, in some instances, we find that the OLS estimates even lie outside the NUTS confidence bands, with the OLS estimate having more extreme movements through the period.
- The OLS and NUTS algorithms estimate for the λ parameter align. We find that large upward moves in this parameter increase the upper confidence band.
- We note that the MSE on unseen data for both NUTS and OLS are small over the period, with the pattern that the values were nearly zero before the COVID pandemic took effect in 2020 and remained high until late 2023 where the MSEs now revert back towards zero.

These results indicate the utility of using Bayesian techniques to calibrate the NS model. This framework can be extended by considering more advanced MCMC techniques and is not limited to the NS model but can also be utilized for the calibration of other term structure models.

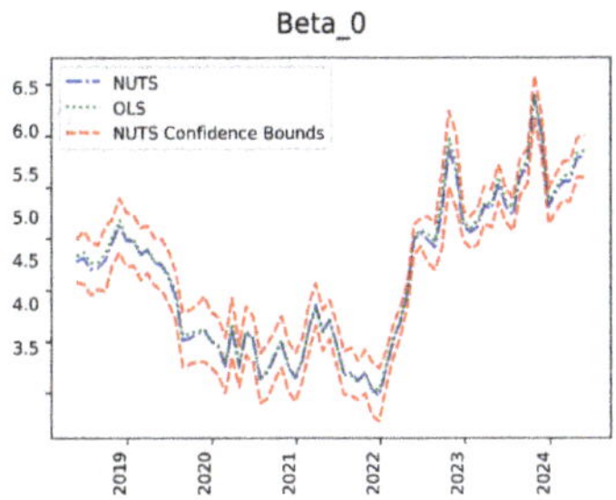

(**a**) Calibrated β_0 parameter through time using NUTS and OLS algorithms. The NUTS algorithm's 1.5 standard deviation confidence intervals are also presented.

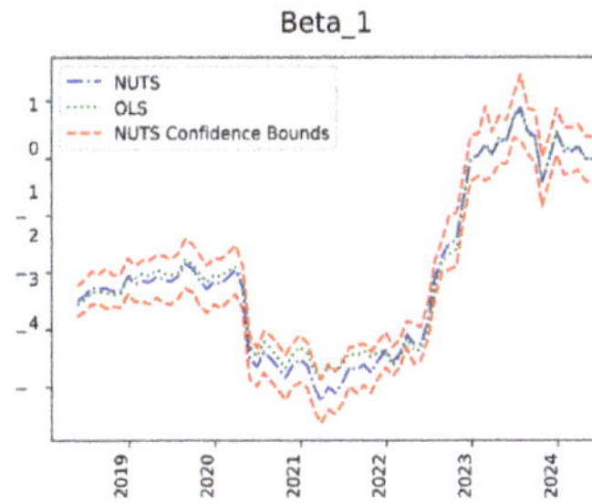

(**b**) Calibrated β_1 parameter through time using NUTS and OLS algorithms. The NUTS algorithm's 1.5 standard deviation confidence intervals are also presented.

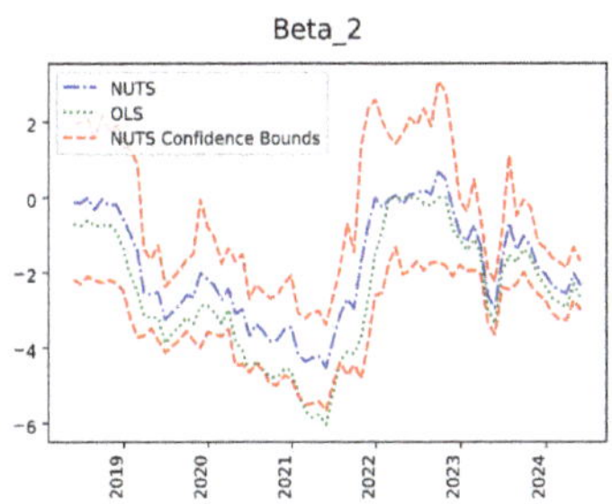

(**c**) Calibrated β_2 parameter through time using NUTS and OLS algorithms. The NUTS algorithm's 1.5 standard deviation confidence intervals are also presented.

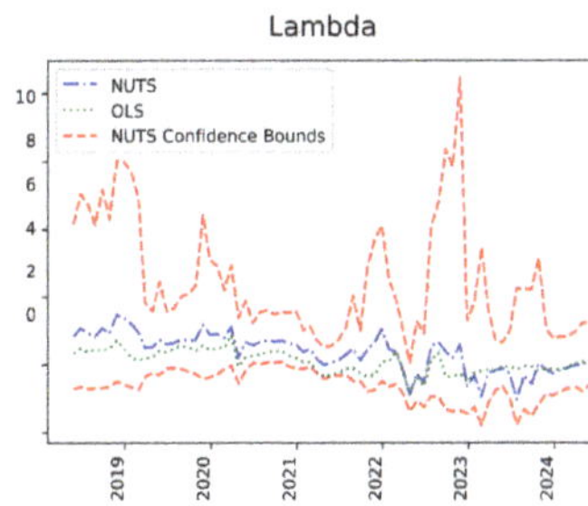

(**d**) Calibrated λ parameter through time using NUTS and OLS algorithms. The NUTS algorithm's 1.5 standard deviation confidence intervals are also presented.

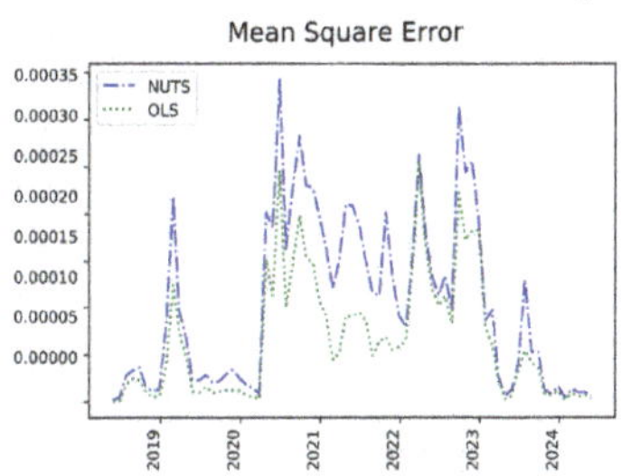

(**e**) Mean Square Error through time calculated on the NUTS and OLS algorithms respectively.

Fig. 11.7 Calibration results on the USA Corporate Bond Yield Curve market data using the NUTS and OLS algorithms between 2018 and 2024

11.6 Conclusion

In this chapter, we explored a first-in-the-literature Bayesian framework for calibrating the Nelson and Siegel (1987) model to local swap and international bond market yield curve data, as well as simulated data. The framework utilized advanced MCMC algorithms, including Hamiltonian Monte Carlo, Separable Shadow hybrid Hamiltonian Monte Carlo, and the No-U-Turns-Sampler.

Our analysis shows that the proposed framework produced results similar to or better than those of OLS-based calibration techniques across various calibration performance metrics. It has the added advantage of producing potentially more stable parameter estimates and the ability to capture uncertainties in the calibrated parameters, which is essential in explaining the parameters' movements over time.

In future work, we aim to extend this analysis to the dynamic NS model which can capture the dynamics of the yield curve through time. Furthermore, we aim to extend this analysis to modeling the term structure of volatilities, as initial studies in that domain have shown promising results. In the next chapter, we consider the task of yield curve model selection using the Nested Sampling approach of Skilling (2004) and its extensions.

References

Afshar, H. M., Oliveira, R., & Cripps, S. (2021). Non-volume preserving Hamiltonian Monte Carlo and No-U-Turn Samplers. In *International conference on artificial intelligence and statistics*. PMLR (pp. 1675–1683).

Andrieu, C., & Thoms, J. (2008). A tutorial on adaptive MCMC. *Statistics and Computing, 18*(4), 343–373.

Annaert, J., Claes, A., Ceuster, D., Marc, J. K., & Zhang, H. (2013). Estimating the spot rate curve using the Nelson-Siegel model: A ridge regression approach. *International Review of Economics & Finance, 27*, 482–496.

Bernadell, C., Coche, J., & Nyholm, K. (2005). Yield curve prediction for the strategic investor. Available at SSRN 701271.

Cox, J. C., Ross, S. A., & Rubinstein, M. (1979). Option pricing: A simplified approach. *Journal of Financial Economics, 7*(3), 229–263.

Diebold, F. X., & Li, C. (2006). Forecasting the term structure of government bond yields. *Journal of Econometrics, 130*(2), 337–364.

Duane, S., Kennedy, A. D., Pendleton, B. J., & Roweth, D. (1987). Hybrid monte carlo. *Physics Letters B, 195*(2), 216–222.

Duffee, G. (2013). Forecasting interest rates. In *Handbook of economic forecasting* (Vol. 2, pp. 385–426). Elsevier.

Gilli, M., Große, S., & Schumann, E. (2010). Calibrating the nelson-siegel-svensson model. Available at SSRN 1676747.

Guo, B., Han, Q., & Zhao, B. (2014). The Nelson-Siegel model of the term structure of option implied volatility and volatility components. *Journal of Futures Markets, 34*(8), 788–806.

Gürkaynak, R. S., Levin, A. T., & Swanson, E. T. (2006). *Does inflation targeting anchor long-run inflation expectations?* UK and Sweden: Evidence from long-term bond yields in the US.

Gürkaynak, R. S., Sack, B., & Wright, J. H. (2007). The US Treasury yield curve: 1961 to the present. *Journal of Monetary Economics, 54*(8), 2291–2304.

Hastings, W. K. (1970). Monte Carlo sampling methods using Markov chains and their applications. *Biometrica, 57*(1), 97–109.

Heide, C., Roosta, F., Hodgkinson, L., & Kroese, D. (2021). Shadow manifold Hamiltonian Monte Carlo. In *International conference on artificial intelligence and statistics*. PMLR (pp. 1477–1485).

Hoffman, M. D., & Gelman, A. (2014). The No-U-turn sampler: Adaptively setting path lengths in Hamiltonian Monte Carlo. *Journal of Machine Learning Research, 15*(1), 1593–1623.

Hölzermann, J. (2021). The Hull-White model under volatility uncertainty. *Quantitative Finance, 21*(11), 1921–1933.

Hull, J., & White, A. (2001). The general Hull-White model and supercalibration. *Financial Analysts Journal, 57*(6), 34–43.

Izaguirre, J. A., & Hampton, S. S. (Nov. 2004). Shadow hybrid Monte Carlo: An efficient propagator in phase space of macromolecules. *Journal of Computational Physics, 200*(2), 581–604. ISSN: 0021-9991. https://doi.org/10.1016/j.jcp.2004.04.016

Kazemie, N. (2014). *Mispricing Due to Nelson-Siegel-Svensson model.*

Kladívko, K., & Rusý, T. (2023). Maximum likelihood estimation of the Hull-White model. *Journal of Empirical Finance, 70*, 227–247.

Lakhany, A., Pintar, A., & Zhang, A. (2021). Calibrating the Nelson-Siegel-Svensson model by genetic algorithm. arXiv preprint arXiv:2108.01760.

Marwala, T., Mbuvha, R., & Mongwe, W. T. (2023). *Hamiltonian Monte Carlo methods in machine learning*. Elsevier.

Mbuvha, R., Boulkaibet, I., & Marwala, T. (2019b). Bayesian automatic relevance determination for feature selection in credit default modelling. In *International conference on artificial neural networks* (pp. 420–425). Springer.

Mbuvha, R., & Marwala, T. (2020). Bayesian inference of COVID-19 spreading rates in South Africa. *PloS One, 15*(8), Article e0237126.

Mbuvha, R., Mongwe, W. T., & Marwala, T. (2021). Separable Shadow Hamiltonian Hybrid Monte Carlo for Bayesian neural network inference in wind speed forecasting. *Energy and A, I*, Article 100108.

Monetary Economic Department. (2005). Zero-coupon yield curves estimated by central banks. In *Technical report 25, bank for international settlements* (Vol. 25). https://www.bis.org/publ/bppdf/bispap25a.pdf

Mongwe, W. T. (Dec. 2015). *Analysis of equity and interest rate returns in South Africa under the context of jump diffusion processes.* Masters Thesis at University of Cape Town. Last Retrieved: 18 March 2021. https://open.uct.ac.za/bitstream/handle/11427/16600/thesis_com_2015_mongwe_wilson_tsakane.pdf?isAllowed=y&sequence=1

Mongwe, W. T., & Malan, K. M (2020). A survey of automated financial statement fraud detection with relevance to the South African context. *South African Computer Journal, 32*(1). https://doi.org/10.18489/sacj.v32i1.777

Mongwe, W. T., Sidogi, T., Mbuvha, R., & Marwala, T. (2022b). Probabilistic inference of south african equity option prices under jump-diffusion processes. In *2022 IEEE symposium on computational intelligence for financial engineering and economics (CIFEr)* (pp. 1–8). IEEE.

Mongwe, W. T. (2021). Adaptively setting the path length for separable shadow Hamiltonian hybrid Monte Carlo. *IEEE Access, 9*, 138598–138607.

Mongwe, W. T. (2022). Shadow Magnetic Hamiltonian Monte Carlo. *IEEE Access, 10*, 34340–34351. https://doi.org/10.1109/ACCESS.2022.3161443

Mongwe, W. T., Mbuvha, R., & Marwala, T. (2021). Adaptive Magnetic Hamiltonian Monte Carlo. *IEEE Access, 9*, 152993–153003. https://doi.org/10.1109/ACCESS.2021.3127931

Mongwe, W. T., Mbuvha, R., & Marwala, T. (2021). Bayesian inference of local government audit outcomes. *Plos One*. https://doi.org/10.1371/journal.pone.0261245

Neal, R. M. (1993). Bayesian learning via stochastic dynamics. In *Advances in neural information processing systems* (Vol. 5, pp. 475–482). Morgan Kaufmann Publishers Inc. ISBN: 1-55860-274-7. http://dl.acm.org/citation.cfm?id=645753.667903

Neal, R. M. et al. (2011). *The No-U-Turn Sampler: Adaptively setting path lengths in Hamiltonian Monte Carlo*. arXiv:1111.4246 [stat.CO]

Neal, R. M., et al. (2011). MCMC using Hamiltonian dynamics. *Handbook of Markov Chain Monte Carlo, 2*(11), 2.

Nelson, C. R., & Siegel, A. F. (1987). Parsimonious modeling of yield curves. *Journal of Business*, 473–489.

Skilling, J. (2004). Nested sampling. In *AIP conference proceedings* (Vol. 735. 1, pp. 395–405). American Institute of Physics.

Svensson, L. E. O. (1995). Estimating forward interest rates with the extended Nelson & Siegel method. *Sveriges Riksbank Quarterly Review, 3*(1), 13–26.

Sweet, C. R., Hampton, S. S., Skeel, R. D., & Izaguirre, J. A. (2009). A separable shadow Hamiltonian hybrid Monte Carlo method. *The Journal of Chemical Physics, 131*(17), Article 174106.

Vasicek, O. (1977). An equilibrium characterization of the term structure. *Journal of Financial Economics, 5*(2), 177–188.

Wahlstrøm, R. R., Paraschiv, F., & Schürle, M. (2022). A comparative analysis of parsimonious yield curve models with focus on the Nelson-Siegel, Svensson and Bliss versions. *Computational Economics*, 1–38.

CHAPTER 12

Static and Dynamic Nested Sampling for Yield Curve Model Selection

12.1 Introduction

Having an appreciation of how the yield curve evolves is critical for various financial problems, including debt structuring, risk management, asset pricing, and portfolio allocation (Nelson & Siegel, 1987; Tavanielli & Laurini, 2023). Furthermore, understanding the yield curve and economic activity in a particular jurisdiction is critical for determining a country's monetary and fiscal policies (Tavanielli & Laurini, 2023). The Nelson and Siegel (1987) model and its extensions are parametric models that are commonly used by portfolio managers and central banks for modeling the yield curve (Department, 2005; Diebold & Li, 2006; Nelson & Siegel, 1987; Svensson, 1995). The original Nelson and Siegel model models the yield curve using three components being the short-term (slope), medium-term (curvature), and long-term (intercept) effects (Department, 2005; Diebold and Li, 2006; Nelson & Siegel, 1987). Thus, under this model, the shape of the yield curve is decomposed into these factor loadings, and this parameterization allows the

Supplementary Information The online version contains supplementary material available at https://doi.org/10.1007/978-3-031-88431-3_12.

W. T. Mongwe et al., *Bayesian Machine Learning in Quantitative Finance*, https://doi.org/10.1007/978-3-031-88431-3_12

Nelson and Siegel model to be flexible enough to capture various shapes of the yield curve (Diebold & Li, 2006; Nelson & Siegel, 1987).

There has been an increase in the number of yield curve models utilized in practice and in the literature (Diebold & Li, 2006; Duffee, 2013; Guo et al., 2014; Hull & White, 2001; Kazemie, 2014; Nelson & Siegel, 1987; Vasicek, 1977). The increase in the number of models used has now brought to the fore the importance of being able to quantify the confidence one has in a specific model, as well as the goodness of fit of a given model when compared to another. This inference problem can be tackled using the frequentist paradigm via cross-validation, for instance, or the Bayesian paradigm, using the Bayesian evidence metric. In this chapter, we explore a first-in-literature approach to calibrating the term structure models under consideration using Bayesian inference and extracting the Bayesian evidence, which we utilize to compare the various models.

Bayesian inference can be implemented for parameter estimation as well as for model selection. With parameter estimation, one is concerned about attaining the most plausible parameters for a given model. Parameter estimation was the focus of the previous chapter. This is usually carried out using sampling approaches such as Markov Chain Monte Carlo (Neal, 1993a) such as the Metropolis-Hastings and Hamiltonian Monte Carlo (HMC) algorithms (Duane et al., 1987; Hastings, 1970) and variational inference techniques (Hinton & Van Camp, 1993; Hoffman et al., 2013). On the other hand, model selection involves calculating the marginal over the parameters likelihood (or the evidence) for each model. This evidence indicates how well a given model fits the observed dataset when compared to another model (Higson et al., 2019; Marwala et al., 2016; MacKay, 1992). The evidence metric itself is not trivial to evaluate analytically and requires numerical methods (Higson et al., 2019; Marwala et al., 2016; Osborne et al., 2012; Russel et al., 2019). This is particularly the case for complex models where the parameter space has a high dimension, such as neural networks. Many techniques have been proposed for calculating the marginal likelihood including Bayesian quadrature (Osborne et al., 2012) and nested sampling (Mthembu et al., 2011; Skilling, 2004).

The Bayesian quadrature approach uses a small number of observations of the likelihood to infer a distribution of the marginal likelihood (Gunter et al., 2014; Osborne et al., 2012). This approach offers improved sample efficiency, which is essential for samples drawn from complex and computationally expensive models. Bayesian quadrature has, however, displayed high variance around the evidence estimate and convergence diagnostics due to variations in the sample observations selected (Gunter et al., 2014).

MacKay (1992) uses the evidence framework in the context of Multi-Layer Perceptrons (MLPs) where the posterior distribution of the parameters was approximated using a Gaussian distribution. This approximation simplifies the calculation of the evidence. The Gaussian approximation has been found to provide inferior evidence estimates due to approximation errors of the Laplace approximation to the true multi-modal posterior (Mbuvha et al., 2017). This leads to trivial or extremely regularized model selection.

The nested sampling approach of Skilling (2006) provides advantages over other evidence approximation techniques in that (1) it transforms the evidence integral into a 1-dimensional integral, thus reducing the computational burden, (2) it calculates the evidence and provides the posterior parameter estimates all in one run at no extra cost. There have been various extensions of this original formulation of nested sampling (Higson et al., 2019). Dynamic nested sampling extends the original nested sampling algorithm of Skilling (2006) by continually varying the number of live points to maximize computation accuracy for a given number of posterior samples (Higson et al., 2019).

In this chapter, we compare various subsets of the Nelson and Siegel model by setting some of the factor loadings to zero and performing model selection on this. We utilize the static and dynamic nested sampling algorithms for this task, which is yet to be considered in the literature. Given that the Nelson and Siegel model has three-factor loadings, it would be interesting to analyze which factors are driving a particular yield curve at a particular point in time. In this chapter, we further extend the original Nelson and Siegel by incorporating automatic relevance determination, which allows us to automatically rank which of the factor loadings are driving a particular yield curve shape at a point in time. We train this model using the No-U-Turn Sampler (NUTS) (Hoffman & Gelman, 2011) algorithm detailed in the previous chapter. The NUTS algorithm is an ideal technique to utilize because it automatically tunes the step size and the path length parameters of the HMC algorithm, making it easy for non-subject matter experts to utilize it (Hoffman & Gelman, 2011).

For our analysis, we consider simulated yield curve data where we know the underlying Nelson and Siegel model parameters that generated the data and a time series of yield curves from the US corporate bond market. We utilize the simulated data to analyze the Bayesian evidence framework for model selection, and we use the time series yield curve data to calibrate our proposed ARD-NS model using the NUTS algorithm. Our results show that our Bayesian evidence approach for model selection can identify which model produced the underlying data. Furthermore, analyzing the importances derived from the ARD-NS model indicates that the medium-term factor loading (which is the curvature component) is the main factor driving the yield curve shape over the period under consideration.

The remainder of this chapter is structured as follows: We first describe the Bayesian models used to model the yield curves in Sect. 12.2; we then detail the Bayesian evidence estimation techniques used in Sect. 12.3; we then present the experiment setup, after which we present the results, discuss them, and provide the conclusion in Sects. 12.4–12.6 respectively.

12.2 Yield Curve Models

In this section, we present the yield curve models that we analyze in this chapter. These models are variations, or subsets, of the Nelson and Siegel (1987) model with some of the factor loading set to zero. We also introduce a new model, which we term the automatic relevance determination Nelson and Siegel (ARD-NS) model.

12.2.1 *Subsets of the Nelson and Siegel Model*

As outlined in the previous chapter, the Nelson and Siegel (1987) model gives the following yield curve function:

$$y_t(\tau) = \beta_0 + \beta_1\left(\frac{1-\exp(-\lambda\tau)}{\lambda\tau}\right) + \beta_2\left(\frac{1-\exp(-\lambda\tau)}{\lambda\tau} - \exp(-\lambda\tau)\right) \tag{12.1}$$

where $\{\beta_0, \beta_1, \beta_2, \lambda\}$ are the parameters of the model, t is the current time (or valuation date in some contexts) and τ is the time period between now and the point of interest on the yield curve. Note that $\beta_0 > 0$ and $\lambda > 0$, and this must be factored into the calibration. In our Bayesian setting, we set the prior distribution to be Gaussian for β_1 and β_2 and LogNormal for β_0 and λ.

This functional form is a convenient and economical three-component exponential approximation, which works very well to model the yield curve, as shown in Diebold and Li (2006). The three factors β_0, β_1, and β_2 are of special interest. The loading on β_0 is 1, a constant that does not approach zero in the limit; therefore, β_0 may be considered a long-term factor. The loading on β_1 is $\left(\frac{1-\exp(-\lambda\tau)}{\lambda\tau}\right)$, a function that starts at 1, however, decays monotonically and rapidly to 0, and hence may be considered as a short-term factor. The loading on β_2 is $\left(\frac{1-\exp(-\lambda\tau)}{\lambda\tau} - \exp(-\lambda\tau)\right)$, which begins at 0, increases, and then converges to zero; therefore, it may be considered as a medium-term factor.

To assess the impact of the factor loadings, we compare the following subsets of the Nelson and Siegel (1987) model, where some of the factor loadings $\{\beta_0, \beta_1, \beta_2\}$ are set to zero:

1. **Model 1**:

$$y_t(\tau) = \beta_0 \tag{12.2}$$

2. **Model 2**:

$$y_t(\tau) = \beta_1\left(\frac{1-\exp(-\lambda\tau)}{\lambda\tau}\right) \tag{12.3}$$

3. **Model 3**:

$$y_t(\tau) = \beta_2\left(\frac{1-\exp(-\lambda\tau)}{\lambda\tau} - \exp(-\lambda\tau)\right) \tag{12.4}$$

4. **Model 4**:

$$y_t(\tau) = \beta_0 + \beta_1\left(\frac{1-\exp(-\lambda\tau)}{\lambda\tau}\right) \tag{12.5}$$

5. **Model 5**:

$$y_t(\tau) = \beta_0 + \beta_2\left(\frac{1-\exp(-\lambda\tau)}{\lambda\tau} - \exp(-\lambda\tau)\right) \tag{12.6}$$

6. **Model 6**:

$$y_t(\tau) = \beta_1\left(\frac{1-\exp(-\lambda\tau)}{\lambda\tau}\right) + \beta_2\left(\frac{1-\exp(-\lambda\tau)}{\lambda\tau} - \exp(-\lambda\tau)\right) \tag{12.7}$$

7. **Model 7**:

$$y_t(\tau) = \beta_0 + \beta_1\left(\frac{1-\exp(-\lambda\tau)}{\lambda\tau}\right) + \beta_2\left(\frac{1-\exp(-\lambda\tau)}{\lambda\tau} - \exp(-\lambda\tau)\right) \tag{12.8}$$

As can be seen, Models 1 to 7 are subsets of the original NS model with some of the factor loadings $\{\beta_0, \beta_1, \beta_2\}$ set to zero. Note that Model 7 is the full NS model.

12.2.2 *Automatic Relevance Determination Nelson and Siegel Model*

In this section, we introduce the automatic relevance determination Nelson and Siegel (ARD-NS) model, an extension of the Nelson and Siegel model that allows us to automatically rank the relevance of each factor loading for the calibrated yield curve. That is, it allows us to know the relative importance of the short-term β_1, medium-term β_2, and long-term β_0 factor loading in an automated manner. The negative log-likelihood $l(\mathrm{D}|\mathbf{w})$ function for this model is given by:

$$l(\mathrm{D}|\mathbf{w} = \{\boldsymbol{\beta_0}, \boldsymbol{\beta_1}, \boldsymbol{\beta_3}, \lambda\}) = \sum_{i}^{N}[y_t(\tau, \{\beta_0, \beta_1, \beta_3, \lambda\}) - y_i]^2 \tag{12.9}$$

where $y_t(\tau, \{\beta_0, \beta_1, \beta_3, \lambda\}) = \beta_0 + \beta_1\left(\frac{1-\exp(-\lambda\tau)}{\lambda\tau}\right) + \beta_2\left(\frac{1-\exp(-\lambda\tau)}{\lambda\tau} - \exp(-\lambda\tau)\right)$, $\mathrm{D} = \{\tau, y\}$ is the data, N is the number of observations and $\mathbf{w} = \{\boldsymbol{\beta_0}, \boldsymbol{\beta_1}, \boldsymbol{\beta_3}, \lambda\}$ are the parameters that need to be estimated. Thus, the target un-normalized posterior log distribution is given as (Mongwe et al., 2021):

$$\ln p(\mathbf{w}|\mathrm{D}) = l(\mathrm{D}|\mathbf{w}) + \ln p(\mathbf{w}|\alpha) + \ln q(\alpha) \tag{12.10}$$

where $\ln p(\mathbf{w}|\alpha)$ is the log of the prior distribution placed on the parameters given the hyperparameters, and $\ln q(\alpha)$ is the distribution of the hyperparameters. Mongwe et al. (2021), Marwala et al. (2023), we model the parameters **w** as having a Gaussian prior with each parameter having zero mean and its own standard deviation or regularization parameter α_i, meaning that we are using an automatic relevance determination (ARD) prior within our framework. The α_i indicates how important the parameter associated with the input feature is. The larger the value of α_i, the more important the input feature is in predicting the expenditures (Mongwe et al., 2021). Thus, this framework automatically ranks the importance of the factor loadings.

Due to the multi-modal and non-convex structure of the ARD loss function, inference of ARD prior hyperparameters is a fundamentally complex inverse problem (MacKay, 1995; Mbuvha et al., 2021; Neal, 1993b). The hyperparameter sampling strategy used in this chapter is to jointly infer the α hyperparameters and the **w** parameters as in Mongwe et al. (2021). Although the effective parameter space is doubled in this approach, compared to the Gibbs sampling strategy described in Mbuvha et al. (2021), MacKay (1995), Neal (1993b) for example, this method has the advantage of producing a more stable exploration across the MCMC methods (Mongwe et al., 2021). As the **w** parameters are assumed to be normally distributed, we select the α hyperparameters to be log-normally distributed to make the joint sampling of parameters and hyperparameters mathematically convenient. In particular, the α_is are assumed to follow a log-normal distribution with mean zero and variance 1. We use the state-of-the-art No-U-Turn Sampler (NUTS) (Hoffman & Gelman, 2014) MCMC algorithm to perform inference on this ARD-NS model.

12.3 Bayesian Evidence Framework

In Bayesian inference, one is interested in estimating the posterior distribution $P(\theta|D, M)$ of a set of parameters θ for a given model M and data D. This inference problem can be written as Bayes theorem:

$$P(\theta|D, M) = \frac{P(D|\theta, M)P(\theta|M)}{P(D|M)} \tag{12.11}$$

where $P(D|\theta, M)$ is the likelihood of the data, $P(\theta|M)$ is the prior for the parameters, and

$$P(D|M) = \int_{\Omega_\theta} P(D|\theta, M)P(\theta|M)d\theta \tag{12.12}$$

is the marginal likelihood (or evidence) for the data given M, where the integral is taken over the entire domain Ω_θ of θ, with θ possibly having a high dimension. It is worth noting that this evidence metric naturally penalizes unnecessarily complex models through the prior distribution. Two models might have the same likelihood, but also have very different degrees of complexity. The evidence metric penalizes the overly complex models in favor of simpler ones and thus naturally embodies Occam's Razor (Bishop, 1997; MacKay, 1992; Rasmussen & Ghahramani, 2001).

For ease of reference, the shorthand notation below will be used in the rest of this chapter (Speagle, 2020):

$$P(\theta_M) = \frac{L(\theta_M)\pi(\theta_M)}{Z_M} \tag{12.13}$$

where $P(\theta_M) := P(\theta|D, M)$ is the posterior, $L(\theta_M) := P(D|\theta, M)$ is the likelihood, $\pi(\theta_M) := P(\theta|M)$ is the prior, $Z_M := P(D|M)$ is the evidence. From the posterior $P(\theta_M)$ one gets the parameter estimates for a given model M, while Z_M allows one to compare models using the Bayes factor (Kass & Raftery, 1995):

$$BF := \frac{Z_{M_1}}{Z_{M_2}} \frac{\pi(M_1)}{\pi(M_2)} \tag{12.14}$$

where $\pi(M_i)$ is the prior belief for model i. Values of the Bayes factor greater than one are considered as evidence in favor of model M_1 and vice versa (Kass & Raftery, 1995). Suppose one has no prior belief that one model is better than another, which is usually the case in practice. In that case, the prior probabilities of all the models are made equal so that comparing models amounts to comparing the model evidence (Kass & Raftery, 1995).

The posterior $P(\theta_M)$ is usually analytically intractable for complicated models. The posterior distribution must then be estimated using numerical methods (Higson et al., 2019; MacKay, 1992; Speagle, 2020). The main focus of this chapter is not on estimating the posterior of the parameters, but rather the focus is on calculating the evidence of a given model. The evidence will be the metric used to compare between different models. We then utilize the estimated posterior $P(\theta_M)$, which is a by-product in the process of estimating the evidence Z_M, to estimate the predictive performance of the model on unseen data.

In the following sections, we present the static (i.e., the classic) and dynamic nested sampling algorithms for calculating the evidence metric Z_M.

12.3.1 Static Nested Sampling

The evidence metric in Eq. 12.12 can be re-formulated as:

$$Z_m = \int_{\Omega_\theta} L(\theta_M)\pi(\theta_M)d\theta. \tag{12.15}$$

This integral can be very high dimensional, depending on the parameter space. The nested sampling algorithm of Skilling (2006) applies a trick of transforming this multidimensional parameter space integral into a one-dimensional integral, after which classical numerical methods such as the trapezoidal rule can be used.

The main idea behind nested sampling is to divide the prior parameter space Ω_θ and order these by the likelihood $L(\theta_M)$. Let the total prior mass be denoted by X, then each unit in this prior mass is $dX = \pi(\theta_M)d\theta$. The likelihood function in the X space is then written as $L(\theta_M) = L(X)$. This formulation transforms the likelihood from a multidimensional function into a function of a single parameter X (Skilling, 2006). The evidence integral then becomes (Skilling, 2006):

$$Z_m = \int_0^1 L(X)dX. \tag{12.16}$$

The steps in the nested sampling algorithm are outlined in Algorithm 12.1. Note that for the models under consideration in this chapter, the likelihood is a Gaussian, i.e., squared error.

Algorithm 12.1: Static Nested Sampling

Data: Training dataset $\{\mathbf{X}^{(i)}, \mathbf{Y}^{(i)}\}$, K live points
Result: Evidence Z_m and posterior distribution of parameters $P(\theta_M)$
begin

1. Sample K parameter values from the prior and evaluate their likelihoods.
2. Order the live points K by their likelihoods
3. Select the live point that results in the lowest likelihood, and increment the evidence by some summation rule
4. Remove the live point with the lowest likelihood from the original K live points
5. Replace it with a new live point sampled from the prior within the remaining prior volume The new live point must have a higher likelihood than the discarded live points likelihood
6. Repeat steps 2 to 5 until some stopping criterion is reached. This could be the desired precision on the evidence or some iteration count.

end

12.3.2 *Dynamic Nested Sampling*

Over the last number of years, the original nested sampling algorithm of Skilling (2006, 2004) has been improved upon. The improvements include the diffusive and dynamic nested sampling algorithms (Brewer et al., 2011; Speagle, 2020), and in this section, we focus on the dynamic nested sampling algorithm (Higson et al., 2019). Higson et al. (2019) propose altering the static nested sampling algorithm outlined in Algorithm 12.1 by continually varying the number of live points K to maximize computation accuracy for a given number of posterior samples, subject to practical limits. This is in contrast to the static nested sampling described above, in which the number of live points K is constant.

The authors show in their work that the dynamic nested sampling method significantly improves calculation accuracy in empirical tests compared to static nested sampling with the same number of samples. They also show that the accuracy of both parameter estimation and evidence calculations can be improved concurrently. Furthermore, unlike in static nested sampling, more accurate results can be obtained by running the dynamic nested sampling algorithm for longer.

The distribution of posterior mass as a function of likelihood is apriori unknown, so for the dynamic nested sampling, we first approximate it with a static nested sampling run using a small constant number of live points K (Higson et al., 2019). The algorithm then iteratively determines the range of likelihoods where adding more live points will maximize calculation accuracy and create an additional thread that runs over these likelihoods (Higson et al., 2019). To lessen the number of times the sampler has to be restarted and the importance needs to be determined, a few more threads (or batches) can be created at each stage if necessary. When the number of samples collected in each batch is small relative to the overall number of samples in the run, Higson et al. (2019) found in empirical testing that employing batches larger than one has minimal influence on efficiency improvements from dynamic nested sampling. Refer to Higson et al. (2019), Speagle (2020) for further details on the dynamic nested sampling algorithm.

12.4 Numerical Experiments

In this section, we present the numerical experiments conducted. We first describe the dataset and then outline the experiments, settings, and performance metrics used.

12.4.1 Experiment Setup And Data Description

Our analysis is based on real-world (for factor loading analysis) and simulated (for model selection) datasets. The simulated data is from Model 4 described above with known parameters being $\{\beta_0 = 0.04, \beta_1 = -0.05, \lambda = 1.3\}$, while the real-world data is the time series of corporate bond yield curves from the US treasury from 1 Jan 2019 to 31 May 2024. We calibrate, using static and dynamic nested sampling, all seven models to the simulated data and perform the model comparison using the Bayesian evidence metric. We then calibrate the ARD-NS model to the real-world data using the NUTS algorithm and analyze the factor loadings through time.

12.4.2 Performance Metrics

The performance metrics used in this chapter are predictive performance on unseen data. The predictive performance metrics used are the Mean Square Error (MSE), Mean Absolute Error (MAE), coefficient of determination (R^2), and Mean Percentage Error (MAPE). For the NUTS algorithm, we set the pre-conditioning matrix $\mathbf{M} = \mathbf{I}$, which is the common approach in practice. We generated five chains with 2000 samples for all the datasets with a burn-in period of 1000. This was sufficient for all the algorithms to converge on all the datasets. We utilize the **dynesty** (Speagle, 2020) Python package for our static and dynamic nested sampling runs with the default settings.

12.5 Results and Discussions

In this section, we present the results and the discussions from the numerical experiments. Table 12.1 shows the log evidence across all the models using the static and dynamic nested sampling algorithms. Tables 12.2 and 12.3 show the predictive performance of the models trained using static and dynamic nested sampling, respectively. Figure 12.1 shows the predictive performance of the models on unseen simulated data from Model 4, while Figs. 12.2, 12.3, 12.4, 12.5, 12.6, 12.7, 12.8, 12.9, 12.10, 12.11, 12.12 and 12.13 shows a summary of the static and dynamic nested runs respectively for Models 4 and 7. Figure 12.14 shows the relative importances of the factor loadings in Model 7 calibrated through time on the US corporate yield curves time series data.

Table 12.1 shows that the static and dynamic nested sampling methods produce similar log evidence metrics across all the models. In addition, we note that the model with the high log evidence is Model 4, meaning that the best model that describes the data is Model 4. This makes sense since the dataset was simulated from this model originally. Furthermore, we note that Models 1, 2, and 3 are the lowest-ranked models. These three models produce constant yield curves as shown in Fig. 12.1 as they incorporate only one-factor loading. We also note that Models 5, 6, and 7 are the next set of models that best capture the underlying data.

Table 12.1 Log evidence on simulated yield market data From Model 4 using the static and dynamic nested sampling algorithms. The entries in **bold** indicate the model that outperforms. The results show that Model 4 has the highest log evidence across both static and dynamic nested sampling methods

Model	*Static nested sampling*	*Dynamic nested sampling*
Model 1	-91.951 +/− 0.133	-91.929 +/− 0.076
Model 2	−106.615 +/− 0.222	−106.559 +/− 0.158
Model 3	−106.250 +/− 0.219	−106.612 +/− 0.152
Model 4	**-23.655 +/− 0.172**	**-23.800 +/− 0.110**
Model 5	-25.416 +/− 0.176	-25.055 +/− 0.110
Model 6	-25.512 +/− 0.177	-25.402 +/− 0.107
Model 7	-26.782 +/− 0.192	-26.852 +/− 0.119

Table 12.2 Predictive performance on simulated yield curve data from Model 4 using static nested sampling. The entries in **bold** indicate the model that outperforms that particular performance metric

Model	R^2	*MSE*	*MAPE*	*MAE*
Model 1	-0.0064029	0.000168	1.929879	0.010900
Model 2	-0.012488	0.0001696	1.8962894	0.01102314
Model 3	−2.525568	0.0005907	0.99554	0.021145
Model 4	0.9998423	2.641148e-08	0.02761311	**0.0001109**
Model 5	0.9808094	3.215827e-06	0.267222	0.00146463
Model 6	-3985.39731	0.6680144	140.25967	0.588773
Model 7	**0.9998634**	**2.289894e-08**	**0.0079024**	0.0001362

Table 12.3 Predictive performance on simulated yield curve data from Model 4 using dynamic nested sampling. The entries in **bold** indicate the model that outperforms that particular performance metric

Model	R^2	*MSE*	*MAPE*	*MAE*
Model 1	-0.006402	0.0001686	1.870011	1.92987
Model 2	-0.0156945	0.000170	1.940044	0.010940
Model 3	-2.55111	0.000595	0.997830	0.0212133
Model 4	**0.99999176**	**1.37963e-09**	**0.003240**	**3.468798e-05**
Model 5	0.980301789	3.300897e-06	0.280548	0.0015040
Model 6	-4105.5842	0.68815	142.2326	0.59926
Model 7	0.99997822	3.6485784e-09	0.0087270	4.246360e-05

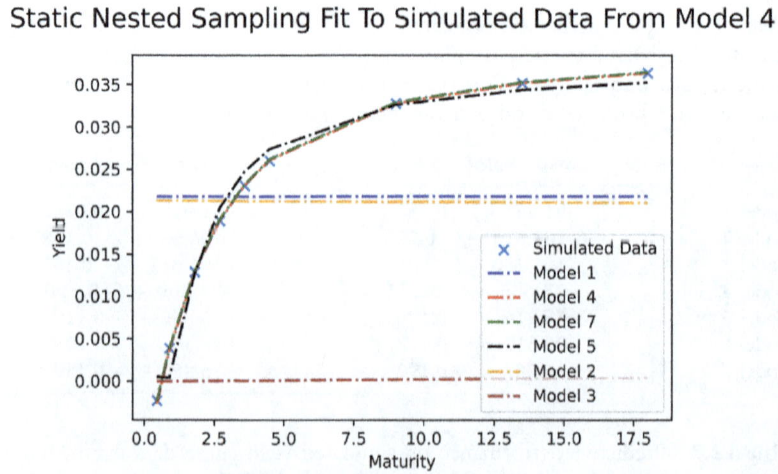

(a) Static nested sampling prediction results across the seven models on unseen data.

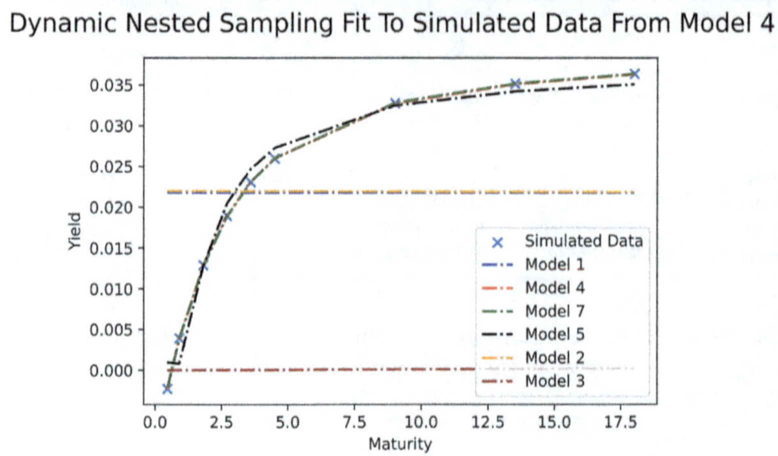

(b) Dynamic nested sampling prediction results across the seven models on unseen data.

Fig. 12.1 Inference results for static and dynamic nested sampling across all seven models on unseen data. The results show that Model 4 and Model 7 can fit the yield curve on unseen data, while the other models cannot reproduce the curve. Note that Model 6 is excluded from the figure as its predictions were far from the target, as shown in Tables 12.2 and 12.3

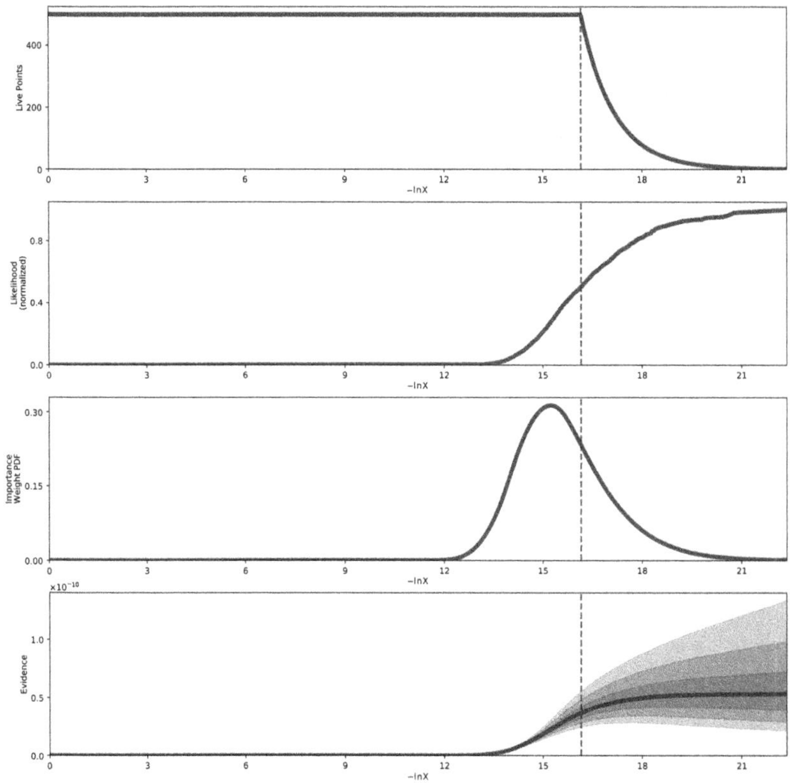

Fig. 12.2 Static nested sampling plot of summary of run on a simulated dataset for Model 4

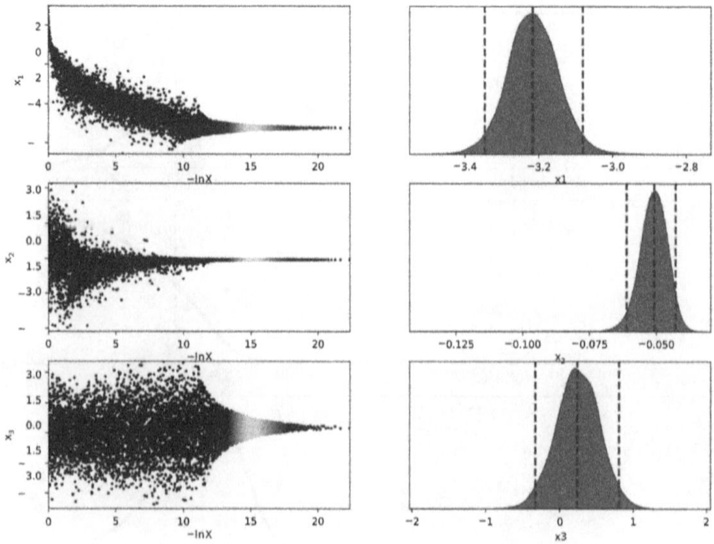

Fig. 12.3 Static nested sampling plot of parameter traces and 1-D marginalized posteriors on simulated for Model 4

However, as the evidence metric penalizes more complex models, these models produce lower evidence compared to Model 4. In particular, as shown in Tables 12.2 and 12.3, Model 7 produces a predictive performance that is comparable only to Model 4 but has lower evidence due to Model 7 having more parameters.

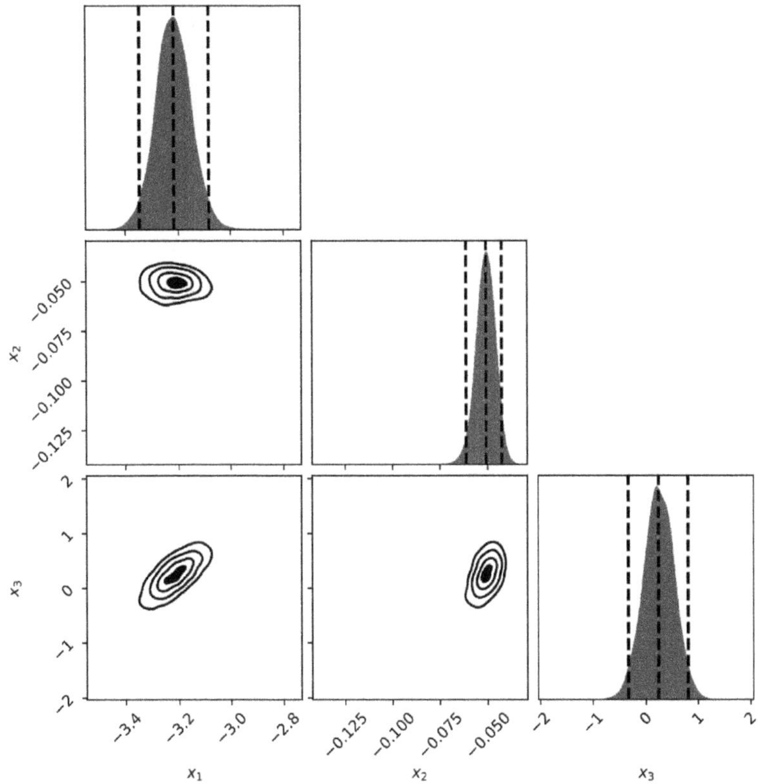

Fig. 12.4 Static nested sampling plot of the 2-D marginalized posteriors on simulated data for Model 4

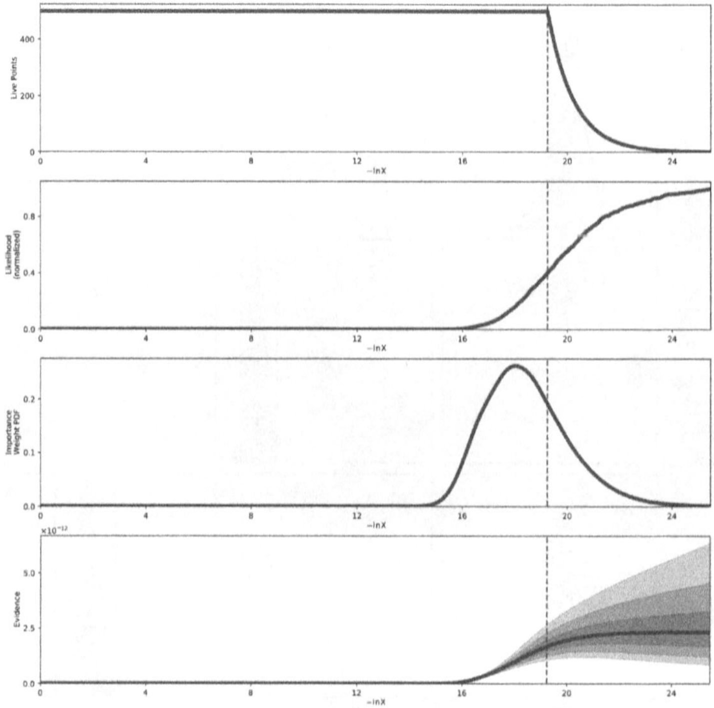

Fig. 12.5 Static nested sampling plot of summary of run on simulated data for Model 7

We note that Model 4 produces the best predictive performance across all the performance metrics when trained using dynamic best sampling, with Model 7 coming in second place. However, when trained using static nested sampling, Model 7 produces the best predictive performance, and Model 4 comes in second place. This shows how similar these models are, except that one is more complex (i.e., has more parameters) than

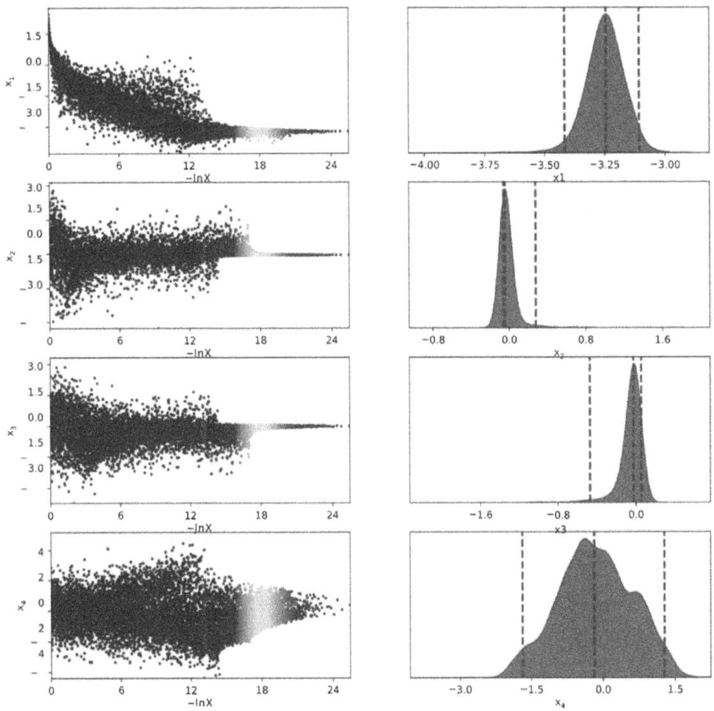

Fig. 12.6 Static nested sampling plot of parameter traces and 1-D marginalized posteriors on simulated data for Model 7

the other. Figures 12.2 to 12.13 show the summary of running the static and dynamic nested sampling algorithms on the closest competing models being Model 4 and Model 7 using static and dynamic nested sampling, respectively. Note that the parameters $\{\beta_0, \beta_1, \beta_2, \lambda\}$ map to $x_i's$ on the static and dynamic nested sampling runs shown in Figs. 12.2 to 12.13. For example, Model 4 parameters $\{\beta_0, \beta_1, \lambda\}$ map to $\{x_1, x_2, x_3\}$ on the static and dynamic nested sampling runs. We further note that using both sampling methods, the inference results for each model are similar.

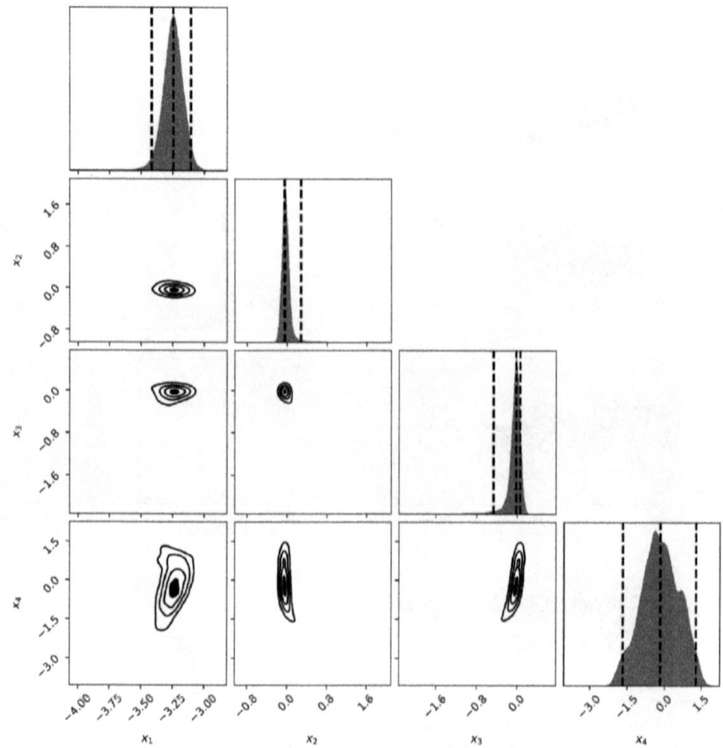

Fig. 12.7 Static nested sampling plot of the 2-D marginalized posteriors on simulated data for Model 7

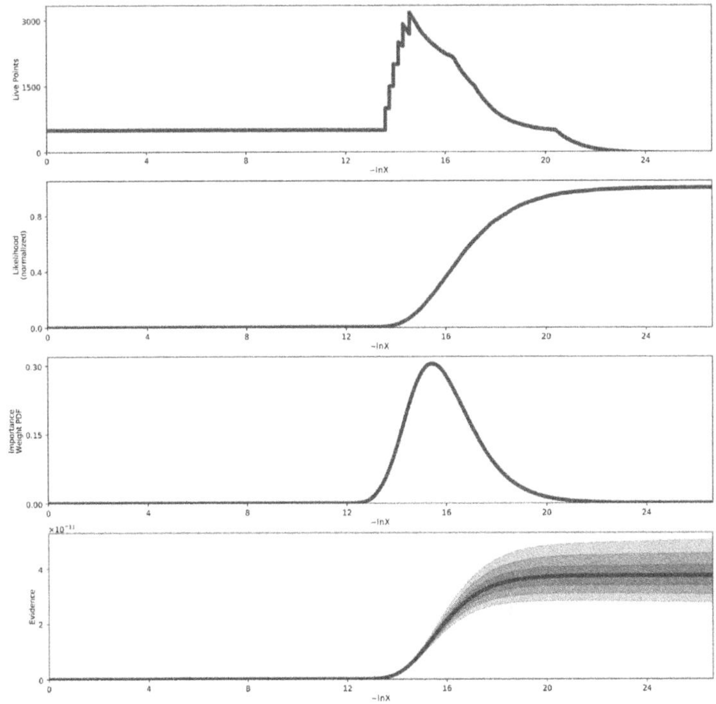

Fig. 12.8 Dynamic nested sampling plot of summary of run on simulated data for Model 4

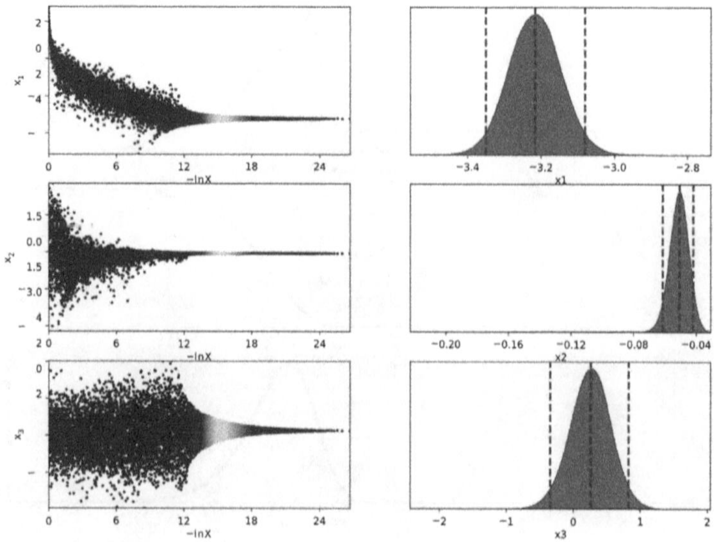

Fig. 12.9 Dynamic nested sampling plot of parameter traces and 1-D marginalized posteriors on simulated data for Model 4

Figure 12.14 shows the resultant importances of the ARD-NS model that we introduced in this chapter. This model was trained using the NUTS MCMC method. The results show that the β_2 factor loading is the main driver of the yield curve, followed by the β_1 factor loading. We also note that the relative influence of each factor varies with time, suggesting that models that capture the temporal nature of the factor loadings, for example, the dynamic (Diebold et al., 2008) model, could also be considered to capture the dynamics of the yield curve through time.

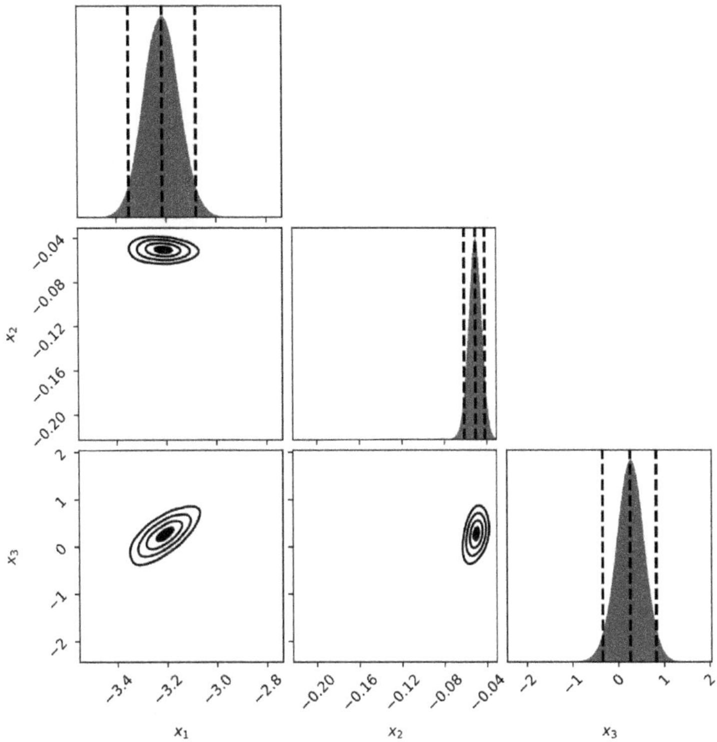

Fig. 12.10 Dynamic nested sampling plot of the 2-D marginalized posteriors on simulated data for Model 4

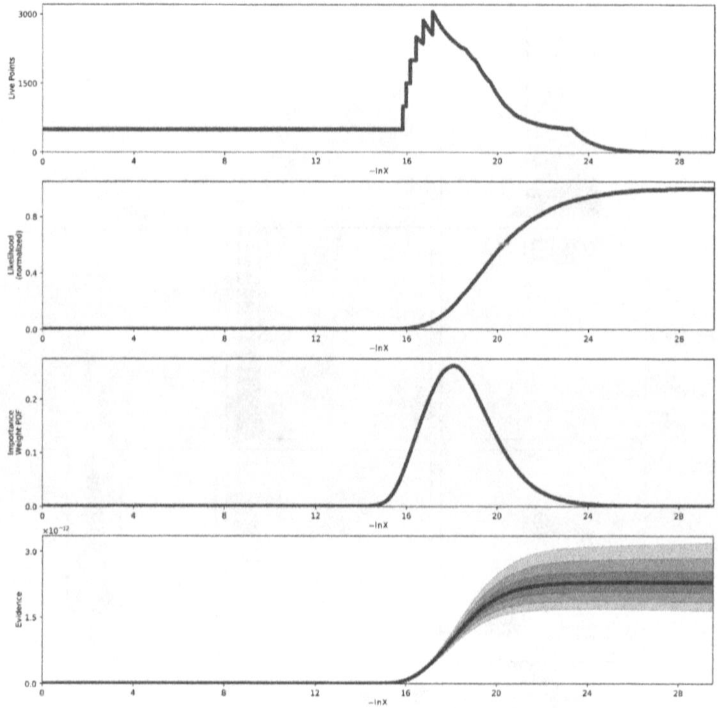

Fig. 12.11 Dynamic nested sampling plot of summary of run on simulated data for Model 7

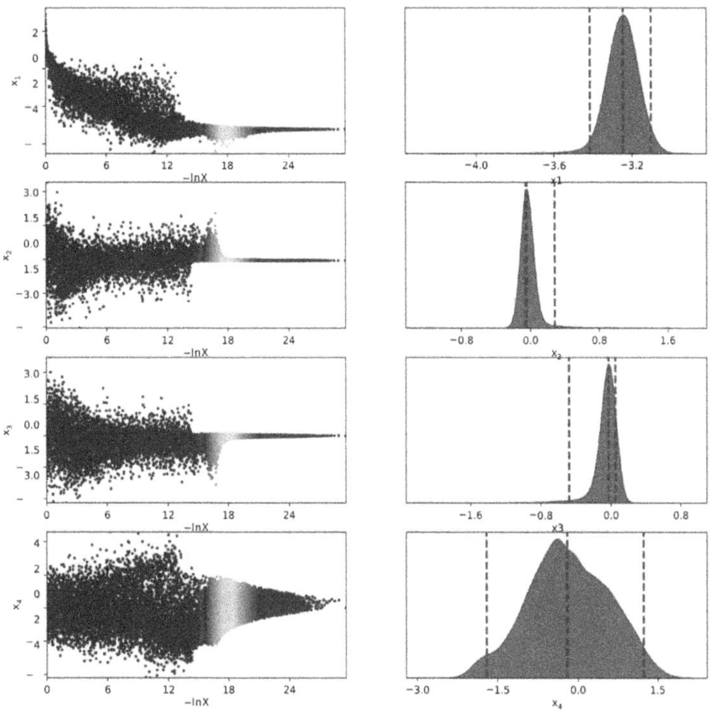

Fig. 12.12 Dynamic nested sampling plot of parameter traces and 1-D marginalized posteriors on simulated data for Model 7

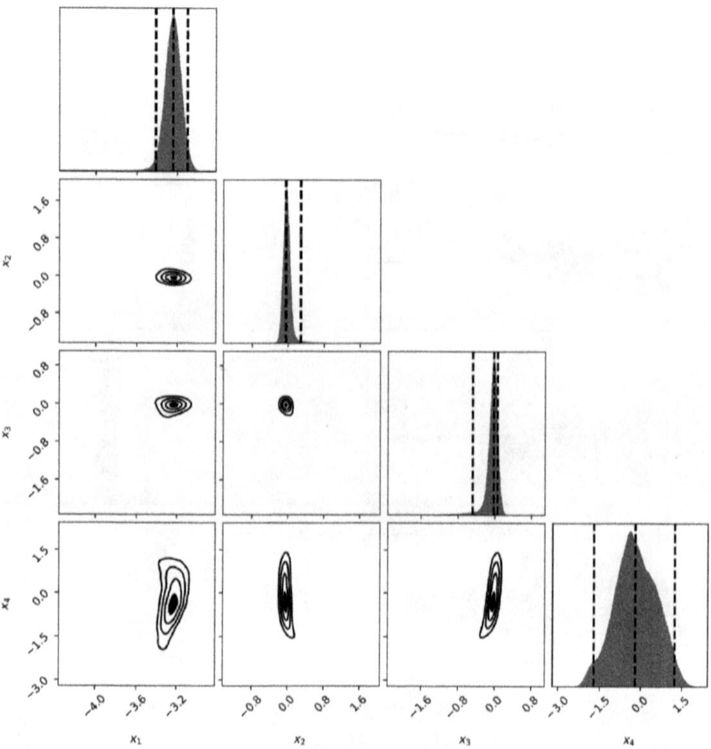

Fig. 12.13 Dynamic nested sampling plot of the 2-D marginalized posteriors on simulated data for Model 7

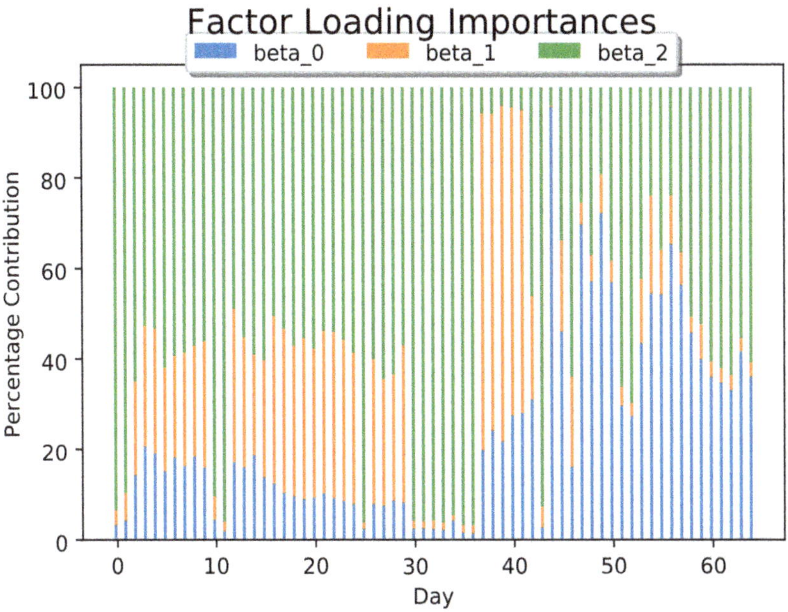

(a)

Fig. 12.14 Factor loadings importance over time between 2019-01-28 and 2024-05-28. The results show the relative importance of the short-term, medium-term, and long-term factors on the yield curve for each day. Note that we exclude the λ parameter from our analysis

12.6 Conclusion

The ability to select between different yield curve models is essential for various stakeholders, such as portfolio managers. This chapter used the Bayesian evidence framework based on static and nested sampling methods to compare the model. Based on simulated yield curve data, we can show that the proposed framework can identify the model that generates the data. Furthermore, we introduce the automatic relevance determination Nelson and Siegel model, trained using the No-U-Turn Sampler algorithm, which allows us to automatically rank which factor loadings are most relevant on a specific yield curve. Our results show through time which factor loadings (that is, short-term, medium-term, and long-term) are important on each day.

The framework we present in this chapter can be extended to incorporate other yield curve models and utilize other evidence calculation methods, such as those based on normalizing flows. In the next chapter, we introduce the Bayesian investment analyst. This framework can be used to predict directional movements in stocks while automatically highlighting which inputs are the most relevant.

References

Bishop, C. M. (1997). Bayesian neural networks. *Journal of the Brazilian Computer Society*, 4. issn: 0104-6500.

Brewer, B. J., Pártay, L. B., & Csányi, G. (2011). Diffusive nested sampling. *Statistics and Computing*, *21*(4), 649–656.

Diebold, F. X., & Li, Canlin. (2006). Forecasting the term structure of government bond yields. *Journal of Econometrics, 130*(2), 337–364.

Diebold, F. X., Li, C., & Yue, V. Z. (2008). Global yield curve dynamics and interactions: a dynamic Nelson-Siegel approach. *Journal of Econometrics, 146*(2), 351–363.

Duane, S., Kennedy, A. D., Pendleton, B. J., & Roweth, D. (1987). Hybrid Monte Carlo. *Physics Letters B, 195*(2), 216–222.

Duffee, G. (2013). Forecasting interest rates. In *Handbook of economic forecasting* (Vol. 2, pp. 385–426). Elsevier.

Gunter, T., Osborne, M. A., Garnett, R., Hennig, P., & Roberts, S. J. (2014). Sampling for inference in probabilistic models with fast Bayesian quadrature. *Advances in Neural Information Processing Systems*, 2789–2797.

Guo, B., Han, Q., & Zhao, B. (2014). The Nelson-Siegel model of the term structure of option implied volatility and volatility components. *Journal of Futures Markets, 34*(8), 788–806.

Hastings, W. K. (1970). Monte Carlo sampling methods using Markov chains and their applications. *Biometrica, 57*(1), 97–109.

Higson, E., Handley, W., Hobson, M., & Lasenby, A. (2019). Dynamic nested sampling: an improved algorithm for parameter estimation and evidence calculation. *Statistics and Computing, 29*, 891–913.

Hinton, G. E., & Van Camp, D. (1993). Keeping the neural networks simple by minimizing the description length of the weights. In *Proceedings of the sixth annual conference on Computational learning theory* (pp. 5–13). ACM.

Hoffman, M. D., & Gelman, A. (2011). *The No-U-turn sampler: Adaptively setting path lengths in Hamiltonian Monte Carlo.* arXiv:1111.4246 [stat.CO].

Hoffman, M. D., Blei, D. M., Wang, C., & Paisley, J. (2013). Stochastic variational inference. *Journal of Machine Learning Research, 14*(5).

Hoffman, M. D., & Gelman, A. (2014). The No-U-turn sampler: adaptively setting path lengths in Hamiltonian Monte Carlo. *Journal of Machine Learning Research, 15*(1), 1593–1623.

Hull, J., & White, A. (2001). The general Hull-White model and supercalibration. *Financial Analysts Journal, 57*(6), 34–43.

Kass, R. E., & Raftery, A. E. (1995). Bayes factors. *Journal of the American Statistical Association, 90*(430), 773–795.

Kazemie, N. (2014). *Mispricing due to Nelson-Siegel-Svensson model.*

MacKay, D. J. C. (1995). Probable networks and plausible predictions—a review of practical Bayesian methods for supervised neural networks. *Network: Computation in Neural Systems, 6*(3), 469–505.

MacKay, D. J. C. (1992). Bayesian interpolation. *Neural Computation, 4*(3), 415–447.

Marwala, T., Boulkaibet, I., & Adhikari, S. (2016). *Probabilistic finite element model updating using Bayesian statistics: applications to aeronautical and mechanical engineering*. Wiley.

Marwala, T., Mbuvha, R., & Mongwe, W. T. (2023). *Hamiltonian Monte Carlo methods in machine learning*. Elsevier.

Mbuvha, R., Jonsson, M., Ehn, N., & Herman, P. (2017). Bayesian neural networks for one-hour ahead wind power forecasting. In *2017 IEEE 6th international conference on renewable energy research and applications (ICRERA)* (pp. 591–596). IEEE.

Mbuvha, R., Mongwe, W. T., & Marwala, T. (2021). Separable shadow Hamiltonian hybrid Monte Carlo for Bayesian neural network inference in wind speed forecasting. *Energy and A, 1*, Article 100108.

Monetary Economic Department. (2005). Zero-coupon yield curves estimated by central banks. *Technical Report 25, Bank for International Settlements* 25. https://www.bis.org/publ/bppdf/bispap25a.pdf

Mongwe, W. T., Mbuvha, R., & Marwala, T. (2021). Bayesian inference of local government audit outcomes. *Plos One*. https://doi.org/10.1371/journal.pone.0261245

Mthembu, L., Marwala, T., Friswell, M. I., & Adhikari, S. (2011). Model selection in finite element model updating using the Bayesian evidence statistic. *Mechanical Systems and Signal Processing, 25*(7), 2399–2412.

Neal, R. M. (1993a). *Probabilistic inference using Markov chain Monte Carlo methods*. Technical report CRG-TR-93-1. University of Toronto, Department of Computer Science.

Neal, R. M. (1993b). Bayesian learning via stochastic dynamics. In *Advances in neural information processing systems* (Vol. 5, pp. 475–482). Morgan Kaufmann Publishers Inc. isbn: 1-55860-274-7. http://dl.acm.org/citation.cfm?id=645753.667903

Nelson, C. R., & Siegel, A. F. (1987). Parsimonious modeling of yield curves. *Journal of Business*, 473–489.

Osborne, M., Garnett, R., Ghahramani, Z., Duvenaud, D. K., Roberts, S. J., & Rasmussen, C. E. (2012). Active learning of model evidence using Bayesian quadrature. *Advances in Neural Information Processing Systems*, 46–54.

Rasmussen, C. E., & Ghahramani, Z. (2001). Occam's razor. *Advances in Neural Information Processing Systems*, 294–300.

Russel, P. M., Brewer, B. J., Klaere, S., & Bouckaert, R. R. (2019). Model selection and parameter inference in phylogenetics using nested sampling. *Systematic Biology, 68*(2), 219–233.

Skilling, J. (2004). Nested sampling. In: *AIP conference proceedings* (Vol. 735. 1, pp. 395–405). American Institute of Physics.

Skilling, J. (2006). Nested sampling for general Bayesian computation. *Bayesian Analysis, 1*(4), 833–859.

Speagle, J. S. (2020). Dynesty: A dynamic nested sampling package for estimating bayesian posteriors and evidences. *Monthly Notices of the Royal Astronomical Society, 493*(3), 3132–3158.

Svensson, L. E. O. (1995). Estimating forward interest rates with the extended Nelson & Siegel method. *Sveriges Riksbank Quarterly Review, 3*(1), 13–26.

Tavanielli, R., & Laurini, M. (2023). Yield curve models with Regime changes: An analysis for the Brazilian interest rate market. *Mathematics, 11*(11), 2549.

Vasicek, O. (1977). An equilibrium characterization of the term structure. *Journal of Financial Economics, 5*(2), 177–188.

CHAPTER 13

A Bayesian Investment Analyst on the Johannesburg Stock Exchange

13.1 Introduction

Over the years, there has been an increase in the coverage of stocks by sell-side analysts across various international stock exchanges (Sidogi et al., 2022). The typical focus is on the blue-chip stocks, with little attention paid to the mid-cap and small-cap stocks. The reports produced by sell-side analysts typically include various elements such as the stock's target price, the earning forecasts, and whether the stock is a buy or a sell (Ahmed & Flint, 2020). Investors use these reports, primarily institutional investors such as pension funds, for their portfolio management decisions. Thus, the evaluation of the accuracy of these reports is critical (Ahmed & Flint, 2020; Park & Park, 2019; Sidogi et al., 2022; Zaremba & Konieczka, 2015).

Sell-side analyst reports are important as they ensure that investors understand the companies they are investing in through the reduction of information asymmetry, as well as keep the management of the companies honest by challenging them on their practices (Ahmed & Flint, 2020; Sidogi et al., 2022). The more analysts that cover a particular

---

Supplementary Information The online version contains supplementary material available at https://doi.org/10.1007/978-3-031-88431-3_13.

W. T. Mongwe et al., *Bayesian Machine Learning in Quantitative Finance*, https://doi.org/10.1007/978-3-031-88431-3_13

company, the more likely that the company's operations are understood by the market—except for exceptional cases such as Steinhoff and Tongard-Hullet, where management was intentionally manipulating the companies' financial accounts (Cronje, 2017). A key disadvantage of the analyst reports is that they sometimes introduce conflicts of interest where the analysts produce reports to align with their economic incentives and that analysts tend to produce forecasts and recommendations that form a consensus with other analysts (Sidogi et al., 2022). These issues reduce the reliability of analyst forecasts. Thus, measuring the accuracy of the analyst's reports is essential.

Various accuracy measures can be used to measure the performance of sell-side reports, including point accuracy and directional accuracy (Ahmed & Flint, 2020). The difference between the target price and the actual price at the conclusion of the prediction horizon is referred to as point accuracy (Ahmed & Flint, 2020). Previous studies have demonstrated that analysts display some optimism in their projections (Ahmed & Flint, 2020). On the other hand, analyst accuracy in predicting the future direction of equity price movement is known as directional forecast accuracy. This metric is critical since many traders base their decisions not on anticipated ultimate price value but rather on expected movement direction (Ahmed & Flint, 2020; Sidogi et al., 2022). Researchers have mostly concentrated on the profitability of buy/sell recommendations, with little attention paid to the directional accuracy of target prices (Ahmed & Flint, 2020; Sidogi et al., 2022). The focus of this chapter is on modeling the directional accuracy of analysts' forecasts.

The South African brokerage industry has seen a rise in the number of sell-side analysts, which has led to an increase in the number of companies and sell-side reports released by different stock analysts (Sidogi et al., 2022). This has led to more stocks on the Johannesburg Stock Exchange being covered, thus reducing the information asymmetry on these stocks. In addition, major financial data vendors such as Bloomberg have also recently begun to capture target price data continuously (Ahmed & Flint, 2020; Sidogi et al., 2022). This has inevitably made it necessary for investors to enhance their investing processes by quickly and impartially processing sell-side data (Barber et al., 2001; Sidogi et al., 2022). This increase in data also increases the potential to reduce the issues and biases of analyst reports by aggregating all the analyst's reports using data-driven techniques such as machine learning.

Few studies utilize machine learning algorithms with sell-side earnings forecast data (Sidogi et al., 2022). In Kua et al. (2022), an iterative filtering algorithm is used to approximate market consensus estimates. This approach enhances the generation of consensus estimates by not merely using the mean consensus estimates. The work of Singh et al. (2021) is one of the closest studies on the subject of data-driven analysis of sell-side forecasts. In their work, stock price prediction uses analyst features, such as analyst ratings. The emphasis of the growing body of research has been on analyst ratings and recommendations (Park & Park, 2019; Zaremba & Konieczka, 2015). The majority of previous research, however, has looked at these results separately rather than considering how the reports' combined results may be used. More recently, using machine learning techniques such as random forests and deep neural network, Sidogi et al. (2022) investigates the possibility of producing better directional forecasts by combining sell-side data reports for FTSE/JSE All Share Index companies. They suggest using an "AI analyst" to help create investment recommendations, including directional forecasts, with little human involvement by utilizing data from sell-side analyst reports. To predict the direction of movement of certain stocks, they use investment signals from sell-side reports as quantitative input features to several machine learning algorithms. This chapter expands on the work of Sidogi et al. (2022) by framing the problem within the Bayesian framework.

The Bayesian inference framework is founded on the Bayes theorem, which outlines how the posterior distribution is obtained from the likelihood and the prior distribution (Mobiny et al., 2021). The first application of Bayesian logistic regression with automated relevance determination (BLR-ARD) for estimating the bidirectional accuracy of sell-side analyst forecasts is presented in this chapter. This framework allows us to quantify uncertainties in our prediction, as well as automatically rank the most relevant features for this task. Our objective is to deduce the posterior distribution of the parameters for the BLR-ARD model. The posterior distribution for the BLR-ARD is not expressible in closed form, necessitating the use of numerical methods to ascertain the posterior (MacKay, 1992). The prevalent methodologies for model training, specifically ascertaining the posterior distribution within the Bayesian paradigm, are variational inference techniques and Markov Chain Monte Carlo (MCMC) algorithms (Hoffman et al., 2013; Hinton & Van Camp,

1993). This chapter uses MCMC methods such as the Metropolis-Adjusted Langevin Algorithm, Hamiltonian Monte Carlo, and Separable Shadow Hamiltonian Hybrid Monte Carlo algorithms to train the BLR-ARD model. We discuss these algorithms in detail later in this chapter.

Our analysis shows that the model outperforms in the industrial and resource sectors, with financial stocks having the lowest bidirectional accuracy. We further find that volatility-related features, as well as the initial and target price, are important features from analyst reports in predicting the direction of the stocks. The results of our analysis can be useful to various stakeholders, especially institutional investors who oversee large portfolios. The results indicate which features in sell-side analyst reports investors can focus on to identify likely instances of outperformance efficiently and thus accurately challenge fund managers' investment strategies.

The remainder of this chapter is structured as follows: We first describe the Bayesian model used to predict the bidirectional accuracy of analyst forecasts in Sect. 13.2; we then detail the Markov Chain Monte Carlo methods used to train the model in Sect. 13.3; we then present the experiment setup, after which we present the results, discuss them, and provide the conclusion in Sects. 13.4 to 13.6 respectively.

13.2 Bayesian Logistic Regression Model

We model the bidirectional accuracy using Bayesian logistic regression. The negative log-likelihood $l(\mathrm{D}|\mathbf{w})$ function for this model is given by (Marwala et al., 2023; Mongwe et al., 2021c):

$$l(\mathrm{D}|\mathbf{w}) = \sum_{i}^{N} y_i \log(\mathbf{w}^T x_i) + (1 - y_i)\log(1 - \mathbf{w}^T x_i) \tag{13.1}$$

where D ={x, y} is the data, N is the number of observations and $\mathbf{w}$ are the parameters that need to be estimated. Thus, the target un-normalized posterior log distribution is given as (Marwala et al., 2023; Mongwe et al., 2021c):

$$\ln p(\mathbf{w}|\mathrm{D}) = l(\mathrm{D}|\mathbf{w}) + \ln p(\mathbf{w}|\alpha) + \ln q(\alpha) \tag{13.2}$$

where $\ln p(\mathbf{w}|\alpha)$ is the log of the prior distribution placed on the parameters given the hyperparameters, and $\ln q(\alpha)$ is the distribution of the hyperparameters. As in Mongwe et al. (2021c), we model the parameters $\mathbf{w}$ as having a Gaussian prior with each parameter having zero mean and its own standard deviation or regularization parameter α_i, meaning that we are using an automatic relevance determination (ARD) prior within our framework.

The α_i indicates how important the parameter associated with the input feature is. The larger the value of α_i, the more critical the input feature is in predicting the bidirectional accuracy of the stock (Mongwe et al., 2021c). Thus, this framework automatically ranks the importance of the input features. The α_i will have low values for irrelevant inputs, which will cause their weights to be driven to decay to values around zero (Mbuvha et al., 2021; Mongwe et al., 2021c). Conversely, essential inputs will have weights with high variances while less important inputs will have low variances (Marwala et al., 2023; Mbuvha et al., 2021). Since the mean for the weight priors is fixed at zero, it follows that weights with high variances can take values far from zero (resulting in a more significant effect). In contrast, those with low variances must take values close to zero (thus reduced effect) (Marwala et al., 2023; Mbuvha et al., 2021).

Due to the multi-modal and non-convex structure of the ARD loss function, inference of ARD prior hyperparameters is a fundamentally hard inverse problem (MacKay, 1995; Marwala et al., 2023; Mbuvha et al., 2021; Mongwe et al., 2021c; Neal, 1993). Through maximizing the Bayesian evidence metric, Mackay (1995) obtains estimates of the ARD hyperparameters, and this is due to the Laplace approximation's simplifying assumptions producing a tractable closed-form calculation of the evidence. On the other hand, Neal (Neal, 2012) deploys an alternating framework of using Hamiltonian Monte Carlo for network weights and Gibbs sampling for ARD hyperparameters from various posteriors such as the Gamma (Mbuvha et al., 2021). This strategy converges to an asymptotically true posterior based on Markov Chain Monte Carlo. However, many design decisions, such as the appropriate prior distribution, are still necessary (Mbuvha et al., 2021). The hyperparameter sampling strategy used in this chapter is to jointly infer the α hyperparameters and the $\mathbf{w}$ parameters as in Mongwe et al. (2021c). Although the effective parameter space is doubled in this approach, compared to the Gibbs sampling strategy, this method produces a more stable exploration across the MCMC methods (Mongwe et al., 2021c). As the $\mathbf{w}$ parameters are assumed to be normally distributed, we select the α hyperparameters to be log-normally distributed to make the joint sampling of parameters and hyperparameters mathematically convenient. In particular, the α_is are assumed to follow a log-normal distribution with mean zero and variance one as in Mongwe et al. (2021c).

13.3 Markov Chain Monte Carlo Algorithms

We present the Markov Chain Monte Carlo (MCMC) methods used to train the Bayesian logistic regression model with an ARD prior. All the MCMC methods were implemented in the Python programming language.

13.3.1 Metropolis-Adjusted Langevin Algorithm

The Metropolis-Adjusted Langevin Algorithm (MALA) enhances the Metropolis-Hastings (MH) method through the use of first-order gradient information of the target posterior. MALA reduces the random walk behavior of MH via the use of Langevin dynamics where the drift component is the derivative of the log of the target posterior, and the diffusive component is Brownian motion which is represented as follows (Gu & Sun, 2020; Marwala et al., 2023; Mongwe et al., 2021d, 2022b):

$$d\mathbf{w}_t = \frac{1}{2} f'(\mathbf{w})dt + dZ_t \tag{13.3}$$

where $\mathbf{w}$ are the parameters, $f'(\mathbf{w})$ is the first derivative of the target $f(\mathbf{w})$ with respect to the parameters, and Z_t is a Brownian motion process at a fictitious time t. The Langevin dynamics in Eq. 13.3 typically cannot be solved analytically, and numerical methods such as the Euler-Maruyama integration scheme are typically used (Marwala et al., 2023)). This, however, introduces errors that can break the detailed balance condition, which would not guarantee that the method would converge to the correct target distribution (Marwala et al., 2023). To rectify this, a Metropolis acceptance step is incorporated into the algorithm to ensure detailed balance (Marwala et al., 2023). The MALA algorithm converges to the stationary distribution at a faster pace than the MH algorithm because it takes into account the density's first-order gradient data, which is represented by $f'(\mathbf{w})$ (Girolami & Calderhead, 2011; Gu & Sun, 2020; Marwala et al., 2023). The samples produced using the MALA method are still highly correlated. Girolami and Calderhead (2011) incorporate second-order gradient information of the target by extending MALA from being on a Euclidean manifold to a Riemannian manifold (Marwala et al., 2023). Despite a corresponding increase in compute time, this approach demonstrated significant gains in the sampling performance of the MALA method (Marwala et al., 2023).

13.3.2 Hamiltonian Monte Carlo

Hamiltonian Monte Carlo (HMC) is a popular MCMC method for performing Bayesian inference and has been utilized in various disciplines such as finance, health, and energy (Duane et al., 1987; Mbuvha & Marwala, 2020; Mbuvha et al., 2021; Mongwe et al., 2021c, 2022b). The method is premised on using Hamiltonian dynamics, which naturally considers the first-order gradient information of the target posterior. The dynamics that underpin HMC are as follows (Marwala et al., 2023, Neal, 1993):

$$\frac{d\mathbf{w}}{\partial t} = \frac{\partial \mathrm{H}(\mathbf{w}, \mathbf{p})}{\partial \mathbf{p}}; \quad \frac{d\mathbf{p}}{\partial t} = -\frac{\partial \mathrm{H}(\mathbf{w}, \mathbf{p})}{\partial \mathbf{w}} \tag{13.4}$$

where $\mathbf{w}$ are the parameters, $\mathbf{p}$ is the auxiliary momentum variable with the same dimensionality as $\mathbf{w}$, and $\mathrm{H}(\mathbf{w}, \mathbf{p})$ is the Hamiltonian—which represents the total energy (i.e., potential energy defined by the target posterior and kinetic energy which is typically captured through a multivariate Gaussian distribution) from this system (Mongwe et al., 2021b, 2022a). This HMC method allows distant proposals, which results in a significant reduction in the autocorrelations of the generated samples (Marwala et al., 2023).

The HMC technique is composed of two steps. The first step integrates Hamiltonian dynamics in Eq. 13.4 typically using the leapfrog integrator (Duane et al., 1987; Marwala et al., 2023; Neal, 1993), and the second step utilizes a Metropolis-Hastings correction to account for the numerical integration errors arising from the first step (Duane et al., 1987; Hastings, 1970; Neal et al., 2011). The parameter and momentum update equations for the leapfrog integration scheme (corresponding to the first step of HMC) are given as follows:

$$\begin{aligned}
\mathbf{p}_{t+\frac{\epsilon}{2}} &= \mathbf{p}_t + \frac{\epsilon}{2}\frac{\partial H(\mathbf{w}_t, \mathbf{p}_t)}{\partial \mathbf{w}} \\
\mathbf{w}_{t+\epsilon} &= \mathbf{w}_t + \epsilon \mathbf{M}^{-1}\mathbf{p}_{t+\frac{\epsilon}{2}} \\
\mathbf{p}_{t+\epsilon} &= \mathbf{p}_{t+\frac{\epsilon}{2}} + \frac{\epsilon}{2}\frac{\partial H\left(\mathbf{w}_{t+\epsilon}, \mathbf{p}_{t+\frac{\epsilon}{2}}\right)}{\partial \mathbf{w}}
\end{aligned} \tag{13.5}$$

where ϵ is the discretization step size and $\mathbf{M}$ is a covariance matrix emanating from the kinetic energy component in $\mathrm{H}(\mathbf{w}, \mathbf{p})$. If the integration of the Hamiltonian dynamics in the first step were solved precisely, the second step would not be required. However, due to the discretization errors, a Metropolis-Hastings acceptance step is typically required where the $\mathbf{w}^*$ proposed by the first step are accepted with probability:

$$\mathrm{P}(\text{accept } \mathbf{w}^*) = \min\left(1, \frac{\exp(-\mathrm{H}(\mathbf{w}^*, \mathbf{p}^*))}{\exp(-\mathrm{H}(\mathbf{w}, \mathbf{p}))}\right). \tag{13.6}$$

The parameters of HMC are the discretization step size ϵ, which is required for the first step in HMC, and the trajectory length, which determines the number of times the integration is performed. The step size parameter is typically set to obtain a user-specified target acceptance rate using the dual averaging method (Hoffman & Gelman, 2014; Marwala et al., 2023) while tuning the trajectory length parameter is a more complex problem (Hoffman & Gelman, 2014). It can further be shown that when the trajectory length parameter is set to 1, the HMC method becomes the MALA method. The overall HMC sampling process follows a Gibbs sampling scheme, where we sample $\mathbf{p}$ auxiliary momentum variable and then sample a new set of parameters $\mathbf{w}$ given the drawn momentum $\mathbf{p}$. This procedure is repeated until the required number of samples are generated (Marwala et al., 2023; Mongwe et al., 2021a, 2021b). The pseudo-code for HMC can be found in Algorithm 3.1 in Chapter 3 of this book.

13.3.3 Separable Shadow Hamiltonian Hybrid Monte Carlo

Although significantly better than MALA, the HMC method still produces auto-correlated samples (Heide et al., 2021; Marwala et al., 2023). This is mainly driven by the fact that the leapfrog integration scheme only preserves the Hamiltonian up to second order $\mathcal{O}(\epsilon^2)$. This causes the change in the Hamiltonian to become large, thus leading to more rejections in the Metropolis-Hastings acceptance step of HMC (Heide et al., 2021; Marwala et al., 2023). There are two possibilities to address this issue; one can either create more accurate (i.e., better than $\mathcal{O}(\epsilon^2)$) integration schemes to integrate the Hamiltonian dynamics, or only run the integration scheme for small step sizes ϵ and short path lengths L—or a combination of these two approaches. However, all these approaches attract longer execution times (Marwala et al., 2023).

It can be shown that when one runs a backward error analysis through the leapfrog integrator, we can derive a modified Hamiltonian (which is called the shadow Hamiltonian) whose energy is better preserved by the leapfrog integrator than the true Hamiltonian (Marwala et al., 2023). By design, the numerical integrator precisely conserves the perturbations of the shadow Hamiltonians. However, as this Hamiltonian is not the true Hamiltonian, we would effectively be sampling from an importance distribution, which we would need to correct so as not to introduce bias in the generated samples (Heide et al., 2021).

At its core, the shadow or modified Hamiltonian is an asymptotic expansion in the powers of the discretization step size ϵ around the Hamiltonian:

$$\tilde{\mathrm{H}} = \mathrm{H} + \epsilon \mathrm{H}_2 + \epsilon^2 \mathrm{H}_3 + \epsilon^3 \mathrm{H}_4 + \dots \tag{13.7}$$

However, to ensure that this expansion does not diverge, a kth order truncation of the expansion is utilized in practice:

$$\begin{aligned} \tilde{\mathrm{H}}^{[k]} &= \mathrm{H} + \epsilon \mathrm{H}_2 + \epsilon^2 \mathrm{H}_3 + \epsilon^3 \mathrm{H}_4 + \dots \\ &= \tilde{\mathrm{H}} + \mathcal{O}(\epsilon^k) \end{aligned} \tag{13.8}$$

Through comparing the associated elements of the Taylor series in terms of ϵ and the extended precise flow of the modified differential equation of the Hamiltonian, the H_k terms can be found. For symplectic integrators like the leapfrog integrator, these altered equations can be considered Hamiltonian (Marwala et al., 2023). This chapter considers a fourth-order truncation of the shadow Hamiltonian under the leapfrog integrator. The fourth-order truncation shadow Hamiltonian is conserved with more accuracy ($\mathcal{O}^4$) than the true Hamiltonian since the leapfrog is second-order accurate ($\mathcal{O}^2$). The fourth-order shadow Hamiltonian for the leapfrog integrator after matching coefficients from the flow and the asymptotic expansion is expressed as:

$$\tilde{\mathrm{H}}^{[4]} = \mathrm{U}(\mathbf{w}) + \mathrm{K}(\mathbf{p}) + \frac{\epsilon^2}{12}\mathrm{K}_{\mathbf{p}}^T\mathrm{U}_{\mathbf{ww}}\mathrm{K}_{\mathbf{p}} - \frac{\epsilon^2}{24}\mathrm{U}_{\mathbf{w}}^T\mathrm{K}_{\mathbf{pp}}\mathrm{U}_{\mathbf{w}} + \mathcal{O}(\epsilon^4) \quad (13.9)$$

where $\mathrm{U}_{\mathbf{w}}$, $\mathrm{U}_{\mathbf{ww}}$, $\mathrm{K}_{\mathbf{p}}$ and $\mathrm{K}_{\mathbf{pp}}$ are Jacobians and Hessians of the potential and kinetic energies respectively. It can be noted that the modified Hamiltonian in Eq. 13.9 is non-separable in terms of the parameter and momentum vectors. This is problematic as it requires potential tuning of additional parameters and momentum acceptance criterion that is computationally expensive (Izaguirre & Hampton, 2004; Marwala et al., 2023; Sweet et al., 2009).

Separable Shadow Hamiltonian Hybrid Monte Carlo (S2HMC) utilizes a processed leapfrog integrator to create a separable Hamiltonian (Sweet et al., 2009). Before passing through the leapfrog integrator, the parameter vector and momenta are pre-processed to minimize computational overhead. The resultant separable Hamiltonian in S2HMC is

$$\tilde{\mathrm{H}}(\mathbf{w}, \mathbf{p}) = \mathrm{U}(\mathbf{w}) + \mathrm{K}(\mathbf{p}) + \frac{\epsilon^2}{24}\mathrm{U}_{\mathbf{w}}^T\mathrm{M}^{-1}\mathrm{U}_{\mathbf{w}} + \mathcal{O}(\epsilon^4) \quad (13.10)$$

The positions and momenta are propagated through the shadow Hamiltonian after performing the reversible mapping $(\hat{\mathbf{w}}, \hat{\mathbf{p}}) = \mathcal{X}(\mathbf{w}, \mathbf{p})$, where $(\hat{\mathbf{w}}, \hat{\mathbf{p}})$ is found through fixed point iterations as:

$$\hat{\mathbf{p}} = \mathbf{p} - \frac{\epsilon}{24}\left[\mathrm{U}_{\mathbf{w}}(\mathbf{w} + \epsilon\,\mathbf{M}^{-1}\hat{\mathbf{p}}) - \mathrm{U}_{\mathbf{w}}(\mathbf{w} - \epsilon\,\mathbf{M}^{-1}\hat{\mathbf{p}})\right] \quad (13.11)$$

$$\hat{\mathbf{w}} = \mathbf{w} + \frac{\epsilon^2\,\mathbf{M}^{-1}}{24}\left[\mathrm{U}_{\mathbf{w}}(\mathbf{w} + \epsilon\,\mathbf{M}^{-1}\hat{\mathbf{p}}) + \mathrm{U}_{\mathbf{w}}(\mathbf{w} - \epsilon\,\mathbf{M}^{-1}\hat{\mathbf{p}})\right] \quad (13.12)$$

After the leapfrog integration is performed, this mapping is reversed using as a post-processing step using following fixed point iterations:

$$\mathbf{w} = \hat{\mathbf{w}} - \frac{\epsilon^2\mathbf{M}^{-1}}{24}\left[\mathrm{U}_{\mathbf{w}}(\mathbf{w} + \epsilon\mathbf{M}^{-1}\hat{\mathbf{p}}) + \mathrm{U}_{\mathbf{w}}(\mathbf{w} - \epsilon\mathbf{M}^{-1}\hat{\mathbf{p}})\right] \quad (13.13)$$

$$\mathbf{p} = \hat{\mathbf{p}} + \frac{\epsilon}{24}\left[\mathrm{U}_{\mathbf{w}}(\mathbf{w} + \epsilon\mathbf{M}^{-1}\hat{\mathbf{p}}) - \mathrm{U}_{\mathbf{w}}(\mathbf{w} - \epsilon\mathbf{M}^{-1}\hat{\mathbf{p}})\right] \tag{13.14}$$

The importance weights are computed after the samples are obtained using the S2HMC technique (Marwala et al., 2023; Mongwe et al., 2021c) to guarantee that the shadow canonical density is used rather than the true density. The differences between the true and shadow Hamiltonians are the basis for determining the importance weights. It is worth noting that S2HMC degenerates to HMC when the shadow Hamiltonian is set to equal the true Hamiltonian. A detailed exposition on S2HMC, HMC, and MALA can be found in Marwala et al. (2023).

13.4 Numerical Experiments

In this section, we present the numerical experiments conducted. We first describe the dataset and then outline the experiments, settings, and performance metrics used.

13.4.1 Data Description

The data utilized in this chapter came from Bloomberg, which is consistent with the approach taken in Ahmed and Flint (2020) and Sidogi et al. (2022). The data consists of sell-side analyst reports on the FTSE/JSE All Share Index companies between January 2004 and June 2018, with the target variable being the bidirectional accuracy from the initial price to the realized closing price over the 12 months. The description of each variable is given below (Ahmed & Flint, 2020; Sidogi et al., 2022):

1. **Firm**—the firm that produces the analyst report.
2. **Target Price**—the target price as set in the analyst report.
3. **Rating**—the stock rating with 1 = Strong Sell, 2 = Sell, 3 = Hold, 4 = Buy, and 5 = Strong Buy.
4. $\mathbf{P_0}$—this is the initial price. That is, it is the price at the issue date of the analyst report.
5. $\mathbf{TP/P_0}$ = ratio of the target price to the initial price.
6. **20d Vol**—rolling 20-day volatility.
7. **Top40 CSV**—monthly Top40 Index cross-sectional volatility.
8. **RelVol**—is the ratio of rolling 20-day volatility and monthly Top40 Index cross-sectional volatility.

9. **DAS**—directional accuracy score, which is based on the classic definition of directional accuracy.
10. **MES**—Met End Score (MES), which is the cumulative number of times an analyst prediction meets the target price at the end of the forecast period.
11. **MAS**—Met Any Score (MAS), which is the cumulative number of times an analyst prediction meets the target price at any time during the forecast horizon.
12. **PAS**—point accuracy score, which is the average absolute point accuracy for an analyst over 12 months.
13. **PTM**—price target momentum, defined as the percentage change in the current issued target price from the previously published target price.
14. **AC**—analyst coverage, which shows the total number of reports for the past 12 months on a specific stock.

The target, a binary variable, has 56% of the instances being the positive class while 44% are the negative class for the period under consideration. The full description of the dataset can be found in Sidogi et al. (2022).

13.4.2 *Experiment Description*

We use analyst reports to fit the Bayesian logistic regression model for the bidirectional stock prediction analysis. We split the data into a train and test set using an 80-20 split. Data normalization was employed using a min-max scaler to obtain the input dataset at the same scale. The full dataset has 29935 analyst reports with corresponding forecast accuracy scores from 11 November 2005 to 29 June 2018. As in Sidogi et al. (2022), we choose between a portion of the analyst dataset and the entire dataset in four separate experiments shown in Table 13.1. The aim of creating these experiments is to assess the performance of the Bayesian investment analyst across the entire JSE universe, as well as the performance in each sector.

When fitting the Bayesian model, we generate a total of 2500 samples, of which 1000 formed the burn-in period where tuning was performed for all the MCMC methods considered in this chapter. The step size parameters of all the methods were tuned using the primal-dual averaging methodology outlined in Hoffman and Gelman (2014) targeting an

Table 13.1 Experiments that we consider in this chapter are based on the sell-side analyst report dataset

Experiment	*Experiment description*	*Number of observations*
1	Using the full dataset	29935
2	Only resource stocks dataset	10522
3	Only financial stocks dataset	7193
4	Only industrial stocks dataset	12220

acceptance rate of 60% for MALA and 80% for both HMC and S2HMC. Note that the path length of HMC and S2HMC was fixed at 15.

13.4.3 Performance Metrics

We evaluate the algorithms' performance by producing trace plots of the un-normalized target posterior distribution, calculating the effective sample sizes of the generated samples, normalizing these effective sample sizes by execution time, and assessing predictive performance on unseen data. The execution time is the duration required to produce the samples following the burn-in period. We employ the multivariate effective sample size metric established by Vats et al. (2019) to measure effective sample size. These performance metrics are described in detail in Chapter 2 of this book.

The Receiver Operating Curve (ROC) and Area Under the ROC are the predictive performance metrics we employ to evaluate the outcomes of the Bayesian analysis. The model's true positives are shown on the y-axis against false positives on the x-axis on the ROC. The Area Under the ROC, or AUC, measures the average rate of misclassifications. When it comes to measuring performance when the costs of misclassifications are unclear, AUC is preferable (Bradley, 1997; Gaganis, 2009; Mongwe & Malan, 2020), which is the case for the bidirectional detection task at hand.

13.5 Results and Discussion

In this section, we present the results and the discussions from the numerical experiments. Table 13.2 shows the performance on unseen data across the three MCMC methods. Tables 13.3, 13.4, and 13.5 show the relative

Table 13.2 Performance on unseen data across the three MCMC methods. The entries correspond to the AUC. The entries in **bold** indicate outperformance on the AUC metric. The higher the AUC, the better the model

Algorithm	*Experiment 1*	*Experiment 2*	*Experiment 3*	*Experiment 4*
MALA	0.618134	0.632456	0.615377	**0.669759**
HMC	**0.618241**	**0.632657**	0.615819	0.668567
S2HMC	**0.618241**	0.632421	**0.616375**	0.668713

ranking of the features across the three MCMC methods and across all four experiments. Figures 13.1, 13.2, and 13.3 show the effective sample size and effective sample size normalized by the execution time for all the experiments and the three MCMC methods. Figures 13.4, 13.5, and 13.6 show the predictive performance on unseen data and the diagnostic trace plots on the negative likelihood of all the experiments and MCMC methods. Figures 13.7, 13.8, 13.9, 13.10, 13.11, and 13.12 show the relative importance of the inputs for all the experiments and across all the MCMC methods.

The results in Table 13.2 show that the models produce similar AUCs in each experiment. We find that HMC and S2HMC outperform on experiments 1 to 3, with MALA outperforming on experiment 4. The results show that industrial stocks, as captured by experiment 4, are where we achieved outperformance across all the MCMC methods. We also performed well in experiment 2, which focused on resource stocks. On the other hand, performance on the financial stocks (represented by experiment 3) is worse than on the complete dataset (captured by experiment 1). These results align with those found in Sidogi et al. (2022).

Figures 13.1, 13.2, and 13.3 show the sampling performance across all the experiments and all the MCMC methods. We find, in general, that the MALA and HMC methods produce similar sampling performance with wide confidence bands in the effective sample size (ESS) and the ESS normalized by execution time. On the other hand, we found that the confidence bands for the ESS and ESS normalized by execution time are narrower for S2HMC—which is related to the shadow Hamiltonian being better conserved by the pre-processed leapfrog integration scheme. We also note that S2HMC produces much lower ESSs on a time-normalized basis due to its long execution time. Figures 13.4, 13.5, and

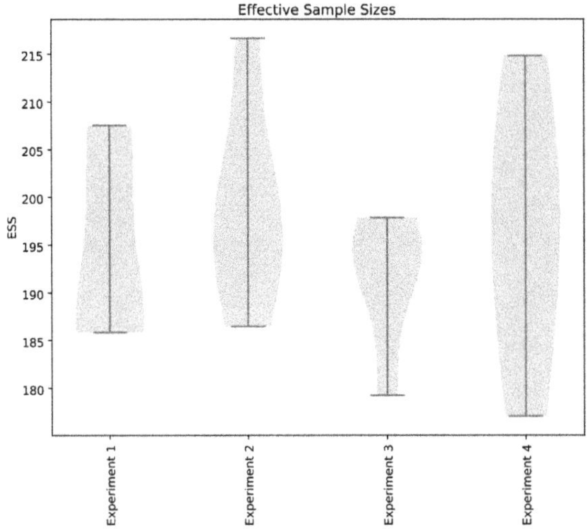

(a) MALA effective sample size across all the experiments.

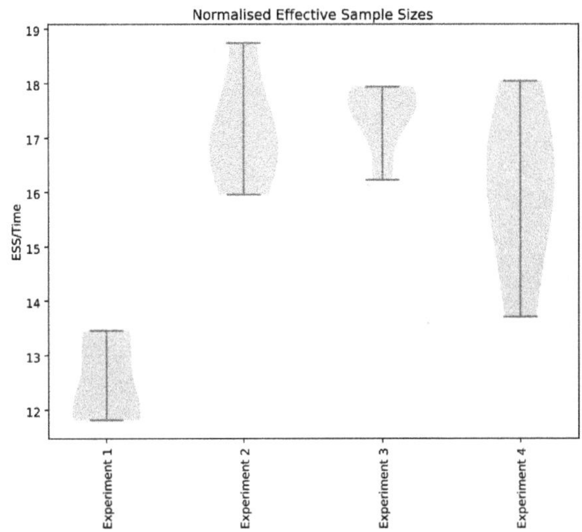

(b) MALA effective sample size normalized by execution time across all the experiments.

Fig. 13.1 Inference results for the Bayesian framework for the MALA algorithm showing the effective sample sizes and effective sample sizes normalized by execution time for the sell-side analyst report dataset

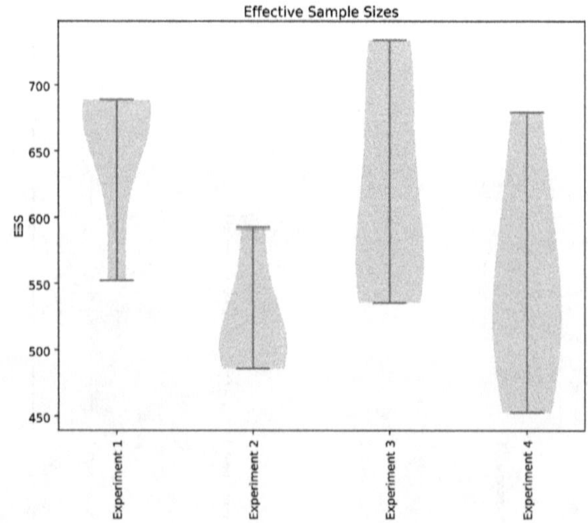

(a) HMC effective sample size across all the experiments.

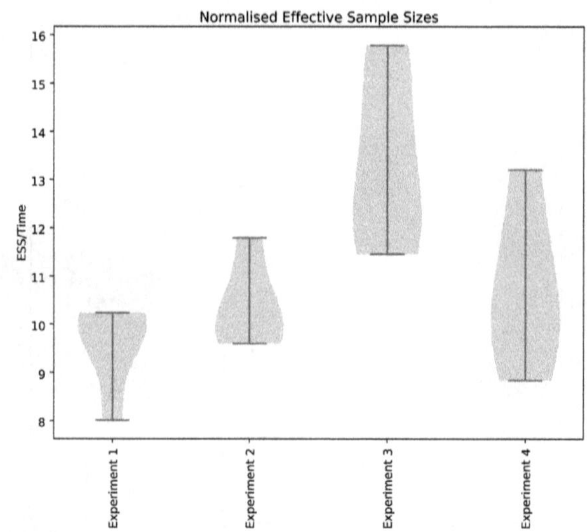

(b) HMC effective sample size normalized by execution time across all the experiments.

Fig. 13.2 Inference results for the Bayesian framework for the HMC algorithm showing the effective sample sizes and effective sample sizes normalized by execution time for the sell-side analyst report dataset

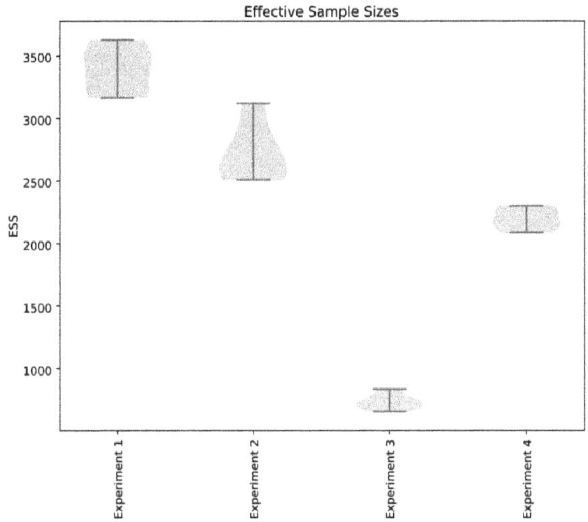

(a) S2HMC effective sample size across all the experiments.

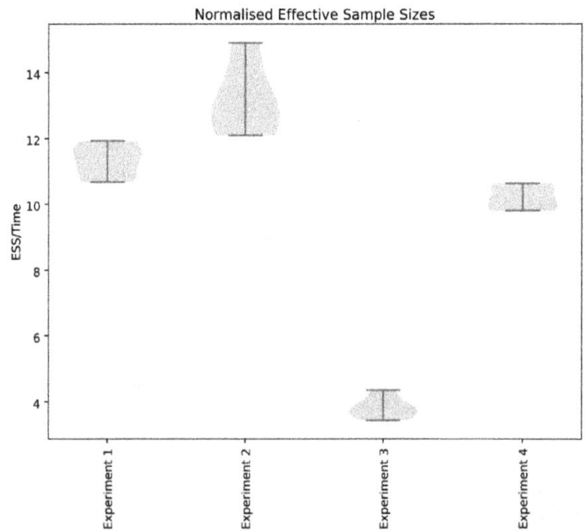

(b) S2HMC effective sample size normalized by execution time across all the experiments.

Fig. 13.3 Inference results for the Bayesian framework for the S2HMC algorithm showing the effective sample sizes and effective sample sizes normalized by execution time for the sell-side analyst report dataset

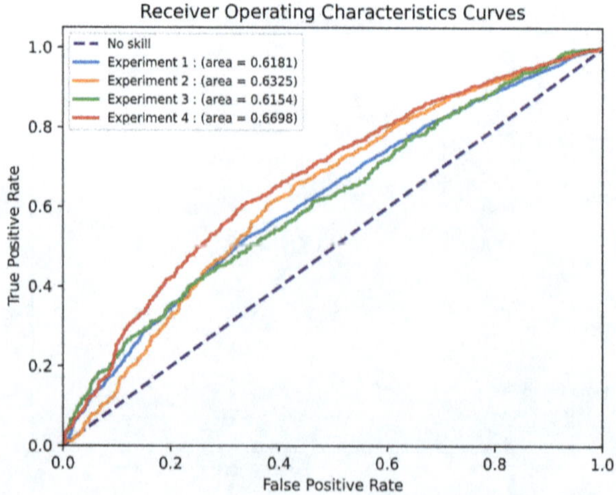

(a) MALA Area under the Receiver Operating Curve across all the experiments.

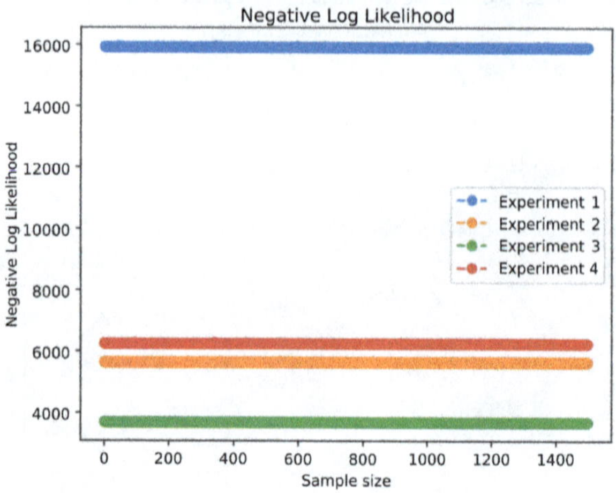

(b) MALA diagnostic negative log-likelihood trace plots across all the experiments.

Fig. 13.4 Inference results for the Bayesian framework for the MALA algorithm across all the experiments showing the diagnostic negative log-likelihood trace plots and the predictive performance based on the Area Under the Receiver Operating Curve (AUC)

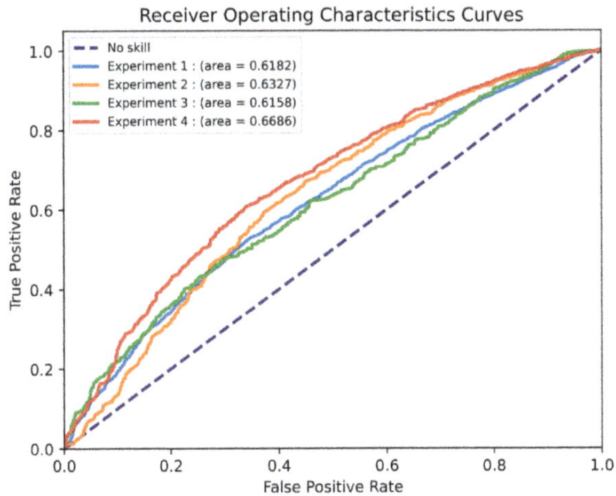

(a) HMC Area under the Receiver Operating Curve across all the experiments.

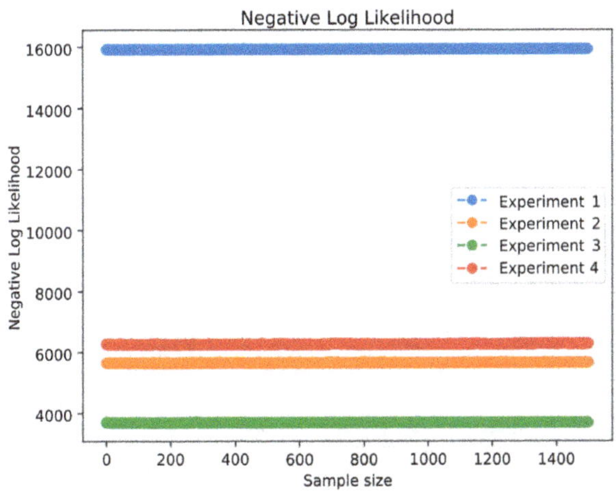

(b) HMC diagnostic negative log-likelihood trace plots across all the experiments.

Fig. 13.5 Inference results for the Bayesian framework for the HMC algorithm across all the experiments showing the diagnostic negative log-likelihood trace plots and the predictive performance based on the Area Under the Receiver Operating Curve (AUC)

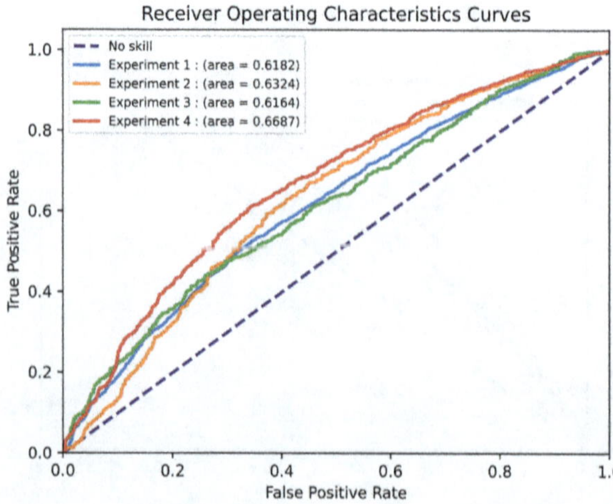

(a) S2HMC Area under the Receiver Operating Curve across all the experiments.

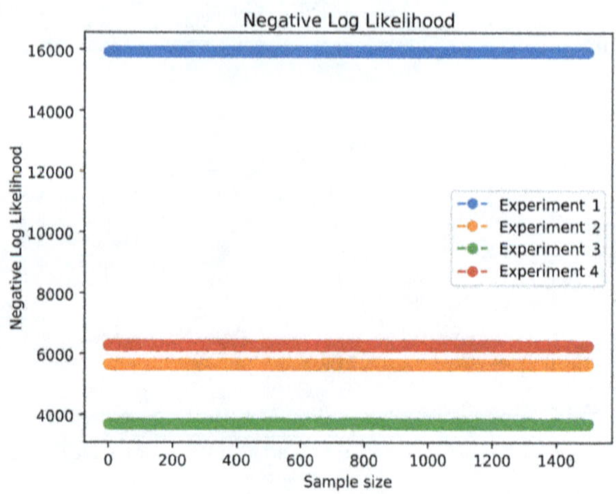

(b) S2HMC diagnostic negative log-likelihood trace plots across all the experiments.

Fig. 13.6 Inference results for the Bayesian framework for the S2HMC algorithm across all the experiments showing the diagnostic negative log-likelihood trace plots and the predictive performance based on the Area Under the Receiver Operating Curve (AUC)

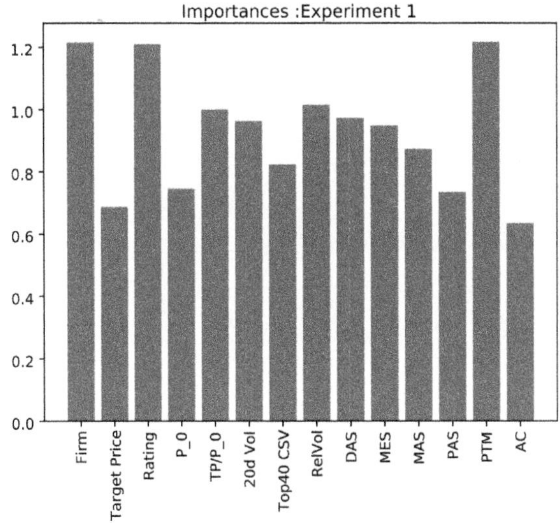

(a) MALA importance's for experiment 1.

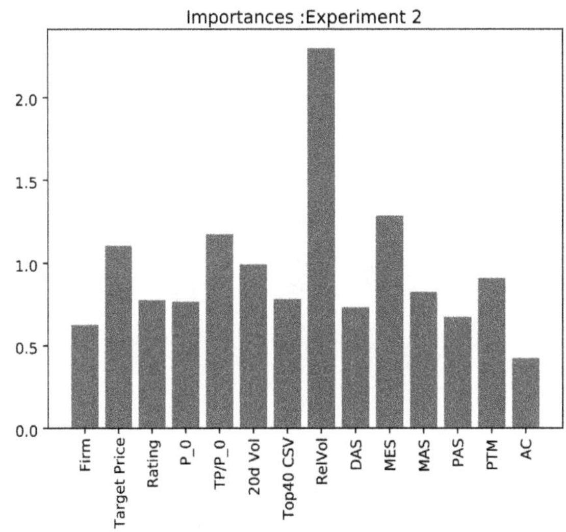

(b) MALA importance's for experiment 2.

Fig. 13.7 Mean posterior importances for experiments 1 and 2 for the MALA method on the sell-side analyst report dataset

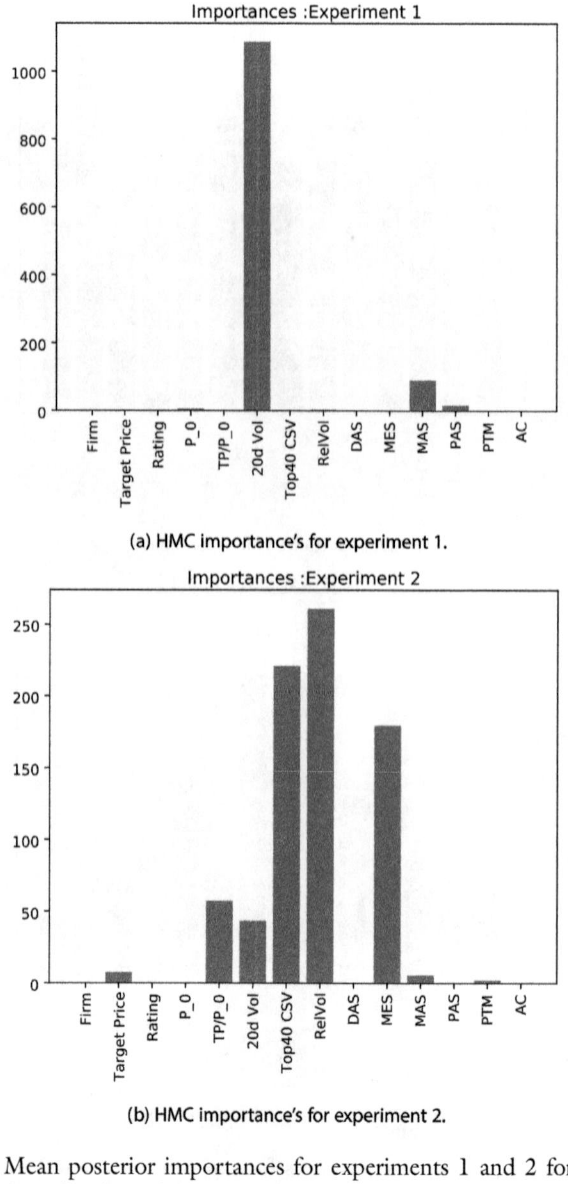

(a) HMC importance's for experiment 1.

(b) HMC importance's for experiment 2.

Fig. 13.8 Mean posterior importances for experiments 1 and 2 for the HMC method on the sell-side analyst report dataset

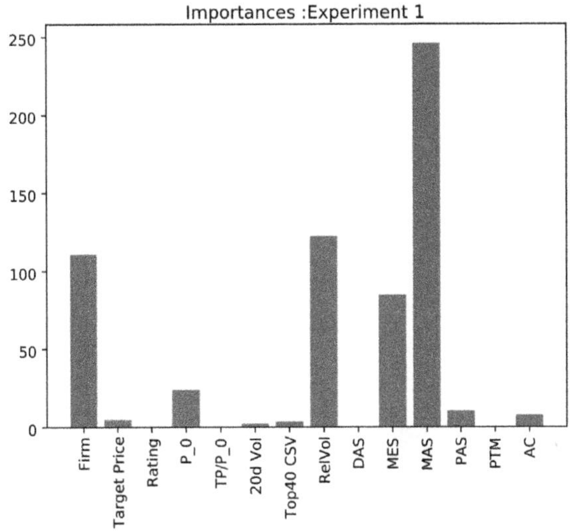

(a) S2HMC importance's for experiment 1.

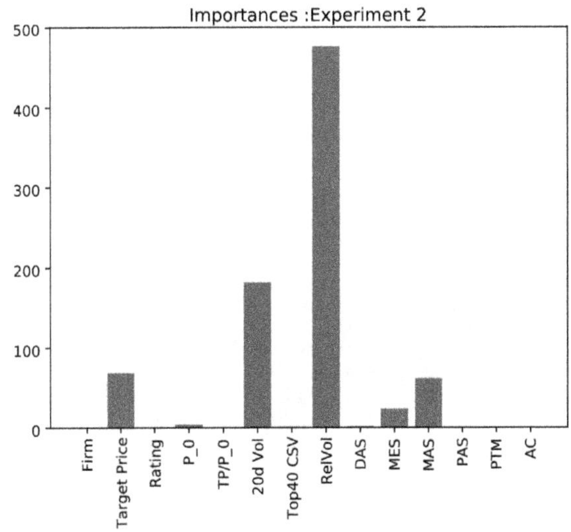

(b) S2HMC importance's for experiment 2.

Fig. 13.9 Mean posterior importances for experiments 1 and 2 across for the S2HMC method on the sell-side analyst report dataset

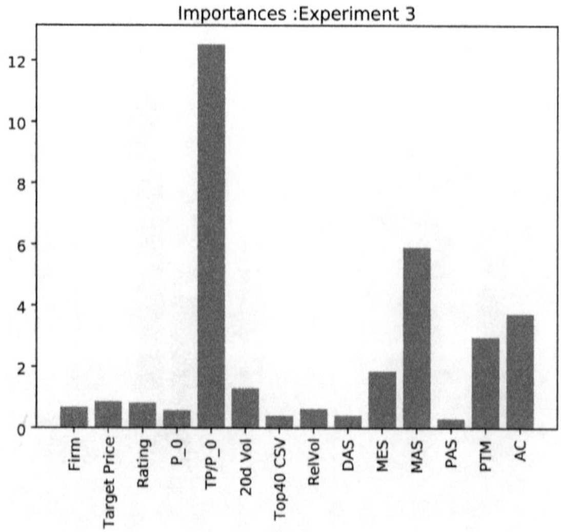

(a) MALA importance's for experiment 3.

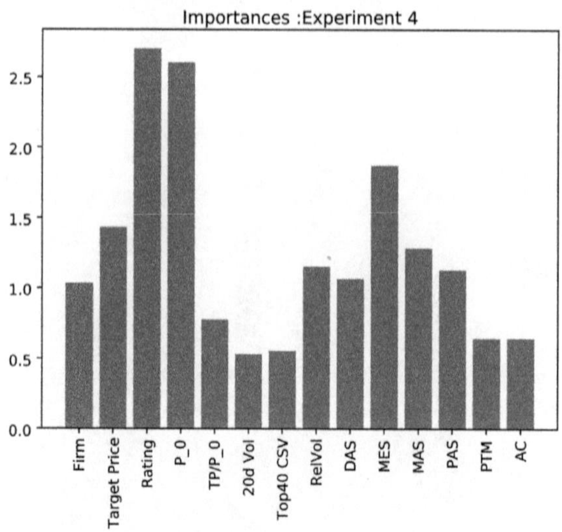

(b) MALA importance's for experiment 4.

Fig. 13.10 Mean posterior importances for experiments 3 and 4 for the MALA method on the sell-side analyst report dataset

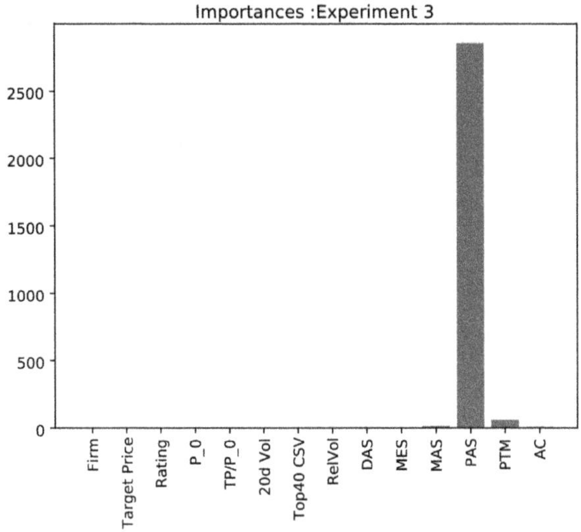

(a) HMC importance's for experiment 3.

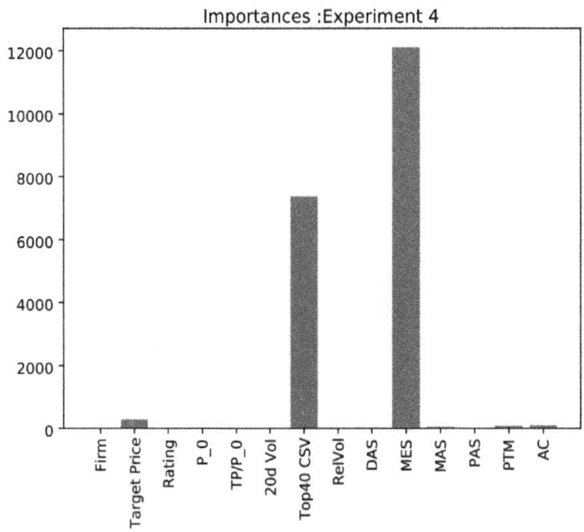

(b) HMC importance's for experiment 4.

Fig. 13.11 Mean posterior importances for experiments 3 and 4 for the HMC method on the sell-side analyst report dataset

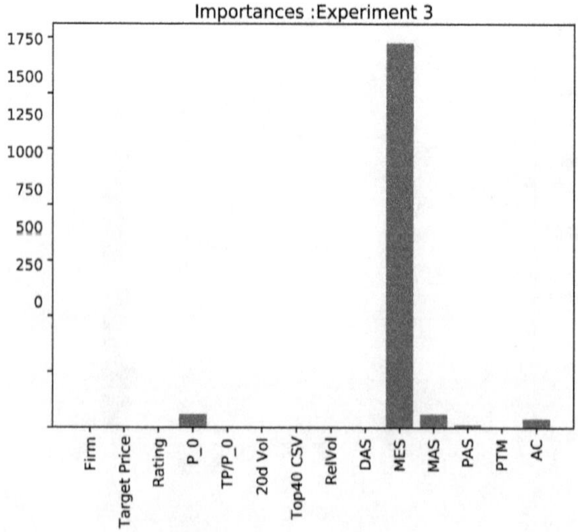

(a) S2HMC importance's for experiment 3.

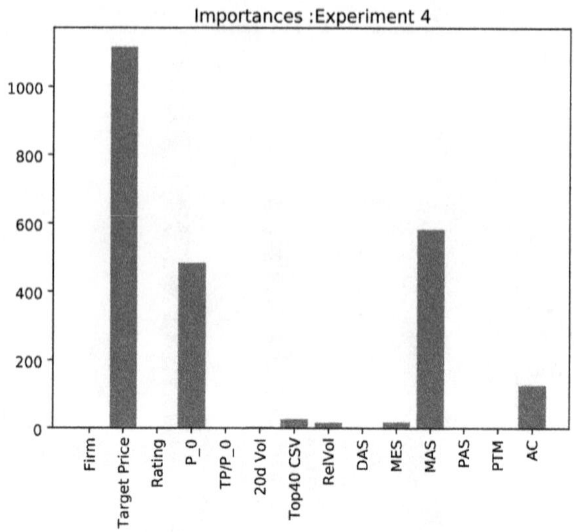

(b) S2HMC importance's for experiment 4.

Fig. 13.12 Mean posterior importance for experiments 3 and 4 for the S2HMC method on the sell-side analyst report dataset

Table 13.3 Ranking of the top five features by MALA. For example, MALA ranks *Firm* as the second most important in Experiment 1, while it ranks *MES* as the third most important in Experiment 4

Ranking	*Experiment 1*	*Experiment 2*	*Experiment 3*	*Experiment 4*
1	*PTM*	*RelVol*	TP/P_0	*Rating*
2	*Firm*	*MES*	*MAS*	P_0
3	*Rating*	TP/P_0	*AC*	*MES*
4	*RelVol*	*TargetPrice*	*PTM*	*TargetPrice*
5	TP/P_0	20*dVol*	*MES*	*MAS*

Table 13.4 Ranking of the top five features by HMC across the four experiments. For example, HMC ranks *MAS* as the second most important in Experiment 1, while it ranks *TargetPrice* as the third most important in Experiment 4

Ranking	*Experiment 1*	*Experiment 2*	*Experiment 3*	*Experiment 4*
1	20*dVol*	*RelVol*	*PAS*	*MES*
2	*MAS*	*Top*40*CSV*	*PTM*	*Top*40*CSV*
3	*PAS*	*MES*	*MAS*	*TargetPrice*
4	P_0	TP/P_0	*AC*	*AC*
5	*RelVol*	20*dVol*	*TargetPrice*	*PTM*

Table 13.5 Ranking of the top five features by S2HMC across the four experiments. For example, S2HMC ranks *RelVol* as the second most important in Experiment 1, while it ranks P_0 as the third most important in Experiment 4

Ranking	*Experiment 1*	*Experiment 2*	*Experiment 3*	*Experiment 4*
1	*MAS*	*RelVol*	*MES*	*TargetPrice*
2	*RelVol*	20*dVol*	*MAS*	*MAS*
3	*Firm*	*TargetPrice*	P_0	P_0
4	*MES*	*MAS*	*AC*	*AC*
5	P_0	*MES*	*PAS*	*Top*40*CSV*

13.6 show that there is convergence across the MCMC method and across all the experiments. This can be seen by the flat diagnostic negative log-likelihood trace plots. In addition, the Area Under the Receiver Operating Curves shows visually the results shown in Table 13.2.

Figures 13.7, 13.8, 13.9, 13.10, 13.11, and 13.12 show the importance of the ranking of each input feature by each MCMC method across all four experiments. The top five features selected by each MCMC method on each experiment are shown in Tables 13.3, 13.4 and 13.5. The results in these tables show that the MCMC methods broadly agree on which features are the most relevant for this task. The critical features vary across the different sectors, with *relative volatility* and *initial price* being most important for the entire dataset, *rolling 20day volatility* and *target price* being critical on the resource stocks; *analyst coverage*, *initial price*, and *target price* being important for financial stocks while the *target price*, *initial price*, *analyst coverage*, and *Top40 index cross-sectional volatility* is essential for industrial stocks. These results could be useful for stakeholders who want to understand the inputs that drive outperformance.

13.6 Conclusion

This chapter introduced the Bayesian investment analyst, which framed the stock prediction problem within a Bayesian framework. This framework utilized data from sell-side analyst reports on stocks listed on the Johannesburg Stock Exchange (JSE) to improve the bidirectional prediction of stock prices. We employ the Bayesian logistic regression with an automatic relevance determination (BLR-ARD) prior distribution model. We train this model using the Metropolis-Adjusted Langevin Algorithm, Hamiltonian Monte Carlo, and Separable Shadow Hamiltonian Hybrid Monte Carlo Markov Chain Monte Carlo (MCMC) techniques.

Our results show that the MCMC methods produce similar predictive performance across the experiments. We further find that we outperform on industrial and resource stocks, with performance on financial stocks being worse than on the entire JSE stock universe. We find that the BLR-ARD model can detect which input features are the more relevant for the stock bidirectional prediction task. The selected features differ for each experiment or industry, showing the importance of tailoring the stock predictions to each industry or sector in the market.

The framework presented in this chapter opens the door for further exploration. The potential for expanding the model by considering more complicated models, such as Bayesian neural networks, instead of Bayesian logistic regression, is an exciting prospect. Furthermore, the idea of training experts in each sector and aggregating the results could significantly improve the model's performance. This could potentially be approached using distributed Gaussian process models, such as the product of expert models.

In the next chapter, we conclude the book and discuss the promising future research directions that could further enhance our understanding of quantitative finance problems when framed within the Bayesian inference framework.

References

Ahmed, S., & Flint, E. (2020). Evaluating equity analyst forecasts in South Africa. *Investment Analysts Journal, 49*(3), 199–214.

Barber, B., Lehavy, R., McNichols, M., & Trueman, B. (2001). Can investors profit from the prophets? Security analyst recommendations and stock returns. *The Journal of Finance, 56*(2), 531–563.

Bradley, A. P. (1997). The use of the area under the ROC curve in the evaluation of machine learning algorithms. *Pattern Recognition, 30*(7), 1145–1159. https://doi.org/10.1016/s0031-3203(96)00142-2

Cronje, J. (2017). *Steinhoff's market cap a mere R20bn as shares drop another 30%.* https://www.fin24.com/Companies/Retail/steinhoff-shares-drop-by-a-fifth-in-early-trade-20171220. Last Retrieved: 15 November 2019.

Duane, S., Kennedy, A. D., Pendleton, B. J., & Roweth, D. (1987). Hybrid monte carlo. *Physics Letters B, 195*(2), 216–222.

Gaganis, C. (2009). Classification techniques for the identification of falsified financial statements: a comparative analysis. *Intelligent Systems in Accounting, Finance & Management, 16*(3), 207–229. https://doi.org/10.1002/isaf.303

Girolami, M., & Calderhead, B. (2011). Riemann manifold langevin and hamiltonian monte carlo methods. *Journal of the Royal Statistical Society: Series B (Statistical Methodology), 73*(2), 123–214.

Gu, M., & Sun, S. (2020). Neural Langevin dynamical sampling. *IEEE Access, 8*, 31595–31605.

Hastings, W. K. (1970). Monte Carlo sampling methods using Markov chains and their applications. *Biometrica, 57*(1), 97–109.

Heide, C., Roosta, F., Hodgkinson, L., & Kroese, D. (2021). Shadow manifold Hamiltonian Monte Carlo. In *International conference on artificial intelligence and statistics*. PMLR (pp. 1477–1485).

Hinton, G. E., & Van Camp, D. (1993). Keeping the neural networks simple by minimizing the description length of the weights. In *Proceedings of the sixth annual conference on Computational learning theory* (pp. 5–13). ACM.

Hoffman, M. D., Blei, D. M., Wang, C., Paisley, J. (2013). Stochastic variational inference. *Journal of Machine Learning Research, 14*(5).

Hoffman, M. D., & Gelman, A. (2014). The No-U-turn sampler: Adaptively setting path lengths in Hamiltonian Monte Carlo. *Journal of Machine Learning Research, 15*(1), 1593–1623.

Izaguirre, J. A., & Hampton, S. S. (2004). Shadow hybrid Monte Carlo: An efficient propagator in phase space of macromolecules. *Journal of Computational Physics, 200*(2), 581–604. isbn: 0021-9991. https://doi.org/10.1016/j.jcp.2004.04.016

Kua, K., & Ignjatovic, A. (2022). Iterative filtering algorithms for computing consensus analyst estimates. In *2022 IEEE symposium on computational intelligence for financial engineering and economics (CIFEr)* (pp. 1–8). IEEE.

MacKay, D. J. C. (1992). A practical Bayesian framework for backpropagation networks. *Neural Computation, 4*(3), 448–472.

MacKay, D. J. C. (1995). Probable networks and plausible predictions—a review of practical Bayesian methods for supervised neural networks. *Network: Computation in Neural Systems, 6*(3), 469–505.

Marwala, T., Mbuvha, R., & Mongwe, W. T. (2023). *Hamiltonian Monte Carlo methods in machine learning*. Elsevier.

Mbuvha, R., & Marwala, T. (2020). Bayesian inference of COVID-19 spreading rates in South Africa. *PloS One, 15*(8), Article e0237126.

Mbuvha, R., Mongwe, W. T., & Marwala, T. (2021). Separable shadow Hamiltonian hybrid Monte Carlo for Bayesian neural network inference in wind speed forecasting. *Energy and A, I*, Article 100108.

Mobiny, A., Yuan, P., Moulik, S. K., Garg, N., Wu, C. C., & Van Nguyen, H. (2021). Dropconnect is effective in modeling uncertainty of bayesian deep networks. *Scientific Reports, 11*(1), 1–14.

Mongwe, W. T., & Malan, K. M. (2020). A survey of automated financial statement fraud detection with relevance to the South African context. *South African Computer Journal, 32*(1). https://doi.org/10.18489/sacj.v32i1.777.

Mongwe, W. T., Mbuvha, R., & Marwala, T. (2021d). Locally scaled and stochastic volatility metropolis-hastings algorithms. *Algorithms, 14*(12). isbn: 1999-4893. https://doi.org/10.3390/a14120351. https://www.mdpi.com/1999-4893/14/12/351.

Mongwe, W. T., Sidogi, T., Mbuvha, R., & Marwala, T. (2022b). Probabilistic inference of south african equity option prices under jump-diffusion processes. In *2022 IEEE symposium on computational intelligence for financial engineering and economics (CIFEr)* (pp. 1–8). IEEE.

Mongwe, W. T., Mbuvha, R., & Marwala, T. (2021). Bayesian inference of local government audit outcomes. *Plos One*. https://doi.org/10.1371/journal.pone.0261245

Mongwe, W. T., Mbuvha, R., & Marwala, T. (2021). Adaptive magnetic Hamiltonian Monte Carlo. *IEEE Access, 9*, 152993–153003.

Mongwe, W. T., Sidogi, T., Mbuvha, R., & Marwala, T. (2021). Adaptively setting the path length for separable shadow Hamiltonian hybrid Monte Carlo. *IEEE Access, 9*, 138598–138607.

Mongwe, W. T., Sidogi, T., Mbuvha, R., & Marwala, T. (2022). Shadow Magnetic Hamiltonian Monte Carlo. *IEEE Access, 10*, 34340–34351.

Neal, R. M. (1993). Bayesian learning via stochastic dynamics. In *Advances in neural information processing systems* (Vol. 5, pp. 475–482). Morgan Kaufmann Publishers Inc. isbn: 1-55860-274-7. http://dl.acm.org/citation.cfm?id=645753.667903

Neal, R. M. (2012). *Bayesian learning for neural networks* (Vol. 118). Springer Science & Business Media.

Neal, R. M., et al. (2011). MCMC using Hamiltonian dynamics. *Handbook of Markov Chain Monte Carlo, 2*(11), 2.

Park, S. J., & Park, K. Y. (2019). Can investors profit from security analyst recommendations?: New evidence on the value of consensus recommendations. *Finance Research Letters, 30*, 403–413.

Sidogi, T., Mongwe, W. T., Mbuvha, R., & Marwala, T. (2022). Fusing sell-side analyst bidirectional forecasts using machine learning. *IEEE Access, 10*, 76966–76974.

Singh, J., & Khushi, M. (2021). Feature learning for stock price prediction shows a significant role of analyst rating. *Applied System Innovation, 4*(1), 17.

Sweet, C. R., Hampton, S. S., Skeel, R. D., & Izaguirre, J. A. (2009). A separable shadow Hamiltonian hybrid Monte Carlo method. *The Journal of Chemical Physics, 131*(17), Article 174106.

Vats, D., Flegal, J. M., Jones, G. L. (2019). Multivariate output analysis for Markov chain Monte Carlo. *Biometrika, 106*(2), 321–337. isbn: 0006-3444. eprint: https://academic.oup.com/biomet/article-pdf/106/2/321/28575440/asz002.pdf.

Zaremba, A., & Konieczka, P. (2015). The profitability of following analyst recommendations on the Polish stock market. *Financial Internet Quarterly" e-Finanse, 11*(1), 22–31.

CHAPTER 14

Conclusions to Bayesian Machine Learning in Quantitative Finance

14.1 Summary of Contributions

The advent of artificial intelligence and the rise of data-driven methods and machine learning techniques are transforming the quantitative finance field. This book explored various domains in quantitative finance and presented the theory and case studies of the potential of machine learning in this space. In particular, we showed that when employing the Bayesian inference framework and consequently Bayesian machine learning—one can then naturally answer questions such as: (1) How can we explain the prediction or output of the models? (2) What is the distribution of the parameters of the model? (3) How do we select between the different models in a statistically principled manner? and (4) Which inputs are most relevant for the task at hand? We applied this framework across the derivative modeling, banking, financial management, insurance, and investments domains. We further provide background to the Bayesian inference framework and Bayesian machine learning in quantitative finance. Our analysis of problems within these quantitative finance domains presented the following insights:

W. T. Mongwe et al., *Bayesian Machine Learning in Quantitative Finance*, https://doi.org/10.1007/978-3-031-88431-3_14

1. **Background to Bayesian inference:** For this theme, we explored the Bayesian paradigm and how this translates to Bayesian machine learning. We discussed some of the advantages and disadvantages of the Bayesian framework and how Bayesian models can be trained and deployed. We also discussed the various performance metrics that can be used to assess the performance of Bayesian machine learning models. We further explored the Bayesian framework and how it can be applied to the various areas of quantitative finance, including derivative modeling, banking, financial management, insurance, and investments. We highlight the impact machine learning is having on the finance industry and the potential benefits of framing problems in quantitative finance within the Bayesian framework.
2. **Derivative modeling:** For this theme, we explored employing the Bayesian inference framework to calibrate complex stochastic models such as the rough Bergomi and the Heston stochastic volatility models. For this task, we utilized single- and multi-output Gaussian processes applied to equity volatility surface data from emerging (South Africa) and developed (Europe) equity markets. The results show that our approach produces similar accuracy to deep neural networks, with the added benefit of showing uncertainty across the volatility surface while requiring fewer hyperparameter configurations. Furthermore, we observe that the Bayesian calibration becomes more specific (i.e., with narrower confidence bands) as we decrease maturity and at lower relative moneyness levels for a given maturity. We further calibrated the Stochastic Alpha Beta Rho model using Markov Chain Monte Carlo algorithms: Metropolis-Adjusted Langevin Algorithm, Hamiltonian Monte Carlo, and Separable Shadow Hamiltonian Hybrid Monte Carlo. Our results show that the proposed approach can fit the volatility skew for each expiry. The empirical findings demonstrate that our method can precisely price the interest-rate volatility skew on both simulated and ZAR swaption data, with the added advantage of producing a distribution of the model predictions and parameters. We find that the Markov Chain Monte Carlo algorithms are reasonably confident (as measured by the width of the confidence bands of the skew) around the at-the-money point but get less confident as we move toward the deep-in and deep-out of the money options. Furthermore, the results show that the methods are more confident in the skew's

right-wing predictions than the skew's left wing. These results could help stakeholders in the generation of volatility stress scenarios, for example. We concluded this derivative modeling theme by tackling the problem of pricing European equity options within the emerging market context using an entirely data-driven approach based on normalizing flows. This approach allowed us to produce arbitrage-free prices without imposing external arbitrage conditions into the loss function, but by instead learning the risk-neutral density directly—which already imposes no-arbitrage conditions—and generating the option prices from this distribution. These results present a new avenue of approaching purely data-driven approaches for option pricing and hedging. Our analysis shows that the mixture of normalizing flow models can reproduce the option prices in a developing economy for various option maturities and moneyless levels. We further find that the options close to expiry require more mixture components than those far from expiry, which raises the question of how to select the optional number of normalizing flow mixture components. The largest errors are typically associated with low strikes, with the error generally reducing with increasing strikes.

3. **Financial management:** For this theme, we utilized Bayesian inference in the context of banking and municipal financial management. In the banking domain, we first explored the problem of modeling credit ratings for corporations. Since generating credit ratings is an intensive process that costs enormous sums of money and is generally performed by large rating agencies, automated means of producing reliable credit ratings are ideal. We utilized sparse and distributed Gaussian processes to predict corporate credit ratings. The sparse and distributed Gaussian processes are more favorable than classical Gaussian processes as they can quickly scale to large datasets. The distributed Gaussian processes that we considered were variations of the product-of-experts distributed Gaussian processes. Our results show that the *debt ratio*, *profit margin-related* metrics, and *return on capital ratio* are the most important financial metrics in determining corporate credit rating. These results could prove helpful for various stakeholders who rely on credit ratings for their decision processes. Within the retail space of a bank, we explored the analysis of defaulted loan recovery rates. For this, we utilized Bayesian inference to detect if there would be any recoveries on non-performing loans. We trained a Bayesian logistic

regression model using Metropolis-Adjusted Langevin Algorithm, Hamiltonian Monte Carlo, and Separable Shadow Hamiltonian Hybrid Monte Carlo Markov Chain Monte Carlo algorithms. We find that the *purpose* of the loan, *home-ownership* status, and the *interest rate* charged on the loan are some of the key features in determining which charged-off account will have recoveries or not. This framework can be easily extended to incorporate more complex models, such as Bayesian deep neural networks. In the munic ipal finance management domain, we considered the problem of model selection in the modeling audit outcomes and the detection of unauthorized expenditures in unaudited financial statements of municipalities. For the audit opinion model selection task, we considered variations for the Bayesian logistic regression model with varying numbers of features or covariates. We then utilized the Bayesian evidence metric to select and compare the various models. The Bayesian evidence was estimated using the harmonic mean estimator, where the target distribution was estimated using normalizing flows. The normalizing flows-based harmonic mean evidence estimator utilizes samples generated from the Metropolis-Adjusted Langevin Algorithm, Hamiltonian Monte Carlo, and No-U-Turn Sampler Markov Chain Monte Carlo methods to learn the target distribution (Mongwe et al., 2021a, 2021c). Our results show that the Bayesian evidence framework can reliably predict which model will outperform on unseen data based on the evidence metric calculated on training data, and we find a positive correlation between evidence on training data and the Area Under the Receiver Operating Curve metric on unseen data. This framework can be easily extended to encapsulate a broader class of models, such as for optimal architecture search for Bayesian neural networks, albeit at an increased computational cost. We conclude this theme on financial management by exploring the utility of Bayesian inference in detecting unauthorized expenditure in South African municipalities. We trained a Bayesian logistic regression model with an automatic relevance determination (BLR-ARD) prior distribution using the Metropolis-Hastings, Metropolis-Hastings Adjusted Langevin Algorithm, Hamiltonian Monte Carlo, and Magnetic Hamiltonian Monte Carlo Markov Chain Monte Carlo methods. The BLR-ARD model allowed us to automatically rank input features that were most relevant to the task at hand. This work provides tools that auditors could use for risk-rating municipal accounts for unauthorized expenditures, and it is easily extendable to other sets of unlawful expenditures, such as irregular and wasteful expenditures.

4. **Insurance and investments:** For this theme, we explored the problems of modeling the likelihood of motor insurance claims occurring, modeling yield curves using the Nelson and Siegel (1987) model, and introducing the Bayesian investment analyst. We infer the motor insurance claims using Bayesian neural networks trained using the Laplace or Gaussian approximation of Mackay (1992), which is a variational inference variant. Furthermore, we examine various architectures of the neural networks—such as deep and wide neural architectures—intending to select between the different models using the Bayesian evidence metric. In addition, each model we consider utilized an automatic relevance determination prior, which allowed us to rank the most relevant inputs. Our results show that the Bayesian evidence metric can select models or the neural network architecture on training data that performs well on unseen data. We find that deeper architectures perform better than wider architectures, highlighting the benefit of adding more layers of non-linearization. We further find that the *claims history*, *type of fuel of vehicle*, *power of the vehicle*, *lapse*, and *number of policies* are the essential features for the claim prediction task. These results could prove helpful to stakeholders as this framework makes the usually black-box neural network models more interpretable to non-expert audiences. We then explore a Bayesian approach to calibrating the seminal Nelson & Siegel (1987) model, widely used by market participants such as central banks and portfolio managers as a yield curve model. We calibrate this model using the Hamiltonian Monte Carlo, the Separable Shadow Hybrid Hamiltonian Monte Carlo, and the No-U-Turn Sampler Markov Chain Monte Carlo methods. Our analysis reveals that our calibration technique gives comparable or better yield curve estimates than ordinary least squares across multiple performance metrics and provides a more comprehensive account of parameter uncertainty, enhancing yield curve estimations' robustness. We then explore using the nested sampling Bayesian

evidence estimation method of Skilling (2004) to select between various nested Nelson and Siegel models. We also introduce the automatic relevance determination Nelson and Siegel (ARD-NS) model, which we train using the No-U-Turn Sampler Markov Chain Monte Carlo technique. This ARD-NS model allows one to automatically rank the short-term, medium-term, and long-term factor loading to determine which one is driving the yield curve at that particular moment in a probabilistically robust manner. Our analysis shows that the evidence framework is robust in detecting the model generating the underlying yield curve data, and results from the ARD-NS model show that the yield curve dynamics are driven mainly by the medium-term (i.e., curvature) factor loading for the period under consideration. This framework can easily be extended to cover a broader class of term structure models. We conclude this insurance and investments theme by considering sell-side analyst reports for stocks on the Johannesburg Stock Exchange (JSE). Through the construction of various experiments, we assess the performance of a Bayesian investment analyst in predicting the bidirectional stock movements of stocks in the industrial, resources, and financial sectors, as well as in the full universe of stocks on the JSE. The Bayesian investment analyst is constructed by training a BLR-ARD model using Markov Chain Monte Carlo methods. Our results show that, across all the Markov Chain Monte Carlo methods considered, the BLR-ARD model has the best performance on the industrial stocks, followed by the resources stocks, with the worst performance being on the financial stocks. Across the four experiments or sectors we consider, the BLR-ARD model outperforms the mean consensus performance of the sell-side analyst's. We further find that the Markov Chain Monte Carlo methods agree on which features are the most relevant for this task. The essential features vary across the different sectors, with *relative volatility* and *initial price* being most important for the entire JSE universe; *rolling 20day volatility* and *target price* being critical on the resource stocks; *analyst coverage*, *initial price*, and *target price* being important for financial stocks while the *target price*, *initial price*, *analyst coverage*, and *Top40 Index cross-sectional volatility* being significant for industrial stocks.

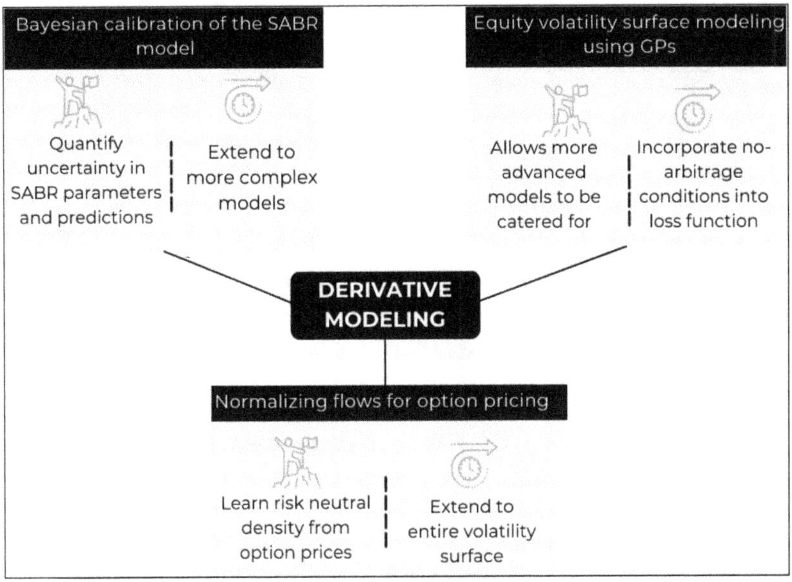

Fig. 14.1 Summary of the contributions and future research directions for the derivative modeling theme covered in this book

These results and insights could help various stakeholders understand the drivers of the results across the various domains of quantitative finance and inform their decisions. In the next section, we discuss the ongoing and future work. Figures 14.1, 14.2, and 14.3 provide a summary of this book's contributions and potential research directions across the themes explored in this book.

14.2 Ongoing and Future Research Directions

This book has highlighted various problems in quantitative finance where the Bayesian framework produced good insights. However, many domains within quantitative finance and other models and algorithms still need to be explored to extend the work presented in this manuscript. A summary of ongoing and future research across the themes covered in this book are:

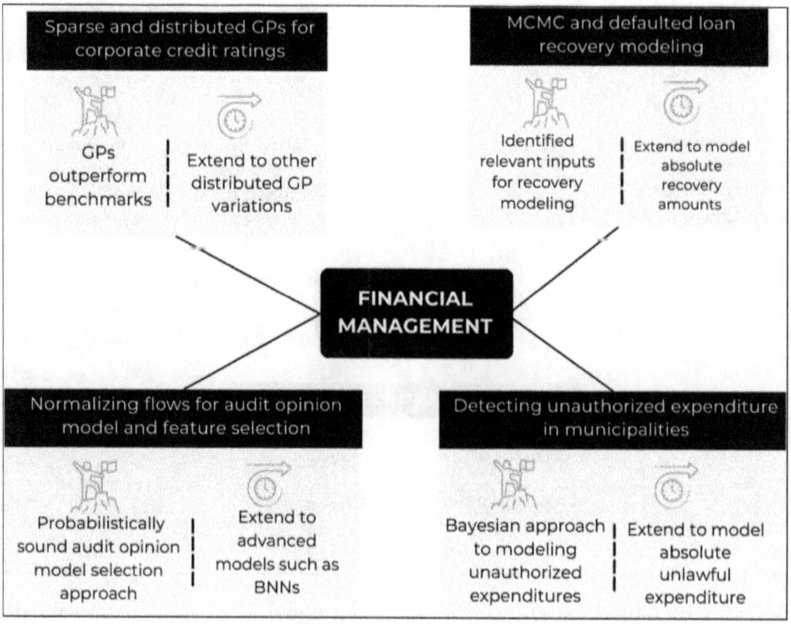

Fig. 14.2 Summary of the contributions and future research directions for the financial management theme covered in this book

- **Derivative modeling:** We used Markov Chain Monte Carlo methods to calibrate the Stochastic Alpha Beta Rho model. We showed the utility of employing the Bayesian framework for this. This work can be enhanced by considering the entire interest-rate volatility surface instead of limiting the data to the 1W into 1Y and 6M into 1Y swaption data as we did in this book. Practitioners could also be interested in comparing other models that can capture the volatility skew, such as jump-diffusion models (Mongwe, 2015; Mongwe et al., 2022). We utilized the single and multi-output Gaussian processes to model the entire volatility surface using rough Bergomi and Heston stochastic volatility models. This work can be improved by ensuring that the inducing points and kernels used for the multi-output GP are not shared. Furthermore, all the models approximated the pricing function without explicitly incorporating no-arbitrage conditions (Sidogi et al., 2022). In future

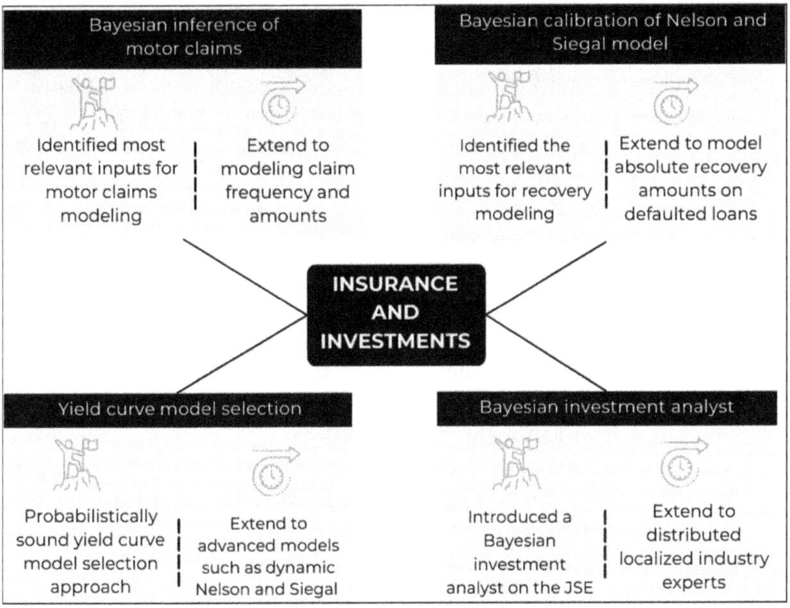

Fig. 14.3 Summary of the contributions and future research directions for the insurance and investment theme covered in this book

work, we plan to incorporate no-arbitrage conditions explicitly. A limitation of the GP approach is the computational complexity of the method; through utilizing start-of-art approaches to scaling GPs, such as distributional GP approaches (Cohen et al., 2020), we aim to address this limitation. We concluded the derivative modeling theme of this book by using a mixture of normalizing flows to learn the risk-neutral density with applications to options on the Johannesburg Stock Exchange. This work can be extended by comparing various techniques to optimally select the number of components in the normalizing flow mixture. Furthermore, it could be interesting to explore jointly modeling the entire option price surface (i.e., across all expiry and strikes) instead of the volatility skew per expiry (Yang & Hospedales, 2023).

- **Financial management:** We successfully utilized sparse and distributed Gaussian processes to model the credit ratings of corporate entities domiciled in the USA. This work can be expanded by considering other distributed Gaussian processes, such as a mixture of experts instead of a product of experts. Furthermore, data from a developing nation such as South Africa could also be utilized to assess the performance of the models. The problem of selecting the number of experts for the distributed Gaussian process model would also be of interest (Cohen et al., 2020). We also used Markov Chain Monte Carlo techniques to train a Bayesian Logistic regression model with automatic relevance determination prior to detect the presence of recoveries in non-performing loans. This work can be extended by considering more complex models like deep neural networks to detect recoveries in defaulted loans. Furthermore, instead of only detecting whether recoveries are present, modeling the actual absolute recovery amount on the defaulted loan using Bayesian techniques would be of interest, and this aspect is yet to be explored in detail in the literature. In the municipal financial management theme, we explored modeling audit opinions using models trained with Markov Chain Monte Carlo methods to perform model selection using the Harmonic mean estimator that utilizes normalizing flows to learn the target posterior. The framework presented in this book can be extended to more complicated models, such as deep neural networks, and by employing more advanced sampling techniques, such as those based on Riemannian manifolds (Marwala et al., 2023; Mongwe et al., 2021b). Furthermore, comparing the model selection results to other Bayesian evidence estimation approaches such as the nested sampling method of Skilling (Skilling, 2004; Speagle, 2020) could also provide interesting insights. We concluded the financial management theme of this book by employing the Bayesian inference framework to detect unauthorized expenditures in South African municipalities using unaudited financial statements. This work can be expanded by considering the case of modeling the absolute value of the unauthorized expenditure and jointly modeling the other unlawful spending, such as fruitless and wasteful expenditures. In addition, we can also explore the added benefit of considering more complex models, such as Bayesian neural networks, for this task.

- **Insurance and investments:** We used the Bayesian inference framework to model the claims in the motor insurance company. For this task, we utilized the Laplace or Gaussian approximation first introduced by Mackay (1992). This approach also allowed us to scale to larger models and select between the different models. This work can be expanded by considering other methods of training the Bayesian neural network, such as Markov Chain Monte Carlo methods, that ensure convergence to the true target posterior. In addition, instead of forecasting whether a claim will occur, we intend to extend the work in this chapter by modeling the absolute value of claims through the analysis of claim frequency and severity. Under the insurance and investments theme, we then explored the Nelson and Siegel yield curve model. We calibrated this model with Markov Chain Monte Carlo techniques and performed a model selection exercise using the nested and dynamic Bayesian evidence estimation techniques. In future work, we aim to extend this analysis to the dynamic Nelson and Siegel model, which can capture the dynamics of the yield curve over time. Furthermore, we aim to extend this analysis to modeling the term structure of volatilities using the Nelson and Siegel model, as initial studies in that domain have shown promising results as shown in Guo et al. (2014). For the model selection aspect, the framework we present in this book can be extended to incorporate other yield curve models beyond variations or subsets of the Nelson and Siegel model. In addition, we plan to utilize other evidence calculation methods, such as those based on normalizing flows and the harmonic mean estimator of the evidence (Polanska et al., 2023). We concluded the insurance and investment theme by introducing the Bayesian investment analyst, trained using Markov Chain Monte Carlo methods, on stocks listed on the JSE. The framework presented in this book opens the door for further exploration. The potential for expanding the approach by considering more complicated models, such as Bayesian neural networks, instead of Bayesian logistic regression, is an exciting prospect (Mbuvha et al., 2021). Furthermore, training experts in each sector and aggregating the results could significantly improve the model's performance. This could potentially be approached using distributed Gaussian process models, such as the product of expert models (Cohen et al., 2020).

- **Other themes:** Machine learning has also been utilized to solve problems within quantitative finance that we did not cover in this book. This includes issues such as hedging options using machine learning (Buehler et al., 2019), predicting stock prices using limit order book data (Sidogi et al., 2023), and the generation of synthetic financial markets data (Sidogi et al., 2022), among other problems. These and other problems are ripe for exploring framing these problems within the Bayesian framework.

As highlighted above and throughout this book, there are various avenues that one can explore to enhance and extend the work presented across the different themes in this book. We look forward to the increased deployment of Bayesian inference frameworks in practice within the quantitative finance domain.

References

Buehler, H., Gonon, L., Teichmann, J., & Wood, B. (2019). Deep hedging. *Quantitative Finance, 19*(8), 1271–1291.

Cohen, S., Mbuvha, R., Marwala, T., & Deisenroth, M. (2020). Healing products of Gaussian process experts. In *International conference on machine learning*. PMLR (pp. 2068–2077).

Guo, B., Han, Q., & Zhao, B. (2014). The Nelson-Siegel model of the term structure of option implied volatility and volatility components. *Journal of Futures Markets, 34*(8), 788–806.

MacKay, D. J. C. (1992). Bayesian interpolation. *Neural Computation, 4*(3), 415–447.

Marwala, T., Mbuvha, R., & Mongwe, W. T. (2023). *Hamiltonian Monte Carlo methods in machine learning*. Elsevier.

Mbuvha, R., Mongwe, W. T., & Marwala, T. (2021). Separable shadow Hamiltonian Hybrid Monte Carlo for Bayesian neural network inference in wind speed forecasting. In *Energy and AI* (p. 100108).

Mongwe, W. T. (2015). *Analysis of equity and interest rate returns in South Africa under the context of jump diffusion processes*. Masters Thesis at University of Cape Town. Last Retrieved: 18 March 2021. https://open.uct.ac.za/bitstream/handle/11427/16600/thesis_com_2015_mongwe_wilson_tsakane.pdf?isAllowed=y&sequence=1

Mongwe, W. T., Mbuvha, R., & Marwala, T. (2021a). Adaptively setting the path length for separable shadow Hamiltonian hybrid Monte Carlo. *IEEE Access, 9*, 138598–138607.

Mongwe, W. T., Sidogi, T., Mbuvha, R., & Marwala, T. (2021b). Antithetic Riemannian manifold and quantum-inspired Hamiltonian Monte Carlo. arXiv preprint arXiv:2107.02070.

Mongwe, W. T., Mbuvha, R., & Marwala, T. (2021c). Bayesian inference of local government audit outcomes. *Plos One*. https://doi.org/10.1371/journal.pone.0261245

Mongwe, W. T., Sidogi, T., Mbuvha, R., & Marwala, T. (2022). Probabilistic inference of south african equity option prices under jump-diffusion processes. In *2022 IEEE symposium on computational intelligence for financial engineering and economics (CIFEr)* (pp. 1–8). IEEE.

Nelson, C. R., & Siegel, A. F. (1987). Parsimonious modeling of yield curves. *Journal of Business*, 473–489.

Polanska, A., Price, M. A., Mancini, A. S., & McEwen, J. D. (2023). Learned harmonic mean estimation of the marginal likelihood with normalizing flows. *Physical Sciences Forum, 9*(1). MDPI, 10.

Sidogi, T., Mongwe, W. T., Mbuvha, R., & Marwala, T. (2022). Creating synthetic volatility surfaces using generative adversarial networks with static arbitrage loss conditions. In *2022 IEEE symposium series on computational intelligence (SSCI)* (pp. 1423–1429). IEEE.

Sidogi, T., Mongwe, W. T., Mbuvha, R., Olukanmi, P., & Marwala, T. (2023). A signature transform of limit order book data for stock price prediction. *IEEE Access*.

Skilling, J. (2004). Nested sampling. In *AIP Conference Proceedings* (Vol. 735, 1, pp. 395–405). American Institute of Physics.

Speagle, J. S. (2020). Dynesty: A dynamic nested sampling package for estimating bayesian posteriors and evidences. *Monthly Notices of the Royal Astronomical Society, 493*(3), 3132–3158.

Yang, Y., & Hospedales, T. H. (2023). Mixture of normalizing flows for european option pricing. In *Uncertainty in artificial intelligence*. PMLR (pp. 2390–2399).

Index

W. T. Mongwe et al., *Bayesian Machine Learning in Quantitative Finance*, https://doi.org/10.1007/978-3-031-88431-3

O

P

Q

R

S

V

Y